GABA AND NEUROPEPTIDES IN THE CNS

HANDBOOK OF CHEMICAL NEUROANATOMY

Edited by A. Björklund and T. Hökfelt

Volume 4:

GABA AND NEUROPEPTIDES IN THE CNS, PART I

Editors:
A. BJÖRKLUND
Department of Histology
University of Lund, Lund, Sweden

T. HÖKFELT
Department of Histology
Karolinska Institute, Stockholm, Sweden

1985

ELSEVIER

Amsterdam – New York – Oxford

ISBN 0 444 90353 4
ISBN SERIES 0 444 90340 2

Library of Congress Cataloging-in-Publication Data
Main entry under title:

GABA and neuropeptides in the CNS.
  (Handbook of chemical neuroanatomy ; v. 4, etc.)
  Includes bibliographies and index.
  1. Neuropeptides–Analysis.   2. GABA–Analysis.
3.Central nervous system–Anatomy.   I. Björklund,
Anders, 1945-   .   II. Hökfelt, Tomas.   III. Series.
[DNLM: 1. Central Nervous System.   2. GABA.   3. Nerve
Tissue Proteins. W1 HA51J v. 4 etc. / WL 104 G112]
QM451.H24   1983 vol. 4, etc.   616.8 s   85-20596
[QP552.N39]   [599′.01′88]
ISBN 0-444-90353-4 (U.S. : pt. 1)

Published by:
Elsevier Science Publishers B.V.
P.O. Box 1126
1000 BC Amsterdam

Sole distributors for the USA and Canada:
Elsevier Science Publishing Co. Inc.
52 Vanderbilt Avenue
New York, NY 10017

Printed in The Netherlands by Casparie – Amsterdam

To
Rolf Luft
Viktor Mutt
and
Bengt Pernow

List of contributors

G.M. ABRAMS
Department of Neurology
College of Physicians and Surgeons
Columbia University
630 West 168th Street
New York, NY 10032
U.S.A.

J. BARRY
Laboratoire d'Histologie
Faculté de Médecine
Place de Verdun
59045 Lille
France

M.J. BROWNSTEIN
Laboratory of Clinical Science
National Institute of Mental Health
Building 10
National Institutes of Health
Bethesda, MD 20205
U.S.A.

P.C. EMSON
MRC Neurochemical Pharmacology Unit
Medical Research Council Centre
Hills Road
Cambridge, CB2 2QH
U.K.

M. GOEDERT
MRC Neurochemical Pharmacology Unit
Medical Research Council Centre
Hills Road
Cambridge, CB2 2QH
U.K.

G.E. HOFFMAN
Department of Anatomy
University of Rochester
School of Medicine and Dentistry
Rochester, NY 14642
U.S.A.

KANG TSOU
Shanghai Institute of Materia Medica
Chinese Academy of Science
Shanghai 200031
China

H. KHACHATURIAN
Mental Health Research Institute
The University of Michigan
205 Washtenaw Place
Ann Arbor, MI 48109
U.S.A.

M.E. LEWIS
Mental Health Research Institute
The University of Michigan
205 Washtenaw Place
Ann Arbor, MI 48109
U.S.A.

J.L. MADERDRUT
Department of Anatomy
Bowman Gray School of Medicine
Winston-Salem, NC 27103
U.S.A.

P.W. MANTYH
MRC Neurochemical Pharmacology Unit
Medical Research Council Centre
Hills Road
Cambridge, CB2 2QH
U.K.

I. MERCHENTHALER
Department of Anatomy
University of North Carolina
111 Swing Building
Chapel Hill, NC 27514
U.S.A.

E. MUGNAINI
Laboratory of Neuromorphology
Department of Biobehavioral Sciences
Box 154, University of Connecticut
Storrs, CT 06268
U.S.A.

G. NILAVER
Department of Neurology
College of Physicians and Surgeons
Columbia University
630 West 168th Street
New York, NY 10032
U.S.A.

W.H. OERTEL
Department of Neurology
Technical University of Munich
Moehlstrasse 28
D-8000 München 80
F.R.G.

M. PALKOVITS
Laboratory of Cell Biology
National Institute of Mental Health
Building 36, Rm 3A-17
National Institutes of Health
Bethesda, MD 20205
U.S.A.

P. PETRUSZ
Department of Anatomy
University of North Carolina
111 Swing Building
Chapel Hill, NC 27514
U.S.A.

V. PICKEL
Laboratory of Neurobiology
Department of Neurology
Cornell University Medical College
1300 York Avenue
New York, NY 10021
U.S.A.

M.V. SOFRONIEW
Department of Human Anatomy
South Parks Road
Oxford, OX1 3QX
U.K.
Present address:
Department of Neurosurgery
Meyer 7-109
The Johns Hopkins Hospital
600 North Wolfe Street
Baltimore, MD 21205
U.S.A.

J.J. VANDERHAEGHEN
Laboratory of Neuropathology and
    Neuropeptide Research
Faculty of Medicine
Free University of Brussels
Queen Elizabeth Medical Foundation
1 J.J. Crocq Avenue
1020 Brussels
Belgium

S.J. WATSON
Mental Health Research Institute
University of Michigan School of
    Medicine
205 Washtenaw Place
Ann Arbor, MI 48109
U.S.A.

S. WRAY
Department of Anatomy
University of Rochester
School of Medicine and Dentistry
Rochester, NY 14642
U.S.A.

E.A. ZIMMERMAN
Department of Neurology
Columbia Presbyterian Hospital
Neurology Institute, Room 216
710 W. 168th Street
New York, NY 10032
U.S.A.

Preface

The first neuroactive peptides to be structurally identified in the central nervous system were vasopressin and oxytocin (Du Vigneaud et al. 1953a,b). At that time, these peptides were viewed as hormones, and the so-called neurosecretory neurons (Bargmann and Scharrer 1951) which produce them were thought to be exceptional in that they secrete their products in an endocrine manner into the bloodstream. The current upsurge of interest in the role of small peptides as transmitter candidates or neuromodulatory compounds dates back to the early 1970's. Of great importance for this development was the discovery by Guillemin, Schally, Vale and their collaborators that the hypothalamic releasing and inhibitory hormones, originally postulated by Harris in 1955 – in terms of their chemistry – belong to the group of small peptides. Thus, thyrotropin releasing hormone (TRH) turned out to be a tripeptide (Bøler et al. 1969; Burgus et al. 1969), the luteinizing hormone releasing hormone (LHRH) a decapeptide (Amoss et al. 1971; Matsuo et al. 1971; Schally et al. 1971), and somatostatin, the growth hormone release inhibiting hormone, a tetradecapeptide (Brazeau et al. 1971).

At about the same time, Leeman and collaborators (Chang et al. 1971) were able to chemically characterize a compound, substance P, which was already discovered in 1931 by Von Euler and Gaddum. Substance P was also found to be a peptide, an undecapeptide. Using radioimmunoassay and immunohistochemistry, it was demonstrated that these peptides occur in neurons not only in the hypothalamus but also in widespread areas of the central nervous system, and in several cases also in peripheral neurons.

These discoveries drew attention to other peptide hormones that had been isolated and structurally characterized much earlier, for example cholecystokinin (CCK), first described by Mutt and Jorpes in 1968. In fact, the demonstration of gastrin/CCK-like immunoreactivity in the brain by Vanderhaeghen and coworkers (1975) showed that a polypeptide which so far had been associated only with endocrine functions in the periphery, could also be present in the central nervous system. These and many other findings were the basis for the growing interest in and formulation of the concept of the brain-gut axis.

During the seventies and eighties, numerous other neuronal peptides have been discovered. Snyder (1980), discussing a possible transmitter role of peptides in the central nervous system, predicted that their number may well be several hundred, and the development since then has supported that prediction. In fact, an important issue has been the realization that families of peptides may exist. One example is the dramatic progress in the field of opioid peptides, starting with the discovery by Hughes, Kosterlitz and collaborators (1975) of two pentapeptides, the enkephalins, with opioid activity in the brain. Thanks to the work of many groups, notably Eipper and Mains and the teams around Chrétien, Goldstein, Herbert and Numa, this research has resulted in less than a decade in a fairly complete knowledge of the precursor molecules not only of these two pentapeptides but also of two other opioid peptide precursors, and the description of a large number of biologically active cleavage products arising from these compounds (see Weber et al. 1983).

Furthermore, evidence has been presented that substance P is not the only tachykinin present in the mammalian nervous system, but that there are several compounds belonging to this peptide family. Thus, substance P and substance K are two peptides coded for by the same gene; in addition, there are other tachykinins (Kangawa et al. 1983; Kimura et al. 1983; Nawa et al. 1983; Minamino et al. 1984; Tatemoto et al. 1985).

New powerful techniques have contributed to these advancements and to the explosive development in the peptide field. Thus, in addition to classical purification methods starting with huge amounts of tissue and purification steps monitored by parallel bioassay, there are now more chemically oriented methods, depending on for example, isolation of peptides containing C-terminal amide groups (Tatemoto and Mutt 1980). The DNA recombinant technology is now rapidly being introduced in the field of neurobiology. The discovery of a calcitonin gene related peptide (CGRP) (Amara et al. 1982; Rosenfeld et al. 1983) with powerful actions in the central and peripheral nervous systems represents a major breakthrough demonstrating the potential of this approach.

The *Neuropeptides* volumes of the *Handbook of Chemical Neuroanatomy* deal with the structural organization of neuropeptide-containing neuronal systems in the CNS, as revealed primarily by the immunohistochemical technique. In the second of the two *Neuropeptide* volumes so far planned, we have also included chapters dealing with peptide receptor localization based on the ligand binding techniques. Peptide distributions in peripheral tissues are covered in the *Peripheral Nervous System* volume of This Series.

The present volume also includes a major chapter by Mugnaini and Oertel on GABA neurons in the CNS as revealed by an antiserum raised against the GABA-synthesizing enzyme, glutamic acid decarboxylase (GAD). This chapter was originally planned for Volume 3, but due to the extensive work the authors had to invest in this chapter – reflecting the vast and complex distribution of the GABAergic system throughout all parts of the CNS – we chose to include it in the present volume. This chapter, which should be studied in conjunction with the chapters by Ottersen and Storm-Mathisen and by McGeer and collaborators in *Volume 3*, gives a unique overview of putative GABAergic neurons in the CNS and contains a wealth of previously unpublished material, including the first complete mapping of GAD in the rat CNS.

The term 'neuropeptide' is as yet poorly defined. The compounds included here share localizational features in that: (1) they are neuron-specific (although they occur in endocrine and paracrine types of cells as well); (2) they are characteristic for defined subsets of neurons, i.e. for some but not all neurons; and (3) they are likely to be secretory products of these neuronal subsets. Functionally, the compounds we now include among the neuropeptides may, on the other hand, turn out to be quite heterogeneous. For some of the most studied peptides, such as vasopressin, oxytocin and the hypophysiotrophic peptides, at least part of their biological properties (in particular their neurohormonal actions) are well known. But even so, the role of neuropeptides in neuronal communication is only beginning to be unraveled. This problem is particularly evident for individual members of the 'peptide families' such as the opioid peptide, substance P or the pancreatic polypeptide families mentioned above. It is possible, or perhaps even likely, that only some of these neuropeptides will turn out to possess neurotransmitter- or neuromodulator-type actions, while others may exert e.g. trophic, metabolic or vascular effects.

Regardless of their function, however, the neuropeptides have become important as chemical 'tags' for the study of neuronal circuitries. Thus, the neuropeptides and the neuropeptide families serve to label subsets of neurons that are, or are likely to be, functionally related, and sensitive and specific antibodies raised against the purified or synthetic compounds are today important tools for selective immunohistochemical visualization of such neuronal subsets. The availability of an increasing repertoire of neuropeptide antisera has in fact been of great importance for the rapid development of chemical neuroanatomy over the last decade.

The immunohistochemical visualization of peptide-containing neurons forms the basis of most chapters in the present volume. While this has proved to be a powerful approach, there are definite interpretational problems inherent to the technique which are important to bear in mind, viz. the shortcomings of the immunological recognition mechanisms which underlie the attachment of the antibodies to antigens in the tissue. Thus, most antibodies used recognize only a small part of a peptide molecule, and it is well known that such antigenic determinant parts may be shared by several different (although sometimes related) peptides. Specificity is therefore frequently a difficult problem in the interpretation of immunohistochemical pictures. In some fields, such as the opioid peptide or the pancreatic polypeptide family, this has been gradually sorted out through the combined use of antibodies directed against different parts of a molecule or against different related molecules. However, in other cases, e.g. the gastrin/ CCK family of peptides or the tachykinin family of peptides, much work obviously remains in order to establish the diversity and identity of immunohistochemically visualized compounds. This elementary feature of antibody-based staining is the reason why most authors chose to characterize their observed material as (peptide)-like immunoreactivity. This is particularly warranted in microscopic material, where high concentrations of antiserum are used and where the tissue most often is exposed to fixatives (such as formaldehyde or glutaraldehyde) which can modify or significantly alter the chemical structure of the compounds under study.

Peptide research has a strong tradition in Sweden. Substance P, in a broad sense one of the best characterized neuronal peptides, was discovered by Von Euler and Gaddum in 1931. Börje Uvnäs and his collaborators have been working since the sixties on the physiology and pharmacology of gastrointestinal hormones. Viktor Mutt and his colleagues have for decades played a leading role in the work of isolating peptides from the gastrointestinal tract and, much based on their discoveries, an intense peptide research has been going on since the beginning of the seventies at Swedish Universities, especially at the Karolinska Institutet and in Lund.

The two volumes *'Neuropeptides in the CNS'* are dedicated to three of the pioneer Swedish scientists who have been of special importance to us and the development in this research area. They are Rolf Luft, Bengt Pernow and Viktor Mutt. Viktor Mutt, Professor of Biochemistry at Karolinska Institutet, has discovered more than a dozen peptides, mainly by isolation from the gastrointestinal tract. Among these peptides are cholecystokinin, vasoactive intestinal polypeptide (VIP), neuropeptide Y, peptide HI and peptide YY. Through his work and extreme generosity, laboratories not only in Sweden but all over the world have benefited greatly and obtained peptides for their research. Uncountable numbers of papers have been published based on peptides provided by Viktor Mutt and his associates.

Initiation of research in a new area is often the result of the insight and foresight of single individuals. Thus, the explosive development of peptide research in Sweden was much dependent on the initiative of Professor Bengt Pernow and Professor Rolf Luft. In the beginning of the 1970's they were among the first to realize the interesting new opportunities that were opening up in the neuropeptide field. Bengt Pernow, Professor of Clinical Physiology at the Karolinska Hospital, wrote his now classical thesis on substance P (Pernow 1953) in the mid fifties, working in Ulf von Euler's laboratory. When Susan Leeman and her collaborators in 1971 sequenced substance P, Pernow realized the full potential of this discovery and initiated a new dynamic phase of substance P research which was then transmitted to many laboratories in Sweden, including our own. He recently summarized the progress in the substance P field in a review article

Preface

in *Pharmacological Reviews* (Pernow 1983). Rolf Luft was the first Professor of Endocrinology in Sweden, and already in the late forties he carried out work related to hypothalamic control of anterior pituitary hormone secretion. As a leading scientist in the field of diabetes, he became interested in somatostatin and initiated work at the Karolinska Institutet on the distribution and functional role of this peptide not only as a hypothalamic hormone but also, surprisingly, with regard to its involvement in the function of the endocrine pancreas (Luft et al. 1974).

It is an honour and pleasure to dedicate the neuropeptide volumes to these three pioneers and friends, who have been of great importance not only for our own research but for biomedical research in Sweden in general.

Lund and Stockholm in July 1985

ANDERS BJÖRKLUND   TOMAS HÖKFELT

References

Amaria SG, Jonas V, Rosenfeld MG, Ong ES, Evans RM (1982): Alternative RNA-processing in calcitonin gene expression generates mRNAs encoding different polypeptide products. *Nature (London), 298,* 240-244.

Amoss M, Burgus R, Blackwell R, Vale W, Fellows R, Guillemin R (1971): Purification, amino acid composition and N-terminus of the hypothalamic luteinizing hormone-releasing factor (LRF) of bovine origin. *Biochem. Biophys. Res. Commun., 44,* 205-210.

Bargmann W, Scharrer B (1951): The site of origin of the hormones of the posterior pituitary. *Am. Sci., 39,* 255-259.

Bøler J, Enzmann F, Folkers K, Bowers CY, Schally AV (1969): The identity of chemical and hormonal properties of the thyrotropin-releasing hormone and pyroglutamyl-histidyl-proline amide. *Biochem. Biophys. Res. Commun., 37,* 705-710.

Brazeau P, Vale W, Burgus R, Ling N, Butcher M, Rivier R, Guillemin R (1973): Hypothalamic polypeptide that inhibits the secretion of immunoreactive pituitary growth hormone. *Science, 179,* 77-79.

Burgus R, Dunn TF, Desiderio D, Guillemin R (1969): Structure moléculaire du facteur hypothalamique hypophysiotrope TRF d'origine ovine: mise en évidence par spectrométrie de masse de la séquence PCA-His-Pro-NH$_2$. *C.R. Acad. Sci. Paris (Ser. D), 269,* 1870-1873.

Chang MM, Leeman SE, Niall HD (1971): Amino acid sequence of substance P. *Nature New Biol., 232,* 86-87.

Du Vigneaud V, Lawler HC, Popenoe EA (1953a): Enzymatic cleavage of glycinamide from vasopressin and a proposed structure for the pressor-antidiuretic hormone of the posterior pituitary. *J. Am. Chem. Soc., 75,* 4880-4881.

Du Vigneaud V, Ressler C, Swan JM, Roberts CW, Katsoyannis PG, Gordon S (1953b): The synthesis of an octapeptide amide with the hormonal activity of oxytocin. *J. Am. Chem. Soc., 75,* 4879-4880.

Harris GH (1955): *Neural Control of the Pituitary Gland.* Edward Arnold, London.

Hughes J, Smith TW, Kosterlitz HW, Fothergill LA, Morgan BA, Morris HR (1975): Identification of two related pentapeptides from the brain with potent opiate agonist activity. *Nature (London), 258,* 577–579.

Kangawa K, Minamino N, Fukuda A, Matsuo H (1983): Neuromedin K: a novel mammalian tachykinin identified in porcine spinal cord. *Biochem. Biophys. Res. Commun., 114,* 533-540.

Kimura S, Okada M, Sugita Y, Kanazawa I, Munekata E (1983): Novel neuropeptides, neurokinin α and β, isolated from porcine spinal cord. *Proc. Jap. Acad., 59,* 101.

Luft R, Efendic S, Hökfelt T, Johansson O, Arimura A (1974): Immunohistochemical evidence for the localization of somatostatin-like immunoreactivity in a cell population of the pancreatic islets. *Med. Biol., 52;* 428-430.

Matsuo H, Arimura A, Nair RMG, Schally AV (1971): Synthesis of the porcine LH and FSH releasing hormone by the solid phase method. *Biochem. Biophys. Res. Commun., 45,* 822-827.

Minamino N, Kangawa, K, Fukuda A, Matsuo H (1984): A novel mammalian tachykinin identified in porcine spinal cord. *Neuropeptides, 4,* 157-166.

Mutt V, Jorpes JE (1968): Structure of porcine cholecystokinin-pancreozymin. I. Cleavage with thrombin and with trypsin. *Eur. J. Biochem., 6,* 156-162.

Nawa H, Hirose T, Takashima H, Ianyama S, Nakanishi S (1983): Nucleotide sequences of cloned cDNAs for two types of bovine brain substance P precursor. *Nature (London), 306,* 32-36.

Pernow B (1953): Studies on substance P: purification, occurrence and biological actions. *Acta Physiol. Scand., 29 (Suppl.),* 1-105.

Pernow B (1983): Substance P. *Pharmacol. Rev., 35,* 85-141.

Rosenfeld MG, Mermod J-J, Amara SG, Swanson LW, Sawchenko PE, Rivier J, Vale WW, Evans RM (1983): Production of a novel neuropeptide encoded by the calcitonin gene via tissue-specific RNA processing. *Nature (London), 304,* 129-135.

Schally AV, Arimura A, Baba Y, Nair RMG, Matsuo J, Redding TW, Debeljuk L, White WF (1971): Isolation and properties of the FSH- and LH-releasing hormone. *Biochem. Biophys. Res. Commun., 43,* 393-399.

Snyder SH (1980): Brain peptides as neurotransmitters. *Science, 209,* 976-983.

Tatemoto K, Mutt V (1980): Isolation of two novel candidate hormones using a chemical method for finding naturally occurring polypeptides. *Nature (London), 285,* 417-418.

Tatemoto K, Lundberg JM, Jörnvall M, Mutt V (1985): Neuropeptide K: isolation, structure and biological activities of a novel brain tachykinin. *Nature (London),* submitted for publication.

Vanderhaeghen JJ, Signeau JC, Gepts W (1975): New peptide in the vertebrate CNS reacting with anti-gastrin antibodies. *Nature (London), 257,* 604-605.

Von Euler US, Gaddum JH (1931): An unidentified depressor substance in certain tissue extracts. *J. Physiol. (London), 72,* 74-87.

Weber E, Evans CJ, Barchas JD (1983): Multiple endogenous ligands for opioid receptors. *TINS, 6,* 333-336.

Contents

Contents

Contents

V. β-ENDORPHIN, α-MSH, ACTH, AND RELATED PEPTIDES –
H. KHACHATURIAN, M.E. LEWIS, KANG TSOU AND S.J. WATSON

Contents

Contents

X. AN ATLAS OF THE DISTRIBUTION OF GABAERGIC NEURONS
   AND TERMINALS IN THE RAT CNS AS REVEALED BY GAD
   IMMUNOHISTOCHEMISTRY – E. MUGNAINI AND W.H. OERTEL

CHAPTER I

Distribution of neuropeptides in the central nervous system using biochemical micromethods

MIKLÓS PALKOVITS AND MICHAEL J. BROWNSTEIN

1. INTRODUCTION

Since the substantive material in this chapter can be found in the maps that we have prepared, the text that follows will be brief and of a general nature. About 3 dozen biologically active peptides have been detected in the central nervous system to date (see Palkovits 1984). Not all of these have been rigorously characterized and only 20 have been mapped extensively in the rat brain (Figs 2–21). The remainder have either been measured in extracts of large brain areas (see Palkovits 1980,1984) or in random assortments of nuclei.

The figures that we present are based on radioimmunoassays (RIAs) of peptides in microdissected ('punched') samples of rat brain, though the distributions of neuropeptides have been measured in the brains of several other species. In our studies we removed each nucleus in its entirety (see Brownstein and Palkovits, *Vol. 2*, This Series). Within certain nuclei, peptides are heterogeneously distributed; however, finer dissections would be needed to reveal this heterogeneity.

Most of the maps presented are based on our own RIA data. We only incorporated data from other workers' studies into our figures when their values were similar. This is because different investigators have obtained somewhat different absolute values when they have determined the concentrations of peptides in brain samples; thus, we used symbols indicating relative peptide levels instead of numerical values. We will not attempt to evaluate differences in tissue preparation, extraction, or assay procedures used in various laboratories, nor will we comment on the specificity of antibodies employed in our studies or those of others. For such a discussion the reader is referred to the original papers (see References).

When no peptide is detected in a particular nucleus, it is possible that the assay used is not sensitive enough to measure what is there; 'non-detectable' should not be equated with 'absent'. Since neuropeptides are synthesized in neuronal perikarya and rapidly transported away, it seems generally true that areas rich in peptide have dense fiber networks.

Each of the peptides mapped in the rat brain to date has its own characteristic distribution pattern. They are shown in Figures 2–21 (p. 10), whereby the various brain nuclei are labeled with their abbreviations in Figure 1 (p. 7). In Table 1 a key is given to the correlation between the actual concentrations of the various peptides in ng/mg protein. Four categories (very high, high, moderate, low) are created and indicated by red symbols in the maps.

Handbook of Chemical Neuroanatomy. Vol. 4: GABA and Neuropeptides in the CNS, Part I.
A. Björklund and T. Hökfelt, editors.
© Elsevier Science Publishers B.V., 1985.

TABLE 1. *Concentrations of neuropeptides (ng peptide/mg protein)*

	Classes			
	Very high	High	Moderate	Low
	Over:		*Between:*	*Less than:*
LH-RH	10	2–10	0.5–2	0.5
TRH	10	2–10	0.5–2	0.5
CRF	10	2–10	0.5–2	0.5
Somatostatin	15	5–15	1–5	1
Oxytocin	100	20–100	1–20	1
Vasopressin	100	20–100	1–20	1
ACTH	5	5–5	0.5–2	0.5
α-MSH	8	3–8	1–3	1
β-Endorphin	10	2–10	0.5–2	0.5
Met-enkephalin	12	4–12	1–4	1
Leu-enkephalin	4	1.5–4	0.5–1.5	0.5
Dynorphin A	0.32	0.22–0.32	0.14–0.22	0.14
Dynorphin B	0.30	0.15–0.30	0.075–0.15	0.075
α-Neo-endorphin	0.60	0.30–0.60	0.15–0.30	0.15
β-Neo-endorphin	0.28	0.20–0.28	0.12–0.20	0.12
VIP	7.5	3–7.5	1–3	1
Cholecystokinin	7.5	5–7.5	2.5–5	2.5
Bombesin	5	2.5–5	1.2–2.5	1.2
Substance P	7.5	2.5–7.5	1–2.5	1
Neurotensin	5	2–5	0.5–2	0.5

2. COMMENTS ON THE DISTRIBUTIONAL MAPS

Neuropeptides are present in all major CNS areas. A list of brain regions with particularly high peptide levels appears in Table 2. The region that is the most rich in neuropeptides in the brain is the median eminence. All of the 20 neuropeptides mapped here are measurable there; 7 of these are present in very high levels (Table 3).

The hypothalamus is the major brain region that is richest in neuropeptides. This region has been extensively studied and mapped with both biochemical and immunohistochemical techniques. *All* neuropeptides identified in the central nervous system are present in the hypothalamus. On the basis of 20 complete biochemical mapping studies, one can conclude that 15 of the 20 neuropeptides are present in *all* hypothalamic nuclei (Table 3). There are 2 major groups of cells where neuropeptides are highly concentrated: the arcuate and paraventricular nuclei. In the preoptic area (mainly in the medial preoptic nucleus) several neuropeptides have been measured in relatively high levels (Table 3).

Neuropeptide-rich extrahypothalamic nuclei include the central amygdala, bed nucleus of the stria terminalis, lateral septal nucleus, midbrain central gray, substantia nigra, parabrachial nuclei and nucleus of the solitary tract (Table 3).

2.1. LUTEINIZING HORMONE RELEASING HORMONE (LH-RH) (*Fig. 2*)

LH-RH is less widely distributed in the brain than other neuropeptides. It is concentrated in the median eminence and supraoptic crest (organum vasculosum laminae terminalis), and only found in significant amounts in the hypothalamus and preoptic area (Palkovits et al. 1974; Samson et al. 1980; Selmanoff et al. 1980; Kerdelhué et al. 1981).

TABLE 2. *Regions with the highest neuropeptide levels*

LH-RH	– median eminence
TRH	– median eminence
CRF	– median eminence
GRF	– median eminence
Somatostatin	– median eminence
Oxytocin	– median eminence
Vasopressin	– median eminence
ACTH	– arcuate nucleus
α-MSH	– arcuate nucleus
β-Endorphin	– central gray matter
Enkephalins	– globus pallidus
Dynorphins	– substantia nigra
VIP	– NIST (dorsal)
CCK	– claustrum
Bombesin	– nucleus of the solitary tract
Substance P	– substantia nigra
Neurotensin	– median eminence

TABLE 3. *Number of neuropeptides in selected brain nuclei (the total number of neuropeptides in this study is 20)*

	Concentrations			
	No. of peptides	Very high	High	Moderate	Low
---	---	---	---	---	---
CORTEX	17	–	2	1	14
STRIATUM	17	–	3	3	11
PALLIDUM	14	2	1	3	9
THALAMUS					
Periventricular nucleus	12	–	2	7	3
LIMBIC					
Central amygdaloid nucleus	16	–	6	8	2
Lateral septum	17	–	3	9	5
Hippocampus	17	–	1	4	12
Bed nucleus of stria terminalis (NIST)	16	1	6	7	2
HYPOTHALAMUS					
Median eminence	20	7	6	5	2
Arcuate nucleus	20	2	8	7	3
Suprachiasmatic nucleus	19	1	6	11	1
Anterior nucleus	20	–	7	10	3
Dorsomedial nucleus	18	–	9	6	3
Paraventricular nucleus	19	2	5	8	4
Ventromedial nucleus	18	–	8	8	2
Periventricular nucleus	18	2	4	10	2
Supraoptic nucleus	15	2	2	5	6
Lateral hypothalamic area (MFB)	18	–	3	9	6
MEDIAL PREOPTIC	19	2	4	10	3
MIDBRAIN					
Substantia nigra	19	3	–	4	12
Central gray matter (SGC)	20	1	6	6	7
PONS					
Parabrachial nucleus	15	1	3	4	7
MEDULLA OBLONGATA					
NTS	18	1	6	6	5
Nucleus spinalis of the Vth	13	–	2	2	9

2.2. THYROTROPIN RELEASING HORMONE (TRH) (*Fig. 3*)

TRH is found in high concentrations in the hypothalamic nuclei and in fairly high amounts in the motor nuclei of the cranial nerves (Brownstein et al. 1974; Kerdelhué et al. 1981; Eskay et al. 1983), in good agreement with immunohistochemical findings (Hökfelt et al. 1975).

2.3. CORTICOTROPIN RELEASING HORMONE (CRF) (*Fig. 4*)

The highest CRF level has been found in the median eminence, more than 10 times greater than that in the brain nuclei. CRF-like immunoreactivity was detected in 32 rat brain areas in concentrations higher than 0.3 ng/mg protein (Palkovits et al. 1985). The RIA data are, in general, fairly consistent with immunohistochemical findings.

2.4. SOMATOSTATIN (*Fig. 5*)

High somatostatin levels have been measured in the median eminence and several hypo-thalamic and preoptic nuclei (Brownstein et al. 1975; Palkovits et al. 1976, 1980). Soma-tostatin is relatively abundant in the amygdaloid nuclei (Epelbaum et al. 1979), and cer-tain lower brainstem regions, like central gray matter in the midbrain, parabrachial nuclei in the pons, and in the nucleus of the solitary tract in the medulla oblongata (Douglas and Palkovits 1982).

2.5. OXYTOCIN (*Fig. 6*)

Oxytocin levels are high in the median eminence and in the magnocellular nuclei. There are only few brain nuclei where oxytocin is detectable by RIA (George et al. 1976; Dog-terom et al. 1978; Hawthorn et al. 1984).

2.6. VASOPRESSIN (*Fig. 7*)

Vasopressin is more widely distributed in the brain than oxytocin (George and Jacobo-witz 1976; Hawthorn et al. 1980,1984; Laczi et al. 1983; Zerbe and Palkovits 1984). Be-side the magnocellular vasopressin system (nucleus supraoptic – paraventricular and median eminence), vasopressin is synthesized in the suprachiasmatic nucleus where high vasopressin levels were detected.

2.7. ACTH (*Fig. 8*)

The level of ACTH is highest in the hypothalamus, but it is only 0.1–1% of the pituitary ACTH content (Krieger et al. 1977; Palkovits et al. 1978). The intrahypothalamic distri-bution of the ACTH is fairly uneven (Mezey et al. 1985). The vast majority of ACTH immunoreactivity in the hypothalamus (and most probably in the brain) is actually CLIP (ACTH(18–39)).

2.8. MELANOCYTE-STIMULATING HORMONES (MSH's)

The presence of α-, β and γ-MSH has been shown in the central nervous system of rat by biochemical and immunohistochemical techniques. By RIA, only the α-*MSH* has been mapped (Fig. 9). α-MSH is concentrated in the hypothalamus, particularly the posterior areas but it is detectable in several brain nuclei (Eskay et al. 1979; O'Donohue et al. 1979; Mezey et al. 1985).

2.9. β-ENDORPHIN (*Fig. 10*)

β-Endorphin is present both in hypothalamic and extrahypothalamic brain areas in various concentrations (Palkovits et al. 1978; Dupont et al. 1980; Dorsa et al. 1981; Kerdelhué et al. 1983; Mezey et al. 1985). The highest β-endorphin levels were measured in the central gray matter, the dorsal raphe nucleus, the median eminence and in the hypothalamic nuclei. Recent evidence indicates the presence of α- and γ-endorphins and their des-tyrosine fragments in rat brain. These peptides have been detected in almost all major brain areas by RIA (Dorsa et al. 1981; Verhoef et al. 1982).

2.10. ENKEPHALINS (*Figs 11, 12*)

The pentapeptides leucine-enkephalin (leu-ENK) and methionine-enkephalin (met-ENK) derive from the precursor pro-enkephalin molecule. It contains 4 copies of met-ENK and single copies of leu-ENK, the heptapeptide met-ENK-Arg^6-Phe^7, and octapeptide met-ENK-Arg^6-Gly^7-Leu^8. The latter 2 are probably native opioid neurotransmitters themselves. The presence and wide distribution of met-ENK-Arg^6-Phe^7 and met-ENK-Arg^6-Gly^7-Leu^8 in the central nervous system have been recently mapped by immunohistochemistry (Williams and Dockray 1983) or RIA (Zamir et al. 1985), respectively. met-ENK (Fig. 11) and leu-ENK (Fig. 12) are widely distributed in the central nervous system. Their ratio varies from 1:1 to 6:1 with an average of 3.5:1. Extraordinarily high concentrations of enkephalins are found in the globus pallidus. High met-ENK levels were measured in the medial preoptic nucleus and the bed nucleus of the stria terminalis (NIST). High leu-ENK concentrations were found in the central amygdala and several hypothalamic nuclei (Hong et al. 1977; Kobayashi et al. 1978; Palkovits et al. 1978; Dupont et al. 1980; Zamir et al. 1985).

2.11. DYNORPHINS (*Figs 13–16*)

Five dynorphin-related peptides, dynorphin A (Fig. 13), Dy(1–9), dynorphin B (Fig. 14), α-neo-endorphin (Fig. 15) and β-neo-endorphin (Fig. 16) have been mapped in the rat brain. Their distributions in the central nervous system are not identical and the ratio of their molar concentrations varies from nucleus to nucleus. Dynorphin A is relatively evenly distributed throughout the brain, while very high concentrations of the other 4 dynorphins were measured in the substantia nigra, the ventral pallidum and the lateral preoptic area (Zamir et al. 1983, 1984a,b,c,).

2.12. VASOACTIVE INTESTINAL POLYPEPTIDE (VIP) (*Fig. 17*)

VIP is present in high concentrations in the suprachiasmatic nucleus and dorsal subdivisions of the bed nucleus of the stria terminalis (NIST). The claustrum, central amygdaloid nucleus, and cerebral cortical regions have relatively high levels as well (Lorén et al. 1979; Palkovits et al. 1981; Eiden et al. 1982; Rostène et al. 1982).

2.13. CHOLECYSTOKININ (CCK) *(Fig. 18)*

CCK is widely distributed throughout the rat brain; it is highly concentrated in the cerebral cortex, telencephalic basal ganglia (caudate-putamen, and the claustrum, nucleus accumbens), amygdala and septal nuclei (Beinfeld et al. 1981; Beinfeld and Palkovits 1981,1982).

2.14. BOMBESIN *(Fig. 19)*

Gastrin-releasing peptide (GRP) has been proposed as the mammalian counterpart of amphibian bombesin. The highest bombesin concentrations were measured in the hypothalamus, especially in the arcuate nucleus, in the midbrain interpeduncular nucleus, and in the medulla oblongata (nucleus of the solitary tract, nucleus tractus spinalis of the Vth nerve (Moody et al. 1981)). (It is worthy of note that many GRP/bombesin antisera cross-react with substance P.)

2.15. SUBSTANCE P *(Fig. 20)*

Substance P is concentrated in certain lower brainstem nuclei (substantia nigra, parabrachial nuclei, nucleus of the solitary tract, nucleus tractus spinalis of the Vth nerve) and the substantia gelatinosa of the spinal cord (Brownstein et al. 1976; Kanazawa and Jessell 1976; Kerdelhué et al. 1981; Douglas et al. 1982).

2.16. NEUROTENSIN *(Fig. 21)*

Neurotensin levels are high in the preoptic area and the median eminence but only moderate in the hypothalamic nuclei. The highest concentrations of extrahypothalamic neurotensin were found in the bed nucleus of the stria terminalis, the accumbens nucleus, mammillary body, lateral septum and the central amygdala (Kobayashi et al. 1977; Emson et al. 1982).

Biochemical mapping of other neuropeptides in the rat brain is rather *ad hoc* and incomplete. Concentrations of growth hormone releasing hormone (GRF), luteinizing hormone (LH), thyrotropin (TSH), growth hormone (GH), pancreatic polypeptides (NPY), secretin, glucagon, insulin, FMRF-amide and delta-sleep inducing peptide (DSIP) in certain rat brain nuclei are summarized and tabulated in a recent review (Palkovits 1984).

Fig. 1. (Section 1–3). These maps have been adapted from a detailed atlas of the rat brain (Palkovits 1980). Serial coronal sections at 300 μm intervals are depicted. They are proportional to one another in size; each section is magnified 5.8 times. White matter is black: nuclei are surrounded by solid lines; larger brain areas are drawn with broken lines. Microdissected areas are circular or quadrangular in shape. The size of the circular punches are 300, 500 or 1000 μm in diameter. Their location has been indicated in Chapter II, *Volume 2* of this Handbook Series.
For abbreviations, see the General Abbreviations List, p. 609.

Figs 2–21. (Section 1–3 of each). Schematic illustration of the distribution of various neuropeptides (see text) as measured by radioimmunoassays. Symbols in red as used in the maps: ■ = very high; ▨ = high; ▨ = moderate, and ▦ = low. Concentrations in ng/mg protein of these categories are given in Table 1.

6

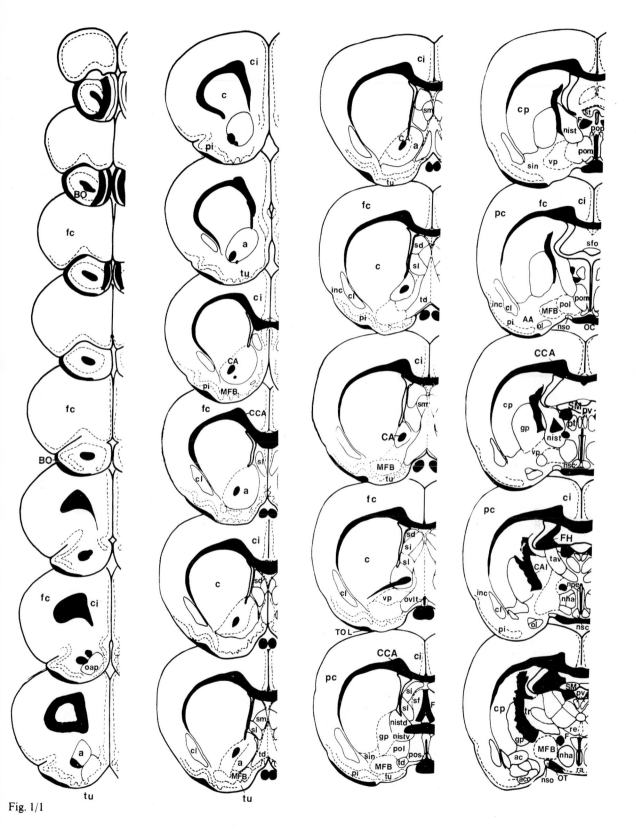

Fig. 1/1

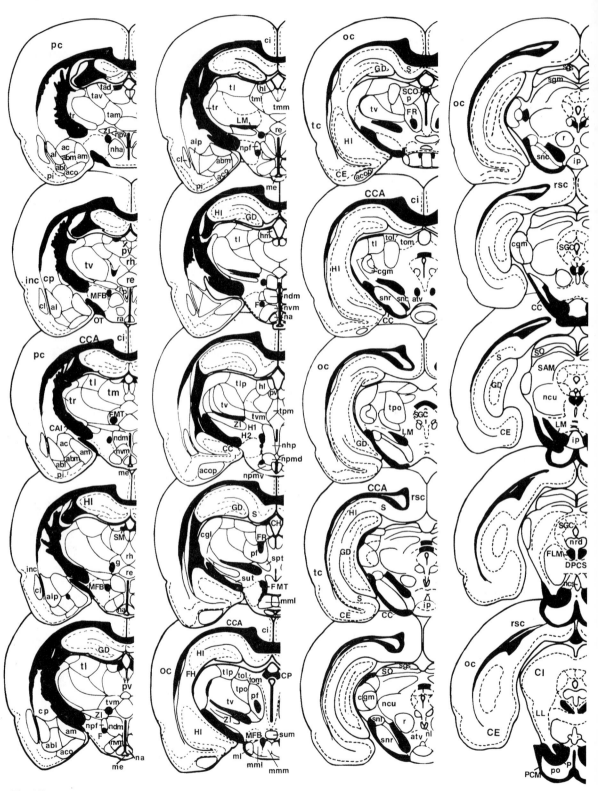

Fig. 1/2

8

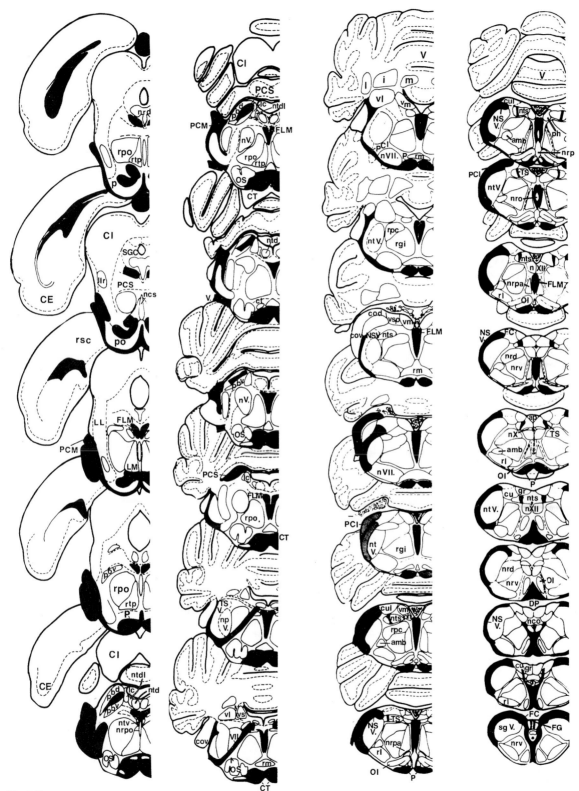

Fig. 1/3

9

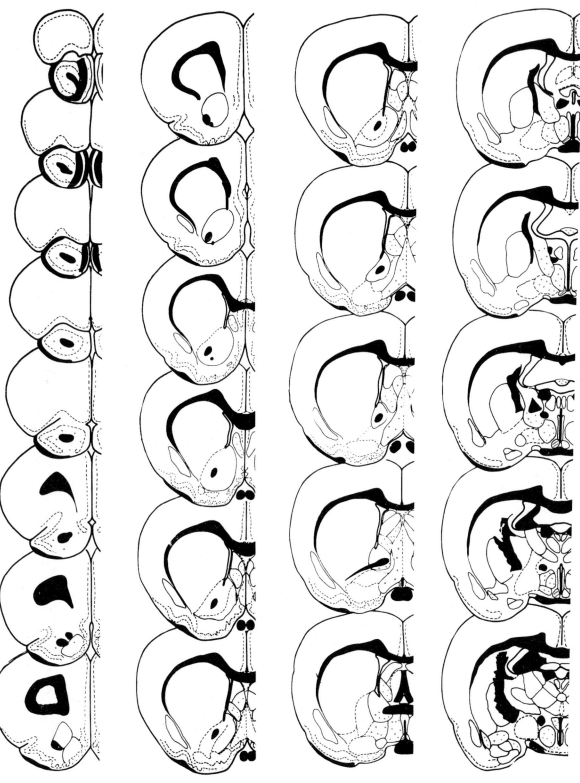

Fig. 2/1

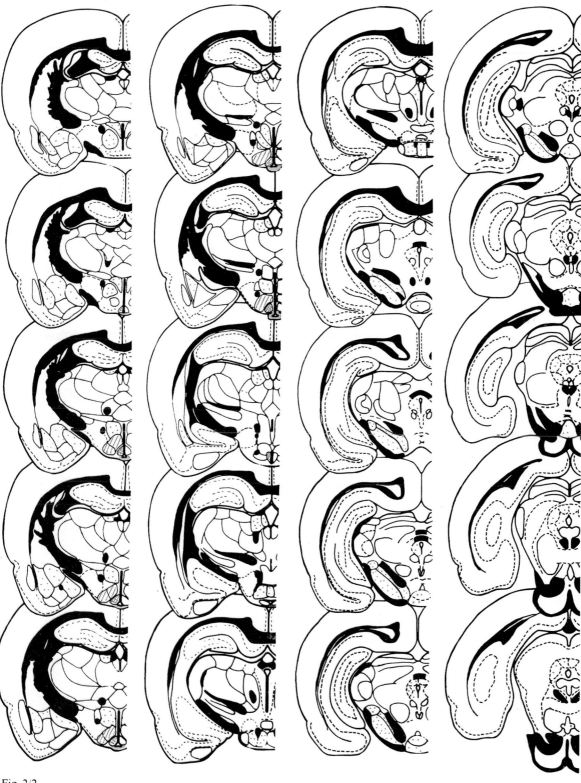

Fig. 2/2

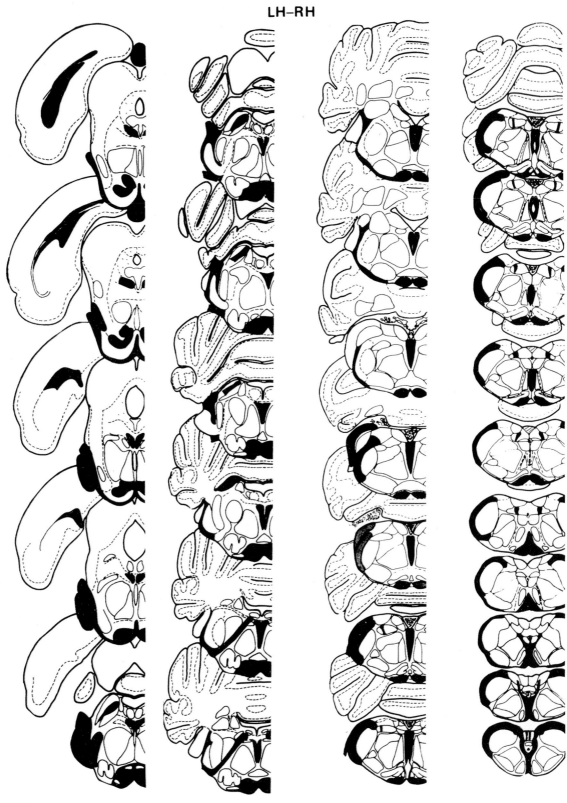

Fig. 2/3

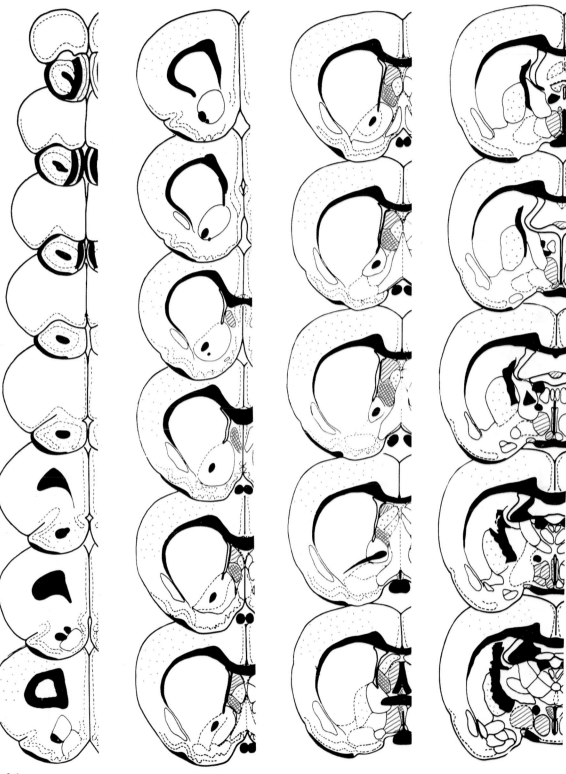

Fig. 3/1

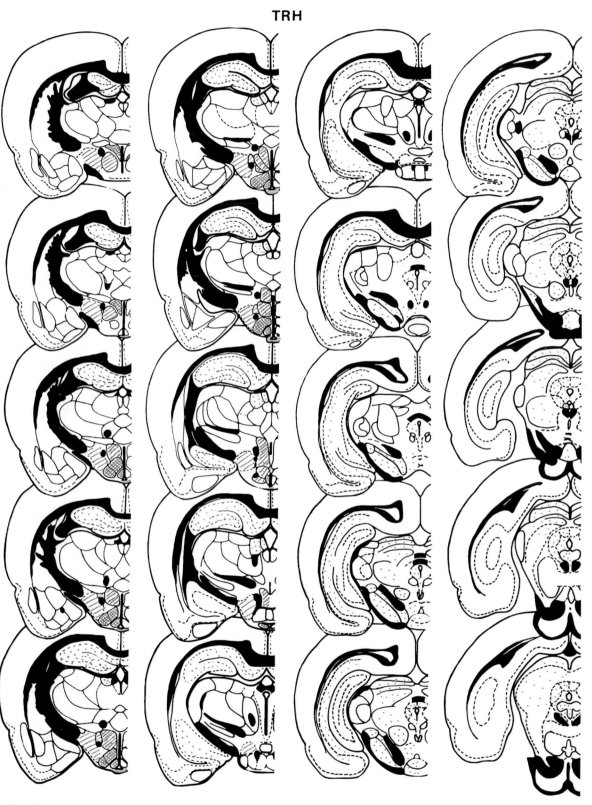

Fig. 3/2

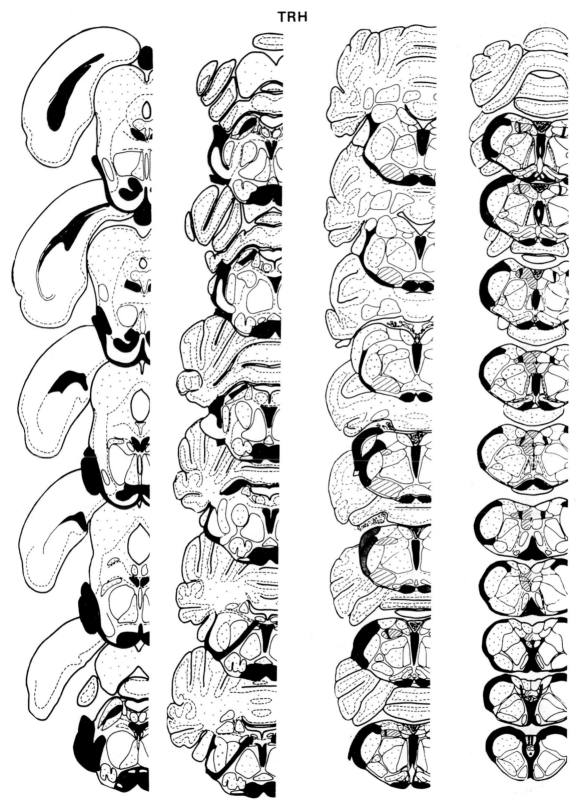

Fig. 3/3

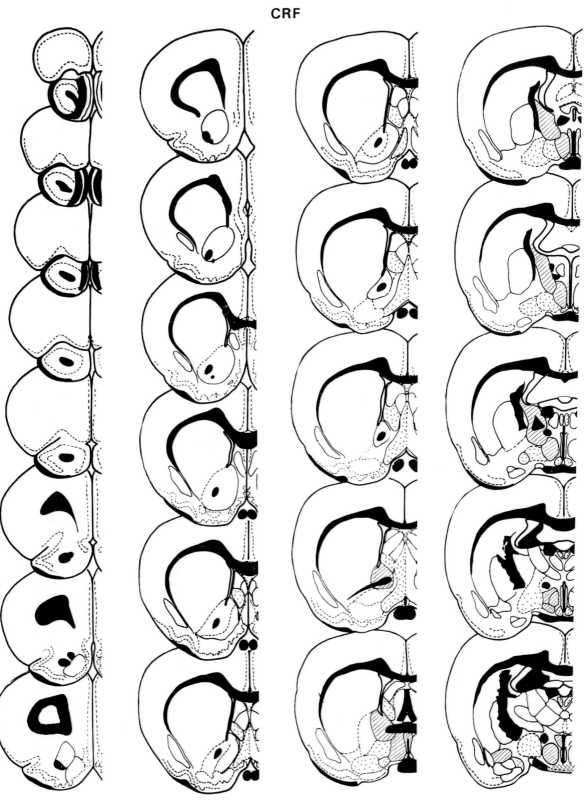

Fig. 4/1

CRF

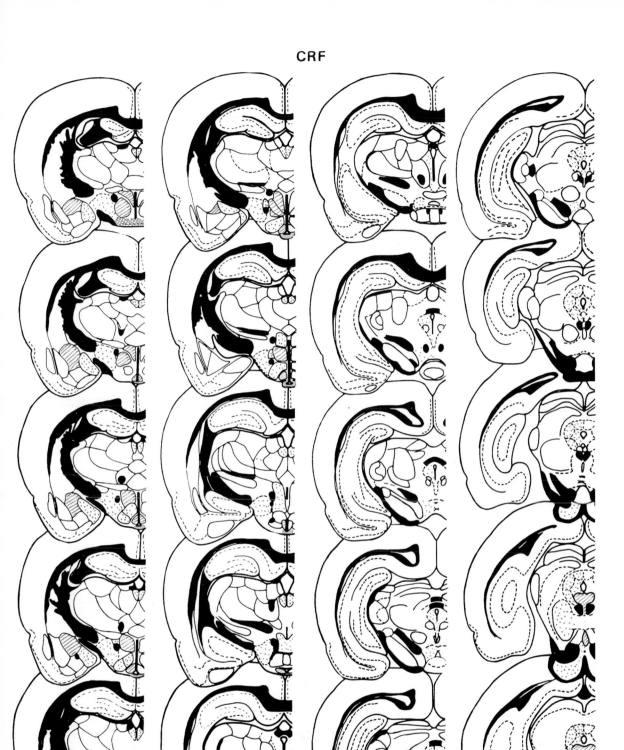

Fig. 4/2

17

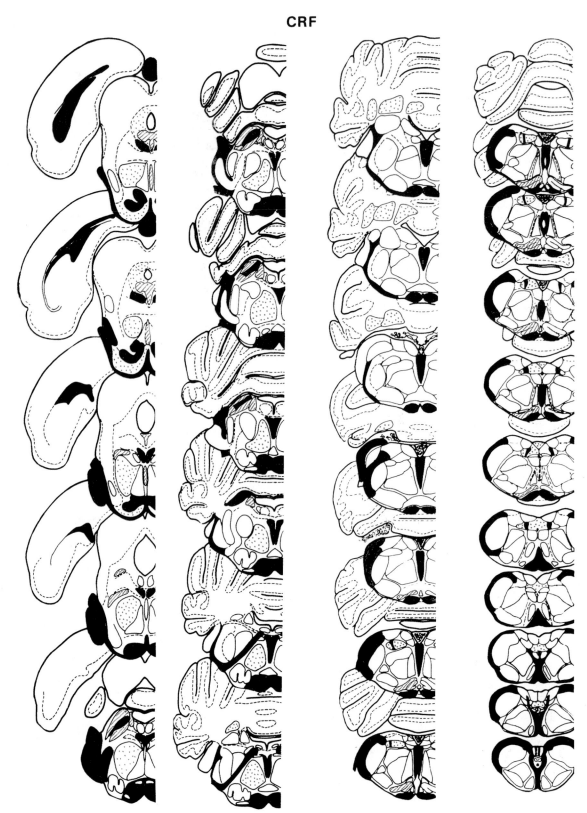

Fig. 4/3

18

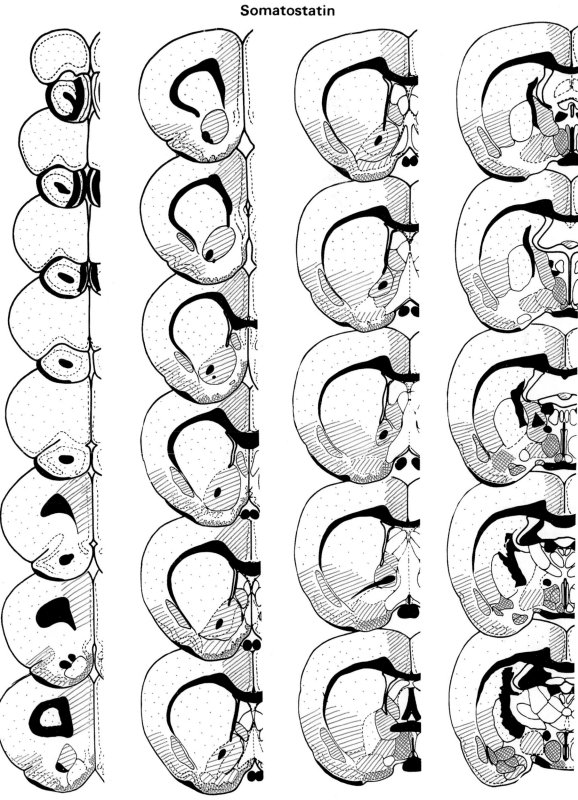

Fig. 5/1

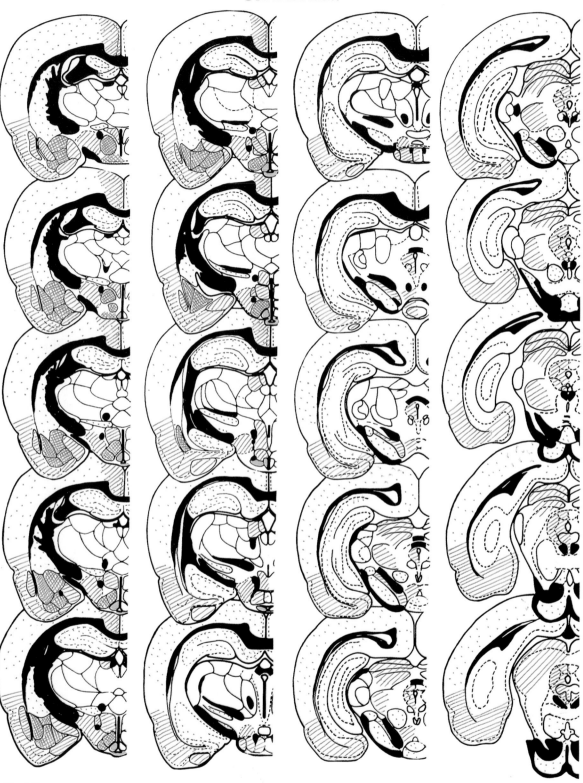

Fig. 5/2

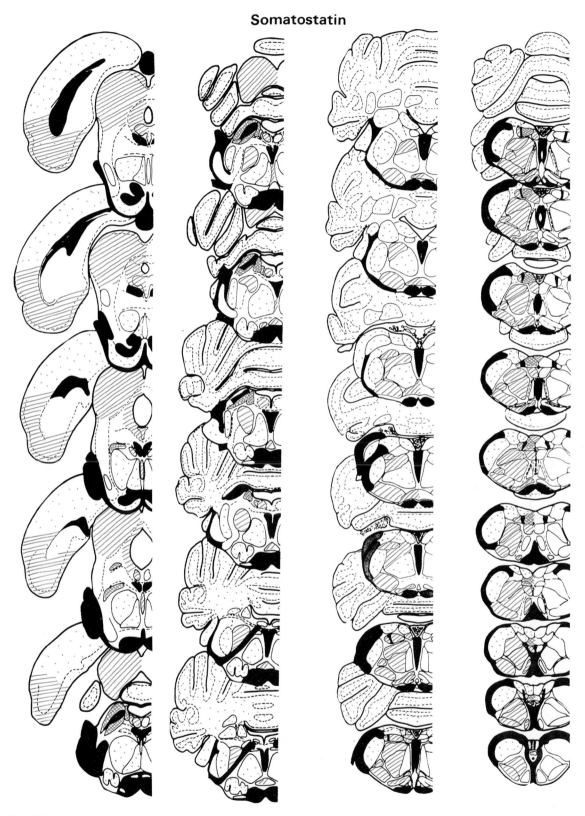

Fig. 5/3

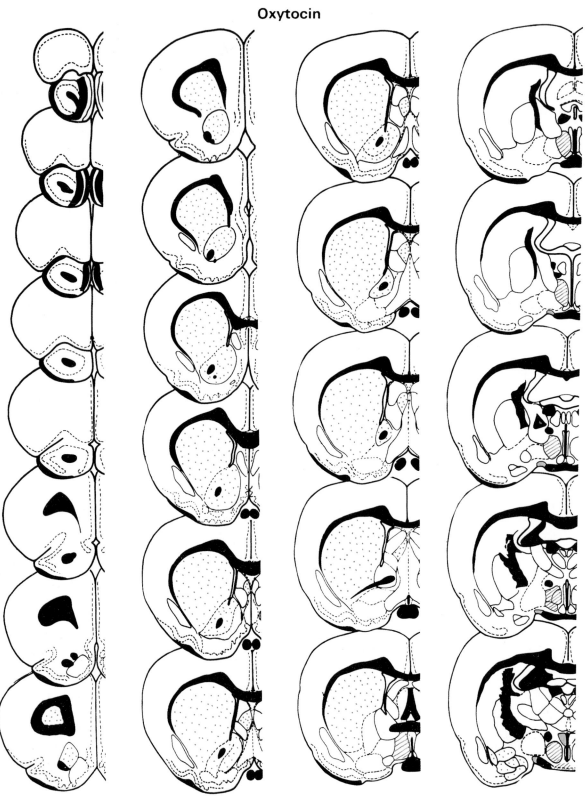

Fig. 6/1

22

Oxytocin

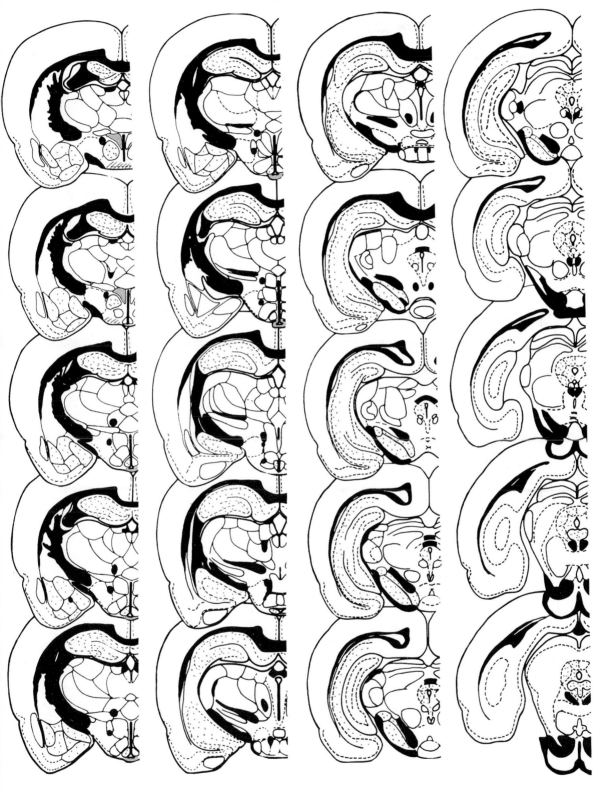

Fig. 6/2

Oxytocin

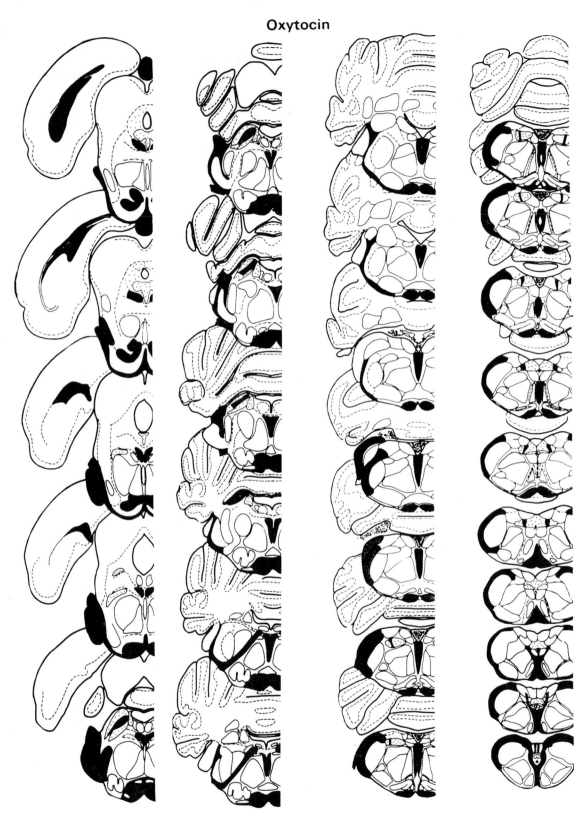

Fig. 6/3

24

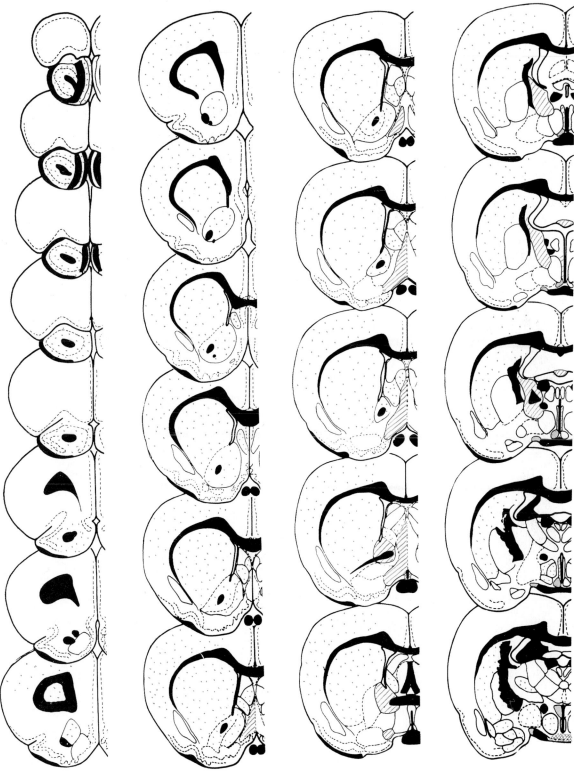

Fig. 7/1

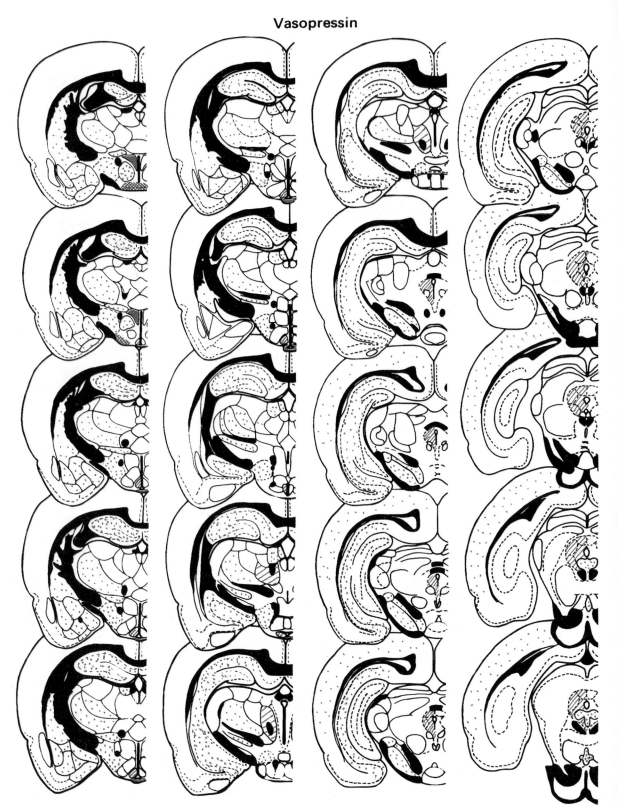

Fig. 7/2

26

Vasopressin

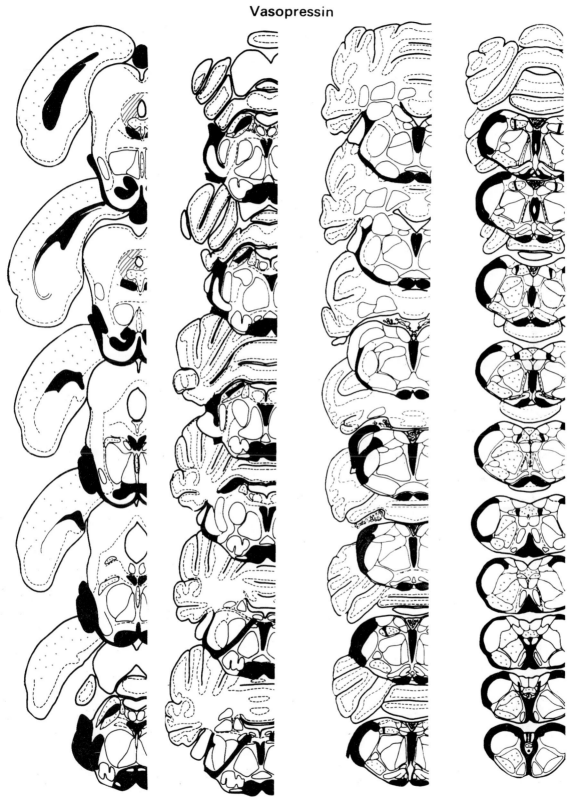

Fig. 7/3

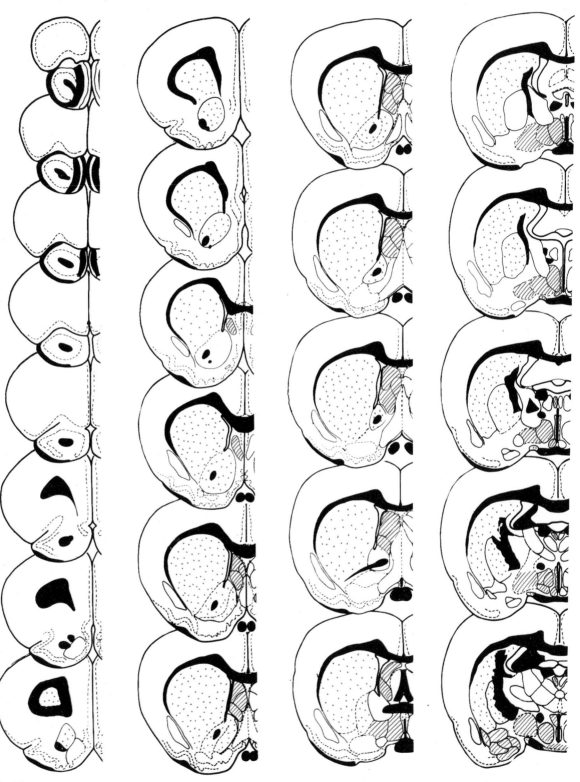

Fig. 8/1

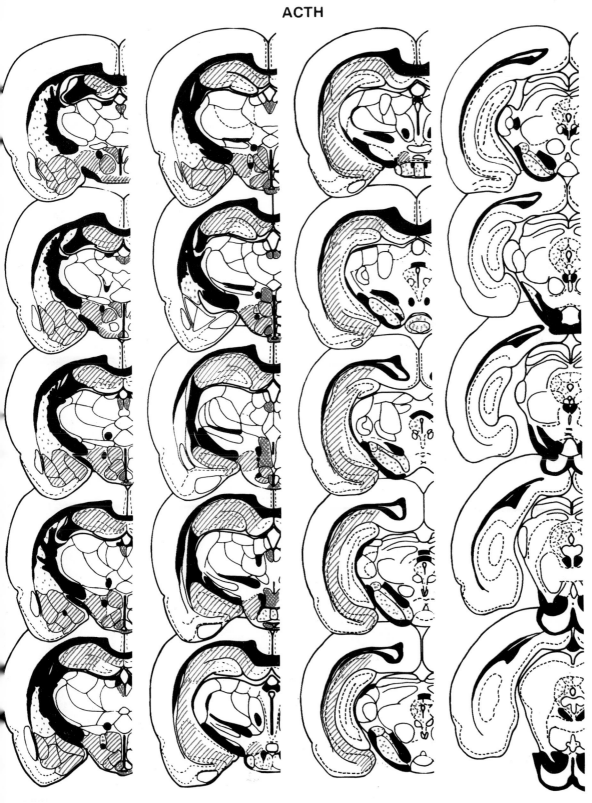

Fig. 8/2

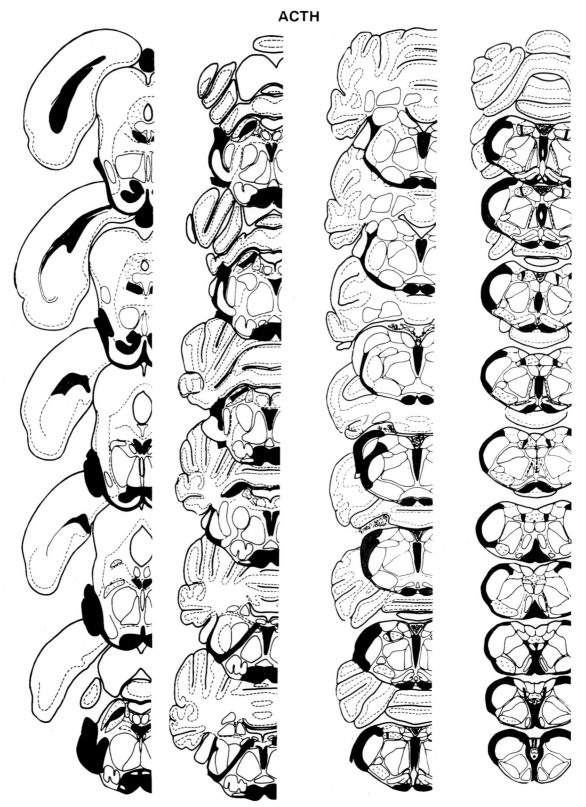

Fig. 8/3

α-MSH

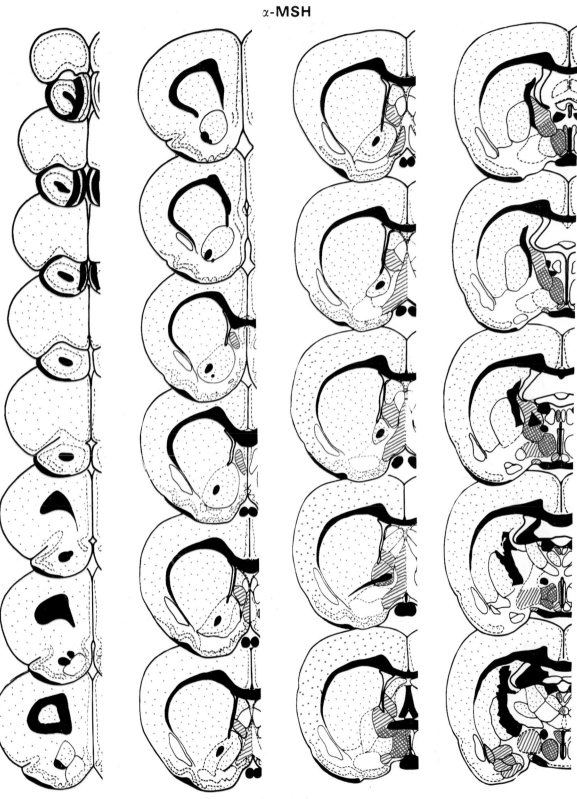

Fig. 9/1

31

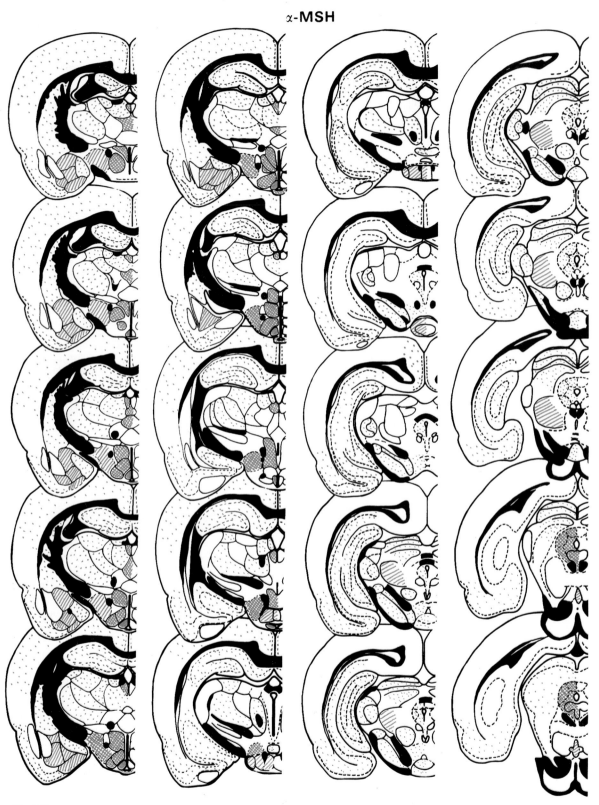

Fig. 9/2

α-MSH

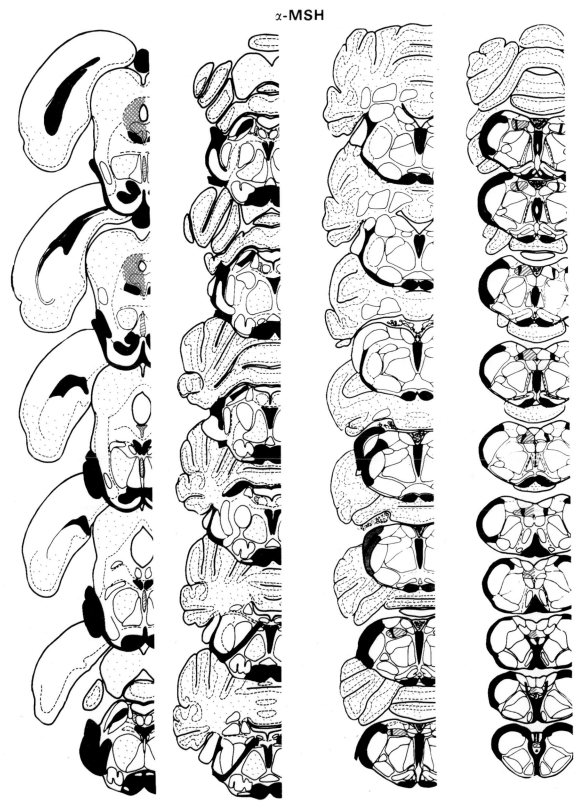

Fig. 9/3

33

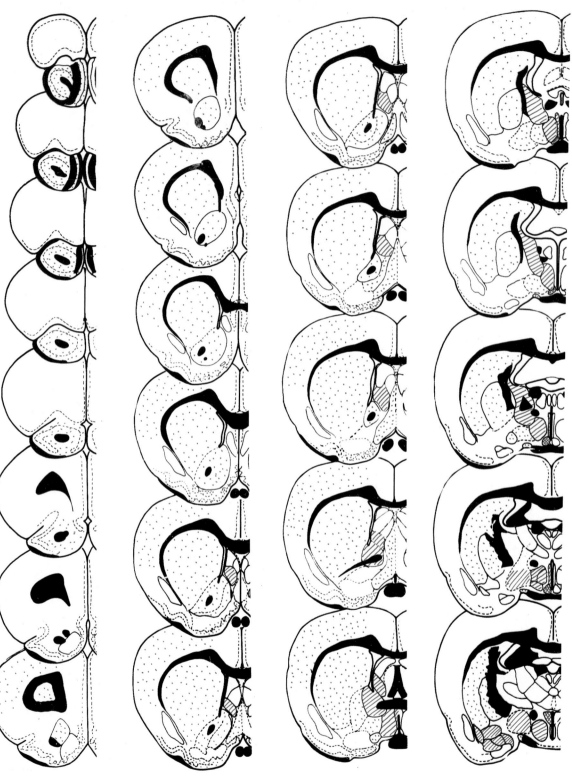

Fig. 10/1

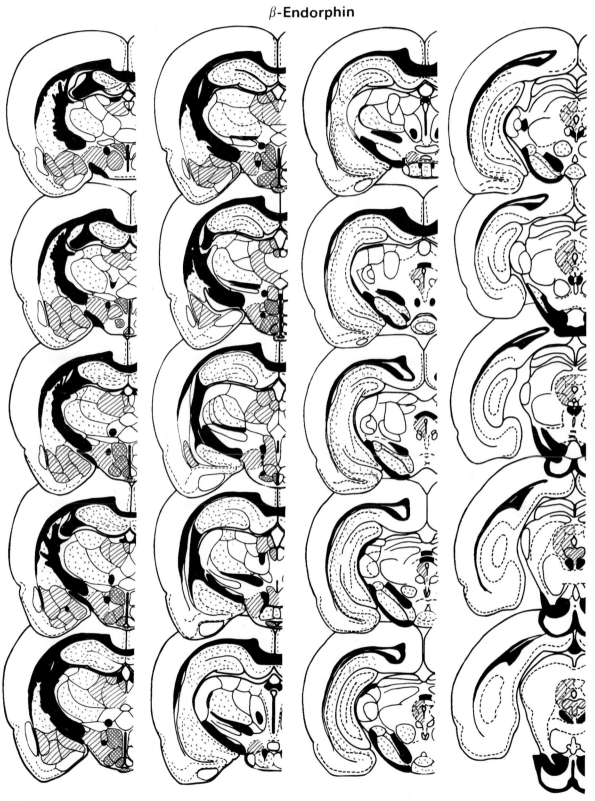

Fig. 10/2

β-Endorphin

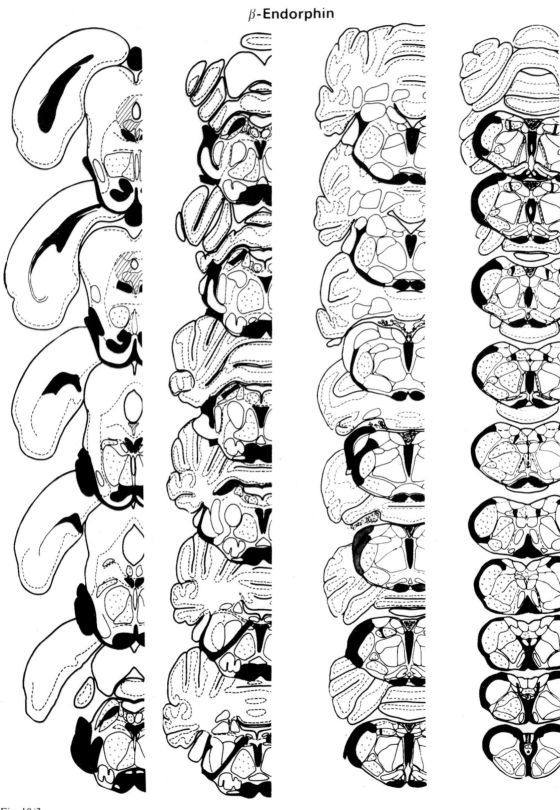

Fig. 10/3

36

Met-enkephalin

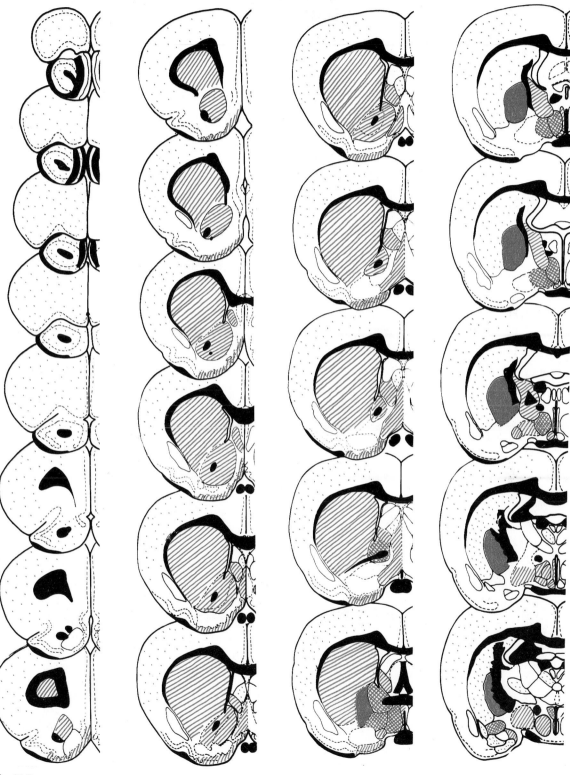

Fig. 11/1

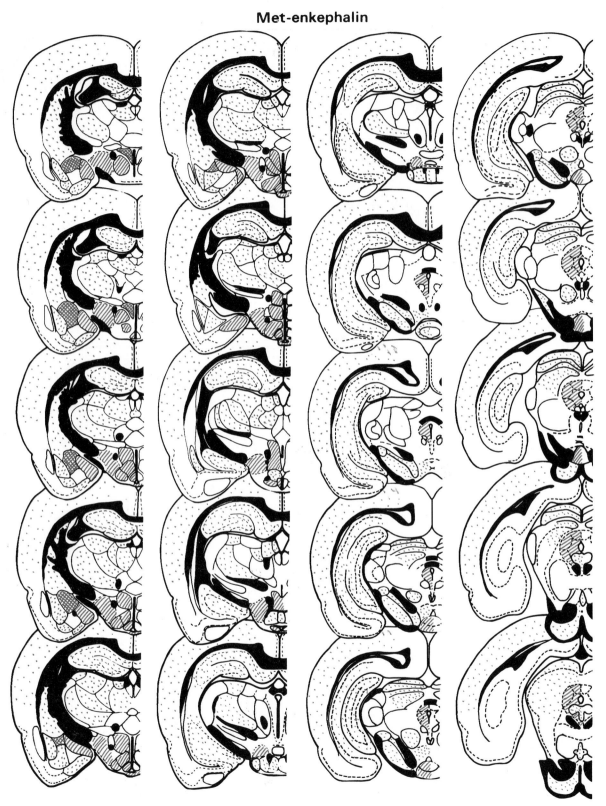

Fig. 11/2

Met-enkephalin

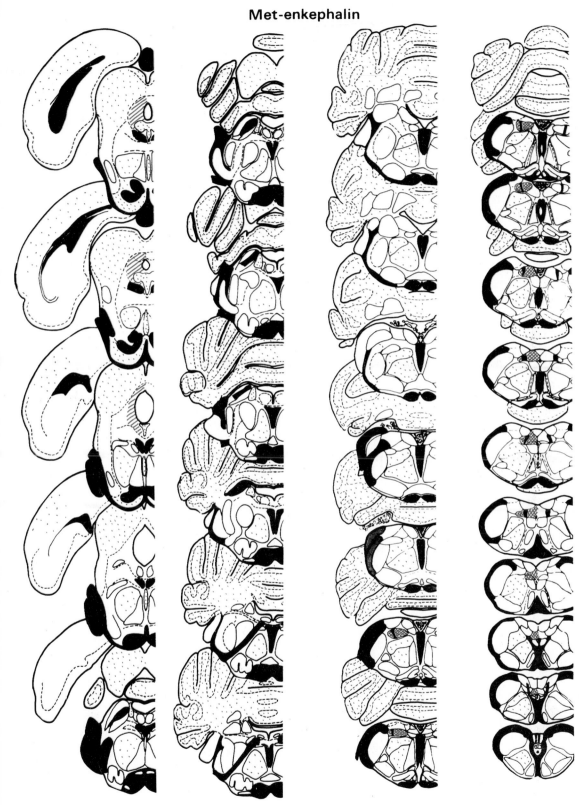

Fig. 11/3

39

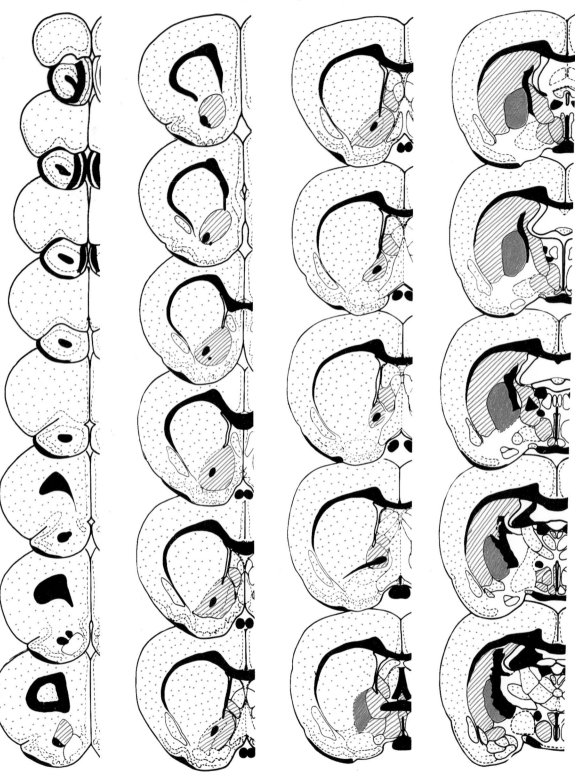

Fig. 12/1

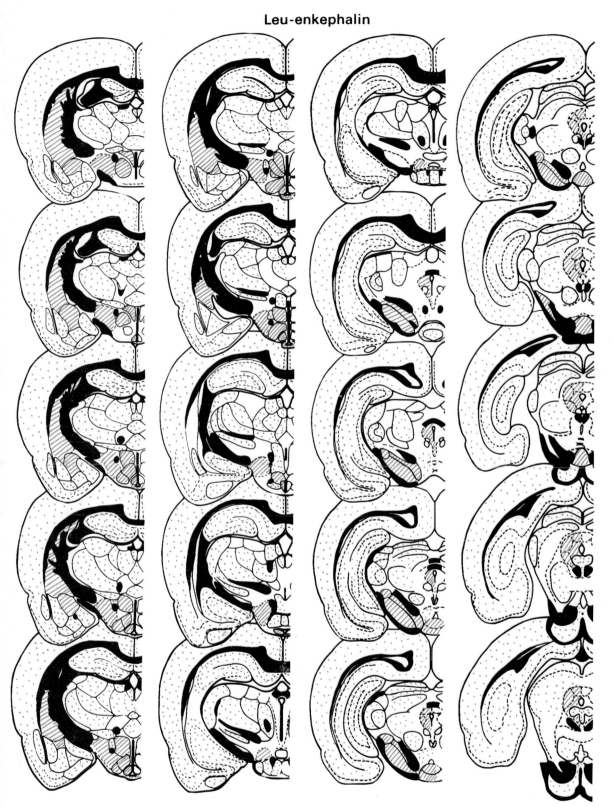

Fig. 12/2

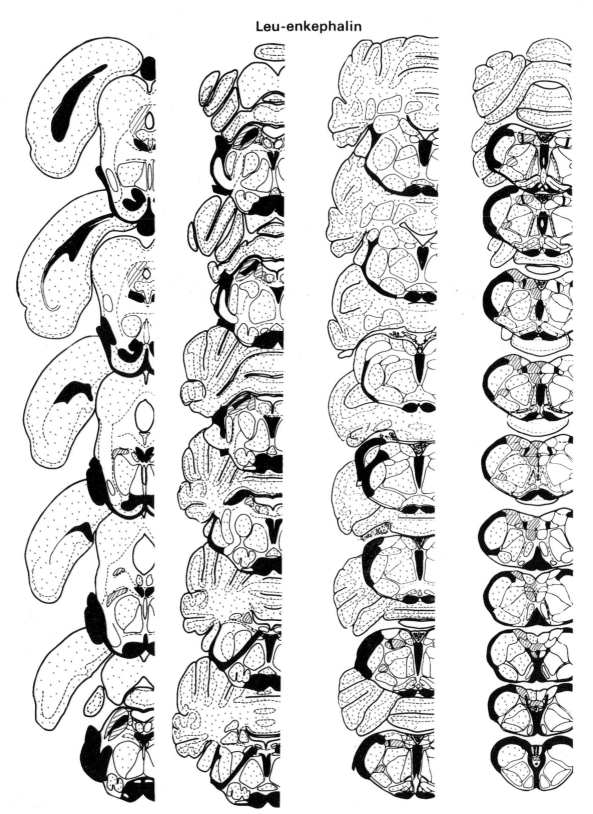

Fig. 12/3

42

Dynorphin A

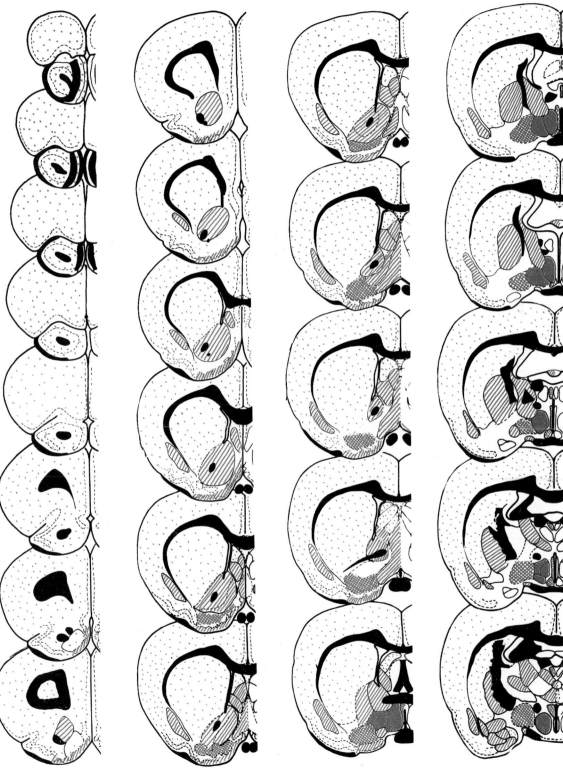

Fig. 13/1

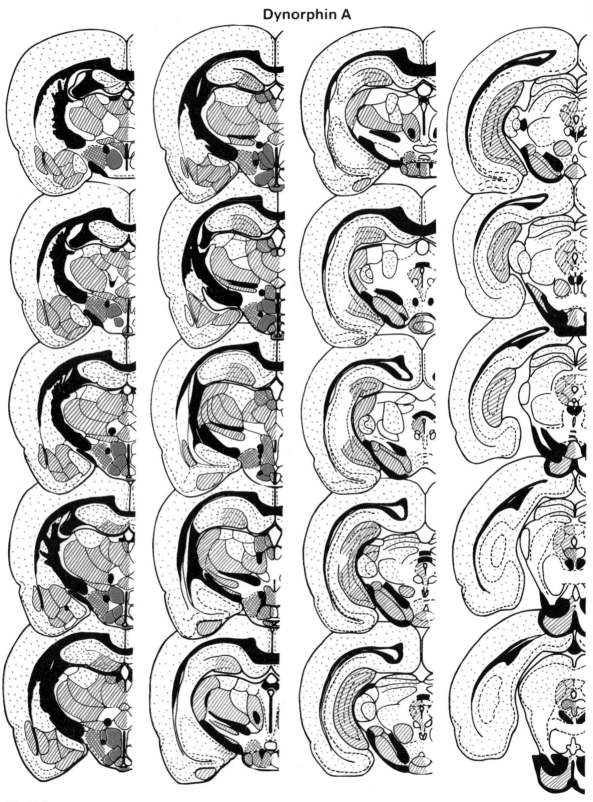

Fig. 13/2

44

Dynorphin A

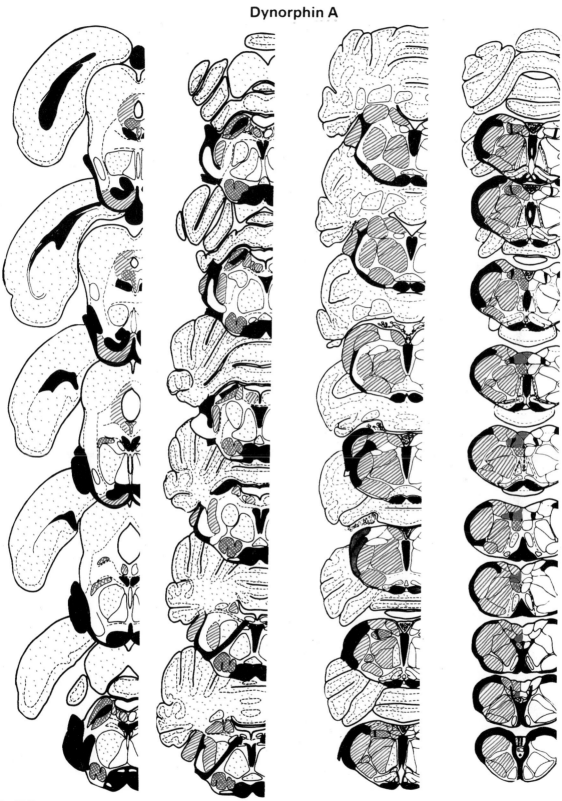

Fig. 13/3

45

Dynorphin B

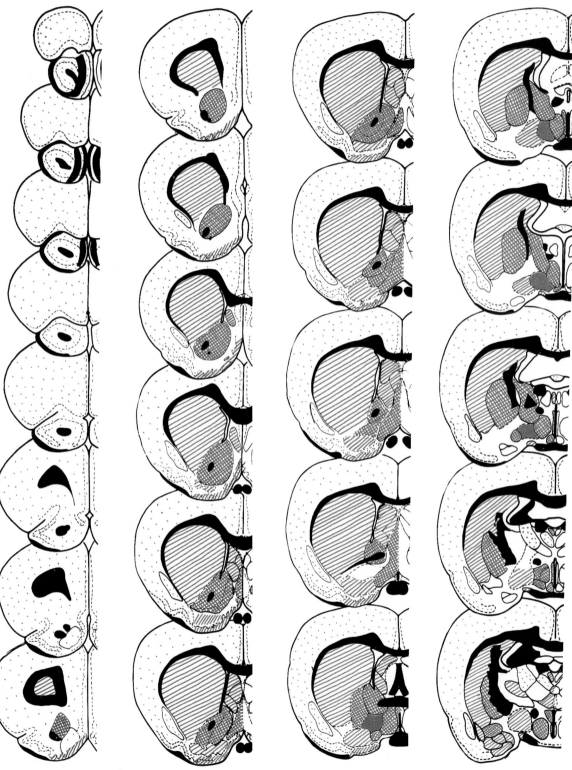

Fig. 14/1

46

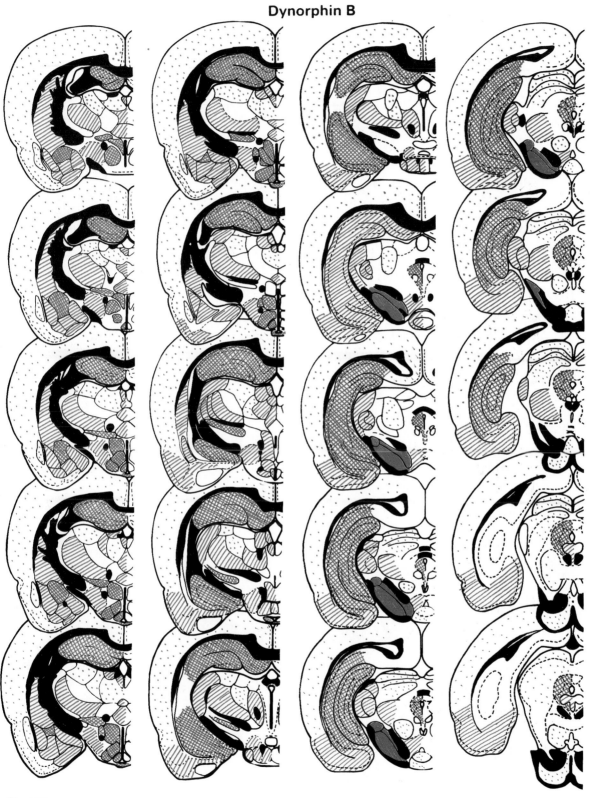

Fig. 14/2

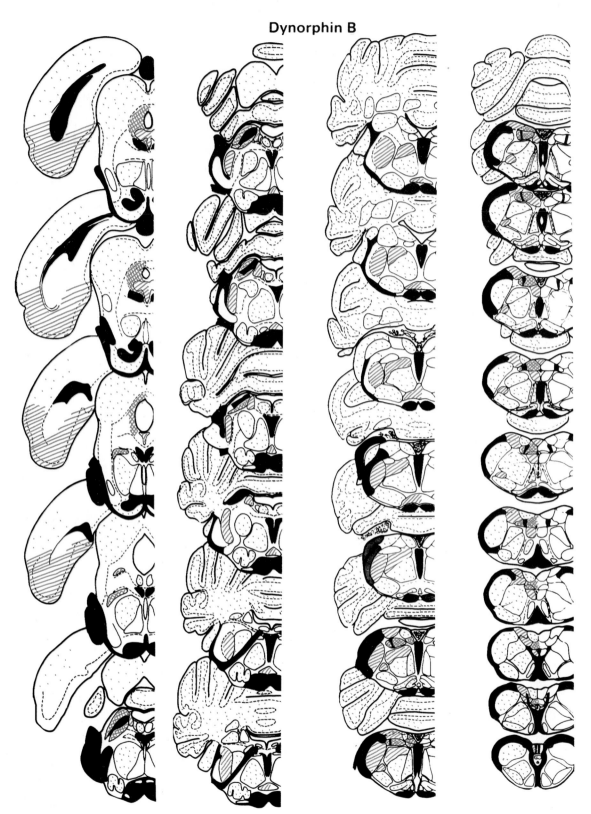

Fig. 14/3

α-Neo-endorphin

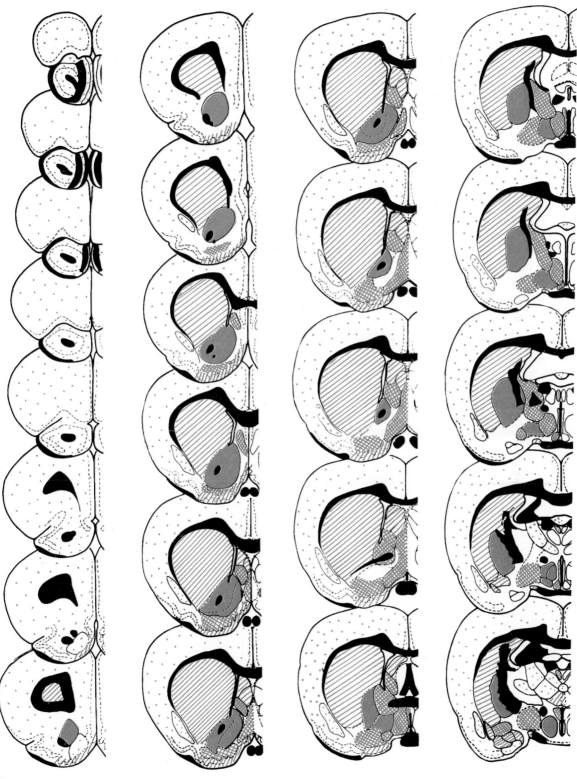

Fig. 15/1

49

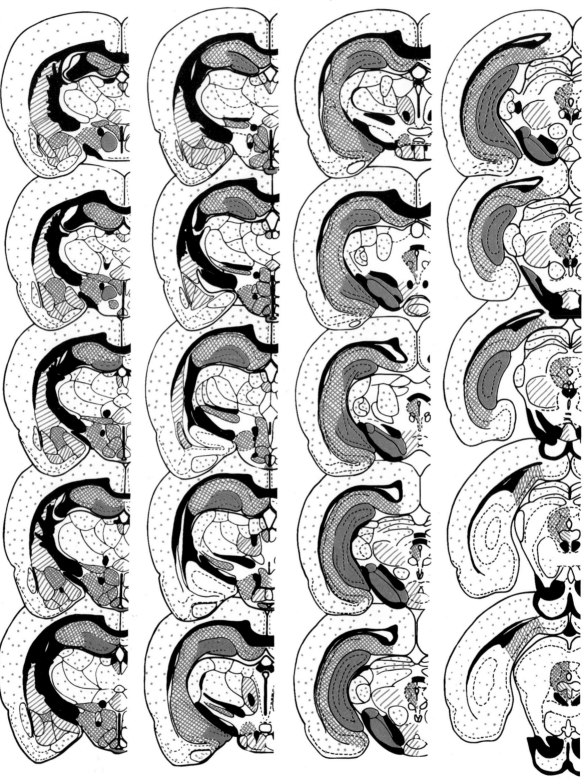

Fig. 15/2

α-Neo-endorphin

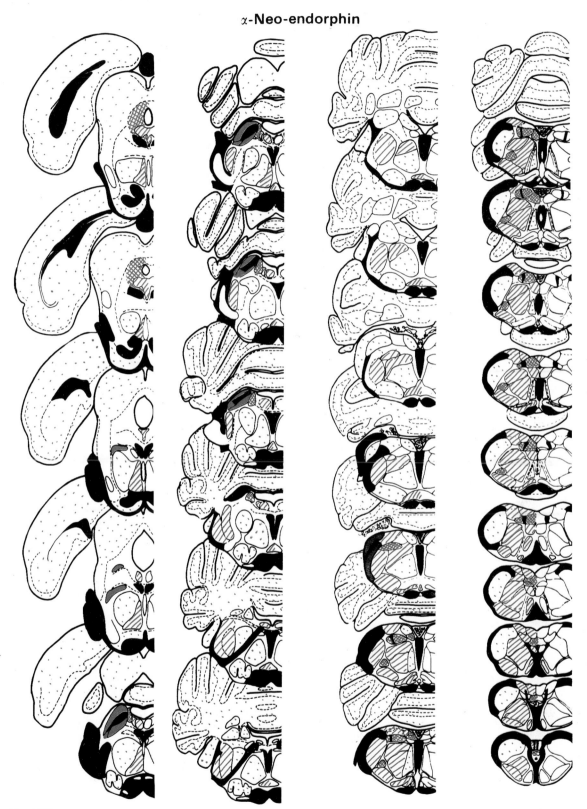

Fig. 15/3

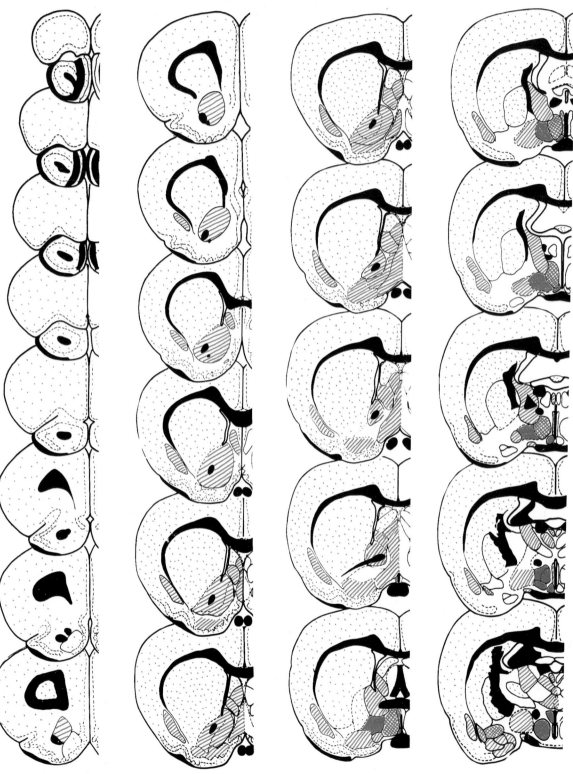

Fig. 16/1

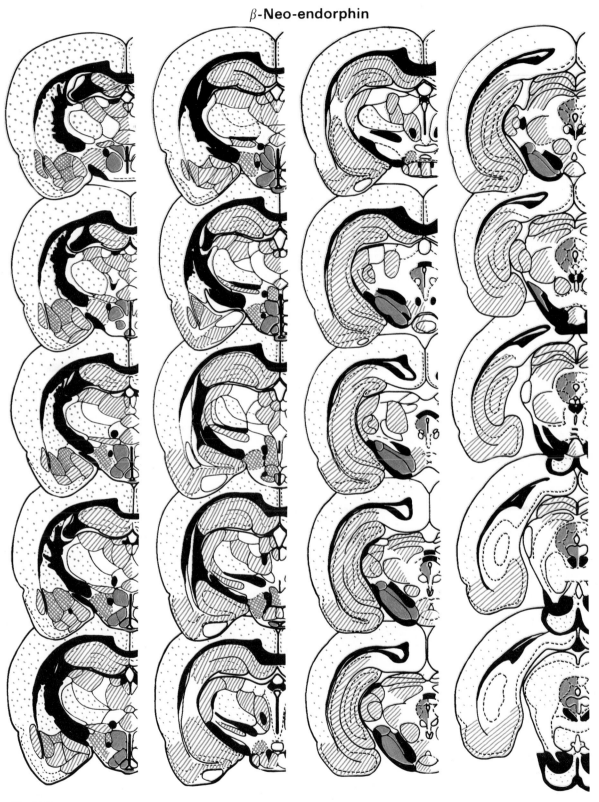

Fig. 16/2

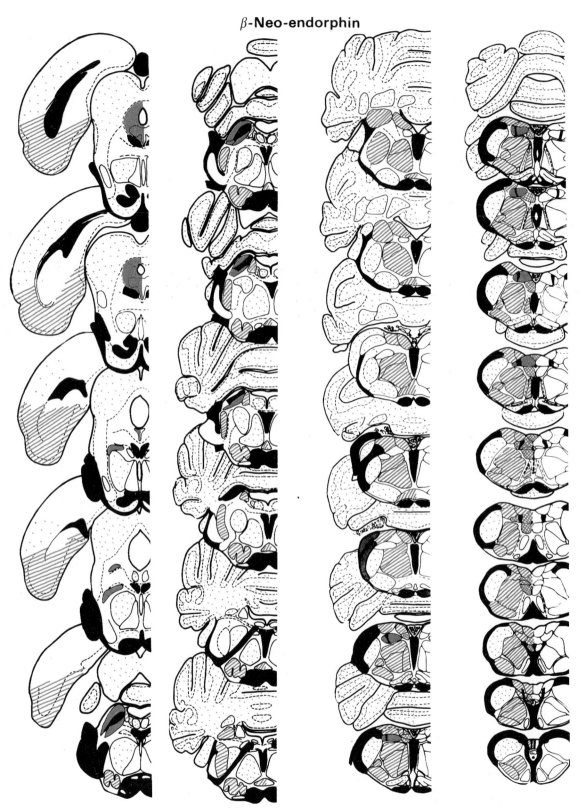

Fig. 16/3

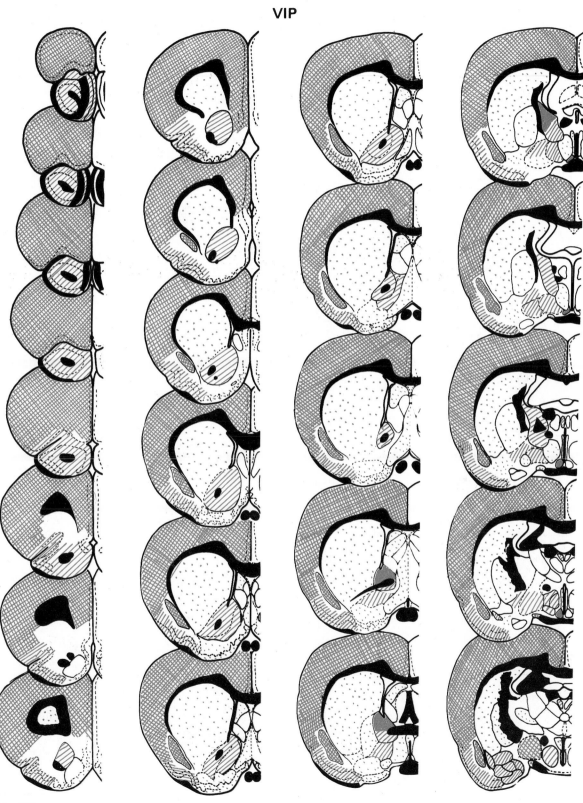

Fig. 17/1

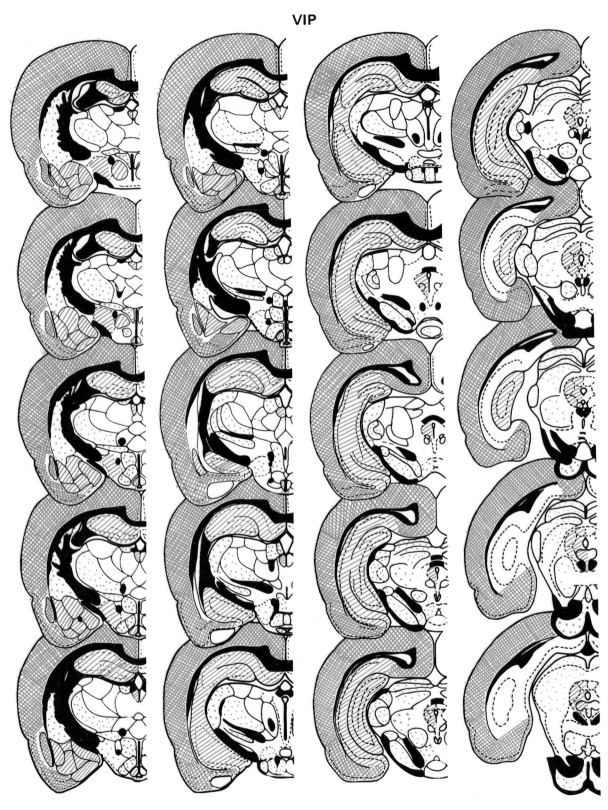

Fig. 17/2

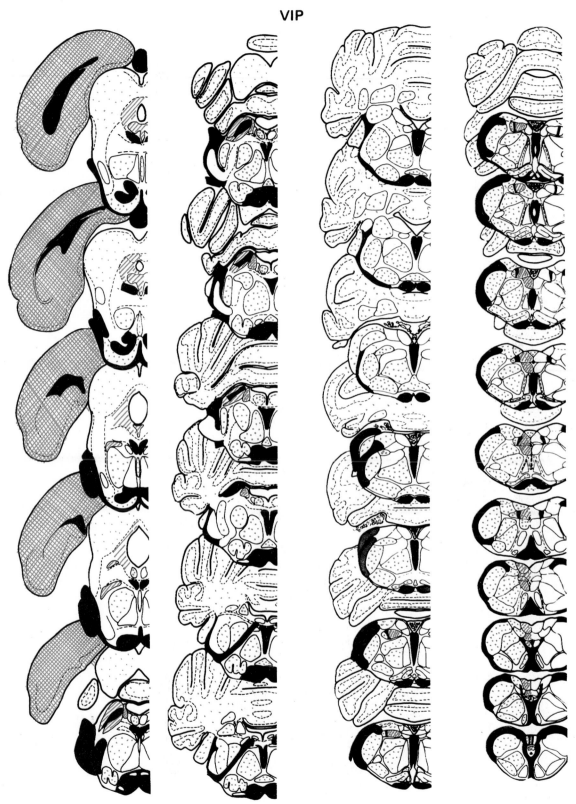

Fig. 17/3

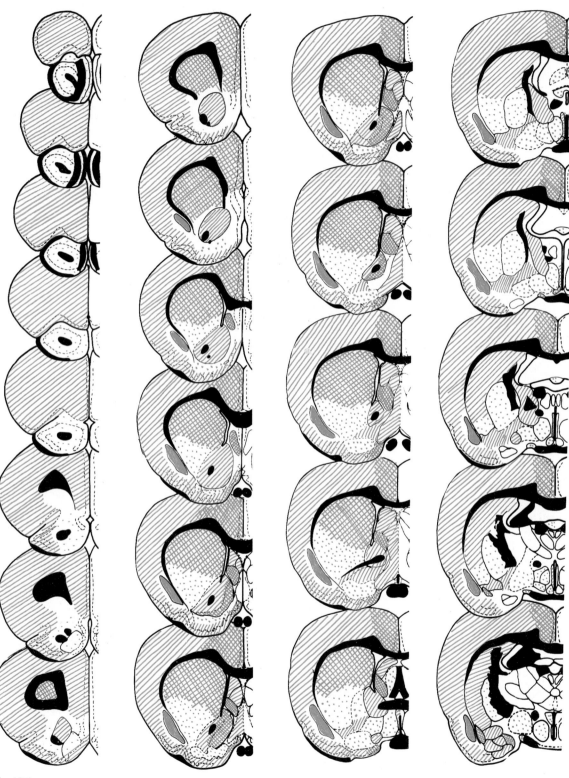

Fig. 18/1

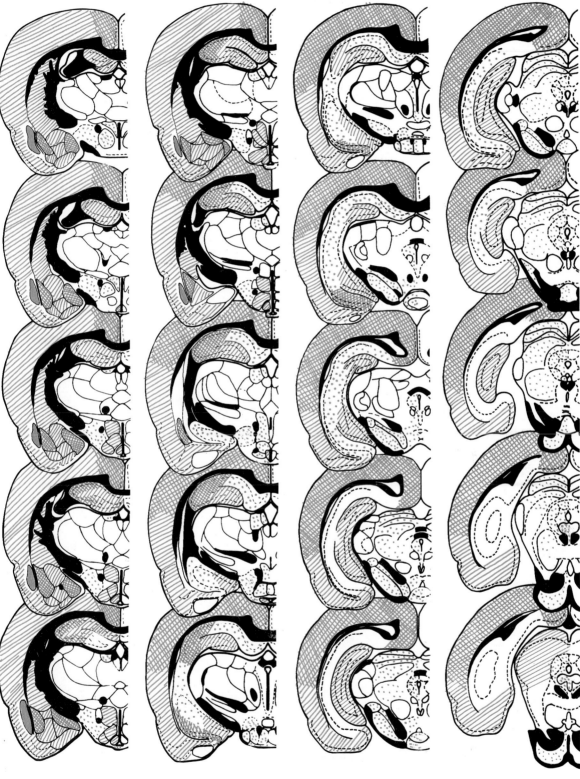

Fig. 18/2

Cholecystokinin

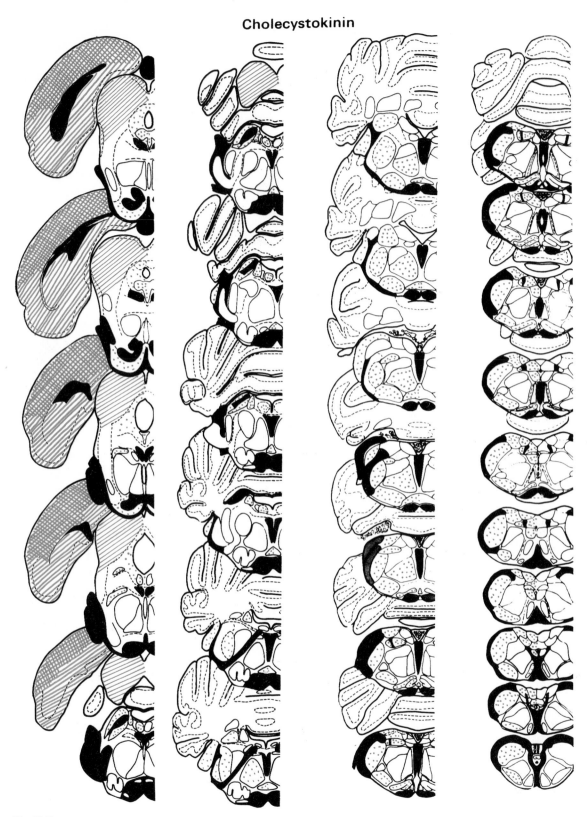

Fig. 18/3

60

Bombesin

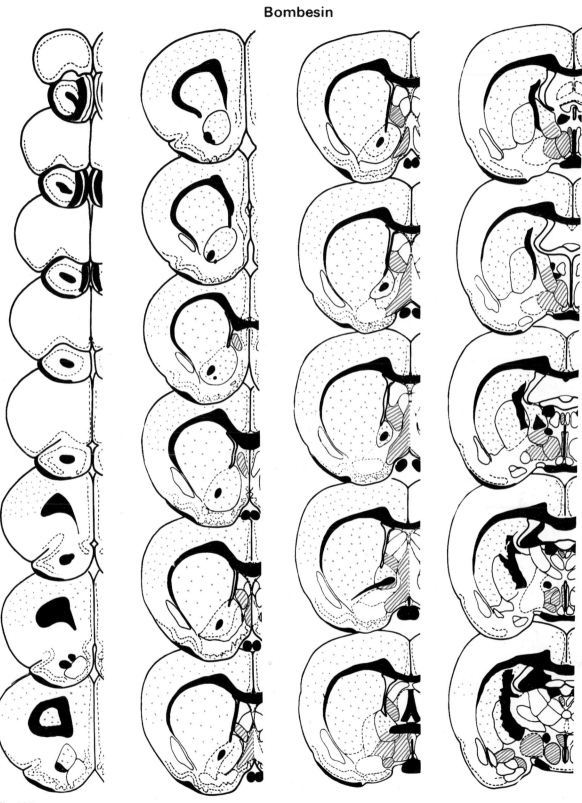

Fig. 19/1

61

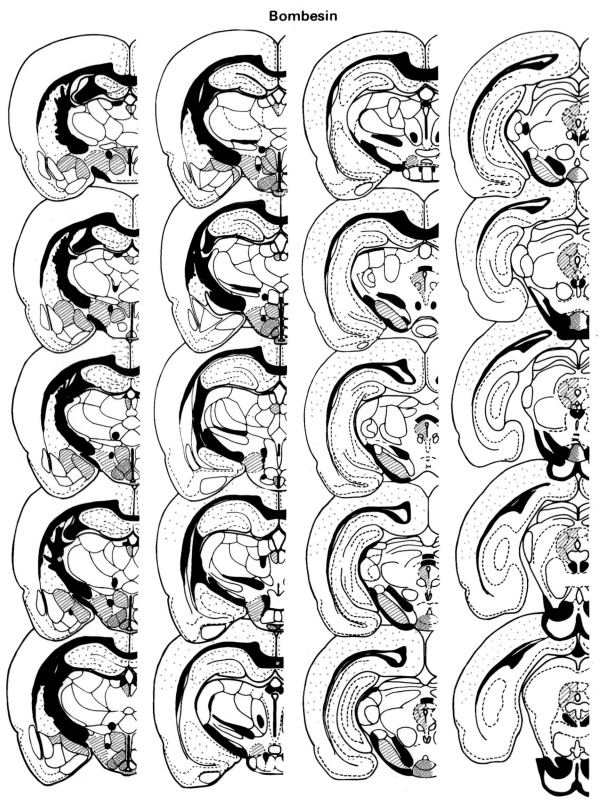

Fig. 19/2

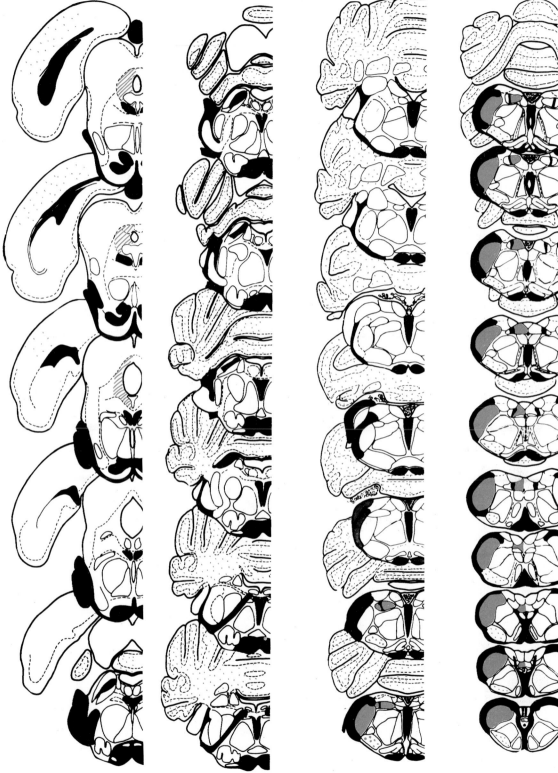

Fig. 19/3

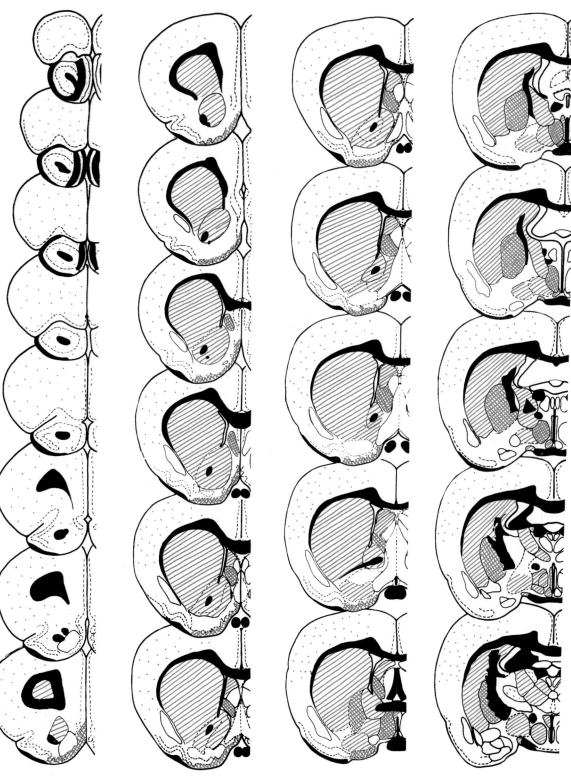

Fig. 20/1

64

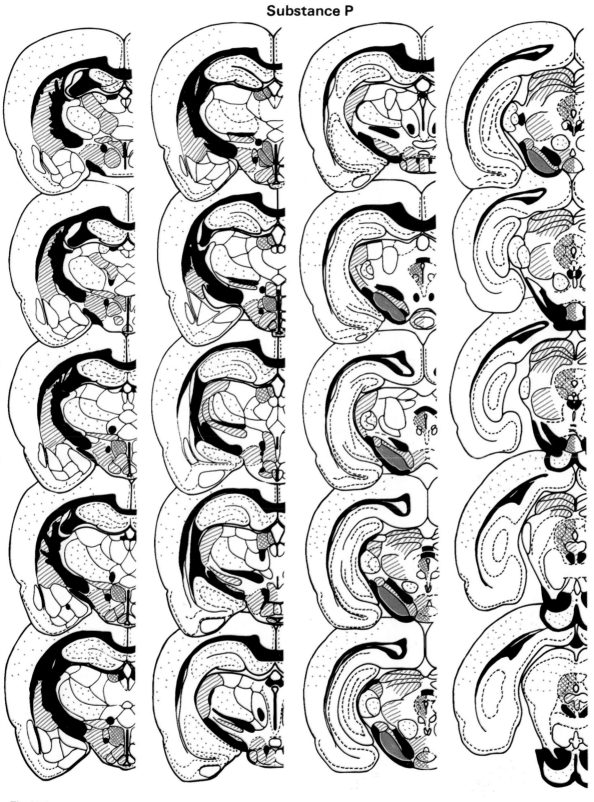

Fig. 20/2

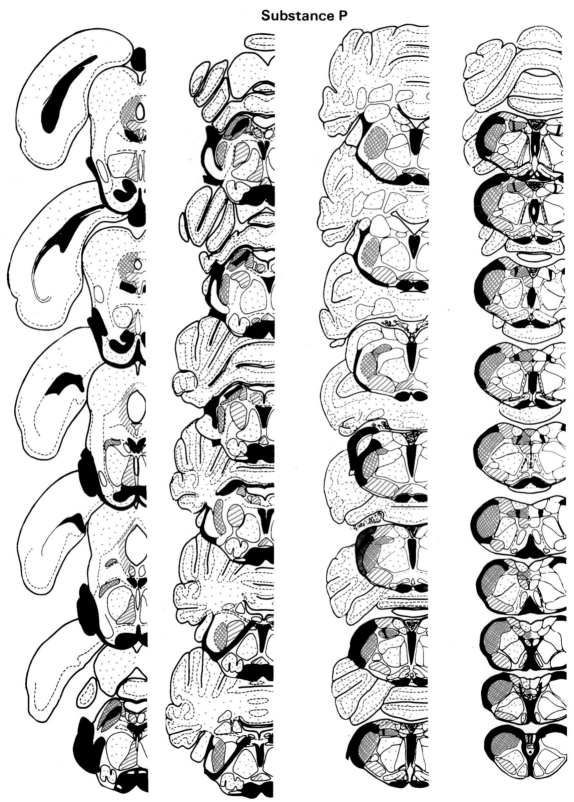

Fig. 20/3

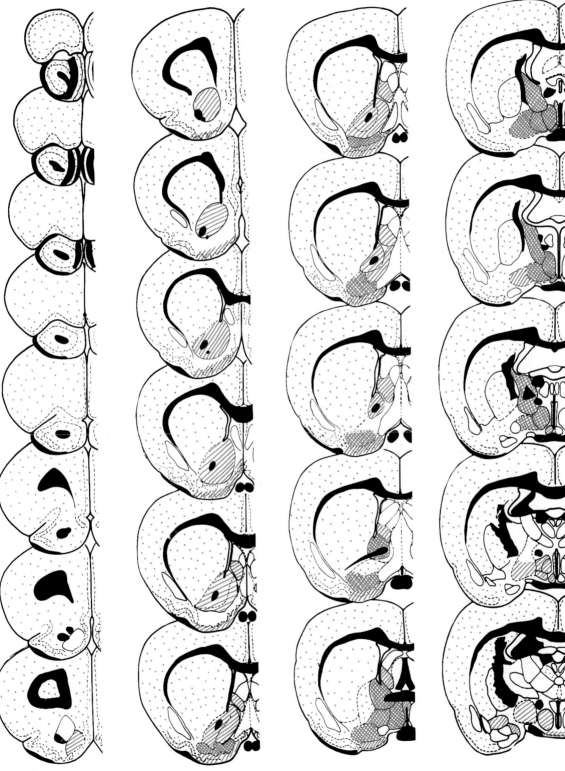

Fig. 21/1

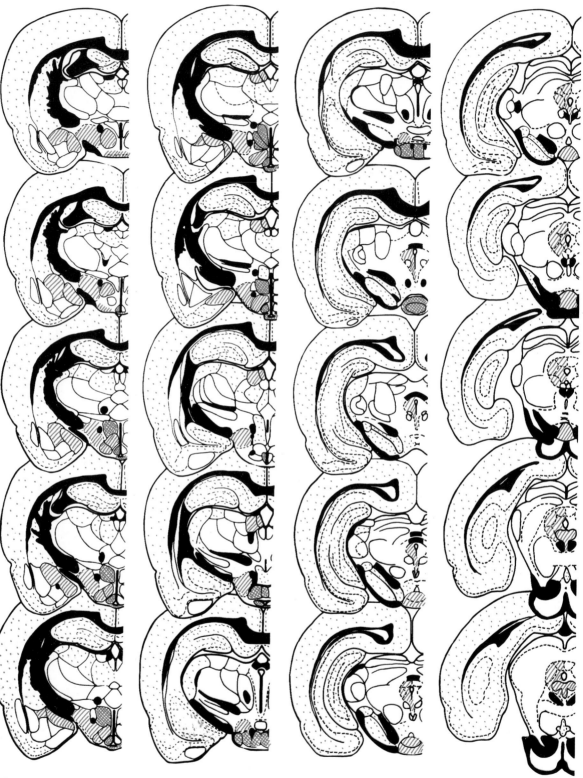

Fig. 21/2

Neurotensin

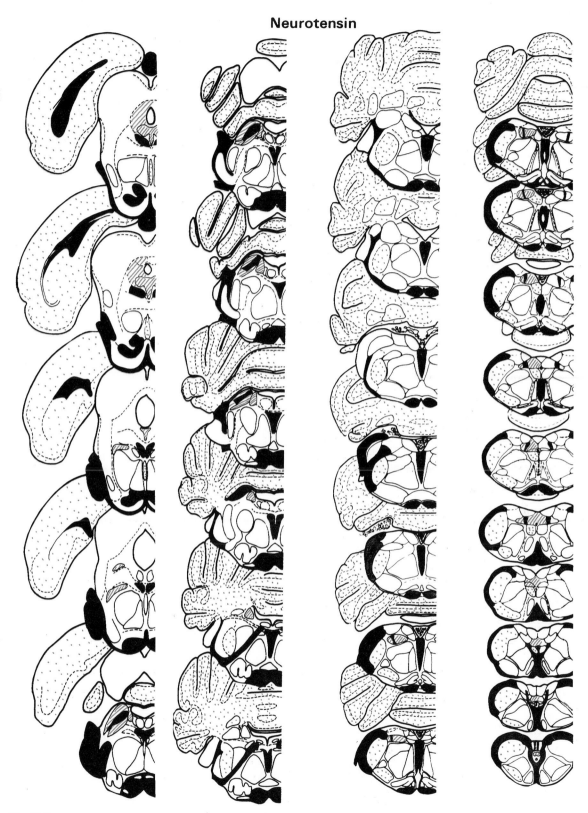

Fig. 21/3

3. REFERENCES

Beinfeld MC, Palkovits M (1981): Distribution of cholecystokinin (CCK) in the hypothalamus and limbic system of the rat. *Neuropeptides, 2,* 123–129.

Beinfeld MC, Palkovits M (1982): Distribution of cholecystokinin (CCK) in the rat lower brain stem nuclei. *Brain Res., 238,* 260–265.

Beinfeld MC, Meyer DK, Eskay RL, Jensen RT, Brownstein MJ (1981): The distribution of cholecystokinin immunoreactivity in the central nervous sytem of the rat as determined by radioimmunoassay. *Brain Res., 212,* 51–57.

Brownstein MJ, Palkovits M, Saavedra JM, Bassiri RM, Utiger RD (1974): Thyrotropin-releasing hormone in specific nuclei of the brain. *Science, 185,* 267–269.

Brownstein M, Arimura A, Sato H, Schally AV, Kizer JS (1975): The regional distribution of somatostatin in the rat brain. *Endocrinology, 96,* 1456–1461.

Brownstein MJ, Mroz EA, Kizer JS, Palkovits M, Leeman SE (1976): Regional distribution of substance P in the brain of the rat. *Brain Res., 116,* 299–305.

Dogterom J, Snijdewint FGM, Buijs RM (1978): The distribution of vasopressin and oxytocin in the rat brain. *Neurosci. Letters, 9,* 341–346.

Dorsa MD, Majumdar AL, Chapman BM (1981): Regional distribution of gamma- and beta-endorphin-like peptides in the pituitary and brain of the rat. *Peptides, 2,* 71–77.

Douglas LF, Palkovits M (1982): Distribution and quantitative measurements of somatostatin-like immunoreactivity in the lower brainstem of the rat. *Brain Res., 242,* 369–373.

Douglas LF, Palkovits M, Brownstein MJ (1982): Regional distribution of substance P-like immunoreactivity in the lower brainstem of the rat. *Brain Res., 245,* 376–378.

Dupont A, Barden N, Cusan L, Mérand Y, Labrie F, Vaudry H (1980): β-Endorphin and met-enkephalins: their distribution, modulation by estrogens and haloperidol, and role in neuroendocrine control. *Fed. Proc., 39,* 2544–2550.

Eiden LE, Nilaver G, Palkovits M (1982) Distribution of vasoactive intestinal polypeptide (VIP) in the rat brain stem nuclei. *Brain Res., 231,* 472–477.

Emson PC, Goedert M, Horsfield P, Rioux F, St Pierre S (1982): The regional distribution and chromatographic characterization of neurotensin-like immunoreactivity in the rat central nervous system. *J. Neurochem., 38,* 992–999.

Epelbaum J, Arancibia LT, Kordon C, Ottensen OP, Ben-Ari Y (1979): Regional distribution of somatostatin within the amygdaloid complex of the rat brain. *Brain Res., 174,* 172–174.

Eskay RL, Giraud P, Oliver C, Brownstein MJ (1979): α-Melanocyte stimulating hormone in the rat brain, evidence that α-MSH containing cells in the rat arcuate region send projections to extrahypothalamic sites. *Brain Res., 1978,* 55–67.

Eskay RL, Long RT, Palkovits M (1983): Localization of immunoreactive thyrotropin releasing hormone in the lower brainstem of the rat. *Brain Res., 277,* 159–162.

George JM, Jacobowitz DM (1976): Localization of vasopressin in discrete areas of the rat hypothalamus. *Brain Res., 93,* 363–366.

George JM, Staples S, Marks BM (1976): Oxytocin content of microdissected areas of the hypothalamus. *Endocrinology, 98,* 1430–1433.

Hawthorn J, Ang VTY, Jenkins JS (1980): Localization of vasopressin in the rat brain. *Brain Res., 197,* 75–81.

Hawthorn J, Ang VTY, Jenkins JS (1984): Comparison of the distribution of oxytocin and vasopressin in the rat brain. *Brain Res., 307,* 289–294.

Hökfelt T, Fuxe K, Johansson O, Jeffcoate S, White N (1975): Distribution of thyrotropin-releasing hormone (TRH) in the central nervous system as revealed with immunohistochemistry. *Eur. J. Pharmacol., 34,* 389–392.

Hong JS, Yang H-Y, Fratta W, Costa E (1977): Determination of methionine enkephalin in discrete regions of rat brain. *Brain Res., 134,* 383–386.

Kanazawa I, Jessell T (1976): Post mortem changes and regional distribution of substance P in the rat and mouse nervous system. *Brain Res., 117,* 362–367.

Kerdelhué B, Palkovits M, Kárteszi M, Reinberg A (1981): Circadian variations in substance P, luliberin (LH-RH) and thyroliberin (TRH) contents in hypothalamic and extrahypothalamic brain nuclei of adult male rats. *Brain Res., 206,* 405–412.

Kerdelhué B, Kárteszi M, Pasqualini C, Reinberg A, Mezey É, Palkovits M (1983): Circadian variations in β-endorphin concentrations in pituitary and in some brain nuclei of the adult male rat. *Brain Res., 261,* 243–248.

Kobayashi RM, Brown M, Vale W (1977): Regional distribution of neurotensin and somatostatin in rat brain. *Brain Res., 126,* 584–588.

Kobayashi RM, Palkovits M, Miller RJ, Chang K-J, Cuatrecasas P (1978): Brain enkephalin distribution is unaltered by hypophysectomy. *Life Sci., 22,* 527–530.

Krieger DT, Liotta A, Brownstein MJ (1977): Presence of corticotropin in limbic system of normal and hypophysectomized rats. *Brain Res., 128,* 575–579.

Laczi F, Gaffori O, De Kloet ER, De Wied D (1983): Differential responses in immunoreactive arginine-vasopressin content of microdissected brain regions during passive avoidance behavior. *Brain Res., 260,* 342–346.

Lorén I, Emson PC, Fahrenkrug J, Björklund A, Alumets J, Håkanson R, Sundler F (1979): Distribution of vasoactive intestinal polypeptide in the rat and mouse brain. *Neuroscience, 4,* 1953–1976.

Mezey É, Kiss JZ, Mueller GP, Eskay R, O'Donohue TL, Palkovits M (1985): Distribution of the pro-opiomelanocortin derived peptides, adrenocorticotropic hormone, α-melanocyte-stimulating hormone and β-endorphin (ACTH, α-MSH, β-END) in the rat hypothalamus. *Brain Res., 328,* 341–360.

Moody TW, O'Donohue TL, Jacobowitz DM (1981): Biochemical localization and characterization of bombesin-like peptides in discrete regions of rat brain. *Peptides, 2,* 75–79.

O'Donohue TL, Miller RL, Jacobowitz DM (1979): Identification, characterization and stereotaxic mapping of intraneuronal α-melanocyte-stimulating hormone-like immunoreactive peptides in discrete regions of the rat brain. *Brain Res., 176,* 101–123.

Palkovits M (1980): *Guide and Map for the Isolated Removal of Individual Cell Groups from the Rat Brain* (Hungarian text). Akadémiai Kiadó, Budapest.

Palkovits M (1984): Distribution of neuropeptides in the central nervous system: a review of biochemical mapping studies. *Prog. Neurobiol., 23,* 151–189.

Palkovits M, Arimura A, Brownstein M, Schally AV, Saavedra JM (1974): Luteinizing hormone-releasing hormone (LH-RH) content of the hypothalamic nuclei in rat. *Endocrinology, 95,* 554–558.

Palkovits M, Brownstein M, Arimura A, Sato H, Schally AV, Kizer JS (1976): Somatostatin content of the hypothalamic ventromedial and arcuate nuclei and the circumventricular organs in the rat. *Brain Res., 109,* 430–434.

Palkovits M, Gráf L, Hermann I, Borvendég J, Ács Zs, Láng T (1978): Regional distribution of enkephalins, endorphins and ACTH in the central nervous system of rats determined by radioimmunoassay. In: Gráf L, Palkovits M, Rónai AZ (Eds), *Endorphins '78,* pp. 187–195. Akadémiai Kiadó, Budapest.

Palkovits M, Kobayashi RM, Brown M, Vale W (1980): Changes in hypothalamic, limbic and extrapyramidal somatostatin levels following various hypothalamic transections in rat. *Brain Res., 195,* 499–505.

Palkovits M, Besson J, Rotsztejn W (1981): Distribution of vasoactive intestinal polypeptide in intact, stria terminalis transected and cerebral cortex isolated rats. *Brain Res., 213,* 455–459.

Palkovits M, Brownstein MJ, Vale W (1985): Distribution of corticotropin-releasing factor in rat brain. *Fed. Proc., 44,* 215–219.

Rostène WH, Léránth Cs, Maletti M, Mezey É, Besson J, Eiden LE, Rosselin G, Palkovits M (1982): Distribution of vasoactive intestinal peptide (VIP) following various brain transections in the rat by radioimmunoassay and electronmicroscopic immunocytochemistry. *Neuropeptides, 2,* 337–350.

Samson WK, McCann SM, Chud L, Dudley CA, Moss RL (1980): Intra- and extrahypothalamic luteinizing hormone-releasing hormone (LHRH) distribution in the rat with special reference to mesencephalic sites which contain both LHRH and single neurons responsive to LHRH. *Neuroendocrinology, 31,* 66–72.

Selmanoff MK, Wise PM, Barraclough CA (1980): Regional distribution of luteinizing hormone-releasing hormone (LH-RH) in rat brain determined by microdissection and radioimmunoassay. *Brain Res., 192,* 421–432.

Verhoef J, Wiegant VM, De Wied D (1982): Regional distribution of α- and γ-type endorphins in rat brain. *Brain Res., 231,* 454–460.

Williams RG, Dockray GJ (1983): Distribution of enkephalin-related peptides in rat brain: immunohistochemical studies using antisera to met-enkephalin and met-enkephalin-Arg[6]-Phe[7]. *Neuroscience, 9,* 563–586.

Zamir N, Palkovits M, Brownstein MJ (1983): Distribution of immunoreactive dynorphin in the central nervous system of the rat. *Brain Res., 280,* 81–93.

Zamir N, Palkovits M, Brownstein MJ (1984a): Distribution of immunoreactive α-neo-endorphin in the central nervous system of the rat. *J. Neurosci., 4,* 1240–1247.

Zamir N, Palkovits M, Brownstein MJ (1984b): Distribution of immunoreactive β-neo-endorphin in discrete areas of the rat brain and pituitary gland: comparison with α-neo-endorphin. *J. Neurosci., 4,* 1248–1252.

Zamir N, Palkovits M, Weber E, Brownstein MJ (1984c): Distribution of immunoreactive dynorphin B in discrete areas of the rat brain and spinal cord. *Brain Res., 300,* 121–127.

Zamir N, Palkovits M, Brownstein MJ (1985) Distribution of immunoreactive met-enkephalin-Arg[6]-Gly[7]-Leu[8] and leu-enkephalin in discrete regions of the rat brain. *Brain Res., 326,* 1–8.

Zerbe RL, Palkovits M (1984): Changes in the vasopressin content of discrete brain regions in response to stimuli for vasopressin secretion. *Neuroendocrinology, 38,* 285–289.

CHAPTER II

General morphological features of peptidergic neurons

VIRGINIA M. PICKEL

1. INTRODUCTION

The concept that neurons within the central nervous system (CNS) may produce peptides or other substances which elicit a response from other cells through humoral release into the bloodstream or through release at synaptic junctions, has been recognized for a number of years (Von Euler and Gaddum 1931; Scharrer and Scharrer 1954). However, isolation of active peptides from the brain, pituitary and other tissues has only been achieved through the exhaustive efforts of a number of investigators in the last few decades (Du Vigneaud 1956; Schalley et al. 1973, 1980; Gainer et al. 1977; Guillemin 1978a). Following isolation, highly sensitive and specific methods were soon developed for detecting small quantities of peptides in homogenates by radioimmunoassay (Yallow 1978) and in sections of tissue by immunocytochemistry (Sternberger 1979). An astounding and continually increasing number of peptides, many of which were originally isolated from peripheral tissues, have now been localized immunocytochemically in the CNS (Gibson et al. 1981; Hökfelt et al. 1980; McCann 1982; Petrusz et al. 1977). The immunocytochemical localization of these peptides makes it feasible to consider the morphological features which may underlie the neurosecretory and transmitter functions in magnocellular and in smaller peptidergic neurons.

Larger peptides such as oxytocin and vasopressin are produced in *magnocellular neurons* of the hypothalamus at a rate which induces morphological changes recognizable with the light and electron microscope (Scharrer and Scharrer 1954; Guillemin 1978b). These neurons have many characteristics of glandular cells including vital staining and specialized relations with blood vessels. For many years after their discovery, the neurosecretory, peptidergic fibers were believed not to be associated with structures other than blood vessels (Knowles 1974). However, in 1967, Bargmann and co-workers first described 'peptidergic synapses' between neurosecretory axons and epithelial cells of the pars intermedia of the pituitary. Since then, numerous immunocytochemical studies have shown that both oxytocin and vasopressin and the associated neurophysins are present in nerve terminals forming conventional synapses within the CNS. These observations further support the concept that peptidergic neuroregulators may modulate certain forms of interneuronal communication and also serve hormonal functions.

In contrast to oxytocin and vasopressin within magnocellular neurons, many other active peptides contain only a few amino acid residues and are produced in small quantities which impart no easily recognizable morphology associated with their secretion. The

Handbook of Chemical Neuroanatomy. Vol. 4: GABA and Neuropeptides in the CNS, Part I.
A. Björklund and T. Hökfelt, editors.
© Elsevier Science Publishers B.V., 1985.

identity of these peptide-containing neurons depends exclusively on the detection of a specific reaction product which indicates the presence of an antigen–antibody reaction. Since this complex may form between longer chains containing the amino acid sequence of smaller peptides, the identity of a reaction product within a cell is spoken of as like-immunoreactivity. Most of the smaller peptides have been immunocytochemically localized in terminals forming axodendritic synapses within the CNS. However, the pluripotentiality with respect to humoral and neural activity has now been demonstrated for the hypophysiotrophic and other peptides (Kozlowski et al. 1976; Moss 1979; Piercey et al. 1981; Tsunoo et al. 1982).

In this chapter, the general light and electron microscopic features of a few representative peptide-containing neurons in brain are comparatively described; whereas, the more detailed consideration of individual peptides is presented in the following chapters. While morphological features cannot be used to identify a peptide-containing neuron exclusive of the reaction product, they may provide a structural basis for interactions between neurons containing neuropeptides and other transmitters in the same or synaptically joined neurons and for the relation of peptide-containing neurons and non-neuronal structures such as glia and blood vessels.

2. LIGHT MICROSCOPY

2.1. REGIONAL DISTRIBUTION

One of the first and most readily apparent basis which might be used for distinguishing the neuropeptide-containing neurons is regional distribution within the central and peripheral nervous systems as detected by biochemical (Brownstein et al. 1975) or immunocytochemical methods (Hökfelt et al. 1977a; Haber and Elde 1982; Ljungdahl et al. 1978; Goldstein et al. 1978). Many peptides have been localized to regions containing first- or second-order sensory neurons such as the substantia gelatinosa of the dorsal horn (Aronin et al. 1981; Barden et al. 1981; Barber et al. 1979; Bennett et al. 1982; DiFiglia et al. 1982; Hunt et al. 1980) or the nuclei of the solitary tracts within the medulla (Gillis et al. 1980; Pickel et al. 1979). In addition to the sensory neurons there is an abundant distribution of peptides within hypothalamic and limbic regions such as the amygdala, habenula and tegmental nuclei (Elde and Hökfelt 1979; Ho and DePalatis 1980; Roberts et al. 1982; Woodhams et al. 1983), within the basal ganglia (Ljungdahl et al. 1978; Pickel et al. 1980), and within the periaqueductal grey (Moss et al. 1981, 1983). Though concentrated in certain regions, the peptide-containing neuronal perikarya and processes have been identified in almost every region of the CNS including the cerebral cortex (Peters et al. 1983). Thus, regional distribution alone does not distinguish the neuropeptide-containing neurons.

2.2. CYTOLOGY

Certain peptidergic neurons have now been characterized in terms of general shape and dendritic branching pattern by using thick sections for light microscopic immunocytochemistry in comparison to silver impregnation. Improvements in penetration of antiserum through thick frozen or Vibratome sections can be achieved by the use of detergents such as Triton X-100 (Hartman 1973). Grzanna et al. (1978) first used this methodology for the production of 'Golgi-like' images for catecholaminergic neurons containing dopamine β-hydroxylase. More recently, similar methodologies have been applied to neurons immunocytochemically labeled for various peptides such as neurotensin. Like many other peptides, neurotensin is widely distributed in the CNS, particularly in the dorsal horn (Carraway and Leeman 1976; Uhl et al. 1977). In thick sections treated for enhanced penetration of antisera, Seybold and Elde (1982) were able to compare the structural features of neurons showing neurotensin-like immunoreactivity (N-LI) within laminae II and III of the dorsal horn (see Fig. 1) with the morphology of silver impregnated (Gobel 1978a,b) and horseradish peroxidase filled (Bennett et al. 1980) neurons within the same region. While some of the neurons showing N-LI appeared to be islet or central cells, the morphological characteristics of islet cells were not limited to neurotensin. Comparative examination of immunoreactivity with horseradish peroxidase filling also led to the suggestion that enkephalin-containing neurons in substantia gelatinosa may be stalked or islet cells (Bennett et al. 1980; Gobel et al. 1980; Sumal et al. 1982). In other regions, such as the nucleus tractus solitarius, the branching pattern and orientation of dendrites of the peptide-containing neurons are not significantly different from those neurons in the same region for which no specific peptide has been identified (Maley et al. 1983). Thus, examination of the dendritic arborizations is essential for the complete characterization of specific peptidergic neurons, but does not morphologically differentiate the peptidergic neurons within a given region.

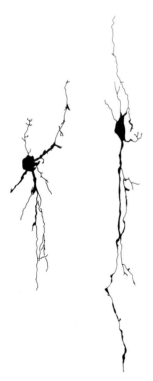

Fig. 1. Camera Lucida tracing of neurotensin-like immunoreactivity in two neurons from laminae III of the dorsal horn of rat. × 600. (Drawings reproduced by permission from V.S. Seybold and R.P. Elde.)

3. ULTRASTRUCTURAL MORPHOLOGY AND NEURONAL INTERACTIONS

3.1. PERIKARYA AND DENDRITES

In most regions of the CNS, the ultrastructural localization of neuropeptides within perikarya and dendrites has been examined only after pre-treatment of animals with colchicine or other blockers of axonal transport (Dube and Pelletier 1979). By diminishing the transport of peptides from their site of synthesis in perikarya to distal terminals, immunoreactivity detected within the cell is significantly enhanced. However, the cytology is also altered by the accumulation of vesicles and other transported material within the soma and by the disruption of microtubules (Morris et al. 1978). Thus, the ultrastructural morphology of peptidergic neurons without colchicine pre-treatment will be described whenever possible in the present account. The objectives are specifically to compare the ultrastructural morphology and peptide localization in neurosecretory neurons of the hypothalamus with smaller peptidergic neurons of the striatum and cerebral cortex in order to highlight common or diversified features of neurons which synthesize and export neuropeptides. Examples chosen for comparison include: oxytocin, vasopressin and neurophysin in the hypothalamus; enkephalin and somatostatin in the neostriatum; and cholecystokinin in the cerebral cortex.

Hypothalamic magnocellular neurons

The magnocellular neurons located within the supraoptic and paraventricular nuclei of the hypothalamus are well characterized by electron microscopy and by the immunocytochemical localization of the polypeptides oxytocin and vasopressin (Palay 1960; Morris et al. 1978; Kozlowski 1983). Many of the ultrastructural features of the perikarya are typically characteristic of the cells of endocrine glands, including a highly infolded nuclear membrane, extensive saccules of endoplasmic reticulum and many dense vesicles having a diameter greater than 150 nm (Palay 1960; Morris et al. 1978; Smith 1971). These neurosecretory granules are considerably larger than the large dense core vesicles (DCV's) of approximately 100 nm that are more typically found in perikarya and terminals throughout the CNS (Fig. 2) (Peters et al. 1976). Utilizing both pre- and post-plastic embedding techniques for peroxidase immunocytochemistry, oxytocin and vasopressin have been localized within the neurosecretory granules of magnocellular neurons (Silverman and Zimmerman 1975; Kozlowski and Nilaver 1983). The precursor peptide neurophysin is also predominately localized to the secretory granules within both perikarya and processes of the hypothalamo-hypophyseal pathway (Kozlowski et al. 1977). However, more recent immunocytochemical evidence suggests that there may be additional non-vesicular pools for neurophysin as well as oxytocin and vasopressin (Kozlowski 1983).

Peptidergic neurons in striatum and neocortex

In contrast to the hypothalamic magnocellular neurons, the cells producing somatostatin, enkephalin and cholecystokinin are smaller, contain few, if any 'neurosecretory' granules and may or may not have an infolded nuclear membrane. However, some of these neurons do have appreciable numbers of coated vesicles and large DCV's within their perikarya and proximal processes. The more detailed cytological features of specific peptidergic neurons in the striatum and cerebral cortex of monkey and rat are described together with a discussion of the possible physiological implications for the localization of peptides within dendrites.

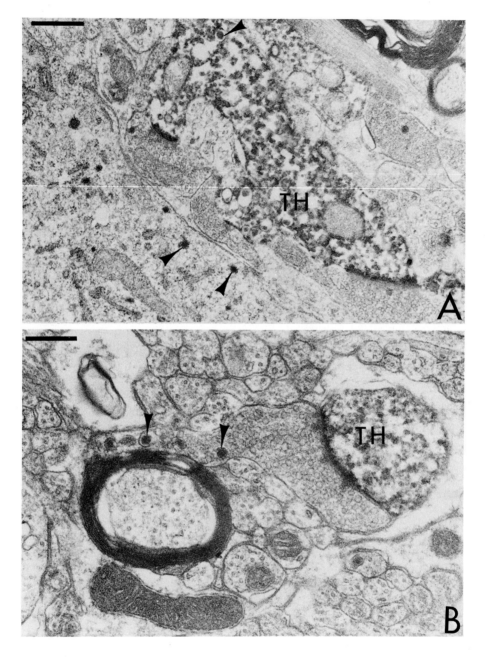

Fig. 2. Electron micrographs showing the distribution of dense core vesicles (arrow heads) in unlabeled peri-karya (A) and terminal (B). In both *A* and *B*, a vesicle containing terminal forms synapses with tyrosine hydroxylase (TH)-labeled dendrite of the A2 catecholamine group. The TH-labeled dendrite in *A* also contains dense core vesicles (arrow head). Bar = 0.2 μm.

Neostriatum

Somatostatin is regionally localized by radioimmunoassay (Brownstein et al. 1975) and cytologically characterized by immunocytochemistry in neurons within the neostriatum (Vincent et al. 1982; Finley et al. 1981; DiFiglia and Aronin 1982; Takagi et al. 1983). Perikarya-containing somatostatin-like immunoreactivity (S-LI) are 10–20 μm in diameter, contain a highly invaginated nucleus and are spindle or fusiform in shape (DiFiglia and Aronin 1982). The reaction product is usually diffusely distributed throughout the cytoplasm of perikarya and processes (Fig. 3; DiFiglia and Aronin 1982). However, greater densities of S-LI may be associated with the Golgi saccules and with scattered dense granular vesicles which could reflect sites of more active synthesis and storage of the prohormone (Johansson 1978; Takagi et al. 1983). Localization of S-LI within dendrites which lack spines, together with measurements of diameter and nuclear configuration, definitively establish that the somatostatin-containing neurons in the neostriatum belong to the medium-aspiney classification (DiFiglia and Aronin 1982).

The morphine-like pentapeptides methionine (Met[5]) and leucine (Leu[5])-enkephalin (Hughes et al. 1975) are similarly well characterized by radioimmunoassay and by immunocytochemistry in regions of the neostriatum-containing opiate receptors (Pert et al. 1975). The neurons showing enkephalin-like immunoreactivity (E-LI) are approximately 20 μm in diameter, contain a round, unindented nucleus and are multipolar (Pickel et al. 1980). As described for somatostatin, the reaction product is diffusely dis-

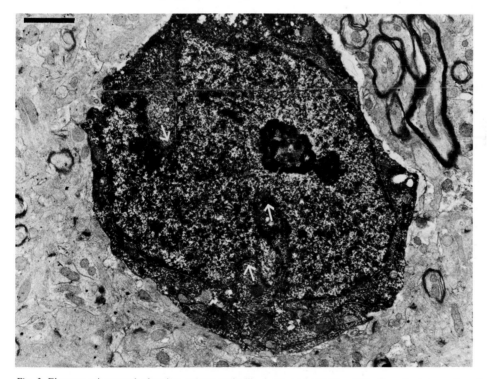

Fig. 3. Electron micrograph showing somatostatin-like immunoreactivity within the cytoplasm and nucleus of medium-sized neuron in the rat caudate nucleus. The medium size and nuclear indentations (white arrows) are characteristic of aspiney neurons. (Micrograph from unpublished material, courtesy of Drs M. DiFiglia and N. Aronin.) Bar = 0.3 μm.

tributed throughout the cytoplasm and dendrites. However, there is not a specific association with the Golgi apparatus and dense granules are rarely detected. The most common vesicular structure within the enkephalin-labeled perikarya are coated or 'alveolate' (Peters et al. 1976) vesicles usually located within the region of the Golgi saccules (Pickel et al. 1980). Coated vesicles are also detected near the post-synaptic specialization of both enkephalin-labeled and unlabeled dendrites within the striatum (Fig. 4) (Pickel et

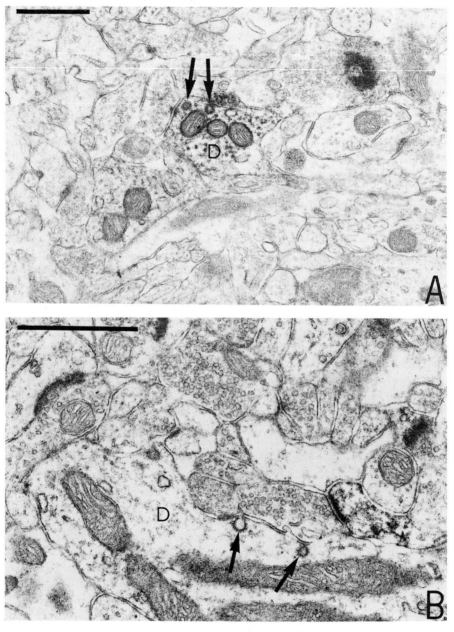

Fig. 4. Ultrastructural demonstration of alveolate vesicles in dendrites in the neostriatum. *A*. Electron micrograph showing 2 alveolate vesicles in a dendrite (D) that is labeled with E-LI. *B*. Electron micrograph showing alveolate vesicles (arrows) in an unlabeled dendrite (D). Bar = 0.1 μm. (Reproduced from Pickel et al. (1980), by courtesy of the Editors of the *Journal of Comparative Neurology*.)

al. 1980). These vesicles may be associated with the transport of materials in dendrites as suggested for saccules of smooth endoplasmic reticulum in many types of neurons. The dendrites showing E-LI are usually post-synaptic to unlabeled axon terminals containing small, round, electron-lucent vesicles and forming asymmetric junctions (Fig. 4) (Pickel et al. 1980). This type of terminal is characteristic for cortical and thalamic afferents to the neostriatum (Hassler et al. 1978; Groves 1980). In contrast to somatostatin-containing neurons, the enkephalin-labeled dendrites exhibit many spines and have the general features ascribed to medium-spiney neostriatal neurons (Pickel et al. 1980). The identification of a neuron as medium aspiney or spiney however, does not necessarily indicate the presence of somatostatin or enkephalin in the respective cells since GABA and other putative transmitters also have been demonstrated in these types of neostriatal neurons (Bolam et al. 1982).

Cerebral cortex

Cholecystokinin (CCK) or the active carboxy terminal octapeptide (CCK-8) is one of a variety of classically defined gastrointestinal peptides recently demonstrated in high concentrations in the cerebral cortex by radioimmunoassay (Beinfeld et al. 1981) and by immunocytochemistry (Innis et al. 1979; Larsson and Rehfeld 1979). The CCK reaction product is diffusely distributed throughout the cytoplasm of neurons which generally have a deeply increscented nucleus comparable to the previously described magnocellular and somatostatin-containing neurons (see Fig. 5) (Hendry et al. 1983).

Cortical neurons showing CCK-LI have a variety of sizes and shapes and are located throughout the cortex. However, most of the perikarya are located in the supragranular layers and are small (10–20 μm) and bipolar (Hendry et al. 1983; Peters et al. 1983). The labeled perikarya and dendrites receive both symmetric and asymmetric synapses which in addition to their dendritic pattern and location, further indicates that they are not pyramidal neurons (Peters et al. 1983).

The predominant localization within bipolar cortical neurons has also been demonstrated for vasoactive intestinal peptide (VIP) (Lorén et al. 1979) and may indicate either a common localization or the presence of 2 gastrointestinal peptides within different populations of bipolar cells (Peters et al. 1983). The possible co-existence of peptides within the same neuron is considered in a separate section.

Dendritic localization

In addition to classifying the neuronal types containing a specific peptide, the dendritic localization suggests that the neuropeptides may be released and/or taken up in dendrites as shown for dopamine in the pars reticulata of the substantia nigra (Geffen et al. 1976). In comparison with dopamine which has been most prominently associated with rough and smooth endoplasmic reticulum in dendrites of the substantia nigra (Wasser et al. 1981; Mercer et al. 1979), enkephalin-containing dendrites in the striatum usually exhibit saccules of endoplasmic reticulum, coated vesicles, and mitochondria with few, if any, synaptic vesicles (Fig. 6). If the neuropeptides are released or taken up in dendrites, additional modulator functions might be postulated (Ralston 1971; Schmitt et al. 1976).

Not only peptides but certain aminopeptidases may be released from dendrites. Greenfield and Shaw (1982) have shown that both acetylcholinesterase and aminopeptidases can be released from the substantia nigra by in vivo infusion of amphetamine.

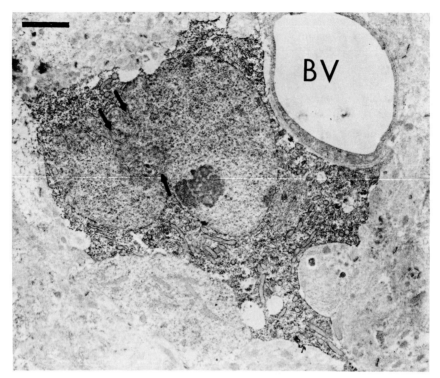

Fig. 5. Localization of CCK-like immunoreactivity in a neuronal perikaryon layer II of the monkey motor cortex. The soma has an irregular contour and lies in proximity to a blood vessel (BV). Most of these neuronal perikarya contain an infolded nucleus (arrows) and receive both symmetric and asymmetric synapses. Bar = 4.0 μm. (Reproduced from Hendry et al. (1983), by courtesy of the Editors of the *Proceedings of the National Academy of Sciences of the USA*.)

The released acetylcholinesterase appears to be unrelated to cholinergic transmission and has been shown to hydrolize substance P (Chubb et al. 1980) and Met- and Leu-enkephalin (Chubb et al. 1982). Like dopamine, acetylcholinesterase also has been localized within the endoplasmic reticulum of dendrites (Kreutzberg et al. 1975; Somogyi et al. 1975). The release of a substance which hydrolizes peptides such as substance P and enkephalin might be a mechanism for terminating their action at presynaptic sites.

3.2. AXON TERMINALS

Synaptic interaction with neurons

Terminals containing immunoreactivity for the neuropeptides form primarily symmetric or asymmetric axodendritic synapses as seen for enkephalin in the neostriatum (Pickel et al. 1980), in substantia gelatinosa (Aronin et al. 1981; Glazer and Basbaum 1981a, b), and in the medial nucleus tractus solitarius (NTS) and locus ceruleus (Pickel et al. 1977); for somatostatin in the neostriatum and dorsal horn, and for substance P in the substantia gelatinosa (De Lanerolle and LaMotte 1980; Barber et al. 1979; DiFiglia et al. 1982). Examples of enkephalin-labeled terminals forming synapses with unlabeled dendrites are shown in Figures 6 and 7A. While the axodendritic synapses are most com-

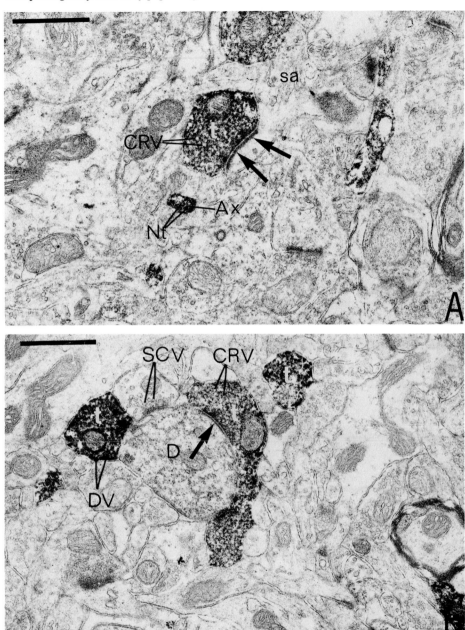

Fig. 6. Immunocytochemical localization of E-LI in axons and axon terminals forming specialized synaptic contacts with dendrites in the neostriatum. *A.* Electron micrograph showing postjunctional plaque (arrows) between an unlabeled dendritic spine that contains a spiney apparatus (sa) and an axon terminal (t) containing E-LI. Small unmyelinated axon (Ax) also shows E-LI and contains neurotubules (Nt). *B.* Electron micrograph showing a synaptic junction (arrow) between an unlabeled proximal dendrite (D) and axon terminals (t) having E-LI. In both *A* and *B*, the labeled axon terminals contain either clear-rimmed vesicles (CRV) or dense vesicles (DV), depending on the density of the reaction product. The vesicles in the labeled terminals are never concentrated near the synaptic density as observed for the small clear vesicles (SCV) in the unlabeled terminal in *B*. Bar = 0.1 μm (Reproduced from Pickel et al. (1980), by courtesy of the Editors of the *Journal of Comparative Neurology.*)

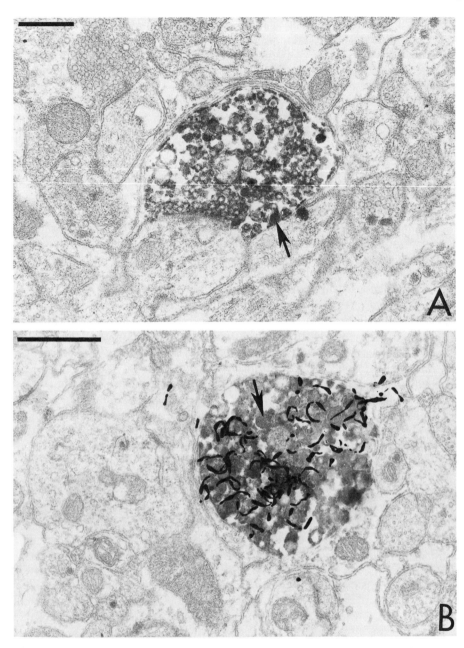

Fig. 7. Electron microscopic localization of serotonin and enkephalin within the same or different axon terminals of the area postrema. *A*. Immunocytochemical localization of enkephalin-like immunoreactivity. Terminal contains both large dense vesicles (arrows) and rimmed small clear vesicles. *B*. Radioautographic localization of ^{3}H-5HT and immunocytochemical localization of enkephalin-like immunoreactivity in the same terminal. Bar = 0.2 μm.

mon, recent studies in the spinal cord, area postrema, and NTS, have demonstrated that the peptide-containing axon terminals may also form axo-axonic synapses (LaMotte and De Lanerolle 1983; Armstrong et al. 1984). Such axo-axonic synapses provide an important morphological correlate for physiological and receptor binding studies (Ninkovic et al. 1981), suggesting that in regions such as the dorsal horn and NTS, enkephalin may inhibit the release of substance P through a direct axonal interaction (Jessell and Iverson 1977). Other possible modes of interaction between the primary afferents, some of which contain substance P, and neurons showing E-LI may also be through convergence on a common dendrite (Hunt et al. 1980; Sumal et al. 1982).

In addition to the axodendritic and axo-axonic synapses, a few synapses between peptide-labeled terminals and neuronal soma have also been reported (Pickel et al. 1980; Sumal et al. 1982). The numerous axodendritic and sparse axo-axonic and axosomatic synapses which have been demonstrated for the neuropeptide-containing neurons are also common features of most neurons in the CNS (Peters et al. 1976; Zhu et al. 1981).

Vesicular localization

As shown for enkephalin in Figure 7A, many axon terminals showing immunoreactivity for neuropeptides contain numerous small, clear (40–60 nm) and a few (1–10) large (70–100 nm) DCV's (Pickel et al. 1979; LaMotte and De Lanerolle 1983). Occasionally very large (130–150 nm) dense vesicles approaching the dimensions of neurosecretory granules have been identified within terminals (Chan-Palay and Palay 1977), and within perikarya of peptidergic neurons (Takagi et al. 1983). The mixed vesicle population has been reported for neuropeptides in a variety of species including rat (Pickel et al. 1977, 1980; Hunt et al. 1980), cat (Glazer and Basbaum 1981a,b), monkey (Aronin et al. 1981), and human (De Lanerolle and LaMotte 1980). However, as illustrated by comparing the terminals showing E-LI in the striatum (Fig. 6) with those in the NTS (Fig. 7A) the relative proportion of the DCV's and small vesicles is highly variable even for the same peptide in different regions (Pickel et al. 1979). Presumably, this difference may reflect local collateral *vs* longer projection pathways, varying cross-reactivities with precursor molecules, or even the number of putative transmitters within the neuron.

The association of neuropeptides with a specific vesicle population has been the subject of considerable controversy. Pickel et al. (1977) reported that substance P-like immunoreactivity (SP-LI) was most prominently associated with the central region of large DCV's. However, Barber and co-workers (1979), using the same antiserum and similar pre-embedding immunocytochemical methods, found SP-LI to be associated with the large DCV's as well as the outer membrane of small clear vesicles, mitochondria and plasmalemma. At least a portion of this discrepancy is methodological. When the immunocytochemical reaction is carried out prior to embedding in plastic (i.e., pre-embedding), the density of the immunoreactivity associated with specific subcellular organelles is greatly influenced by the distance from the surface at which the sections are taken and by the amount of membrane damage evoked by the fixative and solubilizing agents. At depths of 1 μm or less, virtually all membranes within an immunoreactive cell exhibit a dense peroxidase reaction (Fig. 3). Near the surface, we find that substance P, as reported by Barber et al. (1979), and other peptides (e.g., enkephalin; Fig. 7A) show an immunocytochemical reaction product both within the DCV's and rimming most other organelles including the smaller vesicles and mitochondria. However, at greater depths a more selective organelle association is seen, particularly along longitudinal channels such as microtubules and within the DCV's. The localization of peptides within DCV's by the pre-embedding immunocytochemical technique is seriously limited by problems of penetration in well-fixed tissues (Sternberger 1979). For example, we have been unable to detect β-endorphin by the pre-embedding labeling technique in well-fixed tissues employing 0.1–0.2% glutaraldehyde and 4% paraformaldehyde. However, when the glutaraldehyde is omitted many processes in the ventral hypothalamus exhibit a prominent localization of β-endorphin in large DCV's (Fig. 8A). The glutaraldehyde probably maintains the vesicular membrane so intact that the contents are inaccessible to the antisera, or alternatively, the aldehyde may interfere with the antigen–antibody interaction. Use of a post-embedding technique (Sternberger 1979) in which the immunocytochemical reaction is carried out after embedding in plastic partially overcomes the problem of penetration of intact vesicles. All of the vesicles are sectioned and have equal access to the various antisera. In such post-embedding preparations, many peptides have been localized to large DCV's (Pelletier et al. 1977). This does not, however, exclude the possibility that the peptides may also exist free in the cytosol or be contained within the small clear vesicles, since many antigenic sites may be destroyed or lost during the plastic embedding procedure (Kozlowski and Nilaver 1983; Sternberger 1979).

Due to the described limitations of both the pre- and post-embedding techniques, immunocytochemistry cannot be used to unequivocally demonstrate that the neuropeptides are localized to the dense vesicles or to any other organelle. However, the association of peptides with saccules of the Golgi apparatus and dense vesicles within the perikarya (Takagi et al. 1983; Johansson 1978), the accumulation of immunocytochemically labeled DCV's proximal to axonal transections (Fig. 8B; Pickel et al. 1983) and the presence of DCV's in many peptide-containing terminals strongly suggest that the dense vesicles represent at least one synthesis, storage, and transport site for certain neuropeptides (Gilbert 1980). This suggestion is strengthened by recent biochemical studies in which a vesicle population the size of the morphologically identified large DCV shows substance P activity (Floor et al. 1982). If the neuropeptides are contained within DCV's they may be released upon nerve stimulation by exocytosis in a manner analogous to the smaller vesicles or may serve a more modulatory function (Dickinson-Nelson and Reese 1983). Obviously in peptidergic neurons such as the enkephalin-containing cells within the striatum which contain few DCV's in either perikarya or terminals, alternative packaging, transport, and/or possible release must be envisioned.

The localization of peptides in terminals containing mixed or homogeneous vesicle populations may reflect the multiplicity of neurotransmitters identified within the neuron. Immunocytochemistry, radioautography and biochemistry have recently been used to demonstrate the co-localization of different peptides (Dalsgaard et al. 1982) or peptide and monoamines or acetylcholine within the same neuron (Hökfelt et al. 1978; Klein et al. 1982; Chan-Palay et al. 1978; Chan-Palay 1982; Jan et al. 1979; Campbell et al. 1982).

The first evidence for co-existence of transmitters was established using light microscopic immunocytochemistry in adjacent frozen sections to localize substance P and serotonin in certain perikarya in the raphe (Hökfelt et al. 1978; Chan-Palay et al. 1978). The co-existence of these transmitters as well as serotonin and enkephalin in raphe nuclei (Bowker et al. 1981a,b) and in the area postrema (Armstrong et al. 1984) and glutamic acid decarboxylase and motilin in cerebellar Purkinje cells have now been demonstrated with a variety of double labeling techniques (Chan-Palay 1982). Axon terminals showing uptake of ³H-serotonin by radioautography and enkephalin immunoreactivity in rat area postrema contain a mixed vesicle population with a relatively large number of DCV's (Fig. 8; Armstrong et al. 1984). The resolution is not sufficient to distinguish whether there is subcellular compartmentalization of these transmitters. However, in the adrenal medulla and splenic nerve, both noradrenalin and opioid peptides have been associated with the same DCV (Klein et al. 1982; Wilson et al. 1980). In contrast, cholin-

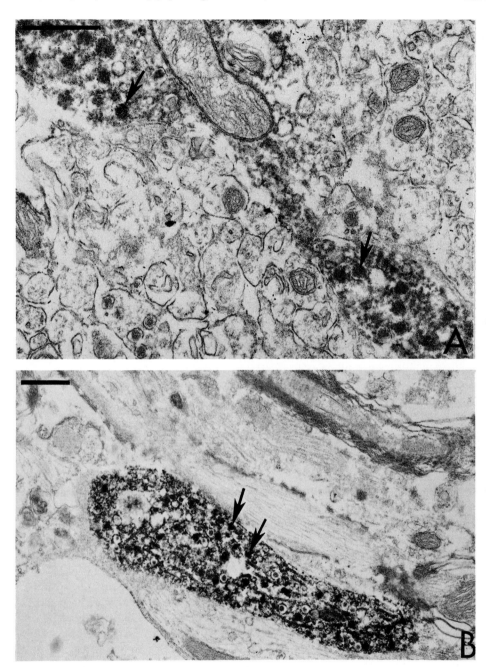

Fig. 8. Electron micrograph showing dense core vesicles (arrows) in immunocytochemically labeled processes. *A. β*-Endorphin in hypothalamic axons of non-colchicine-treated animals. Dense vesicles are detected when tissue is fixed with 4% paraformaldehyde. *B.* Substance P in axons proximal to a cervical spinal transection. Tissue damaged and poorly fixed due to edema and interruption of vasculature in region of transection. Bar = 0.1 μm.

ergic terminals of the frog sympathetic ganglion appear to contain luteinizing hor-mone-releasing hormone (LHRH) in DCV's, whereas acetylcholine is believed to be contained within small clear vesicles (Jan et al. 1979). Thus, the peptides may be within the same or separate storage organelles when they coexist with other transmitters.

4. NON-NEURONAL ASSOCIATIONS

4.1. VASCULAR

Both endocrine and transmitter functions may be mediated by the vascular associations of peptidergic neurons. The *endocrine* property of being released into the circulation for action on more distal target cells (Morris et al. 1978) is now well established for the hypophysiotropic and numerous other peptides including substance P, VIP and CCK (Vale 1978). Many of these peptides are found both in neurons of the CNS and in the gastrointestinal tract which presumably reflects a common neuroectodermal origin (Pearse 1980). While the peptides of the posterior pituitary (oxytocin and vasopressin) are convincingly localized to the large neurosecretory granule (Morris et al. 1978), the localization of smaller peptides such as enkephalin within these granules remains con-troversial (Van Leeuwen et al. 1983; Martin et al. 1983). As seen in enkephalin-contain-ing terminals forming synapses within the CNS, enkephalin in the axons of the pituitary may be more closely associated with the DCV's having a diameter of about 100 nm (Van Leeuwen et al. 1983; Beauvillain et al. 1980).

In addition to the relations between peptidergic axons and the vasculature of the pi-tuitary and median eminence, the neuropeptide containing neurons may be responsible for local alterations of brain–blood composition by exchange of substances between their perikarya and processes and intrinsic blood vessels of the CNS (Chan-Palay 1977). A close apposition is seen between the CCK-labeled neurons and blood vessels within the cerebral cortex (Hendry et al. 1983). In Figure 7 from Hendry et al. (1983), the CCK-labeled perikaryon has many cytoplasmic protrusions and encircles a blood vessel in a manner comparable to an astrocyte (Peters et al. 1976). This neuron can be distin-guished from a glial cell by the presence of axosomatic synapses. No membrane speciali-zations are detected between the CCK-labeled perikaryon and adjacent blood vessel (Hendry et al. 1983).

The putative *transmitter* properties of peptidergic neurons at blood vessels have been most extensively examined for the potent vasodilator, substance P (Barber et al. 1979; Liu-Chen et al. 1982, 1983). Both intrinsic and pial vessels are innervated by axons showing SP-LI. Within the dorsal horn, the SP-LI is found in axons which form a 'bas-ket-line' network around certain intrinsic vessels (Barber et al. 1979). The ultrastructural morphology of these substance P-labeled terminals is similar to the morphology of ter-minals forming neuronal junctions. Both synaptic and vascular terminals have the pre-viously described content of small clear and large DCV's. The vascular processes some-times exhibited close membrane appositions with perivascular glial cells (Barber et al. 1979).

Substance P and other peptides (e.g., neurotensin and VIP) have also been associated with the walls of the internal carotid and basilar arteries and smaller pial vessels (Chan-Palay 1977; Edvinsson 1980; Yamamoto et al. 1983). Based upon the fact that the axons showing SP-LI could be traced only to the level of the arteriole at the termination of the muscle layer, Yamamoto et al. (1983) postulated that substance P acts primarily on vascular smooth muscle. The vasomotor functions of substance P have previously been established by a number of pharmacological studies (Edvinsson and Uddman 1982; Hallberg and Pernow 1975; Furness et al. 1982). However, the relation between the substance-P-containing axons and vascular smooth muscle has not been established by electron microscopy. In addition, most of the substance-P-labeled axons associated with the cerebral vasculature are abolished by trigeminal lesions (Liu-Chen et al. 1982, 1983; Yamamoto et al. 1983), thus suggesting a more sensory function. The non-neuronal association between peptidergic neurons and blood vessels awaits further morphological and physiological clarification.

4.2. VENTRICULAR

The relation between peptidergic neurons and glia or ependymal cells is comparable to the vasculature in that the existing morphological studies are intriguing, but incomplete. The existence of neurono-glial synaptoid contacts has been known for tanycytes in the median eminence for several years (Bargman et al. 1967; Gulder and Wolff 1973). At least some of the neuronal processes contacting tanycytes can be immunochemically labeled for the polypeptide LHRH (Kozlowski 1983). Synaptoid contacts also have been reported for enkephalin-containing axon terminals and glial cells in the median eminence (Beauvillain et al. 1980) and for the astrocytic equivalent, the pituicyte in the pituitary (Van Leeuwen et al. 1983). Other examples of peptide-containing axons and modified glia or ependyma have been shown for substance P in the area postrema (Armstrong et al. 1983). As indicated for the terminals associated with the vasculature, these substance-P-containing terminals have a mixed vesicle population and are apposed to, but show no specialized membrane thickening, at the neuroglial junction. The associations (synaptoid contacts) between astrocytes or other modified glia and peptide-containing terminals suggest that certain peptidergic neurons may regulate uptake or release of substances from blood or cerebrospinal fluid through a glial intermediary.

5. CONCLUSION

The morphological features of peptidergic neurons provide a conceptual framework for understanding how neuropeptides may be synthesized, stored and released alone or with conventional transmitters for direct synaptic actions or more distal humoral effects. With the exception of the neurosecretory granules, the morphology of the characterized neuropeptide-containing neurons is the same as for other neurons whose peptides have not yet been identified.

6. REFERENCES

Armstrong DM, Pickel VM, Reis DJ (1983): Electron microscopic immunocytochemical localization of substance P in the area postrema of rat. *J. Comp. Neurol., 243*, 141–146.

Armstrong DM, Miller RJ, Beaudet A, Pickel VM (1984): Enkephalin-like immunoreactivity in rat area postrema: ultrastructural localization and coexistence with serotonin. *Brain Res., 310*, 269–278.

Aronin N, DiFiglia M, Liotla AS, Martin JB (1981): Ultrastructural localization and biochemical features of immunoreactive leu-enkephalin in monkey dorsal horn. *J. Neurosci., 1*, 561–577.

Barden N, Merand Y, Rouleau D, Moore S, Dockray GJ, Dupont A (1981): Regional distributions of somatostatin and cholecystokinin-like immunoreactivities in rat and bovine brain. *Peptides, 2*, 299–302.

Barber PR, Vaughn JE, Slemmon JR, Salvaterra PM, Roberts E, Leeman SE (1979): The origin, distribution and synaptic relationships of substance P axons in rat spinal cord. *J. Comp. Neurol., 184*, 331–351.

Bargmann W, Lindner E, Andres KH (1967): Über Synapsen an endokrinin Epithelzellen und die Definition sekretorischer Neurone. Untersuchungen am Zwischenlappen der Katzenhypophyse. *Z. Zellforsch., 77*, 282–298.

Beauvillain JC, Tramu G, Corix D (1980): Electron-microscopic localization of enkephalin in the median eminence and adenohypophysis of the guinea-pig. *Neuroscience, 5*, 1705–1716.

Beinfeld MC, Meyer DK, Eskay RL, Jensen RT, Brownstein MJ (1981): The distribution of cholecystokinin immunoreactivity in the central nervous system of the rat as demonstrated by radioimmunoassay. *Brain Res., 212*, 51–57.

Bennett GJ, Abdelmoumene M, Hayashi H, Dubner R (1980): Physiology and morphology of substantia gelatinosa neurons intracellularly stained with horseradish peroxidase. *J. Comp. Neurol., 194*, 809–827.

Bennett GJ, Gobel S, Dubner R (1982): Enkephalin immunoreactive stalked cells and lamina IIb islet cells in cat substantia gelatinosa. *Brain Res., 240*, 162–166.

Bolam JP, Freund TF, Hammond DJ, Smith AD, Somogyi P (1982): Morphological characterization of (³H)GABA-accumulating neurons in the rat neostriatum by Golgi-staining and electron microscopy. *Br. J. Pharmacol., 75, Suppl.*, 46P.

Bowker RM, Steinbusch HWM, Coulter JD (1981a): Serotonin and peptidergic projections to the spinal cord demonstrated by a combined retrograde HRP histochemical and immunocytochemical staining method. *Brain Res., 211*, 412–417.

Bowker RM, Westlund KN, Coulter JD (1981b): Origins of serotonergic and peptidergic projections to the spinal cord. *Anat. Rec., 199*, 35A.

Brownstein RP, Arimura A, Sato H, Schally AV, Kizer JS (1975): The regional distribution of somatostatin in the rat brain. *Endocrinology, 96*, 1456–1461.

Campbell G, Gibbins IL, Morris JL, Furness JB, Costa M, Oliver JR, Beardsley AM, Murphy R (1982): Somatostatin is contained in and released from cholinergic neurons in the heart of the toad *Bufo marinus. Neuroscience, 7*, 2013–2023.

Carraway R, Leeman SE (1976): Characterization of radioimmunoassayable neurotensin in the rat. *J. Biol. Chem., 251*, 7045–7052.

Chan-Palay V (1977): Innervation of cerebral blood vessels by norepinephrine, indoleamine, substance P and neurotensin fibers and the leptomeningeal axons: their roles in vasomotor activity and local alterations of brain blood composition. In: Owman C, Edvinsson L (Eds), *Neurogenic Control of the Brain Circulation*, pp. 39–53. Pergamon Press, Oxford.

Chan-Palay V (1982): Immunocytochemical and radioautographic methods to demonstrate the coexistence of neuroactive substances: cerebellar Purkinje cells have glutamic acid decarboxylase and motilin immunoreactivity, and raphe neurons have serotonin and substance P immunoreactivity. In: Chan-Palay V, Palay SL (Eds), *Neurology and Neurobiology, Vol. I: Cytochemical Methods in Neuroanatomy*, pp. 93–118. Alan R. Liss, New York.

Chan-Palay V, Palay SL (1977): Ultrastructural identification of substance P cells and their processes in rat sensory ganglia and their terminals in the spinal cord by immunocytochemistry. *Proc. Natl Acad. Sci. USA, 74*, 4050–4054.

Chan-Palay V, Jonsson G, Palay SL (1978): Serotonin and substance P coexist in neurons of the rat central nervous system. *Proc. Natl Acad. Sci. USA, 75*, 1582–1586.

Chubb IW, Hodgson AJ, White GH (1980): Acetylcholinesterase hydrolyses substance P. *Neuroscience, 5*, 2065–2072.

Chubb IW, Ranieri E, Hodgson AJ, White GH (1982): The hydrolysis of leu- and met-enkephalin by acetylcholinesterase. *Neurosci. Lett., Suppl., 8*, S39.

Dalsgaard DJ, Vincent S, Hökfelt T, Dockray GJ, Cuello C (1982): Immunohistochemical evidence for coexistence of cholecystokinin and substance P-like peptides in primary sensory neurons. *Soc. Neurosci. Abstracts, 8*, 474.

De Lanerolle NC, LaMotte CC (1980): Light and electron microscopic localization of substance P, met-enkephalin and 5-hydroxytryptamine in the human and monkey spinal cord. *Soc. Neurosci. Abstracts, 6*, 353.

Dickinson-Nelson A, Reese TS (1983): Structural changes during transmitter release at synapses in the frog sympathetic ganglion. *J. Neurosci., 3*, 42.

DiFiglia M, Aronin N (1982): Ultrastructural features of immunoreactive somatostatin neurons in the rat caudate nucleus. *J. Neurosci., 2*, 1267–1272.

DiFiglia M, Aronin N, Leeman SE (1982): Light microscopic and ultrastructural localization of immunoreactive substance P in the dorsal horn of the monkey spinal cord. *Neuroscience, 7*, 1127–1139.

Dube D, Pelletier G (1979): Effect of colchicine on the immunohistochemical localization of somatostatin in the rat brain: light and electron microscopic studies. *J. Histochem. Cytochem., 27*, 1577–1581.

88

Du Vigneaud, V (1956): Hormones of the posterior pituitary gland; oxytocin and vasopressin. *Harvey Lecture Series L 1954–55*, pp. 1–26. Academic Press, New York.

Edvinsson L, Uddmann R (1982): Immunohistochemical localization and dilatory effects of substance P on human cerebral vessels. *Brain Res., 232*, 466–471.

Edvinsson L, Fahrenkrug J, Hanko J, Owman C, Sundler F, Uddman R (1980): VIP (vasoactive intestinal polypeptide)-containing nerves of intracranial arteries in mammals. *Cell Tissue Res., 208*, 135–142.

Elde R, Hökfelt T (1979): Localization of hypophysiotrophic peptides and other biologically active peptides within the brain. *Annu. Rev. Physiol., 41*, 587–602.

Finley JCW, Maderdrut JL, Roger LJ, Petrusz P (1981): The immunocytochemical localization of somatostatin-containing neurons in the rat central nervous system. *Neuroscience, 6*, 2173–2192.

Floor E, Grad O, Leeman SE (1982): Synaptic vesicles containing substance P purified by chromatography on controlled pore glass. *Neuroscience, 7*, 1647–1655.

Furness JB, Parka RE, Della NG, Costa M, Eskay RL (1982): Substance P-like immunoreactivity in nerves associated with the vascular system of guineapigs. *Neuroscience, 7*, 447–459.

Gainer H, Loh YP, Sarne Y (1977): Biosynthesis of neuronal peptides. In: Gainer H (Ed.), *Peptides in Neurobiology*, pp. 183–219. Plenum Press, New York.

Geffen LB, Jessell TM, Cuello AC, Iverson LL (1976): Release of dopamine from dendrites in rat substantia nigra. *Nature (London), 260*, 258–260.

Gibson SJ, Polak JM, Bloom SR, Wall PO (1981): The distribution of nine peptides in rat spinal cord with special emphasis on the substantia gelatinosa and on the area around the central canal (Lamina X). *J. Comp. Neurol., 201*, 65–79.

Gilbert RF (1980): Axonal transport of neuropeptides in the cervical vagus nerve of the rat. *J. Neurochem., 34*, 108–113.

Gillis RA, Helke CJ, Hamilton BL, Norman WP, Jacobowitz DM (1980): Evidence that substance P is a neurotransmitter of baro- and chemoreceptor afferents in nucleus tractus solitarius. *Brain Res., 181*, 476–481.

Glazer EJ, Basbaum AI (1981a): Immunohistochemical localization of leucine-enkephalin in the spinal cord of the cat: enkephalin containing marginal neurons and pain modulation. *J. Comp. Neurol., 196*, 377–389.

Glazer EJ, Basbaum AI (1981b): Serial analysis of leu-enkephalin (ENK) synaptic relationships in cat dorsal horn. *Pain, Suppl. 1*, S133.

Gobel S (1978a): Golgi studies of the neurons in layer I of the dorsal horn of the medulla (trigeminal nucleus caudalis). *J. Comp. Neurol., 180*, 375–394.

Gobel S (1978b): Golgi studies of the neurons in layer II of the dorsal horn of the medulla (trigeminal nucleus caudalis). *J. Comp. Neurol., 180*, 395–414.

Gobel S, Falls WM, Bennett GJ, Abdelmoumene M, Hayashi H, Humphrey H (1980): An EM analysis of the synaptic connections of horseradish peroxidase-filled stalked cells and islet cells in the substantia gelatinosa of adult cat spinal cord. *J. Comp. Neurol., 194*, 781–807.

Goldstein K, Nilsson M, Pernow B, Terenius L, Ganten D, Jeffcoate SL, Rehfeld J, Said S (1978): Distribution of peptide-containing neurons. In: Lipton MA, DiMascio A, Killam KF (Eds), *Psychopharmacology: a Generation of Progress*, pp. 39–66. Raven Press, New York.

Greenfield SA, Shaw SG (1982): Release of acetylcholinesterase and aminopeptidase in vivo following infusion of amphetamine into the substantia nigra. *Neuroscience, 7*, 2883–2893.

Groves PM (1980): Synaptic endings and their postsynaptic targets in the neostriatum: synaptic specializations revealed from analysis of serial sections. *Proc. Natl Acad. Sci. USA, 77*, 6926–6929.

Grzanna R, Molliver ME, Coyle JT (1978): Visualization of central noradrenergic neurons in thick sections by the unlabeled antibody method: a transmitter-specific Golgi image. *Proc. Natl Acad. Sci. USA, 75*, 2502–2506.

Guillemin R (1978a): Peptides in the brain: the new endocrinology of the neuron. *Science, 202*, 390–402.

Guillemin R (1978b): In: Reichlin S, Baldessarini, RJ, Martin JB (Eds), *The Hypothalamus*, pp. 155–194. Raven Press, New York.

Gulder FH, Wolff JR (1973): Neurono-glial synaptoid contacts in the median eminence of the rat: ultrastructure, staining properties and distribution of tanycytes. *Brain Res., 61*, 217–234.

Haber S, Elde R (1982): The distribution of enkephalin immunoreactive fibers and terminals in the monkey central nervous system: an immunohistochemical study. *Neuroscience, 7*, 1049–1095.

Hallberg D, Pernow B (1975): Effect of substance P on various vascular beds in the dog. *Acta Physiol. Scand., 93*, 277–285.

Hassler R, Chung JW, Rinne U, Wagner A (1978): Selective degeneration of two out of the nine types of synapses in cat caudate nucleus after cortical lesions. *Exp. Brain Res., 31*, 67–80.

Hartman BK (1973): Immunofluorescence of dopamine-β-hydroxylase. Application of improved methodology to the localization of the peripheral and central nervous system. *J. Histochem. Cytochem., 21*, 312–332.

Hendry SHC, Jones EG, Beinfeld MC (1983): CCK immunoreactive neurons in rat and monkey cerebral cortex make symmetric synapses and have intimate association with blood vessels. *Proc. Natl Acad. Sci. USA, 80*, 2400–2404.

Ho RH, DePalatis LR (1980): Substance P immunoreactivity in the median eminence of the North American opossum and domestic fowl. *Brain Res., 189*, 565–569.

Hökfelt T, Elde R, Johansson O, Terenius L, Stein L (1977a): The distribution of enkephalin-immunoreactive cell bodies in the rat central nervous system. *Neurosci. Lett., 5*, 25–31.

Hökfelt T, Ljungdahl A, Terenius L, Elde R, Nilsson G (1977b): Immunohistochemical analysis of peptide pathways possibly related to pain and analgesia: enkephalin and substance P. *Proc. Natl Acad. Sci. USA, 74*, 3081–3085.

Hökfelt T, Ljungdahl A, Steinbush H, Verhofstad A, Nilsson G, Brodin E, Pernow B, Goldstein M (1978): Immunohistochemical evidence of substance P-like immunoreactivity in some 5-hydroxytryptamine-containing neurons in the rat central nervous system. *Neuroscience, 3*, 517–538.

Hökfelt T, Johansson O, Ljungdahl A, Lundberg JM, Schultzberg M (1980): Peptidergic neurons. *Nature (London), 284*, 515–521.

Hughes J, Smith TW, Kosterlitz HW, Fothergill LH, Morgan BA, Morris HR (1975): Identification of two related pentapeptides from the brain with potent opiate agonist activity. *Nature (London), 258*, 577–579.

Hunt SP, Kelly JS, Emson PC (1980): The electron microscopic localization of methionine enkephalin within the superficial layers (I and II) of the spinal cord. *Neuroscience, 5*, 1871–1890.

Innis RB, Correa FMA, Uhl GR, Schneider B, Snyder S (1979): Cholecystokinin octapeptide-like immunoreactivity: histochemical localization in rat brain. *Proc. Natl Acad. Sci. USA, 76*, 521–525.

Jan YN, Jan LY, Kuffler SW (1979): A peptide as a possible transmitter in sympathetic ganglia of the frog. *Proc. Natl Acad. Sci. USA, 76*, 1501–1505.

Jessell TM, Iversen LL (1977): Opiate analgesics inhibit substance P release from rat trigeminal nucleus. *Nature (London), 268*, 549–551.

Johansson O (1978) Localization of somatostatin-like immunoreactivity in the Golgi apparatus of central and peripheral neurons. *Histochemistry, 58*, 167–178.

Klein RL, Wilson SP, Dzielak DJ, Yang WH, Viveros OH (1982): Opioid peptides and noradrenaline co-exist in large dense-cored vesicles from sympathetic nerve. *Neuroscience, 7*, 2255–2261.

Knowles F (1974): In: Knowles F, Vollrath L (Eds), *Neurosecretion – The Final Neuroendocrine Pathway*, pp. 3–11. Springer, Berlin.

Kozlowski GP (1983): Comparative ultrastructure of neuropeptide containing cells of the parvo- and magnocellular neurosecretory system. In: Sano U, Ibata Y, Zimmerman EA (Eds), *Structure and Function of Peptidergic and Aminergic Neurons*. Japanese Scientific Society Press, Tokyo.

Kozlowski GP, Nilaver G (1983): Immunoelectron microscopy of neuropeptides – Theoretical and technical considerations. In: Barker JL, McKelvy JF (Eds), *Current Methods in Cellular Neurobiology*. Wiley and Sons, Inc., New York.

Kozlowski GP, Brownfield MS, Hostetter G (1976): Neurosecretory supply to extrahypothalamic structures: choroid plexus, circumventricular organs and limbic structures. In: Kiel WB, Giessen AO, Leningrad AP, Scharrer B (Eds), *Neurosecretion and Neuroendocrine Activity*, pp. 217–235. Springer-Verlag, New York.

Kozlowski GP, Frenk S, Brownfield MS (1977): Localization of neurophysin in rat supraoptic nucleus. *Cell Tissue Res., 179*, 467–473.

Kreutzberg GW, Toth L, Kaiya H (1975): Acetylcholinesterase as a marker for dendritic transport and dendritic secretion. In: Physiology and Pathology of Dendrites. *Adv. Neurol., 12*, 269–281.

LaMotte CC, De Lanerolle N (1983): Substance P, enkephalin and serotonin: ultrastructural basis of pain transmission in primate spinal cord. In: Bonica JJ, Lindblom V, Iggo A (Eds), *Advances in Pain Research and Therapy, Vol. 5*. Raven Press, New York.

Larsson LI, Rehfeld JF (1979): Localization and molecular heterogeneity of cholecystokinin in the cerebral and peripheral nervous system. *Brain Res., 165*, 201–218.

Liu-Chen LY, Dae HH, Moskowitz MA (1982): Pia arachnoid contains substance P projecting from trigeminal neurons: implications for vascular afferent neurotransmission. *Soc. Neurosci. Abstracts, 8*, 474.

Liu-Chen LY, Mayberg M, Moskowitz MA (1983): Immunocytochemical evidence for substance P containing trigeminal-vascular pathway to pial arteries in cats. *Brain Res., 268*, 162–166.

Ljungdahl A, Hökfelt T, Nilsson D (1978): Distribution of substance P-like immunoreactivity in the central nervous system of the rat. I. Cell bodies and nerve terminals. *Neuroscience, 3*, 861–943.

Lorén I, Emson PC, Fahrenkrug J, Björklund A, Alumets J, Hakanson RP, Sundler F (1979): Distribution of vasoactive intestinal polypeptide in the rat and mouse brain. *Neuroscience, 4*, 1953–1976.

Maley B, Mullett T, Elde RP (1983): Nucleus tractus solitarius of cat: a comparison of Golgi impregnated neurons with methionine enkephalin and substance P immunoreactivity. *J. Comp. Neurol., 217*, 405–417.

Martin R, Geis R, Holl R, Schafer M, Voigt KH (1983): Co-existence of unrelated peptides in oxytocin and vasopressin terminals of rat neurohypophyses: immunoreactive methionine⁵-enkephalin-, leucine⁵-enkephalin- and cholecystokinin-like substances. *Neuroscience, 8*, 213–227.

McCann SM (1982): Physiology and pharmacology of LHRH and somatostatin. *Annu. Rev. Pharmacol. Toxicol., 22*, 491–515.

Mercer L, Del Fiacco M, Cuello AC (1979): The smooth endoplasmic reticulum as a possible storage site for dendritic dopamine in substantia nigra neurons. *Experientia, 35*, 101–103.

Morris JF, Nordmann JJ, Dyball REJ (1978) Structure–function correlation in mammalian neurosecretion. *Int. Rev. Exp. Pathol., 18*, 1–95.

Moss RL (1979): Actions of hypothalamic-hypophysiotropic hormones on the brain. *Annu. Rev. Physiol., 41*, 617–631.

Moss MS, Glazer EJ, Basbaum AI (1981): Light and electron microscopic observations of leucine-enkephalin in the cat periaqueductal grey. *Pain, Suppl., 1*, S264.

Moss MS, Glazer EJ, Basbaum AI (1983): The peptidergic organization of the cat periaqueductal grey. I. The distributory of immunoreactive enkephalin-containing neurons and terminals. *J. Neurosci., 3*, 603–616.

Ninkovic M, Hunt SP, Kelley JS (1981): Effect of dorsal rhizotomy on the autoradiographic distribution of opiate and neurotensin receptors and neurotensin like immunoreactivity within the rat spinal cord. *Brain Res., 230*, 111–119.

Palay SL (1960): The fine structure of secretory neurons in the preoptic nucleus of the goldfish. *Anat. Rec., 138*, 417–443.

Pearse, AGE (1980): APUD: concept, tumors, molecular markers and amyloid. *Mikroskopie, 36*, 257–262.

Pelletier G, Dube D, Puviani R (1977): Somatostatin: electron microscope immunohistochemical localization in secretory neurons of rat hypothalamus. *Science, 196*, 1469–1470.

Pert C, Kuhar M, Snyder SH (1975): Autoradiographic localization of the opiate receptor in rat brain. *Life Sci., 16*, 1849–1854.

Petrusz P, Sar M, Grossman GH, Krizer JS (1977): Synaptic terminals with somatostatin-like immunoreactivity in the rat brain. *Brain Res., 137*, 181–187.

Peters A, Palay SL, Webster H de F (1976): *The Fine Structure of the Nervous System: The Neurons and Supporting Cells*. W.B. Saunders Co., Philadelphia, PA.

Peters A, Miller M, Kimerer LM (1983): Cholecystokinin-like immunoreactive neurons in rat cerebral cortex. *Neuroscience, 8*, 431–448.

Pickel VM, Reis DJ, Leeman SE (1977): Ultrastructural localization of substance P in neurons of the spinal cord. *Brain Res., 122*, 534–540.

Pickel VM, Joh TH, Reis DJ, Leeman SE, Miller RJ (1979): Electron microscopic localization of substance P and enkephalin in axon terminals related to dendrites of catecholaminergic neurons. *Brain Res., 160*, 387–400.

Pickel VM, Sumal KV, Beckley SC, Miller RJ, Reis DJ (1980): Immunohistochemical localization of enkephalin in the neostriatum of rat brain: a light and electron microscopic study. *J. Comp. Neurol., 189*, 721–740.

Pickel VM, Miller RJ, Chan J, Sumal KK (1983): Substance P and enkephalin in transected axons of medulla and spinal cord. *Regul. Peptides, 6*, 121–135.

Piercey MF, Dobry PJK, Schroeder LA, Einspahr FJ (1981): Behavioral evidence that substance P may be a spinal cord sensory neurotransmitter. *Brain Res., 210*, 407–412.

Ralston III HJ (1971): Evidence for presynaptic dendrites and a proposal for their mechanism of action. *Nature (London), 230*, 585–587.

Roberts GW, Woodhams PL, Polak JM, Crow TJ (1982): Distribution of neuropeptides in the limbic system of the rat: the amygdaloid complex. *Neuroscience, 7*, 99–131.

Schalley AV, Arimura A, Kastin AJ (1973): Hypothalamic regulatory hormones. *Science, 179*, 341–350.

Schally AV, Huang WY, Chang RCC, Arimura A, Redding TW, Millar RP, Hunkapiller MW, Hood LE (1980): Isolation and structure of prosomatostatin: a putative somatostatin precursor from pig hypothalamus. *Proc. Natl Acad. Sci. USA, 77*, 4489–4493.

Scharrer E, Scharrer B (1954): Hormones produced by neurosecretory cells. *Recent Prog. Hormone Res., 10*, 183–240.

Seybold V, Elde R (1982): Neurotensin immunoreactivity in the superficial laminae of the dorsal horn of the rat. I. Light microscopic studies of cell bodies and proximal dendrites. *J. Comp. Neurol., 205*, 89–100.

Schmitt FO, Dev P, Smith BH (1976): Electrotonic processing of information by brain cells. *Science, 193*, 114–120.

Silverman AJ, Zimmerman EA (1975): Ultrastructural immunocytochemical localization of neurophysin and vasopressin in the median eminence and posterior pituitary of the guinea pig. *Cell Tissue Res., 159,* 291–301.

Smith AD (1971) Summing up: some implications of the neuron as a secreting cell. *Trans. R. Soc. London, B261,* 423.

Somogyi P, Chubb IW, Smith AD (1975): A possible structural basis for the extracellular release of acetyl cholinesterase. *Proc. R. Soc. Britain, 191,* 271–283.

Sternberger, LA (1979): *Immunocytochemistry, 2nd Edition.* John Wiley and Sons, New York.

Sumal KK, Pickel VM, Miller RJ, Reis DJ (1982): Enkephalin-containing neurons in substantia gelatinosa of spinal trigeminal complex: ultrastructure and synaptic interaction with primary sensory afferents. *Brain Res., 248,* 223–236.

Takagi H, Somogyi P, Somogyi J, Smith AD (1983): Fine structural studies on a type of somatostatin-immunoreactive neuron and its synaptic connections in the rat neostriatum: a correlated light and electron microscopic study. *J. Comp. Neurol., 214,* 1–16.

Tsunoo A, Konishi S, Otsuka M (1982): Substance P as an excitatory transmitter of primary afferent neurons in guinea-pig sympathetic ganglia. *Neuroscience, 7,* 2025–2037.

Uhl GR, Kuhar MJ, Snyder SH (1977): Neurotensin: immunohistochemical localization in rat central nervous system. *Proc. Natl Acad. Sci. USA, 74,* 4059–4063.

Vale WW (1978): Distribution, metabolism and pharmacology of peptides. *Neurosci. Res. Program Bull., 16,* 521–534.

Van Leeuwen FW, Pool CW, Sluiter AA (1983): Enkephalin immunoreactivity in synaptoid elements on glial cells in the rat neural lobe. *Neuroscience, 8,* 229–241.

Vincent SR, Skirboll L, Hökfelt T, Johansson O, Lundberg JM, Elde RP, Terenius L, Kimmel J (1982): Coexistence of somatostatin- and avian pancreatic polypeptide (APP)-like immunoreactivity in some forebrain neurons. *Neuroscience, 7,* 439–446.

Von Euler US, Gaddum JM (1931): An unidentified depressor substance in certain tissue extracts. *J. Physiol. (London), 72,* 74–87.

Wasser M, Berod A, Sotelo C (1981): Dopaminergic dendrites in the pars reticulata of the rat substantia nigra and their striatal input. Combined immunocytochemical localization of tyrosine hydroxylase and anterograde degeneration. *Neuroscience, 6,* 2125–2139.

Wilson SP, Klein RL, Chang KJ, Gasparis MS, Viveros OH, Yang WH (1980): Are opioid peptides co-transmitters in noradrenergic vesicles of sympathetic nerves? *Nature (London), 288,* 707–709.

Woodhams PL, Roberts GW, Polak JM, Crow TJ (1983): Distribution of neuropeptides in the limbic system of the rat: the bed nucleus of the stria terminalis, septum, and preoptic area. *Neuroscience, 8,* 677–703.

Yallow RS (1978): Radioimmunoassay: a probe for the fine structure of biologic systems. *Science, 200,* 1236–1245.

Yamamoto K, Matsuyama T, Shiosaka S, Inagaski S, Senba E, Shimizu Y, Ishimoto I, Hayakawa T, Matsumoto M, Tohyama M (1983): Overall distribution of substance P-containing nerves in the wall of the cerebral arteries of the guinea pig and its origins. *J. Comp. Neurol., 215,* 421–426.

Zhu CG, Sandri C, Akert K (1981): Morphological identification of axo-axonic and dendro-dendritic synapses in the rat substantia gelatinosa. *Brain Res., 230,* 25–40.

CHAPTER III

Vasopressin, oxytocin and their related neurophysins*

MICHAEL V. SOFRONIEW

1. INTRODUCTION

1.1. HISTORICAL PERSPECTIVE

In 1895 Oliver and Schäfer first reported the presence of a powerful pressor substance in extracts of the posterior pituitary. Sixty years later, Du Vigneaud and co-workers (1953a,b) isolated and characterized the hormonal principles of the neurohypophysis as the octapeptides vasopressin and oxytocin, vasopressin being responsible for the pressor and antidiuretic, and oxytocin for the oxytocic activities of the gland. These were the first peptides isolated and characterized from neural tissue and their identification lent further credence to the concept of neurosecretion which had developed out of the morphological studies of the Scharrers and Bargmann in the 1930's and 1940's (Bargmann and Sharrer 1951). Our current understanding of posterior pituitary function dates back directly to this concept and in simple terms states that vasopressin and oxytocin are peptides produced by hypothalamic magnocellular neurons which send their processes to the neurohypophysis from which the peptides are released into the blood stream as hormones. Thus, the idea of a neuroendocrine or hormonal function has dominated concepts about these peptides for many years. The past decade has seen a tremendous explosion in the number of peptides identified as being contained within neurons and thought to be involved in neural functions, as described in other chapters in *This Volume*. A large number of these peptides are found simultaneously in several different systems both in the periphery and in the central nervous system (CNS). Particularly common combinations are the presence of the same peptides in the gut and in the CNS, or the presence of the same peptides in peripheral endocrine cells or neuroendocrine neurons and in central neurons. So too, vasopressin and oxytocin, the classical neuroendocrine peptides, have been found distributed throughout the mammalian CNS. This chapter reviews morphological studies on different types of neurons producing vasopressin and oxytocin, the distribution of vasopressin and oxytocin fibers in the mammalian CNS thought to derive from these neurons and will discuss a few functional possibilities.

*Grant support for part of this work was provided by NINCDS (NS06959).

Handbook of Chemical Neuroanatomy. Vol. 4: GABA and Neuropeptides in the CNS, Part I.
A. Björklund and T. Hökfelt, editors.
© Elsevier Science Publishers B.V., 1985.

1.2. BIOSYNTHESIS OF VASOPRESSIN, OXYTOCIN AND THEIR ASSOCIATED NEUROPHYSINS

Before examining the various morphological findings it is helpful to briefly consider the biosynthesis of these peptides. Vasopressin and oxytocin have long been known to have an association with a family of low molecular weight proteins also present in extracts of the neurohypophysis, the neurophysins, prompting speculation about the possibility of a common precursor (Pickering 1976). Gainer and co-workers (Gainer et al. 1977; Russell et al. 1980) succeeded in providing conclusive evidence that the neurophysins are portions of larger precursor proteins from which the peptides and the neurophysins are cleaved. Their findings indicated that there are separate precursors for vasopressin and its associated neurophysin and for oxytocin and its associated neurophysin. Recently, the amino acid sequences of the entire bovine precursors for vasopressin (Land et al. 1982) and oxytocin (Land et al. 1983) have been derived using cloned cDNA. They found that the vasopressin precursor contains one sequence of vasopressin, one sequence of vasopressin-associated neurophysin, and a 39-amino-acid glycoprotein, plus signal sequences. The precursor contains no sequence for oxytocin or any other known peptide. The oxytocin precursor is somewhat shorter, containing one sequence of oxytocin and one of oxytocin-associated neurophysin, plus signal sequences. It contains no sequence for vasopressin or any known peptide. These authors have gone on to demonstrate that the defect in the Brattleboro rat, which has long been known to have the genetic inability to produce vasopressin or its associated precursor (Valtin et al. 1974), is the result of a single base pair deletion in the sequence of the gene in the protein-coding region (Schmale and Richter 1984).

1.3. METHODS OF LOCALIZING VASOPRESSIN, OXYTOCIN OR NEUROPHYSIN

(a) Immunohistochemistry

The descriptions of vasopressin, oxytocin, and neurophysin distribution in the CNS presented in this report are based primarily on our findings using various adaptations of the immunoperoxidase procedure of Sternberger (1979). Where appropriate, the immunohistochemical findings of others will be included, compared or discussed. Detailed descriptions of the variations of the immunohistochemical procedure which we have employed, as well as of the production of the antisera used and of the procedures conducted to verify the specificity of the staining, have been presented previously (Sofroniew et al. 1978, 1979; Sofroniew 1983a; *Vol. 1, This Series, Ch. V*). The principles underlying immunohistochemistry, as well as basic descriptions of the procedures followed, are presented in *Volume 1* of This Series.

   With immunohistochemical staining, vasopressin and oxytocin can readily be distinguished from one another but the different neurophysins usually cannot, unless pretreated antisera against species-homologous neurophysins are used. In the following descriptions, the location of neurophysin is meant to imply the presence of either vasopressin or oxytocin and the relative proportions of vasopressin or oxytocin have been determined by staining specifically for these peptides. Since staining for neurophysin is for various reasons more intense than that for the peptides, it is particularly useful in screening studies or for preparation of survey photomicrographs.

(b) Radioimmunoassay

Radioimmunoassay provides a means of detection of vasopressin or oxytocin in homogenates of brain tissue. A number of studies have examined the distribution of vasopressin, oxytocin or neurophysin in the brains or spinal cords of normal rats (Dogterom et al. 1978a; Glick and Brownstein 1980; Hawthorn et al. 1980; Dorsa and Bottemiller 1982; Lang et al. 1982) and humans (Rossor et al. 1981; Jenkins et al. 1984) by radioimmunoassay of extracted tissue homogenates. Compared with immunohistochemistry, this type of determination allows a more quantitative comparison of different regions but does not allow differentiation of the structures containing the peptides. Thus the results obtained with the two procedures can be used to complement each other. In general, in normal animals, the results obtained with radioimmunoassay are very similar to those obtained with immunohistochemistry. Radioimmunoassay also provides the potential for quantitative comparison of peptide levels in the same region under differing experimental (Van Wimersma Greidanus et al. 1981) or pathological (Rossor et al. 1981) conditions. Where appropriate, results obtained with radioimmunoassay will be included, compared or discussed in the following descriptions.

2. DISTRIBUTION OF NEURONS PRODUCING VASOPRESSIN, OXYTOCIN AND NEUROPHYSIN

Using a histochemical stain commonly employed to identify secretory endocrine cells, Bargmann demonstrated in 1949 (Bargmann 1949) the neurosecretory nature of hypothalamic magnocellular neurons which were thought to project to the posterior pituitary gland. With the advent of immunohistochemical staining procedures, early studies on vasopressin or oxytocin concentrated on these magnocellular hypothalamic neurons. Subsequent immunohistochemical studies, in some cases using methodological or experimental manipulations, revealed a large number of additional parvocellular neurons immunoreactive for vasopressin and to a lesser degree for oxytocin in various sites throughout the brain. The distribution of vasopressin and oxytocin perikarya throughout the rat brain is presented in levels A 9.8–A 3.4, P 1.5–P 2.8 of the Atlas, and summarized in Figure 1 and in Table 1, which also gives the approximate size of the cells in different regions. Figures 2 and 3 compare the size and shape of vasopressin and oxytocin neurons found in various regions. The following description of the distribution of vasopressin and oxytocin neurons is thus, for the sake of clarity, divided into sections on magnocellular and parvocellular neurons. It should be noted that in some cases, such as the hypothalamic paraventricular nucleus or bed nucleus of the stria terminalis, the same nucleus will contain both magno- and parvocellular vasopressin and oxytocin neurons having completely different projections. Unless otherwise stated, all descriptions refer to findings obtained in rats. Some examples of comparative findings from other species will be discussed.

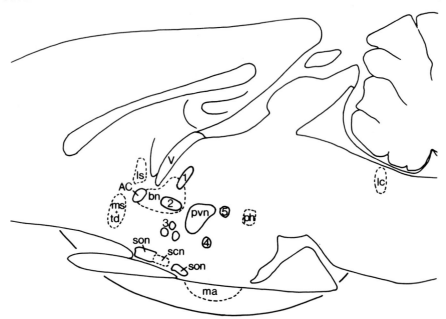

Fig. 1. Sagittal view of the rat brain depicting the approximate topography of the more prominent groups of vasopressin and oxytocin neurons. The numbers 1–5 refer to large groups of so-called accessory magnocellular neurons located outside of the supraoptic (son) and paraventricular (pvn) nuclei, for which there is no generally accepted nomenclature. Number 2 corresponds to the anterior commissural nucleus (acn). In addition, parvocellular vasopressin neurons are present in the regions depicted by dashed lines: bn, bed nucleus of the stria terminalis; lc, locus ceruleus; ls, lateral septum; ma, medial amygdala; ms, medial septum; ph, posterior hypothalamus; scn, suprachiasmatic nucleus; td, nucleus of the diagonal tract (Broca).

TABLE 1. *Mean diameter* of 25 neurons stained for vasopressin or oxytocin in various brain areas*

Area	Mean diameter (μm)	
	Vasopressin	Oxytocin
Septal region (n. septi medialis, n. tractus diagonalis Broca, n. septi lateralis)	16.6	
N. interstitialis stria terminalis	19.2	25.0
Preoptic area and anterior hypothalamus	24.9	24.9
N. suprachiasmaticus	13.7	
N. commissuralis anterior		21.8
N. supraopticus	25.8	25.1
N. paraventricularis pars magnocellularis	25.4	24.2
N. paraventricularis pars caudalis		18.9
Lateral hypothalamus	25.7	24.9
N. amygdaloidius medialis	18.9	
Posterior hypothalamus	17.4	
Locus ceruleus	19.8	

*Calculated from the mean cross-sectional area as measured with a semi-automatic image analysis apparatus.

⟶

Levels OB–SIII/IV. Schematic atlas of frontal sections through the rat brain and spinal cord depicting the distribution of vasopressin and oxytocin neurons and fibers at the various levels shown. The *numbers* of neurons per region per section are indicated by the sizes of the stars as indicated at the beginning of the atlas, and the *sizes* of the neurons in various regions are given in Table 1. The density of fibers in a region is given as either fibers of passage, single fibers or density of 1+ to 4+ using symbols as indicated at the beginning of the Figure. The relative differences between these gradations are shown in Figure 9, and the relative concentrations of vasopressin or oxytocin fibers in various regions are given in Table 2.

For abbreviations, see the General Abbreviations List, p. 609.

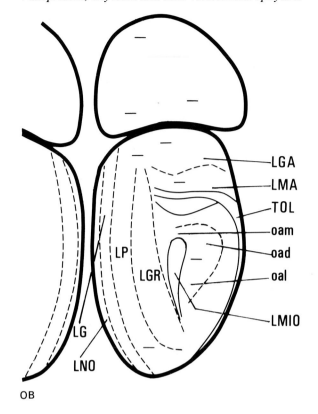

OB

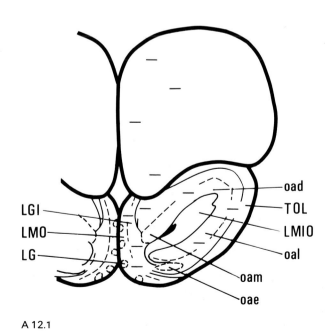

A 12.1

4 +

3 +

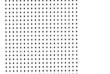

2 +

1 +

— single

axons

★	☆	> 20
★	☆	10 - 20
★	☆	3 - 10
★	☆	1 - 3
VP	OT	

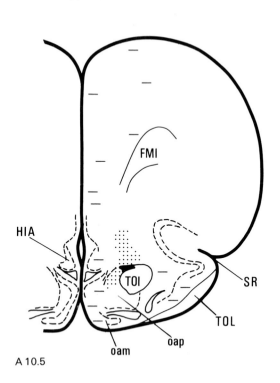

A 10.5

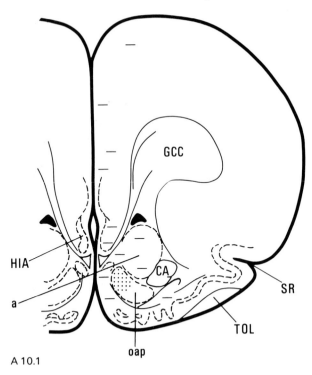

A 10.1

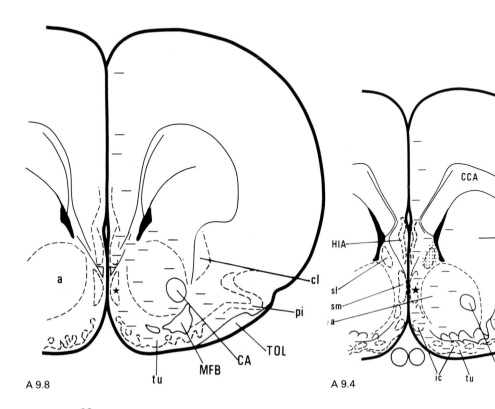

A 9.8

A 9.4

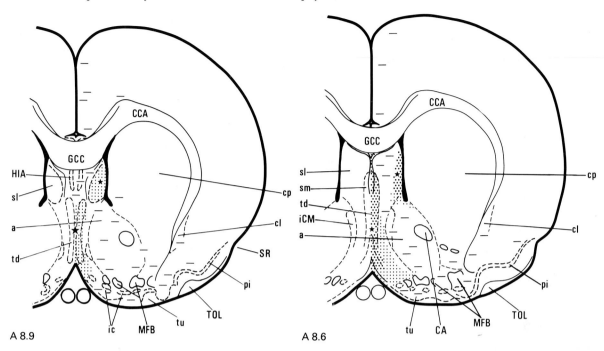

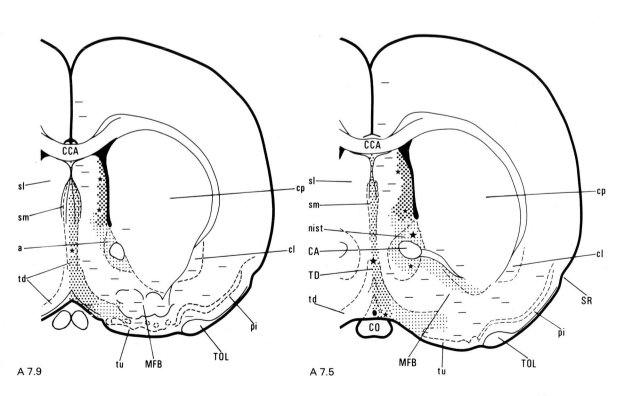

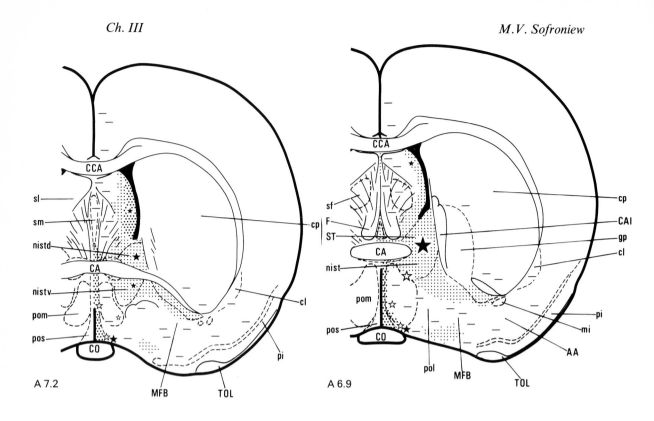

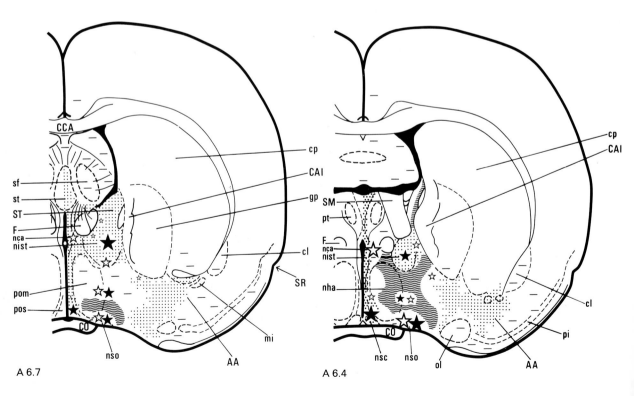

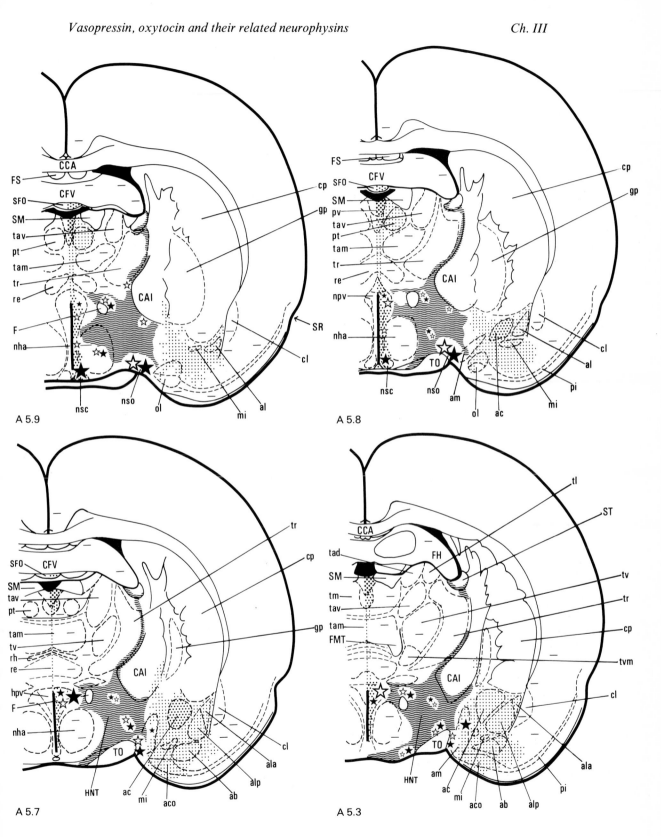

A 5.9

A 5.8

A 5.7

A 5.3

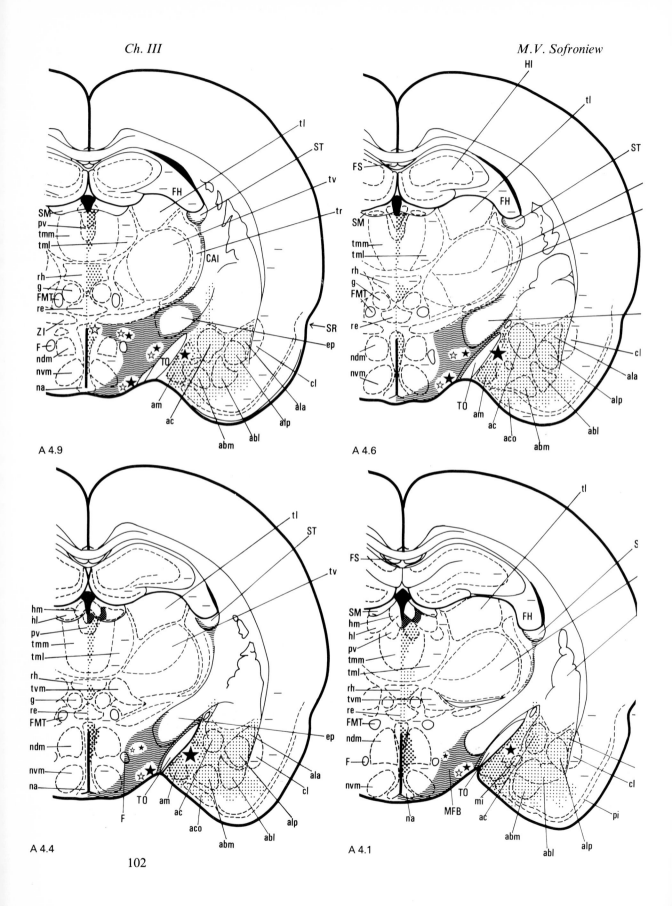

A 4.9

A 4.6

A 4.4

A 4.1

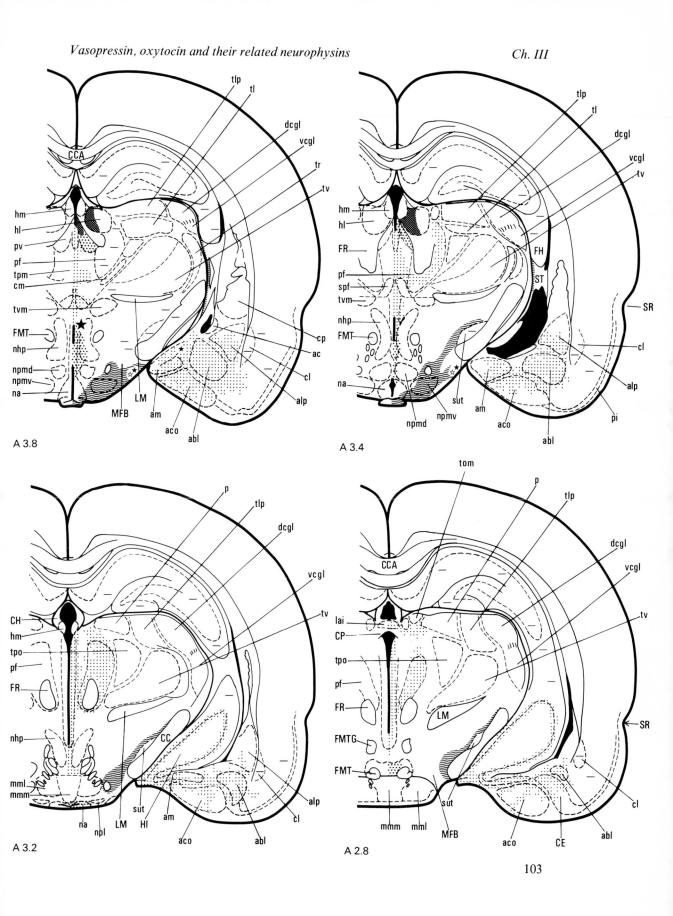

A 3.8

A 3.4

A 3.2

A 2.8

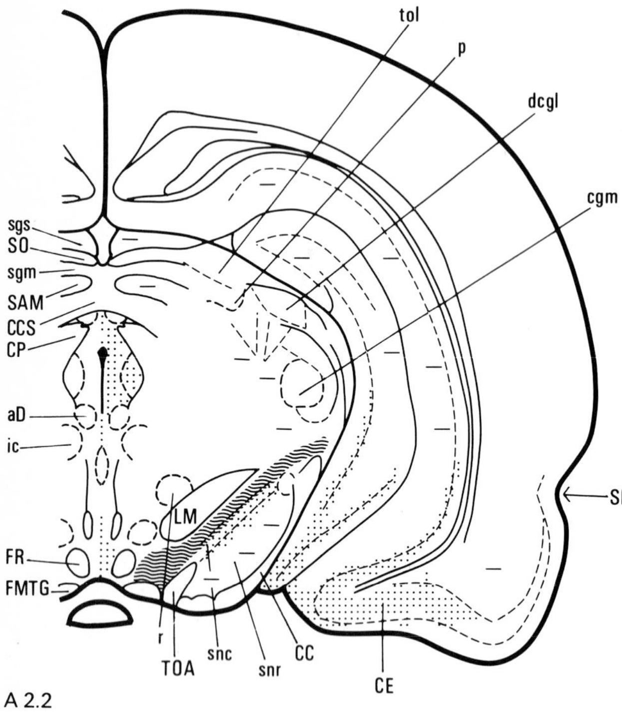

A 2.2

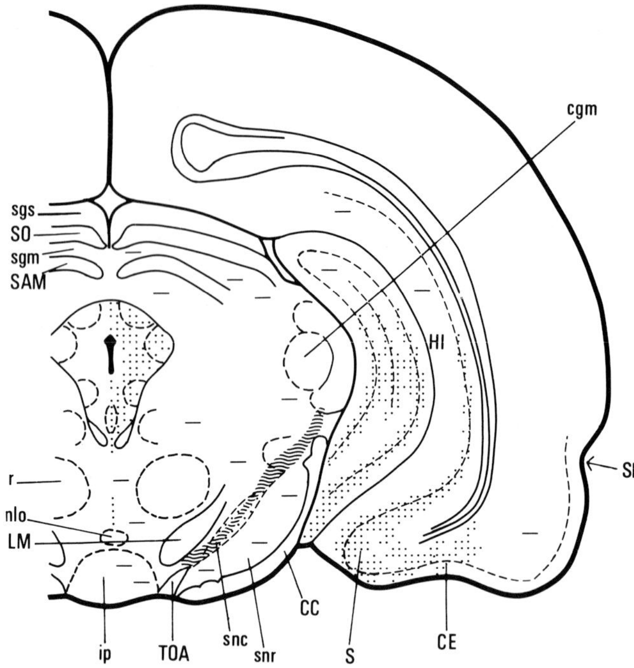

A 1.6

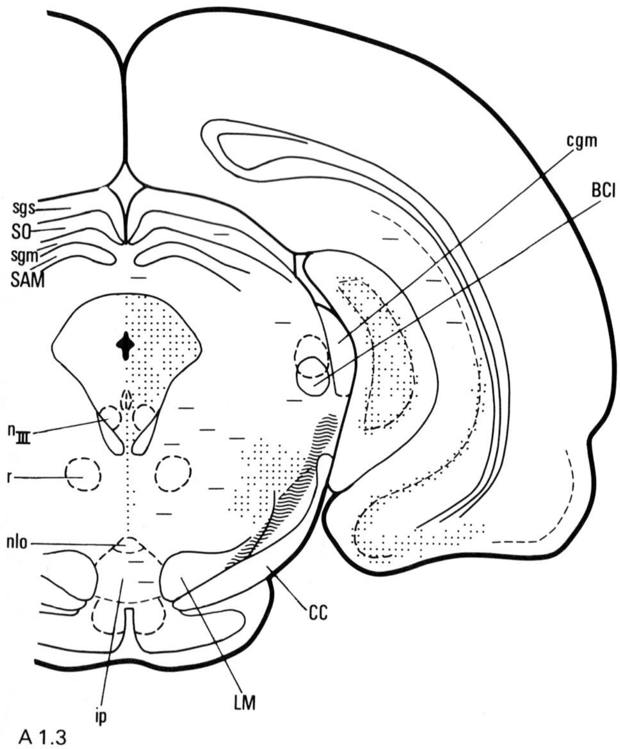

A 1.3

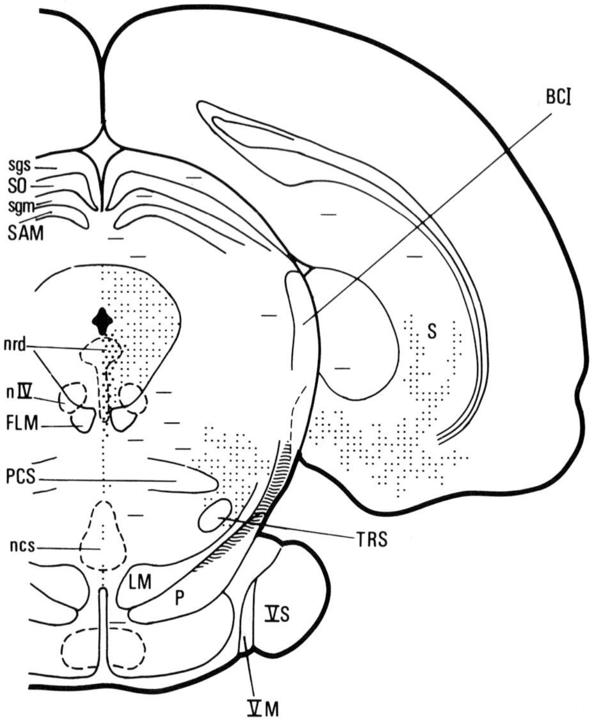

A 0.6

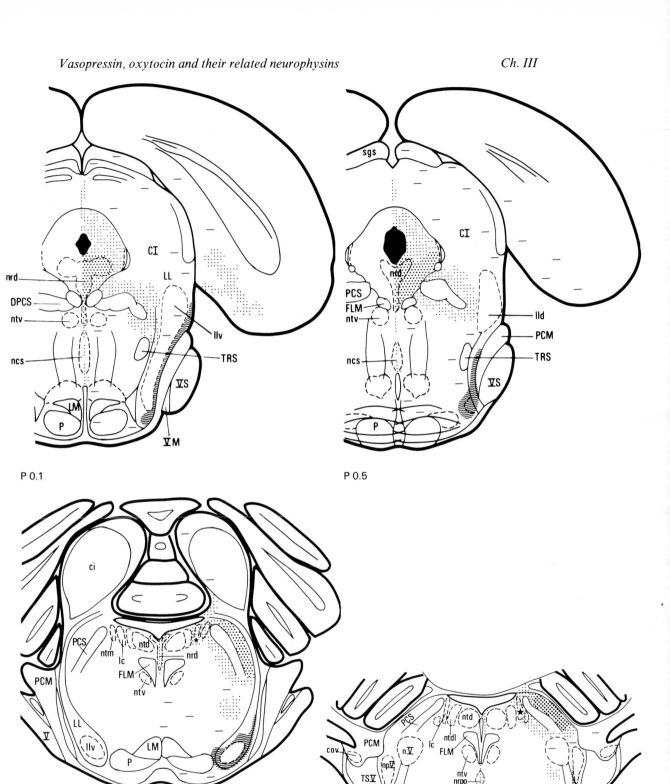

P 0.1

P 0.5

P 1.5

P 2.0

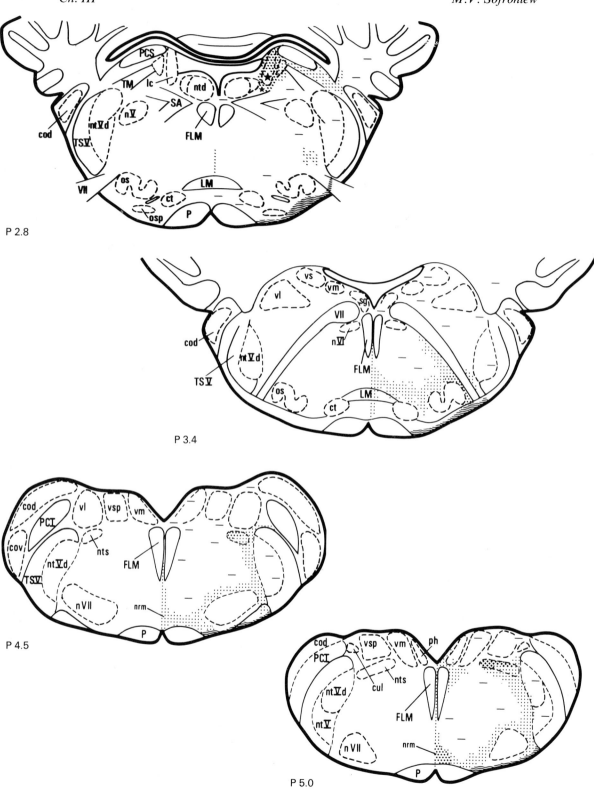

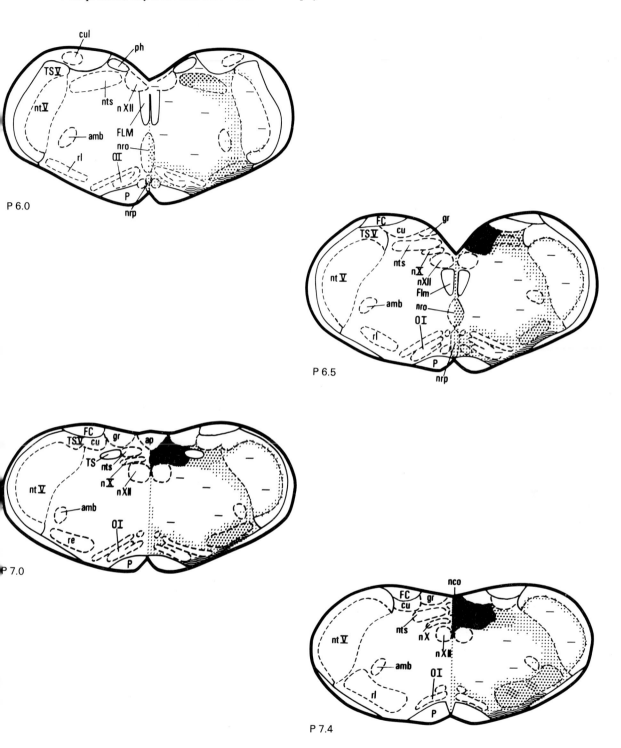

P 6.0

P 6.5

P 7.0

P 7.4

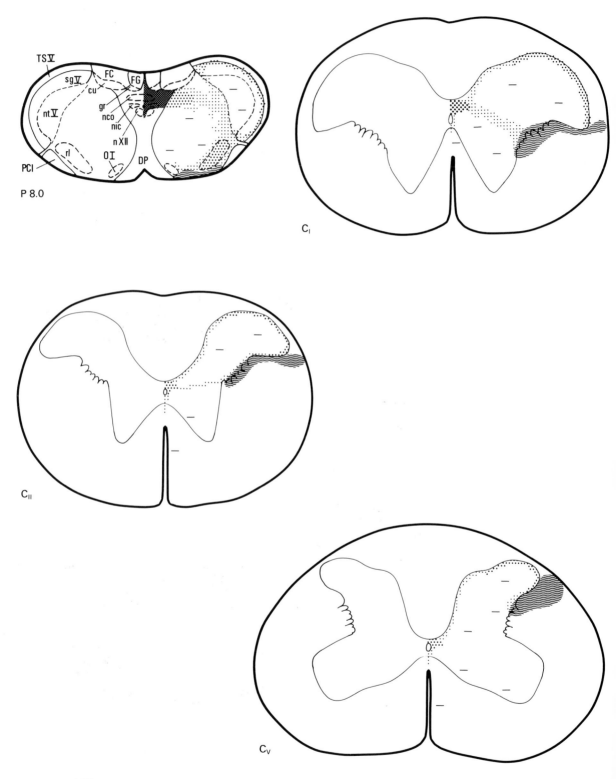

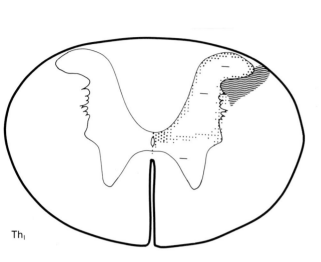

Th$_I$

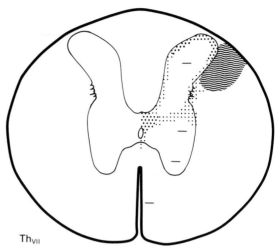

Th$_{VII}$

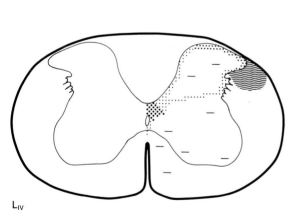

L$_{IV}$

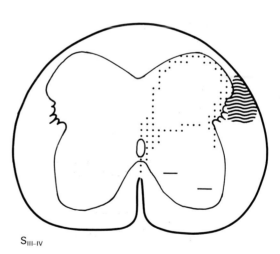

S$_{III-IV}$

2.1. HYPOTHALAMIC MAGNOCELLULAR NEURONS

Immunohistochemical studies have shown that oxytocin and vasopressin are produced in separate magnocellular hypothalamic neurons (Vandesande and Dierickx 1975; Aspeslagh et al. 1976; Van Leeuwen and Swaab 1977) together with their respective associated neurophysins (Vandesande et al. 1975a), in agreement with findings regarding the vasopressin and oxytocin precursors (see section 1.2.). Using an immunohistochemical procedure modified to achieve staining similar to Golgi impregnation, hypothalamic neurons stained for vasopressin, oxytocin or neurophysin exhibit a heterogeneous morphology which varies according to location within the hypothalamus (Sofroniew and Glasmann 1981). Most neurons are simple in appearance, with one or several sparsely branching dendrites and one unbranching axon (Figs 2, 3). The size and shape of perikarya varies considerably, with some being round or oval and some having an elongated spindle shape with short and long diameters of 10–35 μm. Some neurons appear to have 2 axon-like processes, while others have axons which give off short or long collateral branches (Sofroniew and Glasmann 1981; Mason et al. 1984). Some nuclei or groups consist of similarly appearing, others of differently shaped neurons. The paraventricular nucleus is particularly heterogeneous, consisting of a mixture of differently appearing magnocellular as well as parvocellular neurons which are in part intermingled and in

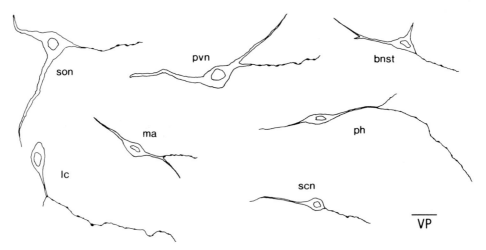

Fig. 2. Camera lucida drawings of representative vasopressin neurons from the various regions indicated, all drawn at the same magnification. For abbreviations, see Figure 1. Scale bar = 25 μm.

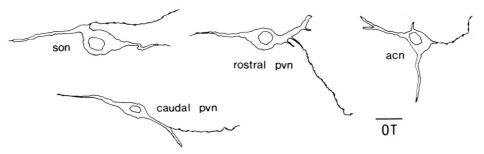

Fig. 3. Camera lucida drawings of representative oxytocin neurons from the various regions indicated, all drawn at the same magnification. For abbreviations, see Figure 1. Scale bar = 25 μm.

part segregated into groups within the nucleus. Another interesting observation is the presence of the peptides in long dendritic processes up to several hundred μm from the cell body (Sofroniew and Glasmann 1981).

Magnocellular vasopressin and oxytocin neurons are clustered in 2 main nuclei, the supraoptic and paraventricular nuclei, as well as in a number of large and small groups scattered throughout the hypothalamus and contiguous regions, the so-called accessory groups (Fig. 4). Although the supraoptic and paraventricular nucleus have traditionally been the focus of attention, the accessory groups contribute a substantial proportion of the vasopressin or oxytocin projections to the neurohypophysis, and are well represented in most mammals including the human.

(a) Supraoptic nucleus

The supraoptic nucleus of the rat consists of 2 main divisions, an anterior and posterior, separated by the optic tract. The posterior division is generally referred to as retrochiasmatic. The anterior division begins rostrally as a few neurons just above the optic chiasm, adjacent to the organum vasculosum of the lamina terminalis (OVLT) (Atlas, A 7.5). Moving caudally, this group swells into a prominent cluster of densely packed neurons abutting the lateral aspect of the optic tract (Figs 4a–e and Atlas, A 7.2–A 5.3). In this *anterior division,* there are roughly equal numbers of oxytocin and vasopressin neurons, with the oxytocin neurons being somewhat more concentrated dorsally, and the vasopressin neurons more ventrally (Swaab et al. 1975; Vandesande and Dierickx 1975; Rhodes et al. 1981). The *retrochiasmatic division* begins roughly where the 2 optic tracts have well separated (A 5.3), and consists of a thin band of neurons stretching from the inner aspect of the optic tract medially (Figs 4d–f). This thin band of cells extends caudally quite far and is still present in the form of a few individual neurons at the most caudal levels of the median eminence (Fig. 4 and Atlas, A 5.3–A 3.4). Although in rats of the Long-Evans strain this division is comprised mostly of vasopressin neurons (Rhodes et al. 1981), in Sprague-Dawley and Wistar rats we find only a slight predominance of vasopressin, with substantial numbers of oxytocin cells.

Most supraoptic nucleus neurons have large perikarya (mean diameter ca. 25 μm), with from 1 to 3 sparsely branching dendrites, which often extend to the ventral aspects of the nucleus and are often varicose in nature and stain intensely for peptide (Sofroniew and Glasmann 1981; Armstrong et al. 1982). Most supraoptic nucleus axons course medially towards the median eminence, and are rarely seen to branch (Sofroniew and Glasmann 1981; Armstrong et al. 1982). The efferent connections of the supraoptic nucleus are considered in more detail in Section 5.1. The afferent connections of the supraoptic nucleus have recently been reviewed in detail (Sawchenko and Swanson 1983; Swanson and Sawchenko 1983).

(b) Paraventricular nucleus

The paraventricular nucleus can, on the basis of cytoarchitectonics as well as other criteria, such as distribution of afferent connections, be divided into a number of subdivisions (Armstrong et al. 1980; Swanson and Kuypers 1980; Swanson and Sawchenko 1983). The relative distributions of magnocellular, as well as parvocellular, vasopressin and oxytocin neurons within these various subdivisions has been described (Sawchenko and Swanson 1982; Armstrong 1985). Here, the distribution of magnocellular neurons will be summarized, while that of parvocellular vasopressin and oxytocin neurons will be described in Section 2.2.d.

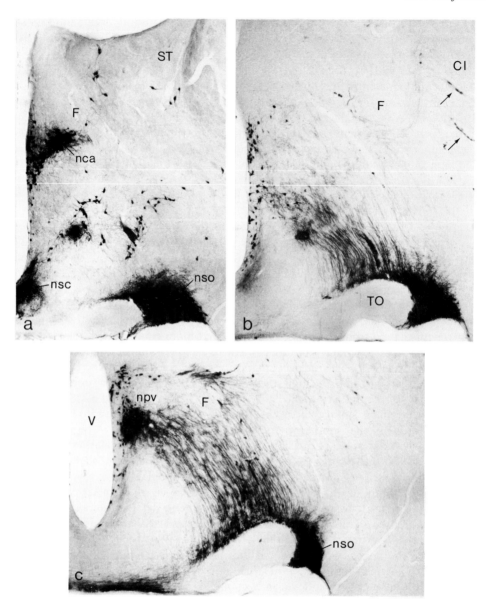

Fig. 4a–f. Series of frontal 100-μm sections stained for neurophysin through the hypothalamus of a normal rat. Magnocellular neurons are present in the supraoptic (nso), paraventricular (npv), and anterior commissural (nca) nuclei, as well as scattered singly or in groups throughout the hypothalamus and contiguous regions. Arrows in *b* indicate groups of magnocellular neurons abutting the internal capsule (CI). A prominent group of parvocellular neurons is present in the suprachiasmatic nucleus (nsc). F, fornix; TO, tractus opticus; V, third ventricle.

The magnocellular portion of the paraventricular nucleus begins in the anterior hypothalamus with a distinct cluster of oxytocin neurons lying near the dorsal aspect of the third ventricle (Fig. 4c and Atlas, A 5.8). There are a number of oxytocin neurons just medial to this cluster lining the wall of the ventricle (Fig. 4c). These neurons are continuous rostrally (Figs 4a–c and Atlas, A 5.9–A 6.4) with neurons in the 'anterior commissu-

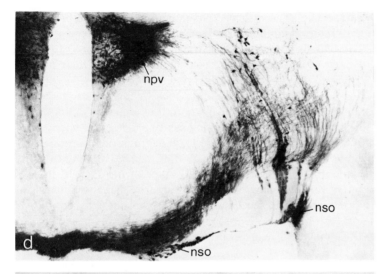

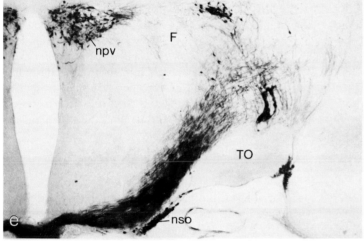

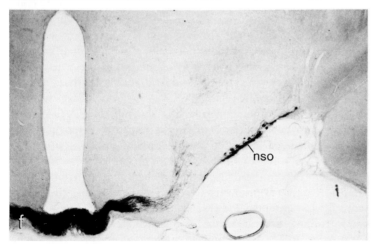

ral nucleus', a group of magnocellular accessory oxytocin neurons described below. Although the neurons in the anterior commissural nucleus have been included in the paraventricular nucleus complex by some authors (Swanson and Sawchenko 1983) we prefer not to since it is clearly separated from the rest of the paraventricular nucleus by a fairly substantial distance (Figs 4a–c and Atlas, A 6.4–A 5.8). Moving caudally from the initial cluster of oxytocin neurons (Fig. 4c and Atlas, A 5.8), the magnocellular portion of the paraventricular nucleus swells laterally until it assumes its characteristic triangular shape (Fig. 4d). At this point one can distinguish two masses of magnocellular neurons, dorsolaterally a cluster of primarily vasopressin neurons, and ventromedially a cluster of primarily oxytocin neurons (Fig. 4d and Atlas, A 5.7). Moving caudally from this point, without an abrupt change in the overall shape of the nucleus, there is a gradual change in the nature of the cells present from primarily magnocellular vasopressin to primarily parvocellular (or mediocellular) oxytocin neurons (Fig. 4e and Atlas, A 5.3–A 4.9). At the same time, the cells become somewhat more loosely packed (Fig. 4e). These parvocellular oxytocin neurons in the paraventricular nucleus are described below.

The morphology of paraventricular nucleus neurons has been studied by Golgi (Armstrong et al. 1980; Van den Pol 1982) and immunohistochemical (Sofroniew and Glasmann 1981) techniques. The magnocellular neurons have a mean cell diameter of about 25 μm and tend to have a simple morphology with few sparsely branching dendrites (Figs 2, 3). Long peptide-containing dendrites, as well as peptide-containing axon collaterals have been observed arising from these neurons (Sofroniew and Glasmann 1981). The efferent connections of these neurons will be considered in Section 5. The afferent connections have been recently examined in detail and are well reviewed (Silverman et al. 1981; Tribollet and Dreifuss 1981; Morris 1983; Sawchenko and Swanson 1983; Swanson and Sawchenko 1983).

(c)   Accessory magnocellular groups

Although it has long been recognized that a substantial proportion of the magnocellular secretory neurons lie outside of the supraoptic nucleus and paraventricular nucleus in various accessory groups (Peterson 1966; Palkovits et al. 1974), these groups have received relatively little attention. In the rat, as many as one-third of the hypothalamic magnocellular vasopressin and oxytocin neurons are located in these accessory groups (Rhodes et al. 1981; Armstrong 1985; personal observations). These neurons are scattered throughout the hypothalamus, often as loose collections of individual neurons, which in some cases form relatively distinct clusters. The location of these neurons is summarized in Figure 4 and in the Atlas, A 7.2–A 4.1. In the rat, major groups consist of: (1) scattered oxytocin neurons in the preoptic region (A 7.2–A 6.9); (2) a large cluster of oxytocin neurons posterior to the anterior commissure (Fig. 4a and Atlas, A 6.7–A 6.4) commonly referred to as the anterior commissural nucleus as named by Peterson (1966); (3) a band of primarily oxytocin neurons lining the ventricular wall in the anterior hypothalamus (Figs 4a–c and Atlas, A 6.4–A 5.8); (4) a number of mixed oxytocin and vasopressin groups and scattered neurons in the mid-portion of the anterior hypothalamus (Figs 4a,b and Atlas, A 6.7–A 5.8); (5) primarily oxytocin neurons along the medial border of the internal capsule and globus pallidus (Figs 4a–c and Atlas, A 6.4–A 5.8); (6) an anterior perifornical group (Fig. 4c and Atlas, A 5.8–A 5.7); (7) a posterior perifornical group (Fig. 4e and Atlas, A 5.3–A 4.9); and (8) numerous neurons in the lateral hypothalamus at somewhat more caudal levels (Figs 4d,e and Atlas, A 5.7–A 4.1).

The function of these dispersed groups is not clear. These neurons exhibit a very heterogeneous morphology, with considerable variation in perikaryal size and shape, in number and ramification of dendrites, and direction and collateralization of axons (Sofroniew and Glasmann 1981). Many of the neurons have long intensely stained peptide-containing dendrites (Sofroniew and Glasmann 1981). Although many of these neurons appear to project to the posterior pituitary others may project elsewhere (see section 4.). In addition, different groups may receive differing afferent input. One example of this may be that certain accessory neurons in the anterior hypothalamus are contacted by somatostatin fibers (Sofroniew and Schrell 1982), while cells in other regions are not. Thus, groups in different locations may release hormone in response to different stimuli.

2.2. PARVO- AND MEDIOCELLULAR NEURONS

Initially, immunohistochemical techniques were used to examine magnocellular hypothalamic vasopressin and oxytocin neurons and their neuroendocrine connections. It became apparent, however, that these peptides were present within neurons and pathways that had no obvious neuroendocrine functions. The initial observation of parvocellular vasopressin and oxytocin neurons was in some cases, such as the suprachiasmatic and paraventricular nuclei, made in untreated animals. In other cases, such as the bed nucleus of the stria terminalis and medial amygdala, colchicine treatment was required to convincingly demonstrate the parvocellular vasopressin neurons. Colchicine is an inhibitor of fast axonal transport (Dahlström 1968; Kreutzberg 1969), and is regularly used in immunohistochemical studies to intensify the staining of neural perikarya which under normal conditions stain only faintly or not at all (Ljungdahl et al. 1978). Lastly, several recent reports indicate that adrenalectomy allows the visualization of a group of parvocellular vasopressin neurons in the paraventricular nucleus (see below). A crucial consideration in assessing the validity of these immunohistochemical observations has been the ability to identify both the peptides vasopressin or oxytocin and their associated neurophysins within the neurons. This identification of 2 distinct portions of the precursor molecule (see 1.2.) strongly suggests production of the peptides by these neurons. In the following description, the distribution of parvocellular (and mediocellular) vasopressin and oxytocin neurons will be summarized, beginning rostrally according to nuclear area. Figures 2 and 3 compare the size and shape of neurons found in various regions.

(a) Septal region

A few scattered vasopressin neurons, from about 4–20 bilaterally per 50-μm section, can be seen in different parts of the septal complex, including the medial septum (Atlas, A 9.8–A 8.6), the lateral septum (A 8.9–A 6.9) and the vertical limb of the diagonal band of Broca (A 8.9–A 7.5) in colchicine-treated rats (Sofroniew 1983b; Van Leeuwen and Caffe 1983; Sofroniew 1985). These cells have a mean diameter of about 16.6 μm (Sofroniew 1985).

(b) Bed nucleus (n. interstitialis) of the stria terminalis

Large numbers of vasopressin neurons are present throughout this nucleus, particularly in its central portions (Figs 5, 6 and Atlas, A 7.5–A 6.4) (Sofroniew 1983b; Van Leeuwen and Caffe 1983; Sofroniew 1985). Although these neurons can sometimes be seen in nor-

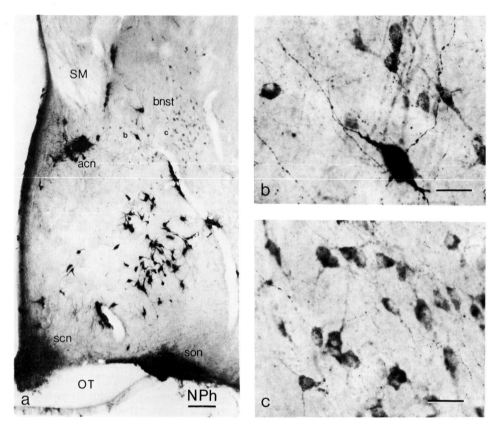

Fig. 5a–c. Frontal 50-μm section stained for neurophysin through the anterior hypothalamus of a rat treated with colchicine. *a.* Survey showing intensely stained masses of neurons in the supraoptic, suprachiasmatic and anterior commissural nuclei and internuclear region. A number of palely stained neurons are present in the bed nucleus of the stria terminalis. Scale bar = 250 μm. *b.* Detail of *a* comparing the size and staining intensity of a magnocellular hypothalamo-neurohypophyseal neuron in the bed nucleus with that of the smaller paler neurons seen as a result of colchicine treatment. Scale bar = 40 μm. *c.* Detail of *a* showing the appearance of neurons found in the bed nucleus following colchicine treatment. Scale bar = 40 μm.

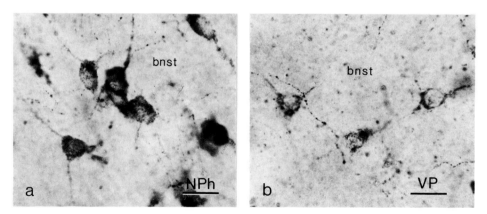

Fig. 6. Oil immersion photomicrographs comparing the appearance of neurons in the bed nucleus of the stria terminalis stained for (a) neurophysin, or (b) vasopressin, subsequent to colchicine treatment in the rat. Scale bars = 25 μm.

mal animals, they are best visualized following colchicine treatment. These cells have a mean diameter of about 19.2 μm (Sofroniew 1985).

(c) Suprachiasmatic nucleus

A dense cluster of vasopressin neurons is concentrated primarily dorsally and medially within this nucleus (Fig. 7), along its entire rostrocaudal extent (Atlas, A 6.7–A 5.8). These neurons are intensely immunoreactive, and can easily be seen in normal animals (Vandesande et al. 1975b; Sofroniew and Weindl 1978b; Van Leeuwen et al. 1978; Sofroniew and Weindl 1980; Van den Pol 1980). These cells have a mean diameter of about 13.7 μm (Sofroniew 1985), and comprise about 17% of the total population of suprachiasmatic nucleus neurons in the rat (Sofroniew and Weindl 1980).

(d) Hypothalamic paraventricular nucleus

In addition to the magnocellular vasopressin and oxytocin neurons described above, the paraventricular nucleus has distinct populations of parvocellular oxytocin and vasopressin neurons. The caudal portion of the nucleus (Fig. 4e) is comprised primarily of small to medium-sized oxytocin neurons (Fig. 3), with relatively few vasopressin neurons (Sofroniew and Schrell 1981; Sawchenko and Swanson 1982), which extend caudally from the main part of the nucleus for some distance (Atlas, A 5.3–A 4.9). These neurons, which are readily stainable in normal animals, have a mean diameter of 18.9 μm (Sofroniew 1985) and are intermingled with some magnocellular neurons (> 25 μm). Other parvocellular vasopressin or oxytocin neurons are scattered throughout the various parvocellular divisions of the paraventricular nucleus (Sawchenko and Swanson 1982). One cluster of parvocellular vasopressin neurons in the medial, central part of the nucleus (A 5.8–A 5.7) is of particular interest. These neurons generally do not stain positively for vasopressin in either normal or colchicine-treated rats, but become visible in adrenalectomized rats (Roth et al. 1982; Tramu et al. 1983; Sawchenko et al. 1984b). These same neurons contain CRF immunoreactivity (Roth et al. 1982; Tramu et al. 1983; Kiss et al. 1984; Sawchenko et al. 1984b), as discussed below.

(e) Posterior hypothalamus

A small group of vasopressin neurons lies clustered in the posterior hypothalamus adjacent to the dorsal aspect of the third ventricle (Atlas, A 3.8). This group has a very narrow rostrocaudal extent, and is generally only visible following colchicine treatment. These cells have a mean diameter of about 17.4 μm (Sofroniew 1985).

(f) Medial amygdala

Large numbers of vasopressin neurons are present in the dorsal portions of this nucleus (Fig. 8) along nearly all of its rostrocaudal extent (Atlas, A 5.7–A 3.8). Although some of these neurons can be seen in normal animals, they are best visualized following colchicine treatment. These cells have a mean diameter of about 18.9 μm (Sofroniew 1985).

(g) Locus ceruleus

A few vasopressin neurons, from 3–8 per 50-μm section can be found in the caudal, ven-

117

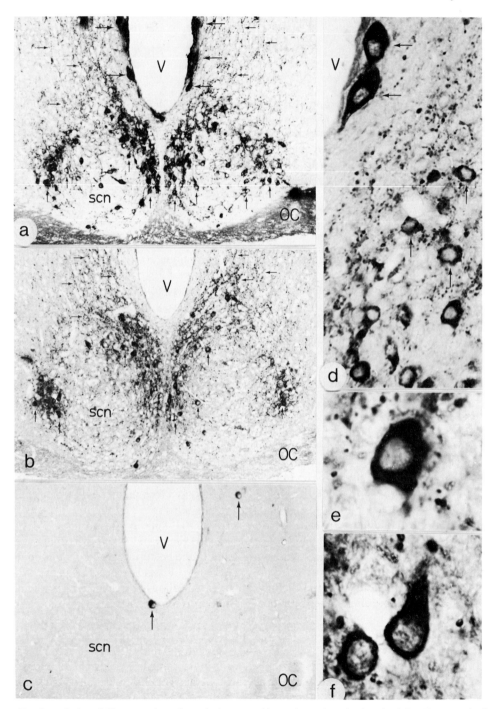

Fig. 7a–c. Series of 10-μm sections through the suprachiasmatic nucleus (scn) stained for (a) neurophysin, (b) vasopressin, and (c) oxytocin. Note that while parvocellular neurons in the scn stain positively for vasopressin and neurophysin, none stain for oxytocin. Arrows in *c* indicate magnocellular oxytocin-positive neurons. *d.* Comparison of parvocellular and magnocellular neurophysin-positive neurons. *e* and *f.* Details of neurophysin- and vasopressin-positive parvocellular neurons. (Reproduced from Sofroniew and Weindl (1978b), by courtesy of the Editors of the *American Journal of Anatomy.*)

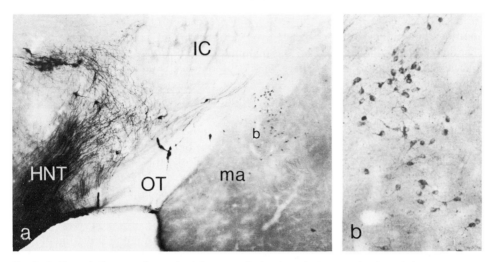

Fig. 8a,b. Frontal 50-μm section stained for neurophysin through the posterior hypothalamus and medial amygdala (ma) of a rat treated with colchicine. *a*. Survey showing the intensely stained magnocellular neurons in the lateral hypothalamus and region of the optic tract (OT), as well as fibers of the magnocellular hypotha-lamo-neurohypophyseal tract (HNT). In addition, numerous lightly stained neurons are visible in the dorsal ma. *b*. Detail of *a* showing the lightly stained neurophysin neurons in the dorsal ma. IC, internal capsule.

tral locus ceruleus and sub-ceruleus (Atlas, P 1.5–P 2.8) in colchicine-treated rats (Caffe and Van Leeuwen 1983; Sofroniew 1985). These cells have a mean diameter of 19.8 μm (Sofroniew 1985).

2.3. COMPARATIVE DIFFERENCES BETWEEN MAMMALIAN SPECIES

The proportion of vasopressin to oxytocin neurons present in the magnocellular su-praoptic nucleus and paraventricular nucleus shows considerable species variation amongst mammals. Regarding the supraoptic nucleus, although there are roughly equal numbers of vasopressin and oxytocin numbers in this nucleus in the rat, in most other mammals vasopressin neurons predominate substantially. These species include the hu-man (Dierickx and Vandesande 1977; Sofroniew et al. 1981), rhesus monkey (Sofroniew et al. 1981; Kawata and Sano 1982), cow (Vandesande et al. 1975a), cat (Reaves and Hayward 1979a), and guinea pig (Sofroniew et al. 1979). The location and structure of the supraoptic nucleus show relatively minor variations. In contrast, the paraventricular nucleus shows considerable species variation not only in the ratio of vasopressin to oxy-tocin neurons, but also in its basic structure and the topographic arrangement of vaso-pressin and oxytocin neurons within this structure. Thus, caution is advised when at-tempting to extrapolate the subdivisions of the paraventricular nucleus which have been well worked out in the rat to other species. The following reports examine the species indicated: human (Dierickx and Vandesande 1977), cow (Vandesande et al. 1975a), cat (Reaves and Hayward 1979a), guinea pig (Sofroniew et al. 1979).

Few studies have dealt with the distribution of vasopressin and oxytocin accessory magnocellular neurons in species other than the rat. In our experience, the exact location of these neurons can show considerable species variation. Nevertheless, such neurons are present in substantial numbers in all mammalian species we have examined, with surprising consistency as to the approximate location of some of the major groups. Even in primates such as the human and rhesus monkey such neurons constitute a major portion of the total population of magnocellular vasopressin and oxytocin neurons.

The suprachiasmatic nuclei of various mammals have been examined for the presence of parvocellular vasopressin neurons. Such neurons were found in all 13 mammalian species examined including the human (Sofroniew and Weindl 1980). In all species these neurons comprised only a portion of the total population of neurons, between 17% and 30% (Sofroniew and Weindl 1980).

Species other than the rat have not yet been examined for the presence of the other parvocellular vasopressin neurons described in various brain regions. Parvocellular oxytocin neurons comparable to those found in the caudal division of the rat paraventricular nucleus are also present in the caudal part of the paraventricular nucleus of the rhesus monkey and human (unpublished observation). It is interesting to note that determination of the vasopressin content of human locus ceruleus by radioimmunoassay yields a much higher content (Rossor et al. 1981) than would be suspected from the relatively sparse number of fibers present there. This and the occasional observation of neurophysin-positive neurons in routine human autopsy specimens of this region (Mai, Berger, Sofroniew, unpublished observation) strongly suggest that vasopressin neurons similar to those found here in the rat are present in the human as well.

2.4. CO-LOCALIZATION OF OTHER SUBSTANCES IN VASOPRESSIN OR OXYTOCIN NEURONS

The concept that neurons may produce and release more than one active agent is expanding in all areas of the peripheral and CNS (see Hökfelt et al. 1980; Chan-Palay and Palay 1984). Co-localization of several different types of neuroactive substances within different populations of vasopressin or oxytocin neurons have been described, including various peptides, amines, and transmitter synthesizing or degrading enzymes. Here brief summaries of several illustrative examples will be presented.

(a) Magnocellular supraoptic and paraventricular nucleus neurons

In addition to vasopressin or oxytocin and their respective neurophysins, all or some of these neurons have been reported to contain immunoreactivity for a large number of peptides and other substances including somatostatin (Dubois and Kolodziejczyk 1975), enkephalin (Sar et al. 1978), angiotensin II (Fuxe et al. 1976; Kilcoyne et al. 1980), renin (Fuxe et al. 1982), glucagon (Tager et al. 1980), CRF (Sawchenko et al. 1984a), cholecystokinin (CCK; Vanderhaeghen et al. 1980), dynorphin (Watson et al. 1982a), and tyrosine hydroxylase (Sofroniew et al. 1984a), as well as histochemical activity for acetylcholinesterase (Koelle 1961; Sofroniew et al. 1984). Although the immunohistochemical observation of co-localization forms a crucial link in the evidence favoring an example of production of more than one substance by the same neurons, it is by no means independently conclusive. Indeed, the large number of substances reported present in magnocellular vasopressin or oxytocin neurons would alone suggest a cautious approach. In some cases the immunohistochemical observations are supported by results obtained with several other techniques, in some cases such additional supporting evidence has not yet been provided, and one case (that of somatostatin) has already been shown to be artifactual. The evidence, both positive and negative, surrounding co-localization in these neurons has recently been reviewed (Sofroniew et al. 1984). In summary, there is substantial evidence that dynorphin is present in magnocellular vasopressin neurons (Watson et al. 1982a; Whitnall et al. 1983), and that both CCK (Beinfeld et al. 1980; Vanderhaeghen et al. 1981) and pro-enkephalin (the enkephalin precursor) (Rossier et al. 1979; Vanderhaeghen et al. 1983) are present in oxytocin neurons. This is not to say that none of the other cases is correct, simply that additional evidence will be required. One of the strong arguments in favor of the co-localization of dynorphin in vasopressin neurons is the persistence of dynorphin staining in the Brattleboro rat (Watson et al. 1982a). This rat has the genetic inability to produce vasopressin (Valtin et al. 1974) and the entire vasopressin precursor. Accordingly, no staining of vasopressin or its associated neurophysin is obtained in the 'vasopressin' neurons of these rats, although the neurons are still present (Sokol et al. 1976; Vandesande and Dierickx 1976). The sequences of the vasopressin (Land et al. 1982) and dynorphin (Kakidani et al. 1982) precursors are known, and neither precursor contains a sequence for the other peptide. Thus, the vasopressin neurons would have to make both precursors. This is in agreement with the Brattleboro rat findings, where the absence of the vasopressin precursor does not affect the staining for dynorphin. This same analogy can be used to test the validity of other examples of reported co-localization in magnocellular vasopressin neurons. The vasopressin precursor contains no sequence for any known peptide other than vasopressin except a carboxy terminal sequence (Land et al. 1982) of unknown function which can also be stained in vasopressin neurons (Watson et al. 1982b). Thus, any peptide truly co-localized in vasopressin neurons should still be stainable within these neurons in Brattleboro rats. If not, it is likely that a nonspecific cross-reaction with a portion of the vasopressin precursor is occurring, as has been documented in the case of somatostatin. Certain somatostatin antisera from various laboratories stain magnocellular vasopressin neurons, in normal but not in Brattleboro rats (see Sofroniew et al. 1984). As expected, this staining was shown to be due to cross-reaction with neurophysin (Dierickx and Vandesande 1979), a portion of the vasopressin precursor. Other cases in which staining is present in normal but not in Brattleboro rats are likewise suspect.

Of major importance when considering co-localization of different peptides within the same neurons, particularly peptides deriving from different precursors as do vasopressin and dynorphin, is whether or not the 2 peptides (and their precursors) are packaged into the same or different secretory granules. Recently, it has been shown that vasopressin and dynorphin are contained within the same granules in the posterior pituitary (Whitnall et al. 1983).

(b) Parvocellular paraventricular nucleus neurons

Vasopressin has long been under investigation as an important factor involved in the control of adenohypophyseal ACTH secretion, and the vasopressin neurons involved in this have been thought to derive from the hypothalamic paraventricular nucleus (see section 5.1.b). Thus, one of the more striking recent examples of co-localization has been the demonstration in several laboratories of CRF and vasopressin immunoreactivities in a subpopulation of parvocellular paraventricular nucleus neurons (Roth et al. 1982; Tramu et al. 1983; Kiss et al. 1984; Sawchenko et al. 1984b). These neurons are located in the medial paraventricular nucleus (see section 2.2.d), and the vasopressin in these neurons can only be immunohistochemically visualized in adrenalectomized animals. The functional implications of this particular example of co-localization are far-reaching. In view of the large amount of information already available on this particular system (see section 5.1.b), this also promises to be an important experimental model for study of the phenomenon of co-localization and the regulation of its expression under different physiological conditions.

(c) Locus ceruleus

The presence of vasopressin neurons in a portion of the locus ceruleus (see section 2.2.g) raises the possibility of co-localization with noradrenalin (Dahlström and Fuxe 1964) within these neurons. A preliminary report of direct immunohistochemical evidence for the co-localization of vasopressin and noradrenalin in certain locus ceruleus neurons has recently been presented (Caffe et al. 1983).

3. DISTRIBUTION OF FIBERS AND TERMINALS

Immunohistochemical techniques were initially applied to study neuroendocrine aspects of vasopressin and oxytocin neurons, confirming the classical pathway from these neurons to the capillaries of the posterior pituitary. During the course of such studies vasopressin, oxytocin and neurophysin fibers were found in areas not directly related to the neuroendocrine pathway, leading to the discovery of an extensive network of such fibers throughout the CNS. The original reports noting the presence of such fibers (Weindl and Sofroniew 1976; Swanson 1977; Buijs 1978; Buijs et al. 1978; Sofroniew and Weindl 1978a,b) have now been extensively confirmed and augmented by a number of reports from different laboratories (Swanson and McKellar 1979; Nilaver et al. 1980; Sofroniew 1980; Sofroniew and Weindl 1981; Petter and Sterba 1982; Phillipson and Gonzalez 1983). The following description of the distribution of vasopressin, oxytocin and neurophysin fibers and terminals in the CNS is based primarily on our own results and is presented according to nuclear areas organized approximately in rostrocaudal sequence. These results are basically in agreement with the findings of others as cited above. The topography of the cumulative distribution of both vasopressin and oxytocin fibers is presented in the Atlas in levels OB, A 12.1–A 0.6, P 0.1–P 8.0 and CI–SIII/IV, and the relative amounts of either vasopressin or oxytocin fibers in particular areas is given in Table 2. Figure 9 shows photomicrographs of the various densities of fibers corresponding to the gradations used in the Atlas.

3.1. FOREBRAIN

(a) Neocortex, claustrum and related areas

Vasopressin and oxytocin fibers have been found selectively in several distinct regions of the neocortex and related areas. These are: medial frontal cortex (Atlas, OB, A 12.1–A 9.8), cingulate cortex (A 9.4–A 5.7), lateral ventral cortical regions in the vicinity of the piriform cortex (A 9.8–A 3.2), and claustrum (A 9.4–A 2.8). The density of fibers in these areas is always light, consisting of single long traversing axons. However, these axons regularly gave rise to numerous short and long collaterals along their routes of passage (Fig. 10), so that the influence of these single axons should not be underestimated. Both oxytocin and vasopressin fibers have been observed. The origin of these fibers is unknown. The medial amygdala is known to project to the medial frontal cortex (Krettek and Price 1977), and this nucleus contains vasopressin neurons. A vasopressin-specific projection, however, remains to be demonstrated.

TABLE 2. *Relative distributions of vasopressin and oxytocin fibers in the rat brain and spinal cord*

Area	Vasopressin	Oxytocin
I. Forebrain		
Olfactory bulb and olfactory nuclei	·	·
Frontal cortex	·	·
N. accumbens	·	·
Claustrum	·	
N. medialis septi	+	·
N. tractus diagonalis Broca	+ +	·
N. lateralis septi	+ + +	·
Tuberculum olfactorium	·	·
N. interstitialis stria terminalis	+	·
Periventricular preoptic area and anterior hypothalamus	+ +	·
N. amygdaloidius anterior, basalis, corticalis and basolateralis	+	+
N. amygdaloidius centralis	+ +	+
N. amygdaloidius medialis	+ +	+
N. periventricularis thalami and mediodorsal thalamus	+ + +	·
Hippocampus	+	+
Entorhinal cortex	+	+
N. habenulae lateralis	+ + + +	
N. rhomboideus	+ +	·
N. medialis thalami pars medialis	+ +	·
N. medialis thalami pars lateralis	·	·
Posterior periventricular hypothalamus	+ + +	·
N. parafascicularis	+	+
N. supramamillaris	·	+
II. Brainstem		
Mesencephalic central gray	+	+
Superior colliculus	·	
Substantia nigra zona compacta	+	+
Substantia nigra zona reticularis	·	·
N. interpeduncularis	·	·
Lateral tegmental reticular formation	+	+
N. raphe dorsalis	+ +	+
Colliculus inferior	·	·
N. parabrachialis ventralis	+	+
N. parabrachialis dorsalis	+ +	+ + +
Locus ceruleus	+ +	+
N. raphe pontis	·	+
N. raphe magnus	+	+ +
N. raphe obscurus	+	+ +
N. tractus solitarius	+ +	+ + + +
N. dorsalis nervi vagi	+ +	+ + + +
N. reticularis lateralis	+	+ +
Substantia gelatinosa trigemini	+	+ +
N. tractus spinalis nervi trigemini	·	·
III. Spinal cord		
Lamina I and II	+	+ +
Lamina III–IX	·	·
Lamina X	+	+ + +
N. intermediolateralis	+	+ +

+, −, + + + + Density 1 + to 4 + of fibers and/or terminals as indicated in Figure 9 and shown in the Atlas sections.

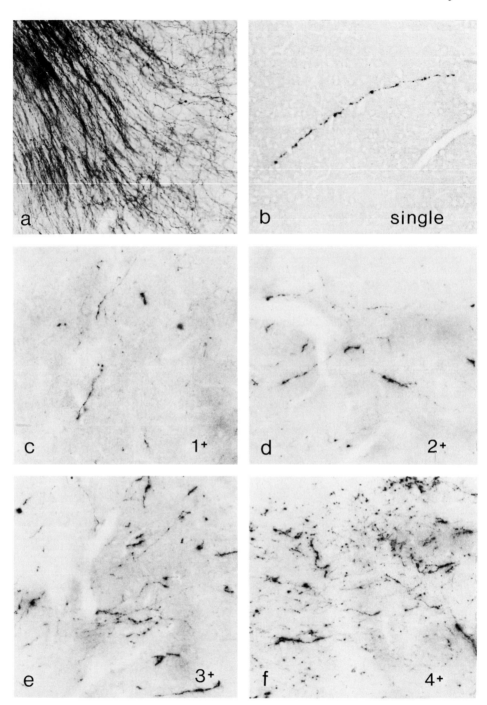

Fig. 9. Comparison of the densities of neurophysin fibers in various regions corresponding to the gradations of density used in Atlas levels OB–SIII/IV. *a.* Fibers of passage in the hypothalamo-neurohypophyseal tract as in level A 5.3. *b.* Single fiber in the frontal cortex as in level A 9.8. *c.* 1+ density of fibers in the brain stem reticular formation as in level P 3.4. *d.* 2+ density of fibers in the locus ceruleus as in level P 2.8. *e.* 3+ density of fibers in the dorsal parabrachial nucleus as in level P 2.0. *f.* 4+ density of fibers in the nucleus tractus solitarius as in level P 7.0.

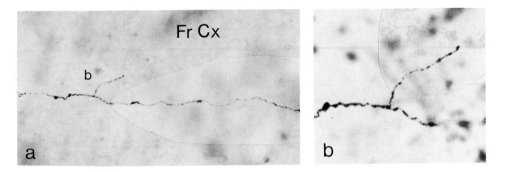

Fig. 10a,b. Survey and detail photomontages of a long single neurophysin fiber which gives off a short collateral in the medial frontal cortex (Fr Cx) of a rat at about the level shown in A 9.8.

(b) Olfactory bulb, olfactory nuclei and olfactory tubercle

Single scattered vasopressin and oxytocin fibers are regularly present in the olfactory bulb (Atlas, OB), in the various divisions of the anterior olfactory nucleus (OB–A 10.1) and in parts of the olfactory tubercle including the islands of Calleja (A 10.1–A 7.5). Except for occasional clusters of fibers (A 10.1), these are generally single axons similar to those seen in the neocortex which give rise to numerous collaterals regularly along their paths. Their origin is unknown.

(c) Septal region

The septal region contains a high density of vasopressin fibers in several of its regions, and some scattered oxytocin fibers as well. In particular, the lateral septal nucleus has a very high density of vasopressin fibers (Fig. 11a and Atlas, A 9.4–A 6.9), and the medial septum and nucleus of the diagonal band (tract) of Broca (both vertical and horizontal limbs) contain a moderate density of vasopressin fibers (A 9.8–A 7.2). The fibers in the lateral septum are continuous with vasopressin fibers in the bed nucleus of the stria terminalis which also contains a moderate density of vasopressin fibers (A 7.5–A 6.4). Single vasopressin fibers are scattered throughout the other parts of the septal region, as are oxytocin fibers. The density of vasopressin fibers in the lateral septum shows a sexual dimorphism. The density is greater in males than in females (De Vries et al. 1981), and is directly related to the levels of circulating androgens such that castration reduces fiber density and steroid substitution restores it (De Vries et al. 1983, 1984). A large portion of the vasopressin fibers in the lateral septum appear to derive from parvocellular vasopressin neurons in the bed nucleus of the stria terminalis (see section 5.). The origin of the other fibers in the region is not clear, although there are scattered vasopressin neurons throughout the area which might give rise to local projections.

(d) Preoptic area and hypothalamus

Continuous rostrally with the fibers in the nucleus of the diagonal band, is a fairly dense band of primarily vasopressin fibers which lines the walls of the third ventricle (Fig. 12) from the level of the lamina terminalis through the posterior hypothalamus and to the central gray of the midbrain (Atlas, A 7.5–A 1.6). This band of fibers is continuous with

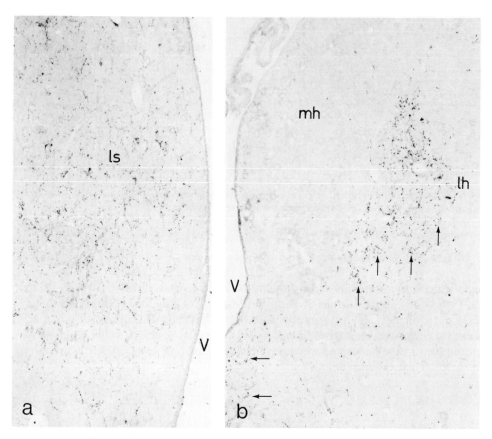

Fig. 11. a. Frontal 10-µm section stained for neurophysin through the lateral septum (ls) of a male rat at about the level shown in A 7.5. *b.* Frontal 10-µm section stained for neurophysin through the lateral habenula (lh) of a male rat at about the level shown in A 3.8. Note the dense clusters of neurophysin fibers. (Reproduced from Sofroniew and Weindl (1978b), by courtesy of the Editors of the *American Journal of Anatomy*.)

vasopressin fibers which ascend to the thalamus at rostral diencephalic levels (Fig. 12 and Atlas, A 6.4–A 5.8). In the posterior hypothalamus at the level of the dorsomedial nucleus, the density of these vasopressin fibers increases markedly and expands into a distinct periventricular cluster suggesting a terminal field (A 4.4–A 3.8). More caudally, there are distinct clusters of intermingled oxytocin and vasopressin fibers in the supramammary region (A 3.2–A 2.8).

In addition, the fibers of the classical hypothalamo-neurohypophyseal tract traverse the hypothalamus from the magnocellular vasopressin and oxytocin neurons to the posterior pituitary (Fig. 4 and Atlas, A 6.7–A 3.4). Some fibers leave this tract to travel dorsally towards the stria terminalis (Fig. 4b).

(e) Thalamus

A dense band of primarily vasopressin fibers ascends into the rostral thalamus from the hypothalamus along the borders of the third ventricle (Fig. 12) and just caudal to this (Atlas, A 6.7–A 5.8). Rostrally, these vasopressin fibers distribute primarily to the mediodorsal thalamus, showing a moderate to heavy density in the periventricular nucleus,

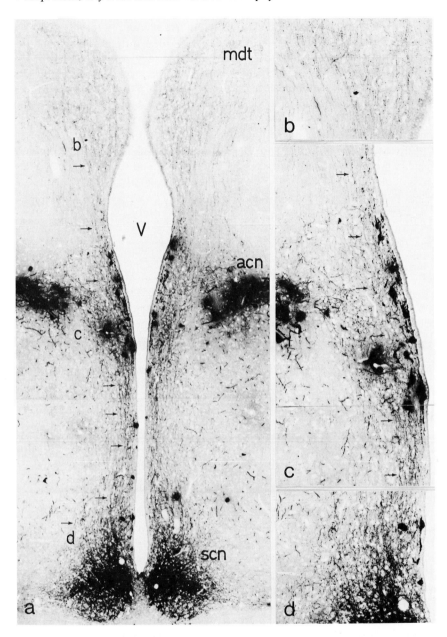

Fig. 12a–d. Survey and details of a frontal 10-μm section stained for neurophysin through the rat diencephalon at about the levels shown in A 6.7–A 6.4. Neurophysin fibers can be traced from the suprachiasmatic nucleus (scn) (arrows) dorsally along the border of the third ventricle (V) to the medial dorsal thalamus (mdt). anc, anterior commissural nucleus. (Reproduced from Sofroniew and Weindl (1981), by courtesy of the Publisher.)

somewhat less in the rostral paratenial nucleus, and scattered fibers in various other regions (A 5.9–A 5.3). These fibers probably derive from the parvocellular vasopressin neurons in the suprachiasmatic nucleus, as suggested by lesion studies and HRP transport (see section 5.2.b). More caudally in the thalamus, vasopressin fibers form clusters in the rhomboid nucleus and other midline regions, and are regularly present in low to moderate density in the centrolateral, parafascicular and other intralaminar nuclei (A 4.9–A 2.8). The origin of these fibers is not certain, although they may also derive from the suprachiasmatic nucleus. Dense clusters of vasopressin fibers are also present in the medial portions of the lateral habenula (Fig. 11b and Atlas, A 4.4–A 3.4). In addition to vasopressin fibers, scattered single oxytocin fibers are present in various regions of the thalamus.

As mentioned above, numerous single axons leave the traditional hypothalamo-neurohypophyseal tract to ascend along the border between the thalamic reticular nucleus and the internal capsule towards the stria terminalis (Fig. 4b and Atlas, A 6.4–A 5.7). Many of these axons appear to enter and retrogradely traverse the stria terminalis (A 5.7–A 3.4). Their destination is not established, but they may be moving from the hypothalamus to the amygdala.

(f) Amygdala

The amygdala contains a widespread distribution of both vasopressin and oxytocin fibers over most of its rostrocaudal extent, ranging in density from low (i.e. single fibers) to fairly heavy in different regions (Atlas, A 6.7–A 2.8). Higher densities of fibers are found in parts of the central nucleus which contains both vasopressin and oxytocin fibers (A 5.7, A 5.8) and most of the medial nucleus which contains primarily vasopressin fibers (A 4.9–A 4.1). The origin of these fibers is not known, although the medial nucleus contains a large number of parvocellular vasopressin neurons which may give rise to local terminals.

(g) Hippocampus and entorhinal cortex

There appear to be 2 pathways by which vasopressin and oxytocin fibers enter the hippocampus, a dorsal and a ventral. Dorsally, fibers pass from the septal region, particularly in the midline, into the fimbria and on to the dorsal hippocampus (Atlas, A 6.9–A 4.6). Ventrally, fibers enter the ventral hippocampus from the rostrally continuous amygdala (A 3.8–A 1.6). The origin of these fibers is not known. The density of fibers is much greater in the ventral part of the hippocampus, although scattered single fibers are present throughout (A 4.6–A 0.6). In contrast to early reports describing only vasopressin fibers (Buijs 1978; Sofroniew 1980), we now find both vasopressin and oxytocin (Fig. 13) fibers in the hippocampus, in similar distributions. The validity of the staining for oxytocin is supported by its presence in Brattleboro rats (Fig. 13a) which are genetically unable to produce vasopressin. Figure 14 shows the distribution of oxytocin fibers in the ventral hippocampus; the fiber density is greatest in the dentate gyrus, but numerous fibers are present in CA1–CA3 as well. Generally, the fibers are close to, and occasionally enter, the pyramidal cell layer (Fig. 13). The distribution of vasopressin is similar. Figure 14 also shows that numerous fibers are present in the subiculum and adjoining entorhinal cortex.

(h) Organum vasculosum of the lamina terminalis (OVLT) and subfornical organ (SFO)

There are numerous vasopressin fibers passing close to or through the *OVLT*, but it is not certain whether these fibers actually make contact with the fenestrated capillaries here. Most of these fibers appear to be of hypothalamic origin as discussed in greater

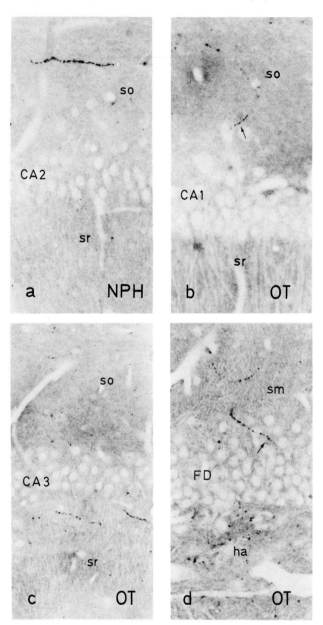

Fig. 13a–d. Horizontal sections stained for (a) neurophysin and (b–d) oxytocin through the ventral hippocampus. *a.* CA2 region of a Brattleboro rat. *b–d.* CA1, CA3, and fascia dentata (FD) regions of a normal rat. ha, hilar area; sm, stratum moleculare; so, stratum oriens; sr, stratum radiatum.

detail in Section 5.1.c. As described above, a number of vasopressin and oxytocin fibers ascend through the septal region, particularly in the midline, to eventually join the fimbria and enter the hippocampus. A number of these fibers, however, ascend through the caudal midline septal region to enter the *SFO* (Atlas, A 6.9–A 5.7) where numerous vasopressin and oxytocin fibers are present around the fenestrated capillaries. The exact origin of these fibers is uncertain, but they may derive from the hypothalamus (see

129

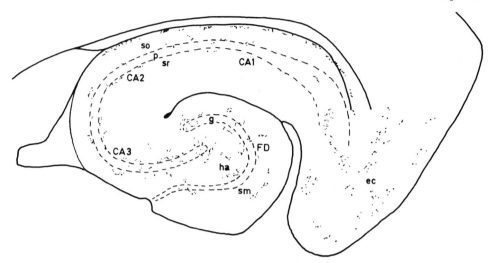

Fig. 14. Camera lucida drawing of a horizontal section through the ventral hippocampus of a normal Sprague-Dawley rat, depicting the location of immunoreactive oxytocin fibers (dots). ec, entorhinal cortex; FD, fascia dentata; g, granule cell layer; ha, hilar area; P, pyramidal cell layer; sm, stratum moleculare; so, stratum oriens; sr, stratum radiatum.

section 5.1.c). Although the SFO has been implicated in regulation of thirst mechanisms, levels of vasopressin in the SFO do not change with the state of hydration (Summy-Long et al. 1984).

(i) Other forebrain areas

The *nucleus accumbens* contains numerous scattered single fibers, both vasopressin and oxytocin, throughout its extent (Atlas, A 10.1–A 7.9). These single fibers often branch and give off collaterals as described above for fibers in the cortex. Occasional fibers, far fewer in number, are also present in the *striatum* (caudate putamen) at various levels. These are generally scattered single fibers which are usually but not always in the ventral portions (A 9.8–A 5.9). Single vasopressin and oxytocin fibers were also regularly present in parts of what constitute the *ventral pallidum, substantia innominata* and *basal nucleus of Meynert* in the rat (A 8.6–A 4.6), the latter of these as defined by the location of magnocellular cholinergic perikarya (Sofroniew et al. 1985). Fibers were more numerous in the rostral parts of the basal nucleus ventral and medial to the anterior commissure (A 7.9–7.2), in the mid-portion of the substantia innominata and ventral pallidum (A 6.7–A 5.9) and in the ventral parts of the caudal basal nucleus (A 5.7–A 4.4).

3.2. BRAINSTEM

(a) Tegmentum and colliculi

Oxytocin and vasopressin fibers descending from the hypothalamus into the brainstem enter the ventral tegmentum by passing from the caudal part of the hypothalamo-neurohypophyseal tract lateral to the fornix and moving laterally and caudally towards the crus cerebri (Atlas, A 3.8–A 3.2). Here the fibers distribute in a thin band just dorsal to and sometimes within the pars compacta of the substantia nigra (A 2.8–A 1.3). Many fibers intermingle with pars compacta neurons, and some fibers pass into the pars reticulata. This same thin band of descending fibers then continues through the entire extent of the brainstem in generally the same lateral ventral location (A 1.3–P 8.0). Numerous single vasopressin and oxytocin fibers in about equal numbers are present in the lateral tegmental reticular formation, particularly in the vicinity of the superior cerebellar peduncle (A 1.3–P 0.1). This region has been referred to as the pedunculopontine tegmental nucleus (Paxinos and Watson 1982). The fibers in this region are continuous with those in the dorsal and ventral parabrachial nuclei (P 0.1–P 2.8). Throughout the tegmentum, scattered single oxytocin and vasopressin fibers are present in the midline, and some fibers enter the interpeduncular nucleus (A 2.2–P 0.5). Other scattered single fibers are present medial to the geniculate nuclei and are scattered throughout the superior and inferior colliculi (A 2.2–P 1.5).

(b) Central gray

Vasopressin and oxytocin fibers enter the mesencephalic central gray via 2 pathways. One is from rostrally and consists of fibers descending along the third ventricle as it narrows to become the cerebral aqueduct (Atlas, A 2.8–A 1.6), and the other is from ventrolaterally and consists of fibers passing from the main ventral bundle of descending fibers described above (A 1.3–P 0.1). Within the mesencephalic central gray, single vasopressin and oxytocin fibers are distributed throughout in roughly equal numbers, with a somewhat higher density ventrally (A 2.2–P 0.5). These fibers are continuous caudally with single fibers in the pontine central gray, which are present only in the midline and are in turn continuous with fibers in the central gray of the medulla and these with fibers in the central gray (lamina X) of the spinal cord (P 1.5–P 8.0).

(c) Raphe nuclei

Virtually all the raphe nuclei contain both vasopressin and oxytocin fibers. The nucleus *raphe dorsalis* (Atlas, A 0.6–P 1.5) contains the highest density, but a number of fibers are also present in the nuclei *raphe pontis* (P 2.0), *raphe magnus* (P 4.5–P 5.0), *raphe obscurus* (Fig. 15 and Atlas, P 6.0–P 6.5), and *raphe pallidus* (P 6.0–P 6.5). The vasopressin and oxytocin fibers are present in about equal numbers in the dorsal raphe nucleus, with a preponderance of oxytocin fibers in the others.

(d) Parabrachial region and locus ceruleus

Oxytocin and vasopressin fibers in the parabrachial region are continuous rostrally with fibers in the lateral tegmental reticular formation (or pedunculopontine tegmental nucleus) as described above. In the parabrachial region, the fibers distribute into both the dorsal and ventral parabrachial nuclei, with a greater density of fibers in the dorsal nucleus (Atlas, P 1.5–P 2.8). Oxytocin fibers clearly predominate over vasopressin in both parabrachial nuclei. The exact origin of these fibers is not known although it is likely that some are of hypothalamic origin. Medially, these fibers are continuous with fibers in the locus ceruleus and surrounding area (P 1.5–P 2.8). Here vasopressin and oxytocin fibers are present in about equal numbers, with perhaps a slight dominance of vasopressin fibers. The exact origin of these fibers is not known, although some may derive from local neurons.

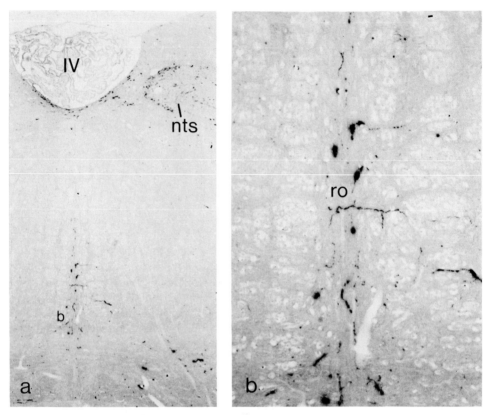

Fig. 15. a. Survey of a frontal 10-μm section stained for neurophysin through the brainstem of a rat. At this level there are prominent clusters of fibers in the nucleus of the solitary tracts (nts), central gray beneath the 4th ventricle (IV) and in the nucleus raphe obscurus (ro). *b.* Detail of *a* showing the fibers in the ro.

(e) Nucleus tractus solitarius and dorsal vagal nucleus

Both oxytocin and vasopressin fibers (Figs 16–18) are present throughout the entire solitary nucleus/dorsal vagal complex, but oxytocin fibers predominate in a ratio of 2:1 or more. The fibers are present through the entire rostrocaudal extent of the solitary nucleus/dorsal vagal complex (Atlas, P 4.5–P 8.0). Rostrally, the fibers are somewhat more dense medially in the complex (Fig. 16 and Atlas, P 4.5–P 6.5), and the greatest density is at the level of the area postrema and just caudal to this (P 7.0–P 8.0). Fibers enter the complex primarily from ventrolaterally, passing from the ventral band of descending fibers described above. These fibers pass through a large part of the lateral reticular formation and some fibers appear to give off collaterals while doing so.

(f) Lateral reticular nucleus

This nucleus, which lies in the ventrolateral part of the medulla oblongata, contains a fairly high density of oxytocin and vasopressin fibers. As in the solitary nucleus/dorsal vagal complex, oxytocin fibers predominate in a ratio of about 2:1. Fibers are present throughout the nucleus (Atlas, P 6.0–P 8.0), generally in a fairly even distribution, with occasional clusters of densely packed fibers (P 7.4).

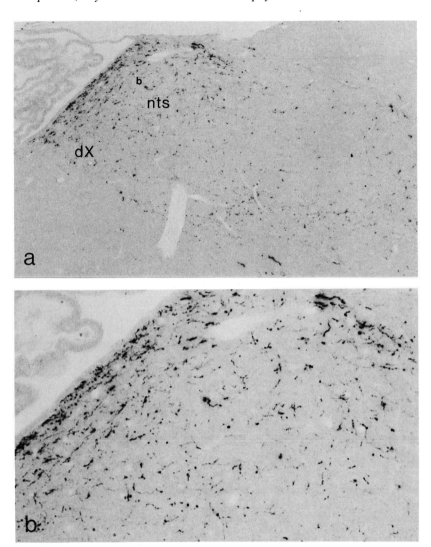

Fig. 16a,b. Survey and detail of a frontal 10-μm section stained for neurophysin through the dorsal medulla of a rat. There is a high density of fibers in the dorsal vagal nucleus (dX) and nucleus of the solitary tract (nts).

(g) Substantia gelatinosa trigemini

Single oxytocin and vasopressin fibers are scattered in the rostral part of the spinal nucleus of the trigeminal nerve, particularly in the lateral aspects and substantia gelatinosa (Atlas, P 2.8–P 6.0). More caudally, these fibers become more numerous and form a thin band of fibers along the entire extent of the substantia gelatinosa (Fig. 19a), with single scattered fibers in the rest of the spinal nucleus (P 6.5–P 8.0). This band of fibers is continuous caudally with fibers extending through the substantia gelatinosa and outer laminae (I–III) of the entire spinal cord. Generally, oxytocin fibers appear to predominate slightly, and the fibers appear to pass into the spinal nucleus from the ventral bundle of descending fibers.

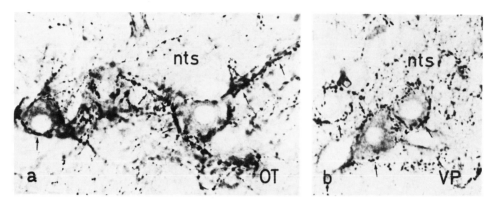

Fig. 17. a. Oxytocin (OT) and *b* vasopressin terminals surrounding the perikarya and lining the dendrites of neurons in the nucleus of the solitary tract (nts). (Reproduced from Sofroniew and Schrell (1982), by courtesy of Editors of the *Journal of Histochemistry and Cytochemistry*.)

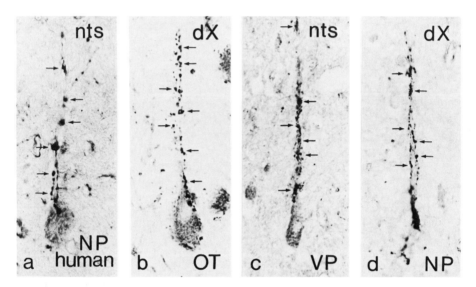

Fig. 18. a. Neurophysin (NP), *b.* oxytocin (OT), *c.* vasopressin (VP), and *d* neurophysin terminals which line the perikarya and dendrites of neurons (counterstained with a Nissl stain) in the human nucleus of the solitary tract (nts) and dorsal vagal nucleus (dX) (taken from a routine autopsy specimen). (Reproduced from Sofroniew (1983d), by courtesy of the Editors of *Trends in Neurosciences*.)

(h) Other brainstem regions

Scattered single vasopressin and oxytocin fibers are present throughout the central reticular core of the brainstem, and in some parts of the reticular formation distinct clusters of vasopressin and oxytocin fibers are regularly present (Atlas, P 1.5–P 8.0). Some of these clusters appear to overlap specific groups of neurons, such as the A5 catecholaminergic group (P 2.8–P 3.4). Fibers are consistently present along the entire rostrocaudal extent of the midline, some are in well-defined raphe nuclei as described above, while others are in regions which could not be readily delineated (P 2.0–P 8.0).

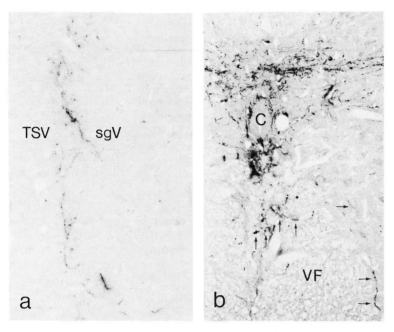

Fig. 19. a. Neurophysin fibers in the marginal zone of the substantia gelatinosa of the spinal nucleus of the trigeminal nerve (sgV) in the rat. Frontal 10-μm section at about the level shown in P 8.0. *b.* Neurophysin fibers in lamina X around the central canal (C) in the upper lumbar spinal cord in the rat. TSV, tractus spinalis trigemini; VF, ventral funiculus. (Reproduced from Sofroniew and Weindl (1981), by courtesy of the Publisher.)

3.3. SPINAL CORD

Oxytocin and vasopressin fibers enter the spinal cord along 2 main pathways. The major pathway is a direct continuation of the bundle of fibers descending ventrolaterally through the brainstem as described above. At the transition of the medulla to the cervical spinal cord this bundle moves dorsolaterally until it occupies a position at the dorsal part of the lateral funiculus, just ventral to and abutting the dorsal horn, where it descends through the rest of the spinal cord (Atlas, P 8.0–SIII/IV). A few fibers also appear to descend in the ventral funiculus. A smaller number of fibers appear to enter the spinal cord in the central gray (lamina X) along the central canal, and pass caudally along the cord for some distance.

Throughout the entire length of the spinal cord, a band of oxytocin and vasopressin fibers is regularly present in *lamina I–III*. Scattered single fibers are present in various parts of the dorsal horn at most levels. A fairly dense cluster of fibers is regularly present at all levels around the central canal in *lamina X* (Fig. 19b and Atlas, CI–SIII/IV). Occasional single fibers are present in the ventral horns at many levels, but more so in lumbar regions. Many fibers are also regularly present throughout the intermediolateral column of preganglionic sympathetic neurons in thoraco-lumbar regions. The density of this innervation varies somewhat from segment to segment, and is greatest in the lower thoracic and upper lumbar levels. Although not shown, fibers are present through the entire extent of the spinal cord, through coccygeal levels and into the filum terminale. In most regions of the spinal cord oxytocin fibers predominate somewhat, but vasopressin fibers are definitely present in all areas.

135

4. NATURE OF TERMINALS IN TARGET AREAS

Axons deriving from vasopressin or oxytocin neurons project to and terminate in both vascular and neural target areas. There is evidence that the nature of the terminals found in these 2 kinds of targets may be somewhat different, and they will be dealt with separately.

4.1. VASCULAR TARGETS

There are 2 vascular targets in which axons of vasopressin or oxytocin neurons are known to terminate, the posterior pituitary and the external zone of the median eminence which contains the hypophyseal portal vessels (see section 5.1.).

In the *median eminence*, the majority of the vasopressin and oxytocin fibers pass through the internal zone to the posterior pituitary. However, a large number of vasopressin, and relatively few oxytocin, fibers leave the internal zone to pass into the external zone. The exact nature of these fibers has not been extensively studied, but the fibers appear at the light microscopic level to surround and contact portal vessels (Parry and Livett 1973; Zimmerman et al. 1973; Dierickx et al. 1976). At the ultrastructural level in the guinea pig, these fibers appear to terminate abutting portal vessels, and contain granules immunoreactive for vasopressin which are smaller than those observed in the posterior pituitary (Silverman and Zimmerman 1975). As described in Section 5.1. these vasopressin fibers derive from the paraventricular nucleus and are thought to be involved in regulation of release of ACTH from the adenohypophysis.

In the *posterior pituitary*, the terminals of neurosecretory axons have been well studied at the ultrastructural level, particularly in connection with the mechanics of the secretory process (Theodosis et al. 1976; Morris and Nordmann 1980; Tweedle 1983). From such studies, it appears that the terminal arborizations of neurosecretory axons within the neural lobe consist of 2 types of dilatations, nerve endings and nerve swellings. Nerve endings contact the perivascular basement membrane and contain both neurosecretory vesicles and microvesicles. In contrast, nerve swellings do not appear to make systematic contact with the perivascular basement membrane and contain neurosecretory granules but not significant numbers of microvesicles (Morris 1976). Newly synthesized granules appear to distribute randomly between nerve swellings or nerve endings according to available space (Chapman et al. 1982), but during acute release, depletion of neurosecretory granules appears to occur primarily from nerve endings (Morris and Nordmann 1980). Less is known about the light microscopic appearance of these terminals and the extent of the terminal arborization, and therefore the number of nerve endings, arising from individual axons. Due to the great density of terminal swellings within the posterior pituitary this question cannot be examined with immunohistochemistry or most other techniques. Golgi studies suggest extensive terminal branching of individual axons (Ramon y Cajal 1966), although this has not been analysed in detail. Interesting information in this regard has recently been obtained from the study of organotypic cell cultures, where supraoptic nucleus and neurointermediate lobe have been co-cultured. In some cases, magnocellular supraoptic nucleus neurons identified immunohistochemically reinnervate the neurointermediate lobe (Sofroniew et al. 1982b, 1983). In these cases, the individual axons give rise to profuse networks of interconnected terminal dilatations suggesting that individual neurons could have a very large number of nerve endings and release a substantial amount of peptide in response to stimulation. It is interesting that this reticular appearance of terminals in a vascular target area is somewhat different from that of terminals in neural areas (Sofroniew, Gähwiler and Dreifuss, in preparation) as described below.

4.2. NEURAL TARGETS

Neural target areas are defined as regions where axons appear to branch extensively and terminate. At the light microscopic level, terminals can often be seen contacting neuronal cell bodies (counterstained with a Nissl stain) or proximal dendrites. In fortunate cases, terminals can be seen lining perikarya or dendrites (Figs 17, 20), even in human specimens (Fig. 18). The nature of the contacts thus visualized is in most cases not certain since light microscopy does not provide adequate resolution. In some areas, vasopressin and oxytocin have been localized in presynaptic structures using immunohistochemistry at the electron microscopic level (Buijs and Swaab 1980; Sterba et al. 1980), but relatively few examples of this were found. Alternatively, vasopressin and oxytocin terminals in certain neural target regions might not form specialized contacts, as has been suggested of various aminergic terminals (Beaudet and Descarries 1978).

Fiber density in target areas generally increases considerably over that seen in the afferent pathways, suggesting fairly extensive terminal arborization. In fortunate specimens, terminal arborizations clearly arising from a single axon can be observed (Sofroniew and Weindl 1978b), which in many cases can be profuse. Such terminal arborization often takes the form of repeated collateralization so as to create the appearance of a cluster of many individual branches (Fig. 20a,b). In other cases, such as the frontal cortex, single main axons may pass for long distances through a target area regularly giving off short collaterals (Fig. 10). Immunohistochemically identified axons of paraventricular nucleus neurons grown in organotypic hypotholamic cultures also exhibit both collaterals in passing and extensive terminal arborization (Sofroniew, Gähwiler and Dreifuss, in preparation). The total arborization arising from single, often very long, axons can be easily and clearly examined. Those axons terminating in neural regions exhibit the same type of terminal arborization, i.e. repeated collateralization, as

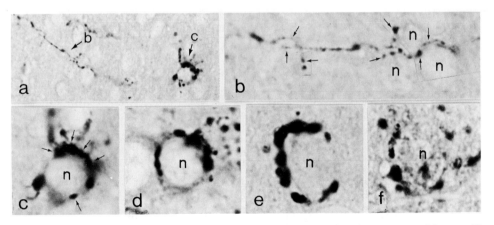

Fig. 20. a. Neurophysin fibers in the lateral septum of the rat. *b.* Detail of *a,* photomontage of the same fiber and its various terminal branches some of which appear to contact local neurons (n). *c.* Detail of *a,* neuron whose soma is almost completely surrounded with neurophysin varicosities (arrows). *d–f.* Additional neurons in the lateral septum whose somata are surrounded by neurophysin (*d, e*) or vasopressin (*f*) varicosities. (Reproduced from Sofroniew and Weindl (1978b), by courtesy of the Editors of the *American Journal of Anatomy.*)

that observed in vivo in neural target areas. This form of terminal arborization is somewhat different from that observed of cultured axons reinnervating a vascular target,
which is reticular in appearance. Together, the in vivo and culture observations suggest
that individual neurons could be responsible for a large number of terminals which in
some cases, such as the frontal cortex, are diffusely spread over a large area. This is
worth remembering in situations where retrograde labeling experiments indicate that
only few neurons of a particular type may project to a given target (Sofroniew and
Schrell 1981; Sawchenko and Swanson 1982). These few neurons might nonetheless give
rise to a fairly extensive innervation.

5. EXPERIMENTALLY ESTABLISHED PROJECTIONS

Given several types of vasopressin and oxytocin neurons distributed in a number of different CNS locations, and an extensive network of vasopressin and oxytocin fibers
throughout the CNS in both neural and vascular target regions, it becomes an important
functional question to establish which neurons give rise to which terminals. This has
been approached using 2 procedures, the placement of lesions in combination with immunohistochemistry, or modified tract-tracing procedures in combination with immunohistochemistry in the same animals. In addition, much can often be inferred, although
not conclusively demonstrated by comparing results of tract-tracing and immunohistochemistry in separate animals. The following description will focus primarily on projections established experimentally using the first 2 procedures. For the sake of clarity vascular and neural projections will be considered separately.

5.1. VASCULAR PROJECTIONS

Vasopressin or oxytocin projections to 2 vascular targets have now been experimentally
established, to the posterior pituitary and to the external zone of the median eminence
which contains the hypophyseal portal capillaries (Fig. 21). These 2 regions will be considered separately. In addition, vasopressin, oxytocin or neurophysin fibers have been
found in various other circumventricular organs, and these will also be discussed.

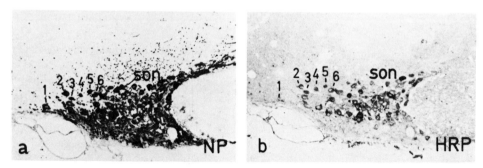

Fig. 21a,b. Neighboring serial 1.5-μm thick sections through the supraoptic nucleus (son) stained for (a) neurophysin (NP) or (b) horseradish peroxidase (HRP) from a rat injected with HRP into the posterior pituitary
48 hr prior to fixation. All neurons in the son transporting HRP from the posterior pituitary also appear
to contain NP, and most neurons in the son containing NP appear to project to the posterior pituitary. The
numbers 1–6 indicate some of the neurons clearly identifiable on both sections. Neurons 2–6 stained positively
for both NP and HRP, while neuron 1 stained only for NP. (Reproduced from Sofroniew et al. (1985), by
courtesy of the Publisher.)

138

(a) Posterior pituitary

The distribution of neurons projecting to the posterior pituitary has been investigated using retrograde transport of HRP (Sherlock et al. 1975; Kelly and Swanson 1980). The distribution depicted (Kelly and Swanson 1980) suggests an almost complete overlap with the distribution of magnocellular vasopressin and oxytocin neurons in the supraoptic nucleus, paraventricular nucleus and various accessory groups as described in Section 2.1. and shown in Figure 4 and in the Atlas, A 7.5–A 3.4. We have examined the distribution of specific vasopressin and oxytocin neurons projecting to the posterior pituitary using a combined tract-tracing and immunohistochemical procedure allowing detection of both the HRP transported and the peptide produced by the same neurons (Sofroniew et al. 1980; Sofroniew 1982, 1983). Following injection of HRP into the posterior pituitary (Sofroniew et al. 1980), we found that all neurons in the supraoptic nucleus which project to the posterior pituitary also contain either vasopressin or oxytocin, and virtually all supraoptic nucleus neurons containing vasopressin or oxytocin project to the posterior pituitary (Fig. 22). In the paraventricular nucleus, in contrast, only magnocellular vasopressin and oxytocin neurons located primarily in the rostral and lateral parts of the nucleus project to the posterior pituitary, while most of the smaller oxytocin or vasopressin neurons lying more caudally in the nucleus appear not to (Sofroniew 1982). In addition, some parvocellular paraventricular nucleus neurons which were HRP-labeled contained neither vasopressin nor oxytocin (Sofroniew 1982). These may have been labeled as the result of spread to the median eminence (Armstrong and Hatton 1980). In addition, we found that most magnocellular neurons in accessory groups as described in Section 2.1.c. projected to the posterior pituitary as summarized in Figure 21.

(b) Median eminence

As described in Section 4.1., the median eminence contains substantial numbers of

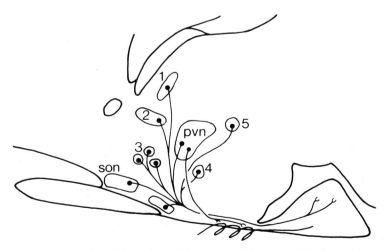

Fig. 22. Sagittal view of the rat hypothalamus and pituitary depicting the vascular projections of hypothalamic vasopressin and oxytocin neurons. Most vasopressin and oxytocin neurons in the supraoptic nucleus (son), rostral paraventricular nucleus (pvn) and various accessory nuclei (1–5, see Fig. 1) project to the posterior pituitary. In addition, some parvocellular vasopressin neurons in the pvn project to the hypophyseal portal capillaries in the median eminence. (Reproduced from Sofroniew (1983b), by courtesy of the Publisher.)

vasopressin fibers in the external zone which contact hypophyseal portal capillaries, and vasopressin is present in very high concentrations in hypophyseal portal blood (Zimmerman et al. 1973). Following adrenalectomy, there is a pronounced increase in the density of vasopressin fibers in the external zone (Fig. 23), and this increase can be blocked by physiologic substitution with pure glucocorticoid, but not with pure mineralocorticoid (Dierickx et al. 1976; Sofroniew et al. 1977; Stillman et al. 1977; Sofroniew 1982). These findings are consistent with an involvement of vasopressin in the hypothalamo-pituitary-adrenal axis, and vasopressin has long been considered a factor involved in control of ACTH release from the anterior pituitary (see Yates and Maran 1974; Gillies and Lowry 1979). The origin of these fibers is thus of considerable interest. Lesion studies in normal and adrenalectomized animals have shown that these vasopressin fibers around portal capillaries derive exclusively from the hypothalamic paraventricular nucleus in both rats (Vandesande et al. 1977) and monkeys (Antunes et al. 1977). Furthermore, retrograde tracing studies show a direct projection from parvocellular neurons in the medial part of the paraventricular nucleus to the external zone (Lechan et al. 1980; Wiegand and Price 1980). These parvocellular neurons are located in precisely that portion of the paraventricular nucleus in which the parvocellular neurons containing both CRF and vasopressin are located (see sections 2.2.d. and 2.4.b.). In these

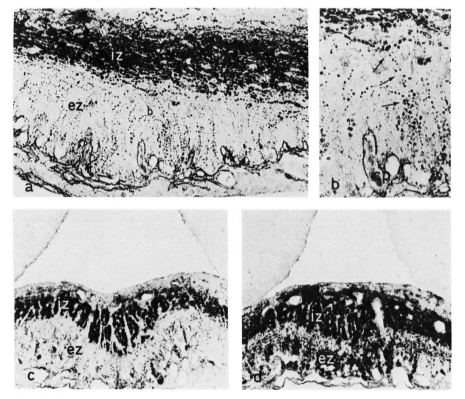

Fig. 23a–d. Rat median eminence stained for neurophysin. *a,b.* Survey and detail of a sagittal section showing fibers in the internal (iz) and external (ez) zones, and that fibers in the ez appear to derive from the iz (arrows). *c,d.* Frontal sections through the median eminence of (c) normal and (d) adrenalectomized rats. Note the pronounced increase of neurophysin in ez fibers following adrenalectomy. (Reproduced from Sofroniew (1982), by courtesy of the Publisher.)

neurons, vasopressin is readily stainable only after adrenalectomy. Thus, adrenalectomy would appear to induce an increase of vasopressin in both the perikarya and terminals of these neurons. Investigation of this well understood system regarding the exact nature of the complementary roles played by vasopressin and CRF in ACTH regulation, and the mechanisms governing the expression of vasopressin in these CRF neurons during different physiologic states promises to reveal much about the purposes underlying co-existence of peptides in the same neurons.

(c) Other circumventricular organs (CVO's)

Although definite projections have not yet been established, there are numerous vaso-pressin or oxytocin fibers either inside or in the vicinity of various CVO's which warrant discussion. Many vasopressin fibers pass close to or through the *organum vasculosum of the lamina terminalis (OVLT)*. The bulk of these fibers appears to originate from the suprachiasmatic nucleus, and a direct vasopressin projection from the suprachiasmatic nucleus to the fenestrated capillaries of the OVLT has been proposed (Hoorneman and Buijs 1982). However, although vasopressin fibers pass close by the OVLT, we could not find many entering the vascular zone to contact the fenestrated capillaries there (Weindl and Sofroniew 1981). In addition, a projection from the suprachiasmatic nucle-us to the permeable blood vessels of the OVLT seems very unlikely since no suprachias-matic nucleus neurons are labeled following intravascular injections of HRP which label all neurons with connections to the vascular system (Broadwell and Brightman 1976). In our preparations it appears that these fibers continue rostrally past the OVLT. In contrast, the *subfornical organ* contains numerous vasopressin and oxytocin fibers in the vicinity of its fenestrated capillaries (Atlas, A 5.9–A 5.7) (Weindl and Sofroniew 1978, 1981). The origin of these fibers is not certain, although they may derive from the hypo-thalamic paraventricular nucleus (Conrad and Pfaff 1976; Silverman et al. 1981). We have seen occasional fibers in the *area postrema*, and fibers in the vicinity of, but not in the *subcommissural organ* (Weindl and Sofroniew 1978). The *pineal gland* deserves consideration in somewhat greater detail. In contrast to reports that the pineal gland produces vasotocin and neurophysin (Pavel 1971; Reinharz et al. 1974), extensive exami-nation in different laboratories has never revealed a pinealocyte specifically immunohis-tochemically stained for these substances although a number of both vasopressin and oxytocin (as well as neurophysin) fibers are occasionally visible (Weindl and Sofroniew 1978; Buijs and Pevet 1980). The precise origin of these fibers is not known, but they appear to be of central derivation, entering via the pineal stock (Weindl and Sofroniew 1978; Buijs and Pevet 1980). Results from 2 laboratories using different highly specific radioimmunoassays indicate that while the pineal gland contains small amounts of vaso-pressin, oxytocin and neurophysin, it contains no vasotocin (Negro-Vilar et al. 1979; Dogterom et al. 1980; Pevet et al. 1980). It thus seems likely that previous reports on the presence of vasotocin in the pineal gland were due to cross-reaction with vasopressin or oxytocin located in nerve fibers of probable central origin, and not in pinealocytes.

5.2. NEURAL PROJECTIONS

Vasopressin and oxytocin fibers and terminals reach a large number of neural targets throughout the CNS, however, the location of the neuronal cell bodies giving rise to the terminals in a particular region has only been established experimentally in a few cases. The following discussion will first consider studies dealing with analysis of projections to a given region, and second, studies of projections arising from a particular set of neurons. Established vasopressin- and oxytocin-specific projections are summarized in Figure 24.

(a) Projections to the medulla oblongata and spinal cord

Neuroanatomical tract-tracing studies have demonstrated direct projections from the hypothalamic paraventricular nucleus to the medulla oblongata and spinal cord (Kuypers and Maiskey 1975; Conrad and Pfaff 1976; Saper et al. 1976; Schober 1978). These caudally projecting neurons are located for the most part, but not exclusively, in the caudal parvocellular portion of the paraventricular nucleus (Ono et al. 1978; Hosoya and Matsushita 1979; Armstrong et al. 1980; Sofroniew and Schrell 1980), while projections to the posterior pituitary arise primarily from lateral and rostral magnocellular portions (Ono et al. 1978; Hosoya and Matsushita 1979; Armstrong et al. 1980). A study using a double tracer procedure indicates that paraventricular nucleus projections to the posterior pituitary or medulla oblongata arise almost exclusively from separate neurons (Swanson and Kuypers 1980), although a few neurons may have projections to both (Zerihun and Harris 1981). These studies all suggest that the vasopressin and oxytocin terminals in the nucleus of the solitary tract, dorsal vagal nucleus and other regions in the brainstem and spinal cord could derive from neurons in the paraventricular nucleus. Conclusive demonstration of this has been provided by studies combining tract-tracing procedures with immunohistochemical analysis of the peptides produced by transporting neurons. These studies (Sofroniew and Schrell 1981; Sawchenko and Swanson 1982) indicate that a number of oxytocin and somewhat fewer vasopressin neurons located primarily in the caudal parvocellular paraventricular nucleus project to the medulla and or spinal cord (Figs 25, 26). In agreement, measurement of oxytocin by radioimmunoassay in the dorsal vagal complex following lesion of the paraventricular nucleus showed a reduction of 100%, while vasopressin was reduced by only 50% (Lang et al. 1983). This suggests that while all oxytocin terminals found in this region may be of paraventricular nucleus origin, the region receives a vasopressin projection

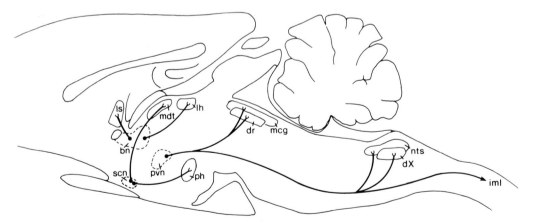

Fig. 24. Sagittal view of the rat brain depicting the major experimentally established vasopressin- or oxytocin-specific projections. Abbreviations: bn, bed nucleus of the stria terminalis; dr, dorsal raphe; dX, dorsal vagal nucleus; iml, intermediolateral nucleus of the spinal cord; lh, lateral habenula; ls, lateral septum; mcg, mesencephalic central gray; mdt, mediodorsal thalamus; nts, nucleus tractus solitarius; ph, posterior hypothalamus; pvn, hypothalamic paraventricular nucleus; scn, suprachiasmatic nucleus.

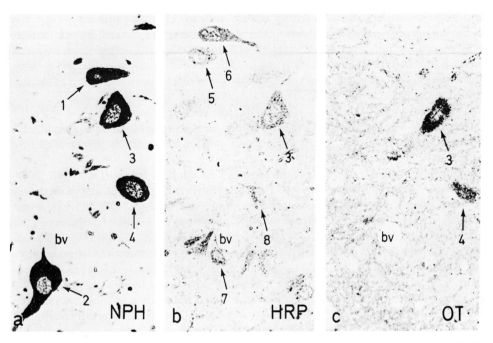

Fig. 25a–c. Serial 1.5-μm frontal sections through the caudal dorsal part of the paraventricular nucleus (at the level shown in Fig. 26c) of a rat injected with horseradish peroxidase (HRP) into the dorsomedial medulla oblongata. Sections were immunohistochemically stained alternately for: *a*, neurophysin (NPH); *b*, HRP; or *c*, oxytocin (OT). *a* and *b* are neighboring sections, between *b* and *c* there is one section not shown which was stained for vasopressin (VP). Neurons 1–4 stained positively for NPH, neurons 3 and 4 also stained for OT, 1 and 2 for VP (not shown). Neuron 3 is an OT/NPH neuron (15–23 μm) which has also transported HRP from the medulla. Neurons 5–8 transported HRP but do not contain NPH or OT (or VP). Note that the HRP contained within neurons 5–8 has not reacted with the diaminobenzidine during staining for OT or NPH. (Reproduced from Sofroniew and Schrell (1981), by courtesy of the Editors of *Neuroscience Letters*.)

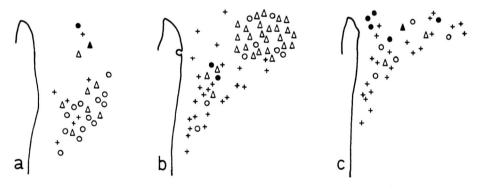

Fig. 26a–c. Schematic frontal drawings of 3 levels of the paraventricular nucleus: *a*, rostral (about A 5.8); *b*, central (about A 5.7); *c*, caudal (about A 5.3) comparing the distribution of neurons containing oxytocin (OT), vasopressin (VP) and/or horseradish peroxidase (HRP); based on immunohistochemical staining of neighboring 1.5-μm sections following injection of HRP into the dorsomedial medulla oblongata. ○ = OT neurons not transporting HRP; △ = VP neurons not transporting HRP; + = HRP neurons not containing VP or OT; ● = OT neurons transporting HRP; ▲ = VP neurons transporting HRP. (Reproduced from Sofroniew and Schrell (1981), by courtesy of the Editors of *Neuroscience Letters*.)

143

from a site in addition to the paraventricular nucleus. The parvocellular vasopressin neurons in the bed nucleus of the stria terminalis (see section 2.2.b.) are likely candidates for such a projection, since similar regions of this nucleus also contain neurons which project to the dorsal vagal region (Sofroniew 1983c; see 5.2.c.). Thus, although the paraventricular nucleus gives rise to a substantial portion of oxytocin and vasopressin projections to the medulla and spinal cord, it may not be the only site to do so.

(b) Projections arising from parvocellular vasopressin neurons in the suprachiasmatic nucleus

In the original studies describing the presence of vasopressin fibers in the CNS, fairly widespread projections were attributed to the parvocellular vasopressin neurons in the suprachiasmatic nucleus (Weindl and Sofroniew 1976; Buijs 1978; Sofroniew and Weindl 1978b). Various experimental studies conducted to examine these have confirmed only some. Both a lesion study (Hoorneman and Buijs 1982) and combined tract-tracing analysis (Schrell et al. 1983; Sofroniew 1983b) show vasopressin projections from suprachiasmatic nucleus neurons to the mediodorsal thalamus, and to the periventricular region near the dorsomedial nucleus in the posterior hypothalamus (Figs 24, 27). The combined tracing study further indicates a light projection to the mesencephalic central gray (Schrell et al. 1983). The other vasopressin projections originally attributed to the suprachiasmatic nucleus, appear at present to be unlikely. We have been unable to consistently find retrogradely labeled neurons in the suprachiasmatic nucleus following injection of tracers into the lateral habenula, lateral septum, hippocampus and medulla oblongata (Schrell and Sofroniew, unpublished observations). Studies using anterograde autoradiographic tracing techniques show suprachiasmatic nucleus projections to a number of regions including the dorsomedial nucleus in the posterior hypothalamus, the mediodorsal thalamus, and mesencephalic central gray (Swanson and Cowan 1975; Berk and Finkelstein 1981; Stephan et al. 1981), in agreement with the experimental studies showing vasopressin projections from the suprachiasmatic nucleus to these sites. In addition, these tracing studies indicate a substantial projection from the supra-

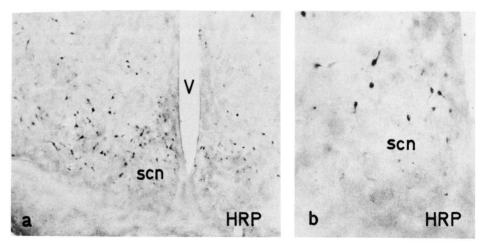

Fig. 27a,b. Survey and detail of neurons in the rat suprachiasmatic nucleus (scn) and surrounding hypothalamus, which have retrogradely transported horseradish peroxidase (HRP) from the mediodorsal thalamus. (Reproduced from Sofroniew (1983b) (from the work of Schrell and Sofroniew), by courtesy of the Publisher.)

chiasmatic nucleus to the paraventricular nucleus (Swanson and Cowan 1975; Berk and Finkelstein 1981; Stephan et al. 1981). A large number of vasopressin fibers originating from the suprachiasmatic nucleus enter the paraventricular nucleus (Sofroniew and Weindl 1978b), suggesting a possible projection, but vasopressin terminals have not yet been ultrastructurally verified in the paraventricular nucleus.

(c) Projections arising from parvocellular vasopressin neurons in the bed nucleus of the stria terminalis (BNST)

Evidence from tract-tracing studies and lesion studies suggests several possible projections for the parvocellular vasopressin neurons in the BNST. Retrograde tract-tracing studies show projections from neurons in those regions of the BNST which contain vasopressin cells to the dorsomedial medulla (Sofroniew 1983c) as well as to the lateral septum (De Vries and Buijs 1983). Following lesions of the BNST, the density of vasopressin fibers was found to decrease considerably in the lateral septum, lateral habenula, nucleus of the diagonal band and anterior amygdala (De Vries and Buijs 1983). A projection from vasopressin neurons in the BNST to these sites thus seems likely.

The origin of the many vasopressin and oxytocin projections to other neural sites is at present unknown. Although most of these projections have been ascribed to paraventricular nucleus neurons by some authors, the large number of vasopressin and to a lesser degree oxytocin neurons in other sites should not be ignored as potential sources.

6. VASOPRESSIN, OXYTOCIN AND NEUROPHYSIN IN CEREBROSPINAL FLUID

Vasopressin, oxytocin, and neurophysin can be detected by both bioassay and radioimmunoassay in mammalian CSF (Cushing and Goetsch 1910; Robinson AG and Zimmerman 1973; Dogterom et al. 1977; Jenkins et al. 1980; Reppert et al. 1981, 1982, 1983; Born et al. 1982; Robinson ICAF 1983). Studies on neurohypophyseal peptides in the CSF, including authenticity as determined chromatographically, basal levels, possible sources, stimuli for release, and clearance have recently been comprehensively reviewed (Robinson ICAF 1983). Here, a brief account of some of these points will be presented.

Basal levels of vasopressin or oxytocin in the CSF are in the low fmol/ml (low pg/ml) range, and generally the CSF levels are slightly lower than plasma levels (Luerssen and Robertson 1980). This ratio of CSF to plasma levels may be reversed in certain pathological states (Jenkins et al. 1980; Robinson ICAF 1983). The authenticity of the vasopressin or oxytocin detected in the CSF has been confirmed by a variety of procedures including bioassay and different forms of chromatography (see Robinson ICAF 1983). There appears to be a definite circadian rhythmicity of vasopressin levels in the CSF (Reppert et al. 1981, 1982, 1983; Perlow et al. 1982; Schwartz et al. 1983), while for oxytocin such a rhythmicity has only been found in primates (Reppert et al. 1983; Perlow et al. 1982). The significance of these circadian differences in peptide level in the CSF is not known, but may be related to the presence of vasopressin neurons in the suprachiasmatic nucleus (Sofroniew and Weindl 1980), which is an important circadian pacemaker (see section 7.8.).

Neither the source nor the functions of vasopressin or oxytocin in the CSF are known. Two possibilities regarding the origin are currently under consideration, either active secretion into the CSF for transport to a distant site of action, or passive diffusion into the CSF from neural sites of action as a means of clearance and eventual degradation. In support of the first possibility, there are peptide-containing processes which contact the ependyma of the 3rd ventricle (Sofroniew and Glasmann 1981). Nevertheless these are not very common, and given the extensive network of vasopressin and oxytocin projections to all areas of the CNS, transport by diffusion through the ventricular system would appear a rather inefficient adjunct. In support of the second possibility, many of the target regions receiving vasopressin and oxytocin projections at various levels of the CNS are either in contact with, or are close to, the ventricular system. Thus the peptides could easily gain access to the CSF by diffusion, and CSF levels may thus reflect release at these target sites. This may represent an important means of clearing the peptides from these sites. Supporting this concept is the rapid rate at which both vasopressin and oxytocin are cleared from the CSF, both have half-times of about 20–25 min in the CSF (Jones and Robinson 1982; Mens et al. 1983), and vasopressin infused into the CSF can appear in the blood in a biologically active form (Clark et al. 1983). Another possible source of the peptides in the CSF is the blood. However, at physiologic levels there appears to be little or no penetration of vasopressin or oxytocin from the vascular system into the CSF (Jenkins et al. 1980; Jones and Robinson 1982; Wang et al. 1982), although a small percent of the peptides will cross if a sufficiently large peripheral concentration (> 100 times normal) is present (Landgraf et al. 1979; Jones and Robinson 1982; Mens et al. 1983).

A number of stimuli which might alter CSF levels of vasopressin or oxytocin have been investigated (see Robinson ICAF 1983). In most cases stimuli releasing the peptides from the neural lobe have no effect on CSF levels. This holds true for dehydration or peripheral osmotic stimulation (Dogterom et al. 1978b; Wang et al. 1982) and suckling (Robinson ICAF and Jones 1982), which have no effect on CSF levels of vasopressin or oxytocin respectively. In contrast, central osmotic stimulation can raise CSF levels of both vasopressin and oxytocin (Barnard and Morris 1982), but this may be due to nonspecific activation of many neurons (Leng et al. 1982; Robinson ICAF 1983). Few stimuli have been found which alter CSF levels of vasopressin or oxytocin (see Robinson ICAF 1983).

The development of specific and sensitive procedures for monitoring CSF levels of vasopressin and oxytocin in humans raises the possibility of future diagnostic application. Increases in CSF levels of vasopressin, oxytocin or neurophysin have been reported in cases of subarachnoid hemorrhage (Jenkins et al. 1980), seizures (Unger et al. 1971), hydrocephalus and raised intracranial pressure (Hammer et al. 1982), bacterial meningitis (Garcia et al. 1981), depression (Legros et al. 1983) and anorexia nervosa (Gold et al. 1983). This last example is of particular interest, since CSF levels of vasopressin which were elevated in anorexics were slowly normalized with weight gain (Gold et al. 1983). As more is understood about the factors governing the release of these peptides into the CSF, monitoring their levels may provide greater diagnostic information.

7. FUNCTIONAL CONSIDERATIONS

Although it is not possible in this context to discuss in detail the many functional considerations surrounding vasopressin and oxytocin neurons and the implications represented by vasopressin or oxytocin projections to various areas in the CNS, some illustrative examples will be considered. Meisenberg and Simmons (1983) have recently reviewed many of the central effects mediated by these peptides.

146

7.1. ELECTROPHYSIOLOGY OF VASOPRESSIN AND OXYTOCIN NEURONS

The electrophysiologic characteristics of hypothalamic magnocellular neurons projecting to the posterior pituitary have been studied in detail for many years, and this subject has been well reviewed (see Hayward 1977; Poulain and Wakerley 1982). Recently, the development of techniques for combining intracellular dye-filling of electrophysiologically studied neurons with immunohistochemical visualization of the substances produced by these neurons (Reaves and Hayward 1979b) has allowed characterization of specifically identified vasopressin or oxytocin magnocellular neurosecretory neurons (Reaves and Hayward 1980; Kayser et al. 1982; Kawata et al. 1983; Reaves et al. 1983; Theodosis et al. 1983; Yamashita et al. 1983a). Reports on the electrophysiology of specific vasopressin or oxytocin neurons with central projections have not yet appeared. Several reports have electrophysiologically examined the connections of the hypothalamic paraventricular nucleus (Pittman et al. 1981; Zerihun and Harris 1981; Thomson 1982; Ferguson et al. 1984; Yamashita et al. 1984).

7.2. RELEASE OF VASOPRESSIN AND OXYTOCIN FROM NERVE TERMINALS

The mechanism by which vasopressin and oxytocin are released from terminals in a vascular target, the posterior pituitary, has been under investigation for many years, and this subject has been well reviewed (Dreifuss 1975; Morris et al. 1978; Nordmann 1983; Theodosis 1983; Tweedle 1983; Castel et al. 1984). Release of peptide probably occurs by exocytosis of the contents of neurosecretory granules and is accompanied by a depletion of granules from the terminals (Dreifuss 1975; Morris et al. 1978; Theodosis 1983; Tweedle 1983). The secretion rate appears to reflect not only the rate, but also the specific firing pattern of neurons, and is closely linked to calcium ion concentration within the terminal (Dreifuss 1975; Morris et al. 1978; Bicknell and Leng 1983; Nordmann 1983; Shaw et al. 1983). The release of vasopressin and oxytocin from central terminals has been much less extensively investigated, but recent studies show that both vasopressin and oxytocin detected by radioimmunoassay can be released from central target areas by potassium stimulation, either in vivo using push-pull cannulae (Disturnal et al. 1984), or in vitro using tissue slices (Buijs and Van Heerikhuize 1982). In addition, stimulation of the hypothalamus in or near the paraventricular nucleus, which is known to send both vasopressin and oxytocin projections to the spinal cord and medulla oblongata (see section 5.2.a.), results in the release of vasopressin and oxytocin as detected by radioimmunoassay into the subarachnoid space of the spinal cord (Pittman et al. 1984) or into the cisterna magna (Jones et al. 1983). Thus, evidence for the release of vasopressin and oxytocin from central terminals is gradually accumulating. Lastly, there is evidence that peripheral release of oxytocin or vasopressin may be dissociated from central release, although in some situations both may occur simultaneously (Burnard et al. 1983; Jones et al. 1983; Epstein et al. 1983; Zerbe and Palkovits 1984).

7.3. AUTHENTICITY OF CENTRAL VASOPRESSIN AND OXYTOCIN

Most reports describing the presence of vasopressin or oxytocin in the CNS tissue are based on immunological techniques, either immunohistochemistry or radioimmunoassay. The possibility of cross-reaction with substances having similar antigenic determinants cannot be excluded when using these procedures. Nevertheless, the immunohistochemical identification of neurophysin as well as vasopressin and oxytocin in the same CNS structures supports the specificity of the findings. Neurophysin is an antigenetically distinct portion of the precursors for these peptides (see section 1.2.). When using 2 different antisera recognizing different portions of the same precursor, a nonspecific cross-reaction against 2 different substances within the same structures would appear to be less likely. In addition, vasopressin-immunoreactive material extracted from a number of different brain sites has been found to be immunologically identical to synthetic vasopressin (Glick and Brownstein 1980; Dorsa and Bottemiller 1983), and analysis of immunoreactive vasopressin extracted from several sites in the rat brain using high-performance liquid chromatography (HPLC) showed AVP to be the predominant, but not exclusive, immunoreactive substance (Dorsa and Bottemiller 1983). Approximately 95% of the immunoreactive vasopressin behaved like synthetic AVP while the remainder probably consists of processing products of vasopressin (Dorsa and Bottemiller 1983) as suggested by the presence of enzymes in synaptosomal membrane preparations which can form biologically active fragments of vasopressin and oxytocin (Burbach et al. 1980; Burbach and Lebouille 1983). A neurophysin-like material has been reported in the cerebellum of scrapie-affected but not normal sheep (Parry and Livett 1976, 1977). Although this is of interest regarding the pathology of this disease, the authenticity of this neurophysin-like substance requires verification by procedures other than immunohistochemistry.

7.4. EVIDENCE FOR CENTRAL VASOPRESSIN AND OXYTOCIN RECEPTORS

At least 3 different receptors have been characterized for vasopressin and oxytocin in peripheral tissues, a vasopressor receptor present on vascular smooth muscle and liver cells, an antidiuretic receptor on renal cells, and an oxytocic receptor on uterine cells (Soloff et al. 1977; Michell et al. 1979; Takhar and Kirk 1981; Jard 1983). These receptors can with varying degrees of selectivity in agonist or antagonist activity be recognized by a number of synthetic analogs of vasopressin and oxytocin (Sawyer et al. 1981; Manning and Sawyer 1983, 1984). The study of central vasopressin or oxytocin receptors which is now beginning, is greatly aided by the wealth of information already available on peripheral receptors and the availability of agonist and antagonist peptides. By using these analogs in electrophysiological studies, a uterine-type oxytocin receptor has been identified on a particular class of interneuron in the rat hippocampus and in the dorsal vagal nucleus (Mühlethaler et al. 1983; Charpak et al. 1984), and an antidiuretic-type receptor has been identified in the guinea pig supraoptic nucleus (Abe et al. 1983). In addition to these electrophysiological studies, binding sites for vasopressin have been identified in several brain areas which contain vasopressin terminals (Baskin et al. 1983; Van Leeuwen and Wolters 1983; Dorsa et al. 1983, 1984), and using synaptosomal membrane fractions from rat hippocampus, a vasopressin binding site has been demonstrated which behaves identically with peripheral antidiuretic-type receptors in displacement studies using synthetic agonists or antagonists (Barberis 1983). Vasopressin binding sites in the medulla appear to be of a different subtype to those in the kidney (Cornett and Dorsa 1985).

7.5. EFFECTS OF VASOPRESSIN AND OXYTOCIN AT THE CELLULAR LEVEL

There is now good evidence that both vasopressin and oxytocin can alter the electrical activity of neurons in various parts of the CNS where fibers containing these peptides are present. These areas include the dorsal vagal nucleus and medulla oblongata (Morris et al. 1980, 1984; Charpak et al. 1984), preganglionic sympathetic neurons in the spinal cord (Gilbey et al. 1982), locus ceruleus (Olpe and Baltzer 1981), hippocampus (Huston and Jakobartl 1977; Mühlethaler et al. 1982, 1983), and lateral septum (Joels and Urban 1983). Nevertheless, these peptides which function as hormones in the periphery might be involved in influencing other aspects of neuronal activity not directly related to synaptic transmission. Biochemical studies have shown that these peptides can cause regionally specific changes in cAMP production (Schneider et al. 1982; Church 1983; Courtney and Raskind 1983), catecholamine turnover (Tanaka et al. 1977; Versteeg et al. 1978, 1979; Delanoy et al. 1982; Gardner et al. 1984), or deoxyglucose uptake (Dunn et al. 1980) in various brain regions.

7.6. NEUROANATOMICAL POTENTIAL FOR INTERACTION WITH OTHER NEUROACTIVE SUBSTANCES

Although it is not possible in this context to discuss the many potential interactions of vasopressin or oxytocin projections with other chemically identified neurons, a few interesting cases of neuroanatomical overlap deserve mention. As mentioned in Section 7.5., vasopressin has been shown to alter catecholamine turnover. In the brainstem and midbrain, areas receiving vasopressin and oxytocin fibers appear to correspond to the location of the A1, A2, A5, A6, A8, and A9 catecholamine neurons (Dahlström and Fuxe 1964; Palkovits and Jacobowitz 1974). These projections may be involved in various aspects of autonomic regulation (see 7.9.). Vasopressin and oxytocin terminals also overlap with cholinergic neurons in the septum, nucleus of the diagonal band and several basal forebrain sites, as well as in the tegmental reticular formation and other brainstem regions (Sofroniew et al. 1982a; Armstrong et al. 1983; Houser et al. 1983; Sofroniew et al. 1985). The significance of this is not clear, but vasopressin and oxytocin interaction with cholinergic neurons in the basal forebrain may be involved in some of the behavioral effects of these peptides (see 7.7.) while interaction in the brainstem may also be involved in autonomic regulation. Vasopressin and oxytocin neurons and their projections overlap with a great many other peptidergic and other identified chemical systems as described in this Handbook. The potential for interaction with these systems is staggering, and can only be alluded to in this context. This will certainly be the basis of much interesting research in the future. In this context it is also interesting to note that vasopressin, oxytocin and neurophysin have recently been reported to be present in the mammalian retina (Gauquelin et al. 1983).

7.7. VASOPRESSIN, OXYTOCIN AND BEHAVIOR

Centrally administered vasopressin or oxytocin induce or modulate several different behaviors. Both peptides affect processes related to memory and learning (De Wied and Versteeg 1979; Le Moal et al. 1981; Van Wimersma Greidanus et al. 1981; Koob and Bloom 1981; De Wied 1983; Doris 1984), not only in experimental animals, but also in clinical trials (Gold et al. 1979; Legros and Gilot 1979; Ferrier et al. 1980;

Weingartner et al. 1981; Koob and Bloom 1982). Specific fragments of vasopressin or oxytocin are also active (Burbach et al. 1983a,b). While vasopressin appears to enhance consolidation and retrieval of memory, oxytocin appears to affect these processes negatively (Bohus et al. 1978; De Wied 1983). In addition, centrally administered oxytocin is capable of inducing maternal behavior in virgin rats (Pedersen and Prange 1979; Pedersen et al. 1982) while centrally administered vasopressin inhibits sexual behavior in female rats (Sodersten et al. 1983). Centrally administered vasopressin or oxytocin also appear to modulate opiate and ethanol addiction (Hoffman et al. 1978; Van Ree and De Wied 1981) as well as rewarded behavior (Schwarzberg et al. 1976). Centrally administered vasopressin has a dipsogenic effect in dogs (Szczepanska-Sadowska et al. 1982) and vasopressin micro-injected into the preoptic area can trigger a complex stereotypic behavior in hamsters (Ferris et al. 1984). In support of these various observations, vasopressin and oxytocin fibers are present in a number of different areas known to be involved in memory and other behavioral processes. These areas include the hippocampus, septal region, amygdala, mediodorsal thalamus, and neocortex.

7.8. VASOPRESSIN, OXYTOCIN AND CENTRAL CARDIOVASCULAR REGULATION

A number of central areas currently thought to be involved in cardiovascular regulation (Palkovits and Zaborszky 1977; Palkovits et al. 1979; Loewy and McKellar 1980) contain vasopressin or oxytocin neurons or receive vasopressin or oxytocin projections. These areas include the paraventricular nucleus, bed nucleus of the stria terminalis, amygdala, raphe nuclei, locus ceruleus, dorsal vagal/solitary nucleus complex and autonomic spinal cord regions. Both vasopressin and oxytocin have well documented peripheral effects on the cardiovascular system acting to dilate or constrict different vascular beds (Nakano 1974), and vasopressin has been strongly implicated as a circulating agent active in both normal control of arterial pressure and certain forms of pathological hypertension (Crofton et al. 1979; Möhring et al. 1980a; Cowley et al. 1982; Cowley and Barber 1983; Brooks et al. 1984). Both anatomical and electrophysiological studies show that hypothalamic vasopressin and oxytocin neurons with vascular projections receive direct input from central areas involved in cardiovascular control (Koizumi and Yamashita 1978; Nakai et al. 1982; Sladek and Sladek 1983; Swanson and Sawchenko 1983; Yamashita et al. 1983b), reciprocal connections appear to exist between oxytocin and vasopressin neurons in the paraventricular nucleus and several brainstem cardiovascular control centers (Van Bogaert et al. 1980; Sofroniew and Schrell 1981; Kannan and Yamashita 1983; Swanson and Sawchenko 1983). In addition, vasopressin levels measured by radioimmunoassay in several forebrain and brainstem sites are elevated in one strain of hypertensive rats (Feuerstein et al. 1981, 1982) and lowered in a different strain of hypertensive rats (Möhring et al. 1980b; Lang et al. 1981). Lastly, central administration of vasopressin, oxytocin or fragments of the peptides affect cardiovascular control mechanisms related to blood pressure regulation (Pittman et al. 1982; Wang et al. 1982; Bohus et al. 1983; Zerbe et al. 1983; Versteeg et al. 1983, 1984). Thus, central vasopressin and oxytocin pathways appear to play an important role in central cardiovascular regulation.

7.9. CENTRAL AUTONOMIC AND NEUROENDOCRINE REGULATION

Although there is little direct evidence that central vasopressin or oxytocin projections are involved in central autonomic or neuroendocrine regulation, morphological evidence suggests that this is likely. Vasopressin and oxytocin neurons or terminal fields are present in a number of areas known to be involved in these functions, including the paraventricular nucleus, amygdala, and various centers in the brainstem and spinal cord (Powley and Laughton 1981; Swanson and Mogenson 1981; Akmayev 1983). More specifically, stimulation of the amygdala has been shown to directly release vasopressin into the circulation (Hayward et al. 1977), and several brainstem areas thought to be involved in the afferent pathway of the milk ejection reflex (Tindal et al. 1967, 1968) receive oxytocin projections. Central administration of vasopressin can reduce peripheral circulating levels of vasopressin. In addition, recent evidence indicates that injection of vasopressin into the lumbar spinal cord, in regions which contain vasopressin terminals, can affect function of the kidney independent of circulating vasopressin (Riphagen and Pittman 1983).

7.10. VASOPRESSIN, OXYTOCIN AND PAIN

Both vasopressin and oxytocin fibers and terminals are present in several central areas involved in pain transmission (see Fields and Basbaum 1978), laminae I–III of the spinal cord, the dorsal raphe nucleus, and the periaqueductal gray, and administration of drugs may alter the levels of peptide found there (Leccese 1983). Furthermore, central administration of vasopressin has an analgesic action which is non-opiate in nature (Berntson and Berson 1980; Berkowitz and Sherman 1982). The role of vasopressin and oxytocin in pain mechanisms seems worthy of further investigation.

7.11. VASOPRESSIN AND FEVER

Several lines of investigation suggest a role for central vasopressin, particularly deriving from terminals in the septum, in maintenance of homeostasis during fever (Kasting et al. 1982). The amount of vasopressin in perfusates of the septal region correlates negatively with body temperature, and vasopressin administered into the septum induces antipyresis (Cooper et al. 1979). Vasopressin levels measured by radioimmunoassay are decreased in the septum and other regions, but increased in the anterior hypothalamus, following exposure to endotoxin (Kasting and Martin 1983), and changes in pattern of immunohistochemical staining in the septum in relation to fever suppression have been noted (Merker et al. 1980). Central administration of vasopressin suppresses prostaglandin-E-induced hyperthermia in rats (Ruwe et al. 1985). The precise effect of vasopressin during fever may vary with species or with cause of fever (Bernardini et al. 1983).

7.12. VASOPRESSIN, SUPRACHIASMATIC NUCLEUS AND BIOLOGICAL RHYTHMS

A number of studies have shown that the suprachiasmatic nucleus receives a direct retinal input (Hendrickson et al. 1972; Moore and Lenn 1972; Mai and Junger 1977), and that lesioning the suprachiasmatic nucleus disrupts the regulation of various biological rhythms (Moore and Eichler 1972; Rusak and Zucker 1979; Van den Pol and Powley 1979). Parvocellular vasopressin neurons make up only the smaller portion of suprachiasmatic nucleus neurons, about 17% in the rat. Furthermore, they are located preferentially in the dorsal and medial portion of the nucleus while the retinal input is preferential to the ventral and lateral portion. Thus, vasopressin neurons might not be involved in suprachiasmatic nucleus regulation of biological rhythms. This indeed seems to be the case, since there seems to be no disturbance of circadian rhythms in Brattleboro rats which have a genetic inability to make vasopressin (Stephan and Zucker 1974; Peterson et al. 1980).

8. SUMMARY AND CONCLUDING REMARKS

Vasopressin and oxytocin are present in fibers throughout the mammalian central nervous system. These fibers derive from neurons scattered in various forebrain as well as brainstem locations. In neural target areas fibers often surround and contact neurons, and in some cases these contacts have been identified as synaptic. In a number of areas vasopressin and oxytocin have been shown to alter the electrical or biochemical activity of neurons. Both peptides appear to be involved in a variety of centrally regulated functions, such as behavior, cardiovascular regulation, nociception, or maintenance of body temperature. Thus these peptides, which were originally characterized as circulating hormones released from the neurohypophysis, can be viewed as having an additional important role in influencing the activity of central neurons through direct projections to those neurons.

9. ACKNOWLEDGMENTS

The author wishes to thank P. Campbell for editorial and B. Archer, A. Barclay and J. Lloyd for photographic assistance.

10. REFERENCES

Abe H, Inoue M, Matsuo T, Ogata N (1983): The effects of vasopressin on electrical activity in the guinea pig supraoptic nucleus in vitro. *J. Physiol. (London), 337*, 607–665.
Akmayev IG (1983): Role of hypothalamic circuitries in neuroendocrine regulations: hypothalamus–endocrine pancreas interactions, a new concept. *Acta Morphol. Hung., 31*, 137–158.
Antunes JL, Carmel PW, Zimmerman EA (1977): Projections from the paraventricular nucleus to the zona externa of the median eminence of the rhesus monkey: an immunohistochemical study. *Brain Res., 137*, 1–10.
Armstrong WE (1985): The supraoptic and paraventricular nuclei. In: Paxinos G, Watson C (Eds), *The Rat Nervous System*. Academic Press, Sydney. In press.
Armstrong WE, Hatton GI (1980): The localization of projection neurons in the rat hypothalamic paraventricular nucleus following vascular and neurohypophysial injections of HRP. *Brain Res. Bull., 5*, 473–477.
Armstrong WE, Warach S, Hatton GI, McNeill TH (1980): Subnuclei in the rat hypothalamic paraventricular nucleus: a cytoarchitectural, horseradish peroxidase and immunocytochemical analysis. *Neuroscience, 5*, 1931–1958.
Armstrong WE, Scholer J, McNeill TH (1982): Immunocytochemical, Golgi and electron microscopic characterization of putative dendrites in the ventral glial lamina of the rat supraoptic nucleus. *Neuroscience, 7*, 679–694.
Armstrong DM, Saper CB, Levey AI, Wainer BH, Terry RD (1983): Distribution of cholinergic neurons in rat brain: demonstrated by the immunocytochemical localization of choline acetyltransferase. *J. Comp. Neurol., 217*, 53–68.
Aspeslagh MR, Vandesande F, Dierickx K (1976): Electron microscopic immuno-cytochemical demonstration of separate neurophysin-vasopressinergic and neurophysin-oxytocinergic nerve fibres in the neural lobe of the rat hypophysis. *Cell Tissue Res., 171*, 31–37.
Barberis C (1983): [³H]Vasopressin binding to rat hippocampal synaptic plasma membrane. Kinetic and pharmacological characterization. *Fed. Eur. Biochem. Soc. Lett., 162*, 400–405.
Bargmann W (1949): Über die neurosekretorische Verknüpfung von Hypothalamus und Neurohypophyse. *Z. Zellforsch. Mikrosk. Anat., 34*, 610–634.
Bargmann W, Scharrer E (1951): The origin of the posterior pituitary hormones. *Am. Scientist, 39*, 255–259.

Barnard RR, Morris M (1982): Cerebrospinal fluid vasopressin and oxytocin: evidence for an osmotic response. *Neurosci. Lett., 29*, 275–279.

Baskin DG, Petracca F, Dorsa DM (1983): Autoradiographic localization of specific binding sites for [³H] [Arg⁸] vasopressin in the septum of the rat brain with tritium-sensitive film. *Eur. J. Pharmacol., 90*, 155–159.

Beaudet A, Descarries L (1978): The monoamine innervation of rat cerebral cortex: synaptic and nonsynaptic axon terminals. *Neuroscience, 3*, 851–860.

Beinfeld MC, Meyer DK, Brownstein MJ (1980): Cholecystokinin octapeptide in the rat hypothalamo-neurohypophysial system. *Nature (London), 288*, 376–378.

Berk ML, Finkelstein JA (1981): An autoradiographic determination of the efferent projections of the suprachiasmatic nucleus of the hypothalamus. *Brain Res., 226*, 1–13.

Berkowitz BA, Sherman S (1982): Characterization of vasopressin analgesia. *J. Pharmacol. Exp. Therap., 220*, 329–334.

Bernardini GL, Lipton JM, Clark WG (1983): Intracerebroventricular and septal injections of arginine vasopressin are not antipyretic in the rabbit. *Peptides, 4*, 195–198.

Berntson GG, Berson BS (1980): Antinociceptive effects of intraventricular or systemic administration of vasopressin in the rat. *Life Sci., 26*, 455–459.

Bicknell RJ, Leng G (1983): Differential regulation of oxytocin- and vasopressin-secreting nerve terminals. In: Cross BA, Leng G (Eds), *The Neurohypophysis: Structure, Function and Control. Progress in Brain Research, Vol. 60*, pp. 333–341. Elsevier, Amsterdam.

Bohus B, Kovacs GL, De Wied D (1978): Oxytocin, vasopressin and memory: opposite effects on consolidation and retrieval processes. *Brain Res., 157*, 414–417.

Bohus B, Versteeg CAM, De Jong W, Cransberg K, Kooy JG (1983): Neurohypophysial hormones and central cardiovascular control. In: Cross BA, Leng G (Eds), *The Neurohypophysis: Structure, Function and Control. Progress in Brain Research, Vol. 60*, pp. 445–458. Elsevier, Amsterdam.

Born J, Geenen V, Legros JJ (1982): Neurophysin II – but not neurophysin I – concentrations are higher in lumbar than in ventricular cerebro-spinal fluid in neurological patients. *Neuroendocrinol. Lett., 4*, 31–35.

Broadwell RD, Brightman MW (1976): Entry of peroxidase into neurons of the central and peripheral nervous systems from extracerebral and cerebral blood. *J. Comp. Neurol., 166*, 257–284.

Brooks DP, Share L, Crofton JT, Rockhold RW, Matsui K (1984): Effect of vertebral artery infusions of oxytocin on plasma vasopressin concentration, plasma renin activity, blood pressure and heart rate and their responses to hemorrhage. *Neuroendocrinology, 38*, 382–386.

Buijs RM (1978): Intra- and extrahypothalamic vasopressin and oxytocin pathways in the rat. Pathways to the limbic system, medulla oblongata, and spinal cord. *Cell Tissue Res., 192*, 423–435.

Buijs RM, Pevet P (1980): Vasopressin- and oxytocin-containing fibres in the pineal gland and subcommissural organ of the rat. *Cell Tissue Res., 205*, 11–17.

Buijs RM, Swaab DF (1980): Immuno-electron microscopical demonstration of vasopressin and oxytocin synapses in the limbic system of the rat. *Cell Tissue Res., 204*, 355–365.

Buijs RM, Van Heerikhuize JJ (1982): Vasopressin and oxytocin release in the brain – a synaptic event. *Brain Res., 252*, 71–76.

Buijs RM, Swaab DF, Dogterom J, Van Leeuwen FW (1978): Intra- and extrahypothalamic vasopressin and oxytocin pathways in the rat. *Cell Tissue Res., 186*, 423–433.

Burbach JPH, Lebouille JLM (1983): Proteolytic conversion of arginine-vasopressin and oxytocin by brain synaptic membranes. Characterization of formed peptides and mechanisms of proteolysis. *J. Biol. Chem., 258*, 1487–1494.

Burbach JPH, De Kloet ER, De Wied D (1980): Oxytocin biotransformation in the rat limbic brain: characterization of peptidase activities and significance in the formation of oxytocin fragments. *Brain Res., 202*, 401–414.

Burbach JPH, Bohus B, Kovacs GL, Van Nispen JW, Greven HM, De Wied D (1983a): Oxytocin is a precursor of potent behaviourally active neuropeptides. *Eur. J. Pharmacol., 94*, 125–131.

Burbach JPH, Kovacs GL, De Wied D, Van Nispen JW, Greven HM (1983b): A major metabolite of arginine vasopressin in the brain is a highly potent neuropeptide. *Science, 221*, 1310–1312.

Burnard DM, Pittman QJ, Veale WL (1983): Increased motor disturbances in response to arginine vasopressin following hemorrhage or hypertonic saline: evidence for central AVP release in rats. *Brain Res., 273*, 59–65.

Caffe AR, Van Leeuwen FW (1983): Vasopressin-immunoreactive cells in the dorsomedial hypothalamic region, medial amygdaloid nucleus and locus coeruleus of the rat. *Cell Tissue Res., 233*, 23–33.

Caffe AR, Van Leeuwen FW, Steinbusch HWM (1983): Co-localization of vasopressin, neurophysin and noradrenalin immunoreactivity in subpopulations of rat locus coeruleus and subcoeruleus. *Soc. Neurosci. Abstracts, 9*, 575.

153

Castel M, Gainer H, Dellman HD (1984): Neuronal secretory systems. *Int. Rev. Cytol., 88*, 303–458.

Chan-Palay V, Palay SL (Eds) (1984): *Coexistence of Neuroactive Substances in Neurons.* John Wiley, New York.

Chapman DB, Morris JF, Valtin H (1982): How do granules distribute between nerve endings and swellings in the neural lobe? Evidence from Brattleboro rats. In: Baertschi AJ, Dreifuss JJ (Eds), *Neuroendocrinology of Vasopressin, Corticoliberin and Opiomelanocortins*, pp. 1–10. Academic Press, New York.

Charpak S, Armstrong WE, Mühlethaler M, Dreifuss JJ (1984): Stimulatory action of oxytocin on neurones of the dorsal motor nucleus of the vagus nerve. *Brain Res., 300*, 83–89.

Church AC (1983): Vasopressin potentiates the stimulation of cyclic AMP accumulation by norepinephrine. *Peptides, 4*, 261–263.

Clark RG, Jones PM, Robinson ICAF (1983): Clearance of vasopressin from cerebrospinal fluid to blood in chronically cannulated Brattleboro rats. *Neuroendocrinology, 37*, 242–247.

Conrad LCA, Pfaff DW (1976): Efferents from medial basal forebrain and hypothalamus in the rat. II. An autoradiographic study of the anterior hypothalamus. *J. Comp. Neurol., 169*, 221–262.

Cooper KE, Kasting NW, Lederis K, Veale WL (1979): Evidence supporting a role for endogenous vasopressin in natural suppression of fever in the sheep. *J. Physiol. (London), 295*, 33–45.

Cornett LE, Dorsa DM (1985): Evidence for arginine[8] vasopressin receptor subtypes. *Endocrinology*, in press.

Courtney N, Raskind M (1983): Vasopressin affects adenylate cyclase activity in rat brain: a possible neuromodulator. *Life Sci., 32*, 591–596.

Cowley AW, Barber BJ (1983): Vasopressin vascular and reflex effects. In: Cross BA, Leng G (Eds), *The Neurohypophysis: Structure, Function and Control. Progress in Brain Research, Vol. 60*, pp. 415–424. Elsevier, Amsterdam.

Cowley AW, Merrill CD, Quillen DW, Skelton MM (1982): Vasopressin enhancement of carotid baroreceptor reflex sensitivity. *Fed. Proc., 41*, 1116.

Crofton JT, Share L, Shade RE, Lee-Kwon WJ, Manning M, Sawyer WH (1979): The importance of vasopressin in the development and maintenance of DOC-salt hypertension in the rat. *Hypertension, 1*, 31–38.

Cushing H, Goetsch E (1910): Concerning the secretion of the infundibular lobe of the pituitary body and its presence in the cerebrospinal fluid. *Am. J. Physiol., 27*, 60–86.

Dahlström A (1968): Effect of colchicine on transport of amine storage granules in sympathetic nerves of rat. *Eur. J. Pharmacol., 5*, 111–112.

Dahlström A, Fuxe K (1964): Evidence for the existence of monoamine-containing neurons in the central nervous system. I. Demonstration of monoamines in the cell bodies of brain stem neurons. *Acta Physiol. Scand., 62, Suppl. 232*, 1–55.

Delanoy RL, Kramarcy NR, Dunn AJ (1982): ACTH[1–24] and lysine vasopressin selectively activate dopamine synthesis in frontal cortex. *Brain Res., 231*, 117–129.

De Vries GJ, Buijs RM (1983): The origin of the vasopressinergic and oxytocinergic innervation of the rat brain with special reference to the lateral septum. *Brain Res., 273*, 307–317.

De Vries GJ, Buijs RM, Swaab DF (1981): Ontogeny of the vasopressinergic neurons of the suprachiasmatic nucleus and their extrahypothalamic projections in the rat brain – presence of a sex difference in the lateral septum. *Brain Res., 218*, 67–78.

De Vries GJ, Best W, Sluiter AA (1983): The influence of androgens on the development of a sex difference in the vasopressinergic innervation of the rat lateral septum. *Dev. Brain Res., 8*, 377–380.

De Vries GJ, Buijs RM, Sluiter AA (1984): Gonadal hormone actions on the morphology of the vasopressinergic innervation of the adult rat brain. *Brain Res., 298*, 141–145.

De Wied D (1983): Central actions of neurohypophysial hormones. In: Cross BA, Leng G (Eds), *The Neurohypophysis: Structure, Function and Control. Progress in Brain Research, Vol. 60*, pp. 155–168. Elsevier, Amsterdam.

De Wied D, Versteeg DHG (1979): Neurohypophyseal principles and memory. *Fed. Proc., 38*, 2348–2354.

Dierickx K, Vandesande F (1977): Immunocytochemical localization of the vasopressinergic and the oxytocinergic neurons in the human hypothalamus. *Cell Tissue Res., 184*, 15–27.

Dierickx K, Vandesande F (1979): Immunocytochemical localization of somatostatin-containing neurons in the rat hypothalamus. *Cell Tissue Res., 201*, 349–359.

Dierickx K, Vandesande F, De Mey J (1976): Identification in the external region of the rat median eminence, of separate neurophysin-vasopressin and neurophysin-oxytocin-containing nerve fibres. *Cell Tissue Res., 168*, 141–151.

Disturnal J, Pittman QJ, Veale WL, Lederis K (1984): Evoked release of arginine vasopressin from rabbit brain. *Proc. Can. Physiol. Soc.*, in press.

Dogterom J, Van Wimersma Greidanus TB, Swaab DF (1977): Evidence for the release of vasopressin and oxytocin into cerebrospinal fluid: measurements in plasma and CSF of intact and hypophysectomized rats. *Neuroendocrinology, 24*, 108–118.

Dogterom J, Snijdewint FGM, Buijs RM (1978a): The distribution of vasopressin and oxytocin in the rat brain. *Neurosci. Lett., 9*, 341–346.

Dogterom J, Van Wimersma Greidanus TB, De Wied D (1978b): Vasopressin in cerebrospinal fluid and plasma of man, dog, and rat. *Am. J. Physiol., 234*, E463–E467.

Dogterom J, Snijdewint FGM, Pevet P, Swaab DF (1980): Studies on the presence of vasopressin, oxytocin and vasotocin in the pineal gland, subcommissural organ and fetal pituitary gland: failure to demonstrate vasotocin in mammals. *J. Endocrinol., 84*, 115–123.

Doris PA (1984): Vasopressin and central integrative processes. *Neuroendocrinology, 38*, 75–85.

Dorsa DM, Bottemiller L (1982): Age-related changes of vasopressin content of microdissected areas of the rat brain. *Brain Res., 242*, 151–156.

Dorsa DM, Bottemiller LA (1983): Vasopressin-like peptides in the rat brain: immunologic and chromatographic behavior and their response to water deprivation. *Regul. Peptides, 6*, 393–403.

Dorsa DM, Majumdar LA, Petracca FM, Baskin DG, Cornett LE (1983): Characterization and localization of ^{3}H-arginine^8-vasopressin binding to rat kidney and brain tissue. *Peptides, 4*, 699–706.

Dorsa DM, Petracca FM, Baskin DG, Cornett LE (1984): Localization and characterization of vasopressin binding sites in the amygdala of the rat brain. *J. Neurosci., 4*, 1764–1770.

Dreifuss JJ (1975): A review on neurosecretory granules: their contents and mechanisms of release. *Ann. NY Acad. Sci., 248*, 184–201.

Dubois MP, Kolodziejczyk E (1975): Centres hypothalamiques du rat secrétant la somatostatine: répartition des péricaryons en 2 systèmes magno et parvocellulaires (étude immunocytologique). *C. R. Acad. Sci. (Paris), 281*, 1737–1740.

Dunn AJ, Steelman S, Delanoy R (1980): Intraventricular ACTH and vasopressin cause regionally specific changes in cerebral deoxyglucose uptake. *J. Neurosci. Res., 5*, 485–495.

Du Vigneaud V, Ressler C, Swan JM, Roberts CW, Katsoyannis PG, Gordon S (1953a): The synthesis of an octapeptide amide with the hormonal activity of oxytocin. *J. Am. Chem. Soc., 75*, 4879–4880.

Du Vigneaud V, Lawler HC, Popenoe EA (1953b): Enzymatic cleavage of glycinamide from vasopressin and a proposed structure for this pressor antidiuretic hormone of the posterior pituitary. *J. Am. Chem. Soc., 75*, 4880–4881.

Epstein Y, Castel M, Glick SM, Sivan N, Ravid R (1983): Changes in hypothalamic and extrahypothalamic vasopessin content of water-deprived rats. *Cell Tissue Res., 233*, 99–111.

Ferguson AV, Day TA, Renaud LP (1984): Connections of hypothalamic paraventricular neurons with the dorsal medial thalamus and neurohypophysis: an electrophysiological study in the rat. *Brain Res., 299*, 376–379.

Ferrier BM, Kennett DJ, Devlin MC (1980): Influence of oxytocin on human memory processes. *Life Sci., 27*, 2311–2317.

Ferris CF, Albers HE, Wesolowski SM, Goldman BD, Luman SE (1984): Vasopressin injected into the hypothalamus triggers a stereotypic behavior in golden hamsters. *Science, 224*, 521–523.

Feuerstein G, Zerbe RL, Ben-Ishay D, Kopin IJ, Jacobowitz DM (1981): Catecholamines and vasopressin in forebrain nuclei of hypertension prone and resistant rats. *Brain Res. Bull., 7*, 671–676.

Feuerstein G, Zerbe RL, Ben-Ishay D, Kopin IJ, Jacobowitz DM (1982): Catecholamines and vasopressin in hindbrain nuclei of hypertension prone and resistant rats. *Brain Res., 251*, 169–173.

Fields HL, Basbaum AI (1978): Brainstem control of spinal pain-transmission neurons. *Annu. Rev. Physiol., 40*, 217–248.

Fuxe K, Ganten D, Hökfelt T, Bolne P (1976): Immunohistochemical evidence for the existence of angiotensin II-containing nerve terminals in the brain and spinal cord of the rat. *Neurosci. Lett., 2*, 229–234.

Fuxe K, Agnati LF, Ganten D, Lang RE, Calza L, Poulsen K, Infantellina F (1982): Morphometric evaluation of the coexistence of renin-like and oxytocin-like immunoreactivity in nerve cells of the paraventricular hypothalamic nucleus of the rat. *Neurosci. Lett., 33*, 19–24.

Gainer H, Sarne Y, Brownstein MJ (1977): Biosynthesis and axonal transport of rat neurohypophysial proteins and peptides. *J. Cell Biol., 73*, 366–381.

Garcia H, Kaplan SL, Feigin RD (1981): Cerebrospinal fluid concentration of arginine vasopressin in children with bacterial meningitis. *J. Pediatr., 98*, 67–70.

Gardner CR, Richards MH, Möhring J (1984): Normotensive and spontaneously-hypertensive rats show differences in sensitivity to arginine-vasopressin as a modulator of noradrenaline release from brainstem slices. *Brain Res., 292*, 71–80.

Gauquelin G, Geelen G, Louis F, Allevard AM, Meunier C, Cuisinaud G, Benjanet S, Seidah NG, Chretien M, Legros JJ, Gharib C (1983): Presence of vasopressin, oxytocin and neurophysin in the retina of mammals, effect of light and darkness, comparison with the neuropeptide content of the neurohypophysis and the pineal gland. *Peptides, 4*, 509–515.

Gilbey MP, Coote JH, Fleetwood-Walker S, Peterson DF (1982): Influence of the paraventriculo-spinal pathway, and oxytocin and vasopressin on sympathetic preganglionic neurones. *Brain Res., 251*, 283–290.

Gillies G, Lowry P (1979): Corticotropin releasing factor may be modulated vasopressin. *Nature (London), 278*, 463–464.

Glick SM, Brownstein MJ (1980) Vasopressin content of rat brain. *Life Sci., 27*, 1103–1110.

Gold PW, Weingartner H, Ballenger JC, Goodwin FK, Post RM (1979): Effects of 1-desamino-8-D-arginine vasopressin on behaviour and cognition in primary affective disorder. *Lancet, 2*, 992–994.

Gold PW, Kaye W, Robertson GL, Ebert M (1983): Abnormalities in plasma and cerebrospinal fluid arginine vasopressin in patients with anorexia nervosa. *N. Engl. J. Med., 308*, 1117–1123.

Hammer M, Sorensen PS, Gjerris F, Larsen K (1982): Vasopressin in the cerebrospinal fluid of patients with normal pressure hydrocephalus and benign intracranial hypertension. *Acta Endocrinol. (Copenhagen), 110*, 211–215.

Hawthorn J, Ang VTY, Jenkins JS (1980): Localization of vasopressin in the rat brain. *Brain Res., 197*, 75–81.

Hayward JN (1977): Functional and morphological aspects of hypothalamic neurons. *Physiol. Rev., 57*, 574–658.

Hayward JN, Murgas K, Pavasuthipaisit K, Perez-Lopez FR, Sofroniew MV (1977): Temporal patterns of vasopressin release following electrical stimulation of the amygdala and the neuroendocrine pathway in the monkey. *Neuroendocrinology, 23*, 61–75.

Hendrickson AE, Wagoner N, Cowan WM (1972): An autoradiographic and electron miscroscopic study of retinohypothalamic connections. *Z. Anat. Entwicklungsgesch., 135*, 1–26.

Hoffman PL, Ritzmann RF, Walter R, Tabakoff B (1978): Arginine vasopressin maintains ethanol tolerance. *Nature (London), 276*, 614–616.

Hökfelt T, Johansson O, Ljungdahl A, Lundberg JM, Schultzberg M (1980): Peptidergic neurones. *Nature (London), 284*, 515–521.

Hoorneman EMD, Buijs RM (1982): Vasopressin fiber pathways in the rat brain following suprachiasmatic nucleus lesioning. *Brain Res., 243*, 235–241.

Hosoya Y, Matsushita M (1979): Identification and distribution of the spinal and hypophyseal projection neurons in the paraventricular nucleus of the rat. A light and electron microscopic study with the horseradish peroxidase method. *Exp. Brain Res., 35*, 315–331.

Houser CR, Crawford GD, Barber RP, Salvaterra PM, Vaughn JE (1983): Organization and morphological characteristics of cholinergic neurons: an immunocytochemical study with a monoclonal antibody to choline acetyltransferase. *Brain Res., 266*, 97–119.

Huston JP, Jakobartl L (1977): Evidence for selective susceptibility of hippocampus to spreading depression induced by vasopressin. *Neurosci. Lett., 6*, 69–72.

Jard S (1983): Vasopressin: mechanisms of receptor activation. In: Cross BA, Leng G (Eds), *The Neurohypophysis: Structure, Function and Control. Progress in Brain Research, Vol. 60*, pp. 383–394. Elsevier, Amsterdam.

Jenkins JS, Mather HM, Ang V (1980): Vasopressin in human cerebrospinal fluid. *J. Clin. Endocrinol. Metab., 50*, 364–367.

Jenkins JS, Ang VTY, Hawthorn J, Rossor MN, Iversen LL (1984): Vasopressin, oxytocin and neurophysins in the human brain and spinal cord. *Brain Res., 291*, 111–117.

Joels M, Urban IJA (1983): Arginine[8]-vasopressin enhances the excitatory responses induced in lateral septal neurons of the rat by excitatory amino acids and electrical stimulation of fimbria-fornix fibers. *Neurosci. Lett., Suppl. 14*, S184 (Abstr.).

Jones PM, Robinson ICAF (1982): Differential clearance of neurophysin and neurohypophysial peptides from the cerebrospinal fluid in conscious guinea pigs. *Neuroendocrinology, 34*, 297–302.

Jones PM, Robinson ICAF, Harris MC (1983): Release of oxytocin into blood and cerebrospinal fluid by electrical stimulation of the hypothalamus or neural lobe in the rat. *Neuroendocrinology, 37*, 454–458.

Kakidani H, Furutani Y, Takahashi H, Noda M, Morimoto Y, Hirose T, Asai M, Inayama S, Nakanishi S, Numa S (1982): Cloning and sequencing analysis of cDNA for porcine α-neo-endorphin/dynorphin precursor. *Nature (London), 298*, 245–249.

Kannan H, Yamashita H (1983): Electrophysiological study of paraventricular nucleus neurons projecting to the dorsomedial medulla and their response to baroreceptor stimulation in rats. *Brain Res., 279*, 31–40.

Kasting NW, Martin JB (1983): Changes in immunoreactive vasopressin concentrations in brain regions of the rat in response to endotoxin. *Brain Res., 258*, 127–132.

Kating NW, Veale WL, Cooper KE (1982): Vasopressin: a homeostatic effector in the febrile process. *Neurosci. Biobehav. Rev., 6*, 215–222.

Kawata M, Sano Y (1982): Immunohistochemical identification of the oxytocin and vasopressin neurons in the hypothalamus of the monkey *(Macaca fuscata)*. *Anat. Embryol., 165*, 151–167.

Kawata M, Sano Y, Inenaga K, Yamashita H (1983): Immunohistochemical identification of lucifer yellow-labeled neurons in the rat supraoptic nucleus. *Histochemistry, 78*, 21–26.

156

Kayser BEJ, Mühlethaler M, Dreifuss JJ (1982): Paraventricular neurones in the rat hypothalamic slice: lucifer yellow injection and immunocytochemical identification. *Experientia, 38,* 391.–393.

Kelly J, Swanson LW (1980): Additional forebrain regions projecting to the posterior pituitary: preoptic region, bed nucleus of the stria terminalis, and zona incerta. *Brain Res., 197,* 1–9.

Kilcoyne MM, Hoffman DL, Zimmerman EA (1980): Immunocytochemical localization of angiotensin II and vasopressin in rat hypothalamus: evidence for production in the same neuron. *Clin. Sci., 59,* 57s–60s.

Kiss JZ, Mezey E, Skirboll L (1984): Corticotropin-releasing factor – immunoreactive neurons of the paraventricular nucleus become vasopressin positive after adrenalectomy. *Proc. Natl Acad. Sci. USA, 81,* 1854–1858.

Koelle GB (1961): A proposed dual neurohumoral role of acetylcholine: its functions at the pre- and postsynaptic sites. *Nature (London), 190,* 208–211.

Koizumi K, Yamashita H (1978): Influence of atrial stretch receptors on hypothalamic neurosecretory neurones. *J. Physiol. (London), 285,* 341–358.

Koob GF, Bloom FE (1982): Behavioral effects of neuropeptides: endorphins and vasopressin. *Annu. Rev. Physiol., 44,* 571–582.

Krettek JE, Price JL (1977): Projections from the amygdaloid complex to the cerebral cortex and thalamus in the rat and cat. *J. Comp. Neurol., 172,* 687–722.

Kreutzberg G (1969): Neuronal dynamics and flow. IV. Blockage of intra-axonal enzyme transport by colchicine. *Proc. Natl Acad. Sci. USA, 62,* 722–728.

Kuypers HGJM, Maiskey VA (1975): Retrograde axonal transport of horseradish peroxidase from spinal cord to brain stem cell groups in the cat. *Neurosci. Lett., 1,* 9–14.

Land H, Schütz G, Schmale H, Richter D (1982): Nucleotide sequence of cloned cDNA encoding bovine arginine vasopressin-neurophysin II precursor. *Nature (London), 295,* 299–303.

Land H, Grez M, Ruppert S, Schmale H, Rehbein M, Richter D, Schütz G (1983): Deduced amino acid sequence from the bovine oxytocin-neurophysin I precursor cDNA. *Nature (London), 302,* 342–344.

Landgraf R, Ermisch A, Hess J (1979): Indications for a brain uptake of labelled vasopressin and oxytocin and the problem of the blood-brain barrier. *Endokrinologie, 73,* 77–81.

Lang RE, Rascher W, Unger T, Ganten D (1981): Reduced content of vasopressin in the brain of spontaneously hypertensive as compared to normotensive rats. *Neurosci. Lett., 23,* 199–202.

Lang RE, Ganten D, Hermann K, Unger T (1982): Distribution of neurophysins in rat brain: radioimmunological measurement and characterization. *Neurosci. Lett., 30,* 279–283.

Lang RE, Heil J, Ganten D, Hermann K, Rascher W, Unger T (1983): Effects of lesions in the paraventricular nucleus of the hypothalamus on vasopressin and oxytocin contents in brainstem and spinal cord of rat. *Brain Res., 260,* 326–329.

Leccese AP (1983): Drug-induced elevation of vasopressin-like immunoreactivity in raphe and septal regions of the mouse CNS. *Neuroendocrinology, 37,* 411.

Lechan RM, Nestler JL, Jacobson S, Reichlin S (1980): The hypothalamic 'tuberoinfundibular' system of the rat as demonstrated by horseradish peroxidase (HRP) microiontophoresis. *Brain Res., 195,* 13–27.

Legros JJ, Gilot P (1979): Vasopressin and memory in the human. In: Peck EJ Jr, Boyd AE III (Eds), *Brain Peptides: A New Endocrinology,* pp. 347–364. Elsevier, Amsterdam.

Legros JJ, Geenen V, Linkowski P, Mendlewicz J (1983): Increased neurophysin-I and neurophysin-II cerebrospinal fluid concentration from bipolar versus unipolar depressed patients. *Neuroendocrinol. Lett., 5,* 201–206.

Le Moal M, Koob GF, Koda LY, Bloom FE, Manning M, Sawyer WH, Rivier J (1981): Vasopressor receptor antagonist prevents behavioural effects of vasopressin. *Nature (London), 291,* 491–493.

Leng G, Mason WT, Dyer RG (1982): The supra-optic nucleus as an osmoreceptor. *Neuroendocrinology, 34,* 75–82.

Ljungdahl A, Hökfelt T, Nilsson G (1978): Distribution of substance P-like immunoreactivity in the central nervous system of the rat. I. Cell bodies and nerve terminals. *Neuroscience, 3,* 861–943.

Loewy AD, McKellar S (1980): The neuroanatomical basis of central cardiovascular control. *Fed. Proc., 39,* 2495–2503.

Luerssen TG, Robertson GL (1980): Cerebrospinal fluid vasopressin and vasotocin in health and disease. In: Wood JH (Ed.), *Neurobiology of Cerebrospinal Fluid, Vol. 1,* pp. 613–623. Plenum Press, New York.

Mai JK, Junger E (1977): Quantitative autoradiographic light- and electron microscopic studies on the retinohypothalamic connections in the rat. *Cell Tissue Res., 183,* 221–237.

Manning M, Sawyer WH (1983): Design of potent and selective in vivo antagonists of the neurohypophysial peptides. In: Cross BA, Leng G (Eds), *The Neurohypophysis: Structure, Function and Control. Progress in Brain Research, Vol. 60,* pp. 367–382. Elsevier, Amsterdam.

Manning M, Sawyer WH (1984): Design and uses of selective agonistic and antagonistic analogs of the neuropeptides oxytocin and vasopressin. *Trends Neurosci., 7,* 6–9.

157

Mason WT, Ho YW, Hatton GI (1984): Axon collaterals of supraoptic neurones: anatomical and electro-physiological evidence for their existence in the lateral hypothalamus. *Neuroscience, 11*, 169–182.

Meisenberg G, Simmons WH (1983): Centrally mediated effects of neurohypophyseal hormones. *Neurosci. Biobehav. Rev., 7*, 263–280.

Mens WBJ, Witter A, Van Wimersma Greidanus TB (1983): Penetration of neurohypophyseal hormones from plasma into cerebrospinal fluid (CSF): half-times of disappearance of these neuropeptides from CSF. *Brain Res., 262*, 143–149.

Merker G, Blähser S, Zeisberger E (1980): The reactivity pattern of vasopressin-containing neurons and its relation to the antipyretic reaction in the pregnant guinea pig. *Cell Tissue Res., 212*, 47–62.

Michell RH, Kirk CJ, Billah MM (1979): Hormonal stimulation of phosphatidylinositol breakdown, with par-ticular reference to the hepatic effects of vasopressin. *Biochem. Soc. Trans., 7*, 861–865.

Möhring J, Glänzer K, Maciel JA, Düsing R, Kramer HJ, Arbogast R, Koch-Weser J (1980a): Greatly en-hanced pressor response to antidiuretic hormone in patients with impaired cardiovascular reflexes due to idiopathic orthostatic hypotension. *J. Cardiovasc. Pharmacol., 2*, 367–376.

Möhring J, Schoun J, Kintz J, McNeill R (1980b): Decreased vasopressin content in brain stem of rats with spontaneous hypertension. *Naunyn-Schmiedeberg's Arch. Pharmacol., 315*, 83–84.

Moore RY, Eichler VB (1972): Loss of a circadian adrenal corticosterone rhythm following suprachiasmatic lesions in the rat. *Brain Res., 42*, 201–206.

Moore RY, Lenn NJ (1972): A retinohypothalamic projection in the rat. *J. Comp. Neurol., 146*, 1–14.

Morris JF (1976): Distribution of neurosecretory granules among the anatomical compartments of the neu-rosecretory processes of the pituitary gland: a quantitative ultrastructural approach to hormone storage in the neural lobe. *J. Endocrinol., 68*, 225–234.

Morris JF (1983): Organization of neural inputs to the supraoptic and paraventricular nuclei: anatomical as-pects. In: Cross BA, Leng G (Eds), *The Neurohypophysis: Structure, Function and Control. Progress in Brain Research, Vol. 60*, pp. 3–18. Elsevier, Amsterdam.

Morris JF, Nordmann JJ (1980): Membrane recapture after hormone release from nerve endings in the neural lobe of the rat pituitary gland. *Neuroscience, 5*, 639–649.

Morris JF, Nordmann JJ, Dyball REJ (1978): Structure–function correlation in mammalian neurosecretion. *Int. Rev. Exp. Pathol., 18*, 1–95.

Morris R, Salt T, Sofroniew MV, Hill RG (1980): Actions of microiontophoretically applied oxytocin, and immunohistochemical localization of oxytocin, vasopressin and neurophysin in the rat caudal medulla. *Neurosci. Lett., 18*, 163–168.

Morris R, Farmery SM, Roberts CJ, Hill RG (1984): The effects of oxytocin and vasotocin analogues, on the responses of rat brainstem neurones to oxytocin. *Neurosci. Lett., 48*, 161–166.

Mühlethaler M, Dreifuss JJ, Gähwiler BH (1982): Vasopressin excites hippocampal neurones. *Nature (Lon-don), 296*, 749–751.

Mühlethaler M, Sawyer WH, Manning MM, Dreifuss JJ (1983): Characterization of a uterine-type oxytocin receptor in the rat hippocampus. *Proc. Natl Acad. Sci. USA, 80*, 6713–6717.

Nakai M, Yamane Y, Umeda Y, Ogino K (1982): Vasopressin-induced pressor response elicited by electrical stimulation of solitary nucleus and dorsal motor nucleus of vagus of rat. *Brain Res., 251*, 164–168.

Nakano J (1974): Cardiovascular responses to neurohypophysial hormones. In: Greep RO, Astwood EB (Eds), *Handbook of Physiology, Section 7: Endocrinology, Vol. IV*, pp. 395–442. American Physiological Society, Washington DC.

Negro-Villar A, Sanchez-Franco F, Kwiatkowski M, Samson WK (1979): Failure to detect radioimmunoas-sayable arginine vasotocin in mammalian pineals. *Brain Res. Bull., 4*, 789–792.

Nilaver G, Zimmerman EA, Wilkins J, Michaels J, Hoffman D, Silverman AJ (1980): Magnocellular hypotha-lamic projections to the lower brain stem and spinal cord of the rat. Immunocytochemical evidence for predominance of the oxytocin-neurophysin system compared to the vasopressin-neurophysin system. *Neuroendocrinology, 30*, 150–158.

Nordmann JJ (1983): Stimulus-secretion coupling. In: Cross BA, Leng G (Eds), *The Neurohypophysis: Struc-ture, Function and Control. Progress in Brain Research, Vol. 60*, pp. 281–304. Elsevier, Amsterdam.

Oliver G, Schäfer EA (1895): On the physiological action of extracts of pituitary body and certain other glan-dular organs. *J. Physiol. (London), 18*, 277–279.

Olpe HR, Baltzer V (1981): Vasopressin activates noradrenergic neurons in the rat locus coeruleus: a micro-iontophoretic investigation. *Eur. J. Pharmacol., 73*, 377–378.

Ono T, Nishino H, Sasaka K, Muramoto K, Yano I, Simpson A (1978): Paraventricular nucleus connections to spinal cord and pituitary. *Neurosci. Lett., 10*, 141–146.

Palkovits M, Jacobowitz DM (1974): Topographic atlas of catecholamine and acetylcholinesterase-containing neurons in the rat brain. II. Hindbrain (mesencephalon, rhombencephalon). *J. Comp. Neurol., 157*, 29–42.

Palkovits M, Zaborszky L (1977): Neuroanatomy of central cardiovascular control. Nucleus tractus solitarii: afferent and efferent neuronal connections in relation to the baroreceptor reflex arc. In: De Jong W, Provoost AP, Shapiro AP (Eds), *Hypertension and Brain Mechanisms. Progress in Brain Research, Vol. 47*, pp. 9–34. Elsevier, Amsterdam.

Palkovits M, Zaborszky L, Ambach G (1974): Accessory neurosecretory cell groups in the rat hypothalamus. *Acta Morphol. Acad. Sci. Hung., 22*, 21–33.

Palkovits M, Mezey E, Zaborszky L (1979): Neuroanatomical evidences for direct neural connections between the brain stem baroreceptor centers and the forebrain areas involved in the neural regulation of the blood pressure. In: Meyer P, Schmitt H (Eds), *Nervous System and Hypertension*, pp. 18–30. Wiley/Flammarion, Paris.

Parry HB, Livett BG (1973): A new hypothalamic pathway to the median eminence containing neurophysin and its hypertrophy in sheep with natural scrapie. *Nature (London), 242*, 63–65.

Parry HB, Livett BG (1976): Neurophysin in the brain and pituitary gland of normal and scrapie-affected sheep. I. Its localization in the hypothalamus and neurohypophysis with particular reference to a new hypothalamic neurosecretory pathway to the median eminence. *Neuroscience, 1*, 275–299.

Parry HB, Livett BG (1977): Neurophysin in the brain and pituitary gland of normal and scrapie-affected sheep. II. Its occurrence in the cerebellum in dystrophic axon terminals with lysosome-lipofuscin accumulation: a possible anomaly of neuronal sulphur-protein metabolism. *Neuroscience, 2*, 53–72.

Pavel S (1971): Evidence for the ependymal origin of arginine vasotocin in the bovine pineal gland. *Endocrinology, 89*, 613–614.

Paxinos G, Watson C (1982): *The Rat Brain in Stereotaxic Coordinates.* Academic Press, Sydney.

Pedersen CA, Prange AJ (1979): Induction of maternal behavior in virgin rats after intracerebroventricular administration of oxytocin. *Proc. Natl Acad. Sci. USA, 76*, 6661–6665.

Pedersen CA, Ascher JA, Monroe YL, Prange AJ (1982): Oxytocin induces maternal behavior in virgin female rats. *Science, 216*, 648–649.

Perlow MJ, Reppert SM, Artman HA, Fisher DA, Seif SM, Robinson AG (1982): Oxytocin, vasopressin and estrogen-stimulated neurophysin: daily patterns of concentration in cerebrospinal fluid. *Science, 216*, 1416–1418.

Peterson RP (1966): Magnocellular neurosecretory centers in the rat hypothalamus. *J. Comp. Neurol., 128*, 181–190.

Peterson GM, Watkins WB, Moore RY (1980): The suprachiasmatic hypothalamic nuclei of the rat. VI. Vasopressin neurons and circadian rhythmicity. *Behav. Neural Biol., 29*, 236–245.

Petter H, Sterba G (1982): Immunocytochemical results indicating neuroendocrine effects on cardiovascular control mechanisms. In: Endroczi E (Ed.), *Neuropeptides and Psychosomatic Processes*, pp. 779–784. Akademiai Kiado, Budapest.

Pevet P, Reinharz AC, Dogterom J (1980): Neurophysins, vasopressin and oxytocin in the bovine pineal gland. *Neurosci. Lett., 16*, 301–306.

Phillipson OT, Gonzalez CB (1983): Distribution of axons showing neurophysin-like immunoreactivity in cortical and anterior basal forebrain sites. *Brain Res., 258*, 33–44.

Pickering BT (1976): The molecules of neurosecretion: their formation, transport, and release. In: Corner MA, Swaab DF (Eds), *Perspectives in Brain Research. Progress in Brain Research, Vol. 45*, pp. 161–179. Elsevier, Amsterdam.

Pittman QJ, Blume HW, Renaud LP (1981): Connections of the hypothalamic paraventricular nucleus with the neurohypophysis, median eminence, amygdala, lateral septum and midbrain periaqueductal gray: an electrophysiological study in the rat. *Brain Res., 215*, 15–28.

Pittman QJ, Lawrence D, McLean L (1982): Central effects of arginine vasopressin on blood pressure in rats. *Endocrinology, 110*, 1058–1060.

Pittman QJ, Riphagen CL, Lederis K (1984): Release of immunoassayable neurohypophyseal peptides from rat spinal cord, in vivo. *Brain Res., 300*, 321–326.

Poulain DA, Wakerley JB (1982): Electrophysiology of hypothalamic magnocellular neurones secreting oxytocin and vasopressin. *Neuroscience, 7*, 773–808.

Powley TL, Laughton W (1981): Neural pathways involved in the hypothalamic integration of autonomic responses. *Diabetologia, 20*, 378–387.

Ramon y Cajal S (1966): *Studies on the Diencephalon* (translated by Ramon-Moliner E), pp. 174–176. Charles C Thomas, Springfield, IL.

Reaves TA, Hayward JN (1979a): Immunocytochemical identification of vasopressinergic and oxytocinergic neurons in the hypothalamus of the cat. *Cell Tissue Res., 196*, 117–122.

Reaves TA, Hayward JN (1979b): Intracellular dye-marked enkephalin neurons in the magnocellular preoptic nucleus of the goldfish hypothalamus. *Proc. Natl Acad. Sci. USA, 76*, 6009–6011.

Reaves TA, Hayward JN (1980): Functional and morphological studies of peptide-containing neuroendocrine cells in goldfish hypothalamus. *J. Comp. Neurol., 193*, 777–788.

Reaves TA, Hou-Yu A, Zimmerman EA, Hayward JN (1983): Supraoptic neurons in the rat hypothalamo-neurohypophysial explant: double-labeling with lucifer yellow injection and immunocytochemical identification of vasopressin- and neurophysin-containing neuroendocrine cells. *Neurosci. Lett., 37*, 137–142.

Reinharz AC, Czernichow P, Vallotton MB (1974): Neurophysin-like protein in bovine pineal gland. *J. Endocrinol., 62*, 35–44.

Reppert SM, Artman HG, Swaminathan S, Fisher DA (1981): Vasopressin exhibits a rhythmic daily pattern in cerebrospinal fluid but not in blood. *Science, 213*, 1256–1257.

Reppert SM, Coleman RJ, Heath HW, Keutmann HT (1982): Circadian properties of vasopressin and melatonin rhythms in cat cerebrospinal fluid. *Am. J. Physiol., 243*, E489–E498.

Reppert SM, Schwartz WJ, Artman HG, Fisher DA (1983): Comparison of the temporal profiles of vasopressin and oxytocin in the cerebrospinal fluid of the cat, monkey and rat. *Brain Res., 261*, 341–345.

Rhodes CH, Morrell JI, Pfaff DW (1981): Immunohistochemical analysis of magnocellular elements in rat hypothalamus: distribution and numbers of cells containing neurophysin, oxytocin, and vasopressin. *J. Comp. Neurol., 198*, 45–64.

Riphagen CL, Pittman QJ (1983): Central action of arginine vasopressin on renal function. *Soc. Neurosci. Abstracts, 9*, 445.

Robinson AG, Zimmerman EA (1973): Cerebrospinal fluid and ependymal neurophysin. *J. Clin. Invest., 52*, 1260–1267.

Robinson ICAF (1983): Neurohypophysial peptides in cerebrospinal fluid. In: Cross BA, Leng G (Eds), *The Neurohypophysis: Structure, Function and Control. Progress in Brain Research, Vol. 60*, pp. 129–146. Elsevier, Amsterdam.

Robinson ICAF, Jones PM (1982): Oxytocin and neurophysin in plasma and CSF during suckling in the guinea pig. *Neuroendocrinology, 34*, 59–63.

Rossier J, Battenberg E, Pittman Q, Bayon A, Koda L, Miller R, Guillemin R, Bloom F (1979): Hypothalamic enkephalin neurones may regulate the neurohypophysis. *Nature (London), 277*, 653–655.

Rossor MN, Iversen LL, Hawthorn J, Ang VTY, Jenkins JS (1981): Extrahypothalamic vasopressin in human brain. *Brain Res., 214*, 349–355.

Roth KA, Weber E, Barchas JD (1982): Immunoreactive corticotropin releasing factor (CRF) and vasopressin are colocalized in a subpopulation of the immunoreactive vasopressin cells in the paraventricular nucleus of the hypothalamus. *Life Sci., 31*, 1857–1860.

Rusak B, Zucker I (1979): Neural regulation of circadian rhythms. *Physiol. Rev., 59*, 449–526.

Russell JT, Brownstein MJ, Gainer H (1980): Biosynthesis of vasopressin, oxytocin, and neurophysins: isolation and characterization of two common precursors (propressophysin and prooxyphysin). *Endocrinology, 107*, 1880–1891.

Ruwe WD, Naylor AM, Veale WL (1985): Perfusion of vasopressin within the rat brain suppresses prostaglandin E-hyperthermia. *Brain Res.*, in press.

Saper CB, Loewy AD, Swanson LW, Cowan WM (1976): Direct hypothalamo-autonomic connections. *Brain Res., 117*, 305–312.

Sar M, Stumpf WE, Miller RJ, Chang KJ, Cuatrecasas P (1978): Immunohistochemical localization of enkephalin in rat brain and spinal cord. *J. Comp. Neurol., 182*, 17–38.

Sawchenko PE, Swanson LW (1982): Immunohistochemical identification of neurons in the paraventricular nucleus of the hypothalamus that project to the medulla or to the spinal cord in the rat. *J. Comp. Neurol., 205*, 260–272.

Sawchenko PE, Swanson LW (1983): The organization of forebrain afferents to the paraventricular and supraoptic nuclei of the rat. *J. Comp. Neurol., 218*, 121–144.

Sawchenko PE, Swanson LW, Vale WW (1984a): Corticotropin releasing factor: co-expression within distinct subsets of oxytocin-, vasopressin-, and neurotensin-immunoreactive neurons in the hypothalamus of the male rat. *J. Neurosci., 4*, 1118–1129.

Sawchenko PE, Swanson LW, Vale WW (1984b): Co-expression of CRF- and vasopressin-immunoreactivity in parvocellular neurosecretory neurons of the adrenalectomized rat. *Proc. Natl Acad. Sci. USA, 81*, 1841–1845.

Sawyer WH, Grzonka Z, Manning M (1981) Neurohypophyseal peptides: designs of tissue-specific agonists and antagonists. *Mol. Cell. Endocrinol., 22*, 117–134.

Schmale H, Richter D (1984): Single base deletion in the vasopressin gene is the cause of diabetes insipidus in Brattleboro rats. *Nature (London), 308*, 705–709.

Schneider DR, Felt BT, Goltman H (1982): Desglycyl-8-arginine vasopressin affects regional mouse brain cyclic AMP content. *Pharmacol. Biochem. Behav., 16*, 139–143.

Schober F (1978): Darstellung der neurosekretorischen hypothalamorhombenzephalen Verbindung bei der Ratte durch retrograden axonalen Transport von Meerrettich-Peroxidase. *Acta Biol. Med. Ger., 37*, 165–167.

Schrell U, Sofroniew MV, Weindl A, Wetzstein R (1983): Analysis of vasopressin projections from the supra-chiasmatic nucleus using combined tracer and peptide immunohistochemistry. *Neurosci. Lett. Suppl. 14*, S334 (Abstr.).

Schwartz WJ, Coleman RJ, Reppert SM (1983): A daily vasopressin rhythm in rat cerebrospinal fluid. *Brain Res., 263*, 105–112.

Schwarzberg H, Hartmann G, Kovacs GL, Telegdy G (1976): Effect of intraventricular oxytocin and vaso-pressin on self-stimulation in rats. *Acta Physiol. Acad. Sci. Hung., 47*, 127–131.

Shaw FD, Dyball REJ, Nordmann JJ (1983): Mechanisms of inactivation of neurohypophysial hormone re-lease. In: Cross BA, Leng G (Eds), *The Neurohypophysis: Structure, Function and Control. Progress in Brain Research, Vol. 60*, pp. 305–317. Elsevier, Amsterdam.

Sherlock DA, Field PM, Raisman G (1975): Retrograde transport of horseradish peroxidase in the magnocel-lular neurosecretory system of the rat. *Brain Res., 88*, 403–414.

Silverman AJ, Zimmerman EA (1975): Ultrastructural immunocytochemical localization of neurophysin and vasopressin in the median eminence and posterior pituitary of the guinea pig. *Cell Tissue Res., 159*, 291–301.

Silverman AJ, Hoffman DL, Zimmerman EA (1981): The descending afferent connections of the paraventri-cular nucleus of the hypothalamus (PVN). *Brain Res. Bull., 6*, 47–61.

Sladek JR, Sladek CD (1983): Anatomical reciprocity between magnocellular peptides and noradrenaline in putative cardiovascular pathways. In: Cross BA, Leng G (Eds), *The Neurohypophysis: Structure, Func-tion and Control. Progress in Brain Research, Vol. 60*, pp. 437–444. Elsevier, Amsterdam.

Sodersten P, Henning M, Melin P, Ludin S (1983): Vasopressin alters female sexual behaviour by acting on the brain independently of alterations in blood pressure. *Nature (London), 301*, 608–610.

Sofroniew MV (1980): Projections from vasopressin, oxytocin and neurophysin neurons to neural targets in the rat and human. *J. Histochem. Cytochem., 28*, 475–478.

Sofroniew MV (1982): Vascular and neural projections of hypothalamic neurons producing neurohypophyseal or ACTH-related peptides. In: Baertschi AJ, Dreifuss JJ (Eds), *Neuroendocrinology of Vasopressin, Corti-coliberin and Opiomelanocortins*, pp. 73–86. Academic Press, New York.

Sofroniew MV (1983a): Golgi-like immunoperoxidase staining of neurons producing specific substances or of neurons transporting exogenous tracer proteins. In: Cuello AC (Ed), *Immunohistochemistry*, pp. 431–447. John Wiley, New York.

Sofroniew MV (1983b): Morphology of vasopressin and oxytocin neurones and their central and vascular projections. In: Cross BA, Leng G (Eds), *The Neurohypophysis: Structure, Function and Control. Progress in Brain Research, Vol. 60*, pp. 101–114. Elsevier, Amsterdam.

Sofroniew MV (1983c): Direct reciprocal connections between the bed nucleus of the stria terminalis and dor-somedial medulla oblongata: evidence from immunohistochemical detection of tracer proteins. *J. Comp. Neurol., 213*, 399–405.

Sofroniew MV (1983d): Vasopressin and oxytocin in the mammalian brain and spinal cord. *Trends Neurosci., 6*, 467–472.

Sofroniew MV (1985): Vasopressin- and neurophysin-immunoreactive neurons in the septal region, bed nucle-us of the stria terminalis, medial amygdala, posterior hypothalamus and locus coeruleus in colchicine-treated rats. *Neuroscience*, in press.

Sofroniew MV, Glasmann (1981): Golgi-like immunoperoxidase staining of hypothalamic magnocellular neu-rons that contain vasopressin, oxytocin or neurophysin in the rat. *Neuroscience, 6*, 619–643.

Sofroniew MV, Schrell U (1980): Hypothalamic neurons projecting to the rat caudal medulla oblongata, ex-amined by immunoperoxidase staining of retrogradely transported horseradish peroxidase. *Neurosci. Lett., 19*, 257–263.

Sofroniew MV, Schrell U (1981): Evidence for a direct projection from oxytocin and vasopressin neurons in the hypothalamic paraventricular nucleus to the medulla oblongata: immunohistochemical visualization of both the horseradish peroxidase transported and the peptide produced by the same neurons. *Neurosci. Lett., 22*, 211–217.

Sofroniew MV, Schrell U (1982): Long-term storage and regular repeated use of diluted antisera in glass stain-ing jars for increased sensitivity, reproducibility, and convenience of single- and two-color light micro-scopic immunocytochemistry. *J. Histochem. Cytochem., 30*, 504–511.

Sofroniew MV, Weindl A (1978a): Extrahypothalamic neurophysin-containing perikarya, fiber pathways and fiber clusters in the rat brain. *Endocrinology, 102*, 334–337.

Sofroniew MV, Weindl A (1978b): Projections from the parvocellular vasopressin- and neurophysin-contain-ing neurons of the suprachiasmatic nucleus. *Am. J. Anat., 153*, 391–430.

Sofroniew MV, Weindl A (1980): Identification of parvocellular vasopressin and neurophysin neurons in the suprachiasmatic nucleus of a variety of mammals including primates. *J. Comp. Neurol., 193*, 659–675.

Sofroniew MV, Weindl A (1981): Central nervous system distribution of vasopressin, oxytocin and neurophysin. In: Martinez JL, Jensen RA, Messing RB, Rigter H, McGaugh JL (Eds), *Endogenous Peptides and Learning and Memory Processes*, pp. 327–369. Academic Press, New York.

Sofroniew MV, Weindl A, Wetzstein R (1977): Immunoperoxidase staining of vasopressin in the rat median eminence following adrenalectomy and steroid substitution. *Acta Endocrinol. (Copenhagen), Suppl. 212*, 72 (Abstr.).

Sofroniew MV, Madler M, Müller OA, Scriba PC (1978): A method for the consistent production of high quality antisera to small peptide hormones. *Fresenius Z. Anal. Chem., 290*, 163.

Sofroniew MV, Weindl A, Schinko I, Wetzstein R (1979): The distribution of vasopressin-, oxytocin- and neurophysin-producing neurons in the guinea pig brain. I. The classical hypothalamo-neurohypophyseal system. *Cell Tissue Res., 196*, 367–384.

Sofroniew MV, Schrell U, Weindl A, Wetzstein R (1980): Hypothalamic accessory magnocellular vasopressin, oxytocin and neurophysin neurons projecting to the neurohypophysis in the rat. *Soc. Neurosci. Abstracts, 6*, 456.

Sofroniew MV, Weindl A, Schrell U, Wetzstein R (1981): Immunohistochemistry of vasopressin, oxytocin and neurophysin in the hypothalamus and extrahypothalamic regions of the human and primate brain. *Acta Histochem. Suppl. 24*, 79–95.

Sofroniew MV, Eckenstein F, Thoenen H, Cuello AC (1982a): Topography of choline acetyltransferase-containing neurons in the forebrain of the rat. *Neurosci. Lett., 33*, 7–12.

Sofroniew MV, Gähwiler BH, Dreifuss JJ (1982b): Cultured hypothalamic vasopressin (AVP), oxytocin (OT) and neurophysin (NPH) neurons examined by Golgi-like immunoperoxidase staining. *Neuroscience, 7, Suppl.*, S198–199 (Abstr.).

Sofroniew MV, Macmillan FM, Eckenstein F, Schrell U, Joh T, Gähwiler BH, Dreifuss JJ, Cuello AC (1983): Immunohistochemical approaches to the study of neuroendocrine and related neurones. *Q. J. Exp. Physiol., 68*, 435–447.

Sofroniew MV, Eckenstein F, Schrell U, Cuello AC (1984): Evidence for colocalization of neuroactive substances in hypothalamic neurons. In: Chan-Palay V, Palay S (Eds), *Coexistence of Neuroactive Substances in Neurons*, pp. 73–90. John Wiley, New York.

Sofroniew MV, Campbell PE, Cuello AC, Eckenstein F (1985): Central cholinergic neurons visualized by immunohistochemical detection of choline acetyltransferase. |In:| Paxinos G, Watson C (Eds), *The Rat Nervous System*. Academic Press, Sydney. In press.

Sokol HW, Zimmerman EA, Sawyer WH, Robinson AG (1976): The hypothalamic-neurohypophysial system of the rat: localization and quantitation of neurophysin by light microscopic immunocytochemistry in normal rats and in Brattleboro rats deficient in vasopressin and a neurophysin. *Endocrinology, 98*, 1176–1188.

Soloff MS, Schroeder BT, Chakraborty J, Pearlmutter AF (1977): Characterization of oxytocin receptors in the uterus and mammary gland. *Fed. Proc., 36*, 1861–1866.

Stephan FK, Zucker I (1974): Endocrine and neural mediation of the effects of constant light on water intake of rats. *Neuroendocrinology, 14*, 44–60.

Stephan FK, Berkley KJ, Moss RL (1981): Efferent connections of the rat suprachiasmatic nucleus. *Neuroscience, 6*, 2625–2641.

Sterba G, Naumann W, Hoheisel G (1980): Exohypothalamic axons of the classic neurosecretory system and their synapses. In: McConnell PS, Boer GJ, Romijn HJ, Van den Poll NE, Corner MA (Eds), *Adaptive Capabilities of the Nervous System. Progress in Brain Research, Vol. 53*, pp. 141–158. Elsevier, Amsterdam.

Sternberger LA (1979): *Immunocytochemistry*. John Wiley, New York.

Stillman MA, Recht LD, Rosario SL, Seif SM, Robinson AG, Zimmerman EA (1977): The effects of adrenalectomy and glucocorticoid replacement on vasopressin and vasopressin-neurophysin in the zona externa of the median eminence of the rat. *Endocrinology, 101*, 42–49.

Summy-Long JY, Keil LC, Hernandez L, Emmert S, Chee O, Severs WB (1984): Effects of dehydration and renin on vasopressin concentration in the subfornical organ area. *Brain Res., 300*, 219–229.

Swaab DF, Nijveldt F, Pool CW (1975): Distribution of oxytocin and vasopressin in the rat supraoptic and paraventricular nucleus. *J. Endocrinol., 67*, 461–462.

Swanson LW (1977): Immunohistochemical evidence for a neurophysin-containing autonomic pathway arising in the paraventricular nucleus of the hypothalamus. *Brain Res., 128*, 346–353.

Swanson LW, Cowan WM (1975): The efferent connections of the suprachiasmatic nucleus of the hypothalamus. *J. Comp. Neurol., 160*, 1–12.

Swanson LW, Kuypers HGJM (1980) The paraventricular nucleus of the hypothalamus: cytoarchitectonic subdivisions and organization of projections to the pituitary, dorsal vagal complex, and spinal cord as demonstrated by retrograde fluorescence double-labeling methods. *J. Comp. Neurol., 194*, 555–570.

Swanson LW, McKellar S (1979): The distribution of oxytocin- and neurophysin-stained fibers in the spinal cord of the rat and monkey. *J. Comp. Neurol., 188*, 87–106.

Swanson LW, Mogenson GJ (1981): Neural mechanisms for the function of autonomic, endocrine, and somatomotor responses in adaptive behavior. *Brain Res. Rev., 3*, 1–34.

Swanson LW, Sawchenko PE (1983): Hypothalamic integration: organization of the paraventricular and supraoptic nuclei. *Annu. Rev. Neurosci., 6*, 269–324.

Szczepanska-Sadowska E, Sobocinska J, Sadowski B (1982): Central dispogenic effect of vasopressin. *Am. J. Physiol., 242*, R372–R379.

Tager H, Hohenboken M, Markese J, Dinerstein RJ (1980): Identification and localization of glucagon-related peptides in rat brain. *Proc. Natl Acad. Sci. USA, 77*, 6229–6233.

Takhar APS, Kirk CJ (1981): Stimulation of inorganic phosphate incorporation into phosphatidylinositol in rat thoracic aorta mediated through V1-vasopressin receptors. *Biochem. J., 194*, 167–172.

Tanaka M, Versteeg DHG, De Wied D (1977): Regional effects of vasopressin on rat brain catecholamine metabolism. *Neurosci. Lett., 4*, 321–325.

Theodosis DT (1983): Intracellular membrane movements associated with hormone release in magnocellular neurones. In: Cross BA, Leng G (Eds), *The Neurohypophysis: Structure, Function and Control. Progress in Brain Research, Vol. 60*, pp. 273–279. Elsevier, Amsterdam.

Theodosis DT, Dreifuss JJ, Harris MC, Orci L (1976): Secretion-related uptake of horseradish peroxidase in neurohypophysial axons. *J. Cell Biol., 70*, 294–303.

Theodosis DT, Legendre P, Vincent JD, Cooke I (1983): Immunocytochemically identified vasopressin neurons in culture show slow, calcium-dependent electrical responses. *Science, 221*, 1052–1054.

Thomson AM (1982): Responses of supraoptic neurones to electrical stimulation of the medial amygdaloid nucleus. *Neuroscience, 7*, 2197–2205.

Tindal JS, Knaggs GS, Turvey A (1967): The afferent path of the milk-ejection reflex in the brain of the guinea pig. *J. Endocrinol., 38*, 337–349.

Tindal JS, Knaggs GS, Turvey A (1968): Preferential release of oxytocin from the neurohypophysis after electrical stimulation of the afferent path of the milk-ejection reflex in the brain of the guinea pig. *J. Endocrinol., 40*, 205–214.

Tramu G, Croix C, Pillez A (1983): Ability of the CRF immunoreactive neurons of the paraventricular nucleus to produce a vasopressin-like material. *Neuroendocrinology, 37*, 467–469.

Tribollet E, Dreifuss JJ (1981) Localization of neurones projecting to the hypothalamic paraventricular nucleus area of the rat: a horseradish peroxidase study. *Neuroscience, 6*, 1315–1328.

Tweedle CD (1983): Ultrastructural manifestations of increased hormone release in the neurohypophysis. In: Cross BA, Leng G (Eds), *The Neurohypophysis: Structure, Function and Control. Progress in Brain Research, Vol. 60*, pp. 259–272. Elsevier, Amsterdam.

Unger H, Pommrich G, Beck R (1971): Oxytocin contents in pathological cerebrospinal fluid in man. *Experientia, 27*, 1486.

Valtin H, Stewart J, Sokol HW (1974): Genetic control of the production of posterior pituitary principles. In: Greep RO, Astwood EB (Eds), *Handbook of Physiology, Section 7: Endocrinology, Vol. IV*, pp. 131–171. American Physiological Society, Washington DC.

Van Bogaert A, Mees U, De Schepper J (1980): Influence de l'excitation du noyau paraventriculaire hypothalamique sur les caractéristiques électriques et contractiles du myocarde chez le chien. *Arch. Mal. Coeur, 73*, 1179–1184.

Van den Pol AN (1980): The hypothalamic suprachiasmatic nucleus of rat: intrinsic anatomy. *J. Comp. Neurol., 191*, 661–702.

Van den Pol AN (1982): The magnocellular and parvocellular paraventricular nucleus of rat: intrinsic organization. *J. Comp. Neurol., 206*, 317–345.

Van den Pol AN, Powley T (1979): A fine-grained anatomical analysis of the role of the rat suprachiasmatic nucleus in circadian rhythms of feeding and drinking. *Brain Res., 160*, 307–326.

Vanderhaeghen JJ, Lotstra F, De Mey J, Gilles C (1980): Immunohistochemical localization of cholecystokinin and gastrin-like peptide in the brain and hypophysis of the rat. *Proc. Natl Acad. Sci. USA, 77*, 1190–1194.

Vanderhaeghen JJ, Lotstra F, Vandesande F, Dierickx K (1981): Coexistence of cholecystokinin and oxytocin-neurophysin in some magnocellular hypothalamo-hypophyseal neurons. *Cell Tissue Res., 221*, 227–231.

Vanderhaeghen JJ, Lotstra F, Liston DR, Rossier J (1983): Proenkephalin, [Met]enkephalin, and oxytocin immunoreactivities are colocalized in bovine hypothalamic magnocellular neurons. *Proc. Natl Acad. Sci. USA, 80*, 5139–5143.

Vandesande F, Dierickx K (1975): Identification of the vasopressin producing and of the oxytocin producing neurons in the hypothalamic magnocellular neurosecretory system of the rat. *Cell Tissue Res., 164*, 153–162.

Vandesande F, Dierickx K (1976): Immuno-cytochemical demonstration of the inability of the homozygous

Brattleboro rat to synthesize vasopressin and vasopressin-associated neurophysin. *Cell Tissue Res., 165,* 307–316.

Vandesande F, Dierickx K, De Mey J (1975a): Identification of the vasopressin-neurophysin II and the oxyto-cin-neurophysin I producing neurons in the bovine hypothalamus. *Cell Tissue Res., 156,* 189–200.

Vandesande F, Dierickx K, De Mey J (1975b): Identification of the vasopressin-neurophysin producing neu-rons of the rat suprachiasmatic nuclei. *Cell Tissue Res., 156,* 377–380.

Vandesande F, Dierickx K, De Mey J (1977): The origin of the vasopressinergic and oxytocinergic fibres of the external region of the median eminence of the rat hypophysis. *Cell Tissue Res., 180,* 443–452.

Van Leeuwen F, Caffe AR (1983): Vasopressin-immunoreactive cell bodies in the bed nucleus of the stria terminalis of the rat. *Cell Tissue Res., 228,* 525–536.

Van Leeuwen F, Swaab DF (1977): Specific immunoelectronmicroscopic localization of vasopressin and oxy-tocin in the neurohypophysis of the rat. *Cell Tissue Res., 177,* 493–501.

Van Leeuwen F, Wolters P (1983): Light microscopic autoradiographic localization of [^{3}H]arginine-vasopres-sin binding sites in the rat brain and kidney. *Neurosci. Lett., 41,* 61–66.

Van Leeuwen F, Swaab DF, De Raay C (1978): Immunoelectronmicroscopic localization of vasopressin in the rat suprachiasmatic nucleus. *Cell Tissue Res., 193,* 1–10.

Van Ree JM, De Wied D (1981): Vasopressin, oxytocin and dependence on opiates. In: Martinez JL, Jensen RA, Messing RB, Rigter H, McGaugh JL (Eds), *Endogenous Peptides and Learning and Memory Proces-ses,* pp. 397–411. Academic Press, New York.

Van Wimersma Greidanus TB, Bohus B, De Wied D (1981): Vasopressin and oxytocin in learning and memo-ry. In: Martinez JL, Jensen RA, Messing RB, Rigter H, McGaugh JL (Eds), *Endogenous Peptides and Learning and Memory Processes,* pp. 413–427. Academic Press, New York.

Versteeg DHG, Tanaka M, De Kloet ER (1978): Catecholamine concentration and turnover in discrete re-gions of the brain of the homozygous Brattleboro rat deficient in vasopressin. *Endocrinology, 103,* 1654–1661.

Versteeg DHG, De Kloet ER, Van Wimersma Greidanus T, De Wied D (1979): Vasopressin modulates the activity of catecholamine containing neurons in specific brain regions. *Neurosci. Lett., 11,* 69–73.

Versteeg CAM, Cransberg K, De Jong W, Bohus B (1983): Reduction of a centrally induced pressor response by neurohypophyseal peptides: the involvement of lower brainstem mechanisms. *Eur. J. Pharmacol., 94,* 133–140.

Versteeg CAM, De Jong W, Bohus B (1984): Arginine^8-vasopressin inhibits centrally induced pressor respon-ses by involving hippocampal mechanisms. *Brain Res., 292,* 317–326.

Wang BC, Share L, Crofton JT (1982): Central infusion of vasopressin decreased plasma vasopressin concen-tration in dogs. *Am. J. Physiol., 243,* E365–E369.

Watson SJ, Akil H, Fischli W, Goldstein A, Zimmerman E, Nilaver G, Van Wimersma Greidanus TB (1982a): Dynorphin and vasopressin: common localization in magnocellular neurons. *Science, 216,* 85–87.

Watson SJ, Seidah NG, Chretien M (1982b): The carboxy terminus of the precursor to vasopressin and neu-rophysin: immunocytochemistry in rat brain. *Science, 217,* 853–855.

Weindl A, Sofroniew MV (1976): Demonstration of extrahypothalamic peptide secreting neurons. *Pharma-kopsychiatrie, 9,* 226–234.

Weindl A, Sofroniew MV (1978): Neurohormones and circumventricular organs. In: Scott DE, Kozlowski GP, Weindl A (Eds), *Brain–Endocrine Interaction. III. Neural Hormones and Reproduction,* pp. 117–137. Karger, Basel.

Weindl A, Sofroniew MV (1981): Relation of neuropeptides to mammalian circumventricular organs. In: Martin JB, Reichlin S, Bick KL (Eds), *Neurosecretion and Brain Peptides,* pp. 303–320. Raven Press, New York.

Weingartner H, Gold P, Ballenger JC, Smallberg SA, Summers R, Rubinow DR, Post RM, Goodwin FK (1981): Effects of vasopressin on human memory functions. *Science, 211,* 601–603.

Whitnall MH, Gainer H, Cox BM, Molineaux CJ (1983): Dynorphin-A-(1–8) is contained within vasopressin neurosecretory vesicles in rat pituitary. *Science, 222,* 1137–1139.

Wiegand SJ, Price JL (1980): Cells of origin of the afferent fibers to the median eminence in the rat. *J. Comp. Neurol., 192,* 1–19.

Yamashita H, Inenaga K, Kawata M, Sano Y (1983a): Phasically firing neurons in the supraoptic nucleus of the rat hypothalamus: immunocytochemical and electrophysiological studies. *Neurosci. Lett., 37,* 87–92.

Yamashita H, Kannan H, Inenaga K, Koizumi K (1983b): The role of neurones in the supraoptic and para-ventricular nuclei in cardiovascular control. In: Cross BA, Leng G (Eds), *The Neurohypophysis: Struc-ture, Function and Control. Progress in Brain Research, Vol. 60,* pp. 459–468. Elsevier, Amsterdam.

Yamashita H, Inenaga K, Koizumi K (1984): Possible projections from regions of paraventricular and su-praoptic nuclei to the spinal cord: electrophysiological studies. *Brain Res., 296,* 373–378.

Yates FE, Maran JW (1974): Stimulation and inhibition of adrenocorticotropin release. In: Greep RO, Astwood EB (Eds), *Handbook of Physiology, Section 7: Endocrinology, Vol. IV*, pp. 367–404. American Physiological Society, Washington DC.

Zerbe RL, Palkovits M (1984): Changes in the vasopressin content of discrete brain regions in response to stimuli for vasopressin secretion. *Neuroendocrinology, 38*, 285–289.

Zerbe RL, Kirtland S, Faden AI, Feuerstein G (1983): Central cardiovascular effects of mammalian neurohypophyseal peptides in conscious rats. *Peptides, 4*, 627–630.

Zerihun L, Harris M (1981): Electrophysiological identification of neurones of paraventricular nucleus sending axons to both the neurohypophysis and the medulla in the rat. *Neurosci. Lett., 23*, 157–160.

Zimmerman EA, Carmel PW, Husain MK, Ferin M, Tannenbaum M, Frantz AG, Robinson AG (1973): Vasopressin and neurophysin: high concentrations in monkey hypophyseal portal blood. *Science, 182*, 925–927.

CHAPTER IV

LHRH-containing systems

J. BARRY, G.E. HOFFMAN AND S. WRAY

1. INTRODUCTION

1.1. LHRH IMMUNOCYTOCHEMISTRY

The purification of luteinizing hormone-releasing hormone (LHRH), the determination of its chemical formula (Amos et al. 1971; Schally et al. 1971) and its synthesis (Matsuo et al. 1971; Monahan et al. 1971; Sievertsson et al. 1971) have enabled the preparation of specific anti-LHRH sera and the immunocytochemical study of LHRH-containing neurons: for reviews, see Barry (1979b), Krisch (1980a), Knigge et al. (1980) and Hoffman (1983).

LHRH decapeptide (pyroGlu-His-Trp-Ser-Tyr-Gly-Leu-Arg-Pro-Gly.NH_2) is poorly antigenic and has been generally coupled with carrier proteins or adsorbed on various substrates (Al_2O_3, polyvinylpyrrolidone (PVP)) to form effective immunogenic complexes (see Table 1). For the preparation of immunosera, their purification (gammaglobulin isolation, saturation or removal of antibodies to carrier proteins), the details of the immunocytochemical procedures used (fluorescein-labeled antibody technique; peroxidase-labeled antibody technique; peroxidase-antiperoxidase (PAP) technique), their advantages, pitfalls and criteria of specificity refer to *Volume 2* of This Series.

From 1973 to 1979 most of the studies on LHRH neurons were performed on tissues prepared according to classical histological techniques, with acidic fixatives and paraffin embedding (Barry 1979b). Under these conditions there was a noticeable loss of tissue LHRH (Goldsmith and Ganong 1975) particularly during acidic fixation, alcohol dehydration and paraffin embedding (Hoffman et al. 1978a; Joseph et al. 1981) and in all vertebrates investigated, it was easier to characterize LHRH terminals than preterminal fibers and LHRH fibers than LHRH perikarya (Barry 1979b; Hoffman et al. 1978b; Nozaki and Kobayashi 1979). It was first supposed by Barry et al. (1973a,b) that this may be due to insufficient perikaryal concentration, to proximal concealment of LHRH through intracellular bonding, or synthesis in the form of non-reactive prohormone, as shown later by Millar et al. (1977), or even (a very remote possibility, now thought to be unlikely) to axonal synthesis. Some improvement in cell localization in the guinea pig was observed after castration and colchicine treatment (Barry et al. 1973a,b) or injection with serotonin (Léonardelli et al. 1974), melatonin (Barry et al. 1974), or sulpiride (NH_2SO_2 benzamide) (Léonardelli et al. 1978). There was variable success of these same treatments in other species (Baker et al. 1975; Flerkó et al. 1978; Goldsmith and Ganong 1975; King and Gerall 1976; King et al. 1974; Kordon et al. 1974; Léonardelli et al. 1973a; Sétáló et al. 1975, 1976a). A few years later it was shown that in some species (mouse, rat, pheasant), only Arimura's 743 antiserum detected perikaryal LHRH

Handbook of Chemical Neuroanatomy. Vol. 4: GABA and Neuropeptides in the CNS, Part I.
A. Björklund and T. Hökfelt, editors.
© Elsevier Science Publishers B.V., 1985.

TABLE 1. *Main anti-synthetic LHRH sera*

Authors	Immunogens	References
Dubois	LHRH(His[2]?)-HSA	Barry et al. (1973a), Dubois (1976)
Kerdelhué	LHRH(His[2]?)-guinea pig Ig	Calas et al. (1974), Kordon et al. (1974)
Kerdelhué	LHRH adsorbed on Al$_2$O$_3$	Kerdelhué et al. (1973)
Arimura(710)	LHRH(Gly[10])-BSA	Arimura et al. (1975), Sétáló et al. (1975)
Arimura(743,744)	LHRH(Glu[1])-HSA	Arimura et al. (1975), Sétáló et al. (1976a)
Arimura(442)	LHRH adsorbed on PVP	Barry and Carette (1975a,b)
Niswender(38)	LHRH(Tyr[5])-BSA	Zimmerman et al. (1974)
Nett, Niswender(42)	LHRH(His[2],Tyr[5])-BSA	Nett et al. (1973), McNeill et al. (1976)
Sternberger(B)	LHRH(Tyr[5])-HRP	Alpert et al. (1975), Knigge et al. (1978)
Alpert	LHRH-TGB	Alpert et al. (1976)
Baker, Dermody(154)	LHRH-limpet hemocyanin	Baker and Dermody (1976)
Barry(21,22)	LHRH adsorbed on PVP	Barry (1976a)
Sorrentino(E,F)	LHRH(His[2],Tyr[5])-BSA	Hoffman et al. (1978b)
Barry(44)	LHRH(His[2]?)-BSA	Barry (1980a), Jennes and Stumpf (1980b), Münz et al. (1981)

HSA, human serum albumin. Ig, immunoglobulin. BSA, bovine serum albumin. PVP, polyvinylpyrrolidone.

(King et al. 1974; Knigge et al. 1980) and that other anti-LHRH sera were not able to characterize the prohormonal form (Hoffman et al. 1978a; King et al. 1978). This pattern of cell reactivity led to labeling the LHRH cells as 'narrowly reactive' (Hoffman et al. 1978b).

At the same time, a number of laboratories using Sorrentino 'F' antiserum thought to be specific for LHRH-like immunoreactivity described reactive perikarya (Type I of Hoffman et al. 1978a) in the arcuate nucleus of various species, including rat and mouse (Hoffman et al. 1978a; Knigge et al. 1978; Silverman 1976; Sternberger and Hoffman 1978). Some months later, Clayton and Hoffman (1979a) reported that this serum contains two populations of antibodies, one with anti-LHRH activity, the other having anti-ACTH(1–24) activity which was responsible for the characterization of Type I neurons. Upon re-evaluation, the arcuate nucleus was essentially devoid of LHRH cells.

Since 1979, the use of perfusion with neutral fixatives (as Zamboni's formaldehyde) and sectioning with cryostat or vibrating microtomes for unembedded tissues have enabled the demonstration of LHRH perikarya with most anti-LHRH sera even in untreated animals of species that were thought to have 'narrowly reacting' cells (Burchanowski et al. 1979; Burchanowski and Sternberger 1980; Hoffman and Gibbs 1982; Jennes and Stumpf 1980c; Joseph et al. 1981; Knigge et al. 1980; Witkin et al. 1982). Vibratome sections have revealed a greater quantity of reactive LHRH and fibers than paraffin-embedded sections in addition to increases in the number of cells stained (up to 800 in the golden hamster (Jennes and Stumpf 1980b), 1600 in the rat (Wray and Hoffman 1983) or 2400 in the baboon (Marshall and Goldsmith 1980)).

LHRH detected in the median eminence (ME) or the organum vasculosum laminae terminalis (OVLT) is chromatographically and biologically similar to synthetic LHRH (Samson et al. 1980). Perikaryal LHRH is probably incorporated into a 'big' prohormone (King et al. 1978; Millar et al. 1977) in the rat and is sensitive to hydrolysis by brain enzymes (King et al. 1978). Alternatively, LHRH may be present in protein-LHRH complexes which are dissociated by lowering the pH and re-associating at neutral pH (Shin and Howitt 1977). It seems that the C-terminus of hypothalamic LHRH provides affinity for hormone binding to various anti-LHRH antibodies (Piekut and Knigge 1981) and that binding of the prohormone or protein occurs at the N-terminal (Knigge et al. 1978).

Vertebrate gonadotrophin-releasing hormone (GnRH) displays some heterogeneity, particularly in birds where it is not chemically identical to synthetic LHRH (Hattori et al. 1980; Jackson 1971; King and Millar 1979). However, anti-LHRH sera generated against the synthetic peptide sequenced from pig hypothalamic specifically react with bird LHRH and can be used for its detection in avian brains as well as lower vertebrates.

2. THE ATLAS OF RAT LHRH

For preparation of the accompanying Atlas, the Vibratome technique was employed since it revealed the most LHRH cells (approximately 1600) in the adult rat (Wray and Hoffman 1983). Since the general patterns of LHRH immunoreactivity are not different in male and female animals, material from both sexes was used to collect data for the plates. Each plate was drawn from a 50-μm section matched to the level of the Atlas. The general lack of high density of LHRH cells and fibers led to the use of literal representation of cells and axons at each level. Except for the ME (Krisch 1980a; Silverman and Desnoyers 1976), OVLT (Krisch 1980a) amygdala (Krisch 1980a) and olfactory bulb (Phillips et al. 1980), LHRH axons have only been studied at the light microscopic level in the rat. Thus, it is not yet known whether synaptic contacts are present in many of the regions containing varicose LHRH axons. Therefore, all levels in which LHRH axons or cells are present are included in the Atlas, and no attempt is made do distinguish between axons coursing through a brain area and those making contact in that area.

The selectivity of the immunoreactive structures was determined by use of the standard absorption test. Synthetic LHRH in concentrations of 0.5–1.0 μg/ml of diluted antisera was added to the anti-LHRH antibody just prior to incubation of the serum with the tissue. Staining of all structures bearing LHRH-like immunoreactivity was *completely* blocked by this procedure. Furthermore, the LHRH patterns were identical when different LHRH antibodies were used.

Atlas of the rat LHRH.
For abbreviations, see the General Abbreviations List, p. 609.

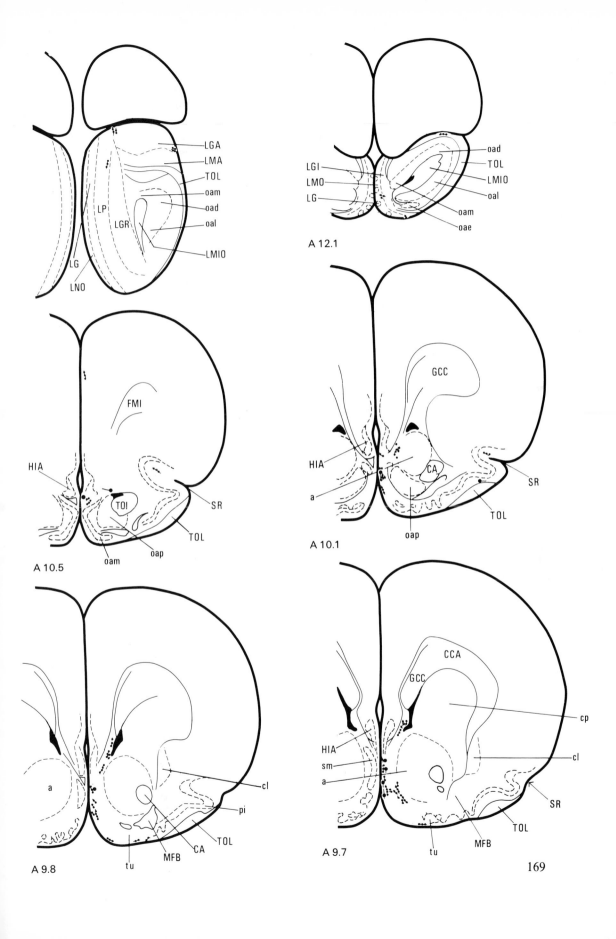

A 12.1

A 10.5

A 10.1

A 9.8

A 9.7

169

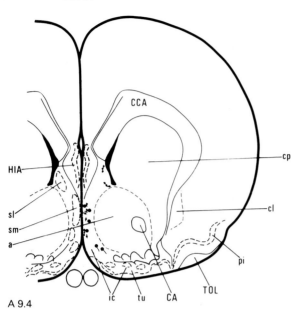

A 9.4

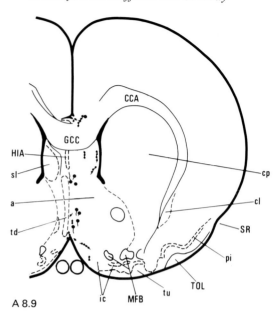

A 8.9

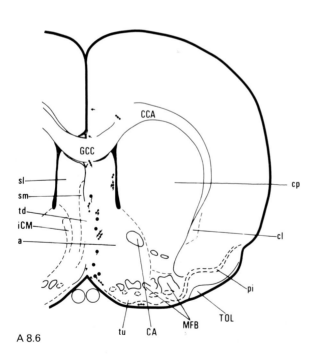

A 8.6

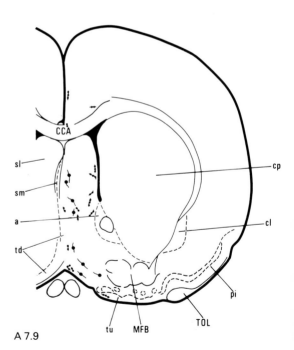

A 7.9

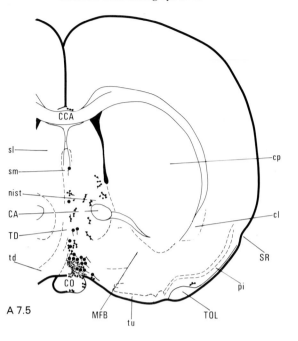

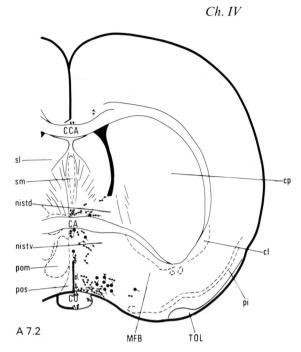

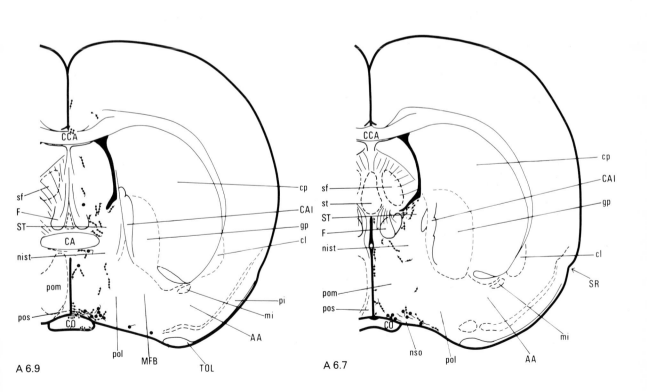

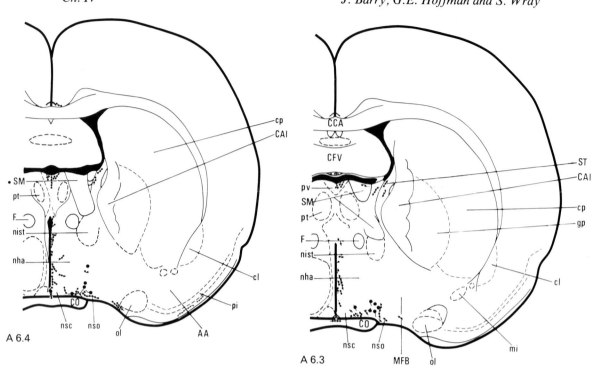

A 6.4

A 6.3

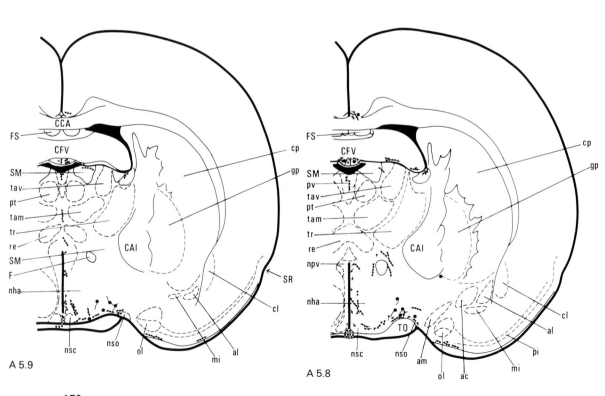

A 5.9

A 5.8

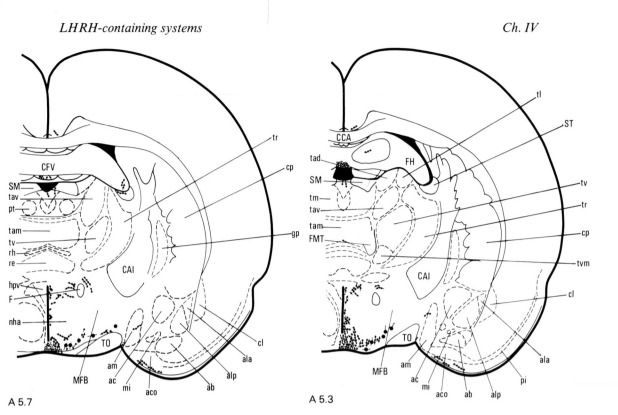

A 5.7

A 5.3

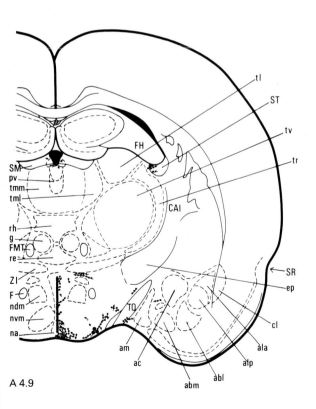

A 4.9

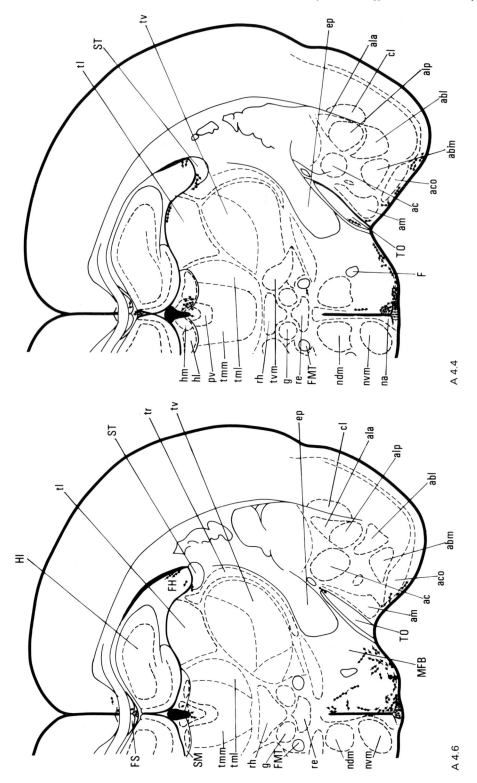

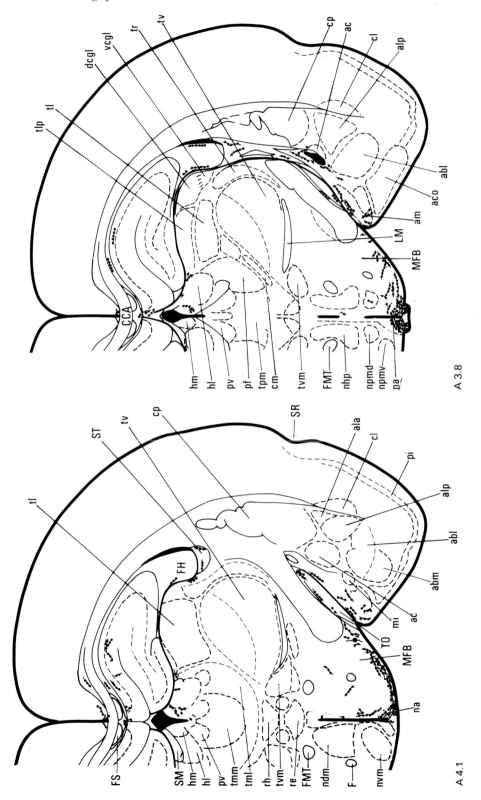

A 3.8

A 4.1

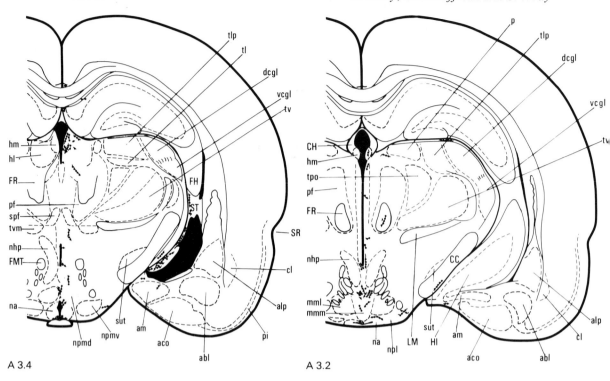

A 3.4

A 3.2

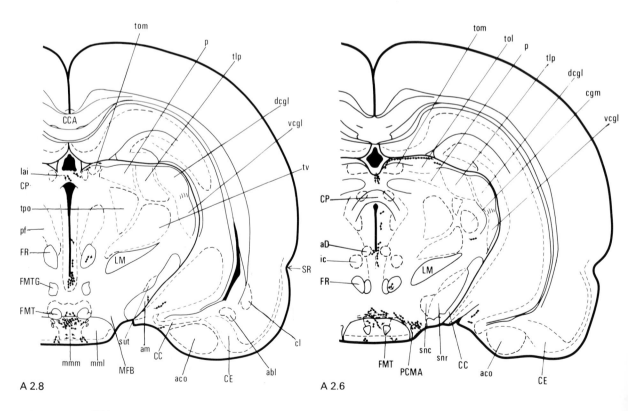

A 2.8

A 2.6

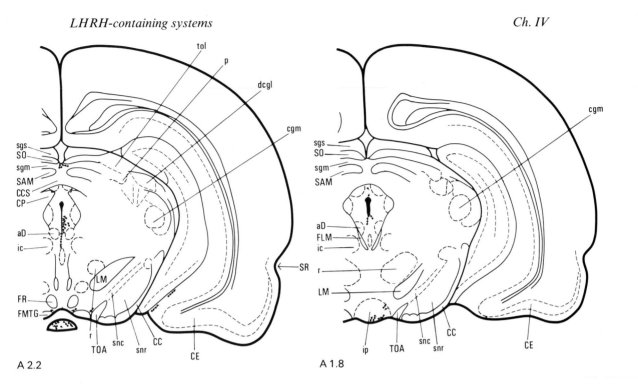

A 2.2

A 1.8

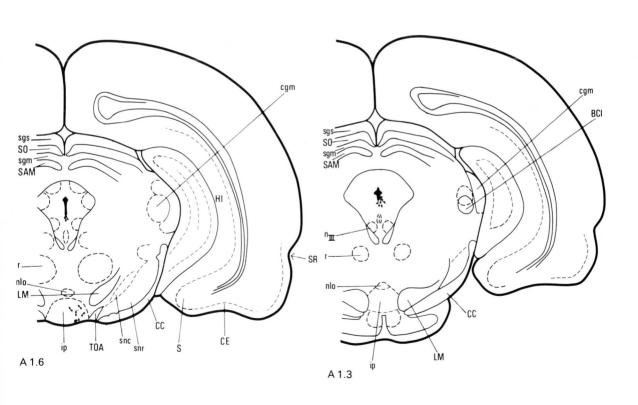

A 1.6

A 1.3

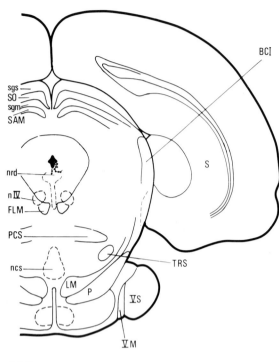

A 0.6

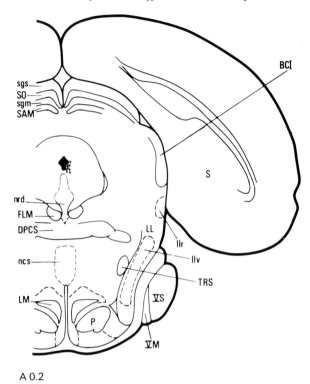

A 0.2

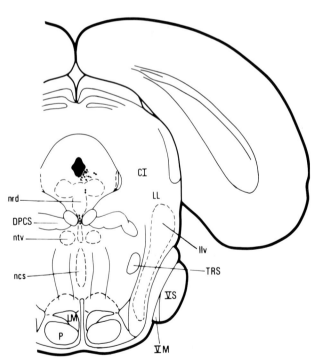

P 0.1

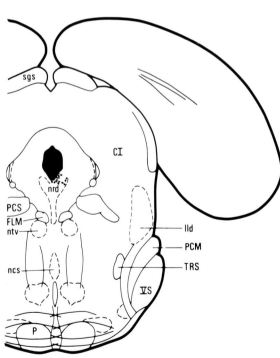

P 0.5

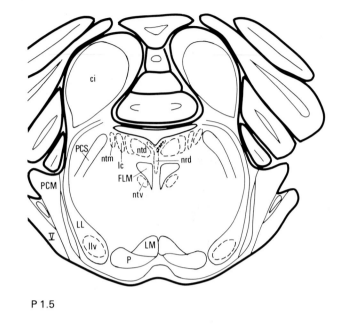

P 1.5

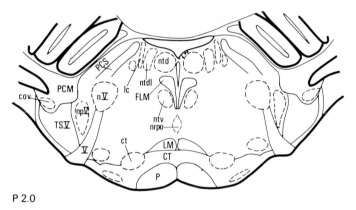

P 2.0

3. LHRH CELLS

3.1. MORPHOLOGY OF REACTIVE LHRH PERIKARYA

For reasons discussed in the first section, the characterization of reactive LHRH perikarya was difficult and controversial, particularly between 1973 and 1978 with some additional confusion resulting from the use of Sorrentino 'F' antiserum.

Mammals

LHRH perikarya were first observed in mammalian species having 'broadly reacting'
cells as determined in paraffin sections (i.e. the cells could be stained with many of the
available LHRH antisera): guinea pig (Barry et al. 1973a,b); cat and dog (Barry and

Dubois 1975); rabbit (Barry 1976a; Flerkó et al. 1978; Hoffman et al. 1978b); Cercopithecus (Barry et al. 1975); *Cebus apella* (Barry and Carette 1975a,b); squirrel monkey (Barry and Carette 1975a,b; Mazzuca 1977); Rhesus monkey (Barry et al. 1975; Hoffman 1976; Zimmerman and Antunés 1976); and garden dormouse (Richoux and Dubois 1976). After many unsuccessful attempts LHRH perikarya were identified in the rat (Flerkó et al. 1978; Hoffman 1976; Hoffman and Gibbs 1982; King and Gerall 1976; Kozlowski and Hostetter 1978; Krisch 1978; Sétáló et al. 1975; Wilkes et al. 1979). Then, reactive perikarya were described in human fetuses (Bloch 1977; Bugnon et al. 1976, 1977b; Paulin et al. 1977) and adults (Barry 1976b, 1977); in the mouse (Hoffman 1976, Hoffman et al. 1978a, 1982); sheep (Barry 1980a; Dees et al. 1981b; Hoffman et al. 1978b); Galago and Tupia (Barry 1980a); hamster (Hoffman 1983; Jennes and Stumpf 1980b); baboon (Marshall and Goldsmith 1980); and pony (Dees et al. 1981a). In these species, the ability to detect perikarya can vary according to the technique, sex, physiological or experimental conditions. The cytoplasm is frequently finely granular with a non-reactive nucleus (Fig. 1). Their dimensions depend in part on the angle of section and the species: 10–30 μm in guinea pig, dog, rabbit, cat; 20–40 μm in primates and man; 10–15 μm in rat. The shape of the perikarion is generally fusiform, oval or round, smooth-contoured, rarely tri- or tetrapolar. In the rat, at least, more sensitive techniques have revealed the presence of spine-like processes on 60–70% of the neurons (Wray and Hoffman 1982). The dendrites, one or two, rarely more, are slightly branched if at all. Some dendrites can be followed for 2000 μm or more as is seen in Vibratome sections of murine brains (Bennett-Clarke and Joseph 1982; Burchanowski et al. 1979; Hoffman 1983; Hoffman and Gibbs 1982) and monkey brains (Marshall and Goldsmith 1980) where processes can be traced for 200–500 μm (even in paraffin sections) and where only 4–5% of the cells are tripolar. In thick Vibratome sections and under favorable conditions in paraffin sections the emergence of the axon from the cell body or the base of a dendrite can be observed and it is possible to follow its course.

Birds

In birds, reactive perikarya have been found in the mallard duck (Bons et al. 1977, 1978a,b; McNeill et al. 1976; Oksche 1978); chicken and pheasant (Hoffman et al. 1978a); Japanese quail (Oksche 1978); and domestic hen (Sterling and Sharp 1982).

Reptiles and amphibians

In reptiles, reactive perikarya have been found only in the snake *Elaphe climacophora* (Nozaki and Kobayashi 1979). LHRH cells have been characterized in several amphibian species: toad (Doer-Scott and Dubois 1975); Xenopus (Doer-Scott and Dubois 1976; Nozaki and Kobayashi 1979); *Rana catesbeiana* and *Cynopus pyrrhogaster ensicauda* (Nozaki and Kobayashi 1979).

Fig. 1. LHRH perikarya in mammals. A. *Cebus apella,* MBH, × 350. B. Dog, AHA. C. Dog, AN. D. Dog, APO. E. Squirrel monkey, OVLT. F. Guinea pig, AHA. G. Squirrel monkey, OVLT. B–F × 900. a: axon; d: dendrite. (Barry, personal documents.) H. Human fetus, 24 weeks old. Electron microscopy of glutaraldehyde fixed hypothalamus. The same LHRH body identified by immunocytology (peroxidase-antiperoxidase complex) on a semi-thin section (insert) and stained with lead citrate and uranyl acetate on the adjacent thin section. (Reproduced from Bugnon et al. (1978), by courtesy of the Publisher.)

For abbreviations not explained in this Chapter, please see the General Abbreviations List on p. 609.

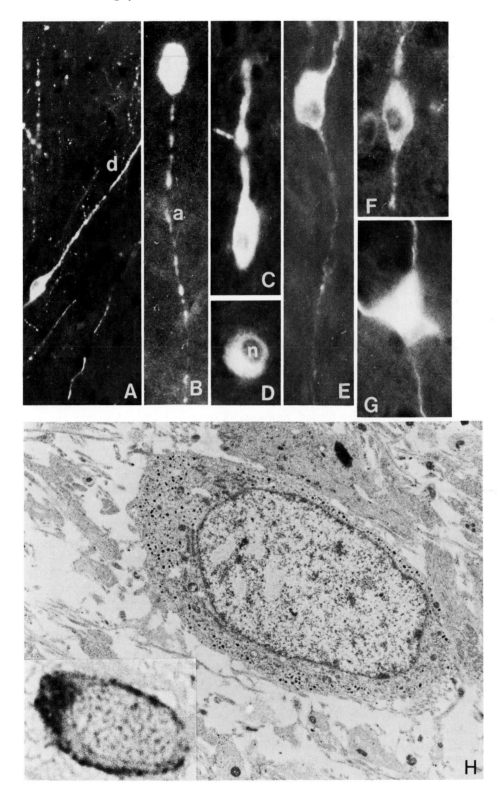

Fishes

In fishes, reactive perikarya have been detected in some species, chiefly: *Salmo gairdneri* (Goos and Murathanoglu 1977); *Xiphophorus maculatus* (Schreibman et al. 1979) and *Entosphenus japonica,* where reactive perikarya were detected with anti-Tyr-BSA-LHRH serum but not with anti-Gly[10]-BSA-LHRH serum (Nozaki and Kobayashi 1979).

Ultrastructure of LHRH cells

The electron microscopic studies of LHRH perikarya (Fig. 1H) have been chiefly performed in the rat (Hoffman 1983; Kozlowski et al. 1980; Krisch 1978, 1980a, b); man (Bugnon et al. 1977a, c); squirrel monkey (Mazzuca 1977) and baboon (Marshall and Goldsmith 1980). They have shown peripheral or scattered reactive granules (70–95 μm in rat, 90–130 μm in squirrel monkey) sometimes associated with dictyosomes, large flattened and parallel-oriented ergastoplasmic cisternae, often an invaginated nuclear membrane, a large nucleolus, microtubules and presynaptic endings. Many of these cells or their processes are in close contact with the basement membrane of brain capillaries in rodents (Hoffman 1983).

3.2. TOPOGRAPHY OF REACTIVE LHRH PERIKARYA

Mammalian

In rat, the topography of LHRH neurons at first was difficult to specify, for histological, histochemical, and antisera-related problems (Clarke 1977; Clayton and Hoffman 1979a; Hoffman and Gibbs 1982; Joseph et al. 1981; Knigge et al. 1978). However, these problems are now resolved. LHRH neurons are chiefly concentrated in the preoptic area (POA), septum (nucleus triangularis septi, medial septal nucleus), and anterior hypothalamic area (AHA), extending laterocaudally, through the medial forebrain bundle (MFB) up to the retrochiasmatic area (Bennett-Clarke and Joseph 1982; Elkind-Hirsch et al. 1981; Hoffman 1983; Hoffman and Gibbs 1982; Hoffman et al. 1978b; Ibata et al. 1979a; Kawano and Daikoku 1981; King et al. 1980; Krisch 1978, 1980b; Sétáló et al. 1976a) (Fig. 2). This topography is similar to that found in mouse (Clayton and Hoffman 1979b; Hoffman 1983; Hoffman et al. 1982) and hamster (Hoffman 1983; Jennes and Stumpf 1980b). Other illustrations can be found in the reviews of Barry (1979b, 1980a), Hoffman (1983), Knigge et al. (1980) and Nozaki and Kobayashi (1979).

In the guinea pig (Barry 1976b; Barry et al. 1973a,b), reactive perikarya are widely scattered in the septo-preoptic area (SPOA), anterior hypothalamic area (AHA), supra- and retrochiasmatic area and, sometimes, in the arcuate nucleus (AN) where they are always few in number but can be increased by 1-(metahydroxyphenyl)-2-aminopropanol tartrate or sodium dimethylthiocarbonate (Léonardelli and Dubois 1974). This topography was later confirmed by many investigators (Hoffman et al. 1978b; Nozaki and Kobayashi 1979; Sétáló et al. 1976a; Silverman 1976; Silverman and Desnoyers 1976; Silverman and Zimmerman 1978b; Weindl and Sofroniew 1978). Some perikarya are more easily observed in fetuses during the last days of fetal life and neonates (Barry and Dubois 1974d) or females towards the end of gestation (Barry and Dubois 1974b). In cat, LHRH neurons are mainly found in the SPOA (Barry and Dubois 1974c; Flerkó et al. 1978; Nozaki and Kobayashi 1979) but in dogs they are much more numerous,

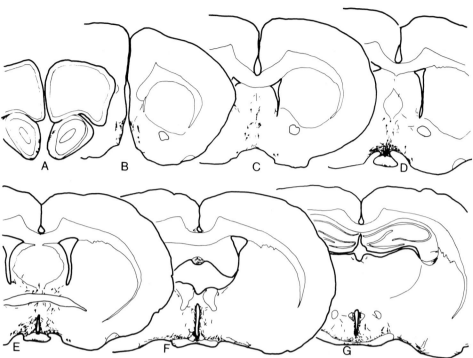

Fig. 2. LHRH cell body localization in the rat brain. A. LHRH cell bodies are first seen along the medial surface of the caudal olfactory bulb. B. LHRH cell bodies maintain a midline position at the level of separation of the frontal lobes. The cells and fibers are associated with the medial olfactory tract. C. At the rostral septum, LHRH cells are scattered in the N. diagonal band of Broca, and ventromedial portion of the medial septum. D. At the level of the OVLT, the majority of LHRH cells lie along the lateral borders of the OVLT in the region where the POA and septum join. E. Within the POA, the LHRH cells lie in the ventral boundary of the medial and lateral POA's. A few cells are also observed in the N. triangularis septum. F. Within the anterior hypothalamus at the level of the suprachiasmatic nuclei, LHRH cells retain a ventrolateral position. LHRH cells are rarely seen within the suprachiasmatic nucleus. Note an occasional LHRH cell is found in the cingulate cortex. G. The most caudal extent of the LHRH field is the region of the retrochiasmatic area. The LHRH cells in this region are mainly found in the ventrolateral hypothalamus just medial to the supraoptic nuclei. (Reproduced from Hoffman (1983), by courtesy of the Publisher.)

particularly in the prepubertal period, and widely scattered through the SPOA, pericommissural and suprachiasmatic area, as well as through the mediobasal hypothalamus (MBH), including the post infundibular eminence and the premammillary region (Barry and Dubois 1974c; Flerkó et al. 1978; Hoffman et al. 1978b). In Rhesus monkey (Barry et al. 1975; Silverman et al. 1977; Young and Kuhar 1980) and Cercopithecus (Barry et al. 1975), reactive perikarya are scattered through the MBH and pericommissural area. In *Cebus apella* (Barry and Carette 1975a,b) and squirrel monkey (Barry and Carette 1975a,b; Hoffman et al. 1978b), positive perikarya are mainly concentrated in the retrochiasmatic, infundibular, post infundibular and premammillary areas, in the lamina terminalis (LT) and the pericommissural region. In the baboon (Marshall and Goldsmith 1980), the greatest number and density of LHRH neurons are observed in the medial preoptic area (MPOA) but most of the neurons presumed to directly influence adenohypophysis are in the MBH. In the rabbit (Barry 1976a; Flerkó et al. 1978), reactive perikarya are also concentrated in the MBH, AHA, suprachiasmatic region and SPOA. In sheep (Hoffman et al. 1978b) they are scattered from the SPOA to the AN and the premammillary area with a few cells extending to the ventromedial nucleus

(Dees et al. 1981b). In the equine brain (Dees et al. 1981a), perikarya are found in the LT, AN and periventricular nucleus. In Galago and Tupia (Barry 1980a) they are mainly concentrated in the MPOA, AHA and LT but not routinely found in the MBH. In the hamster (Hoffman 1983; Jennes and Stumpf 1980b) they are scattered through the SPOA and the anterior and central parts of the ventral hypothalamus. In the human fetus (Barry 1977; Bloch 1977; Bugnon et al. 1976, 1977b) and adult (Barry 1976b, 1977), immunoreactive perikarya have their greatest concentration in the MBH, MPOA and LT.

Birds

In birds, reactive perikarya have been observed in the dorsal region of the preoptic nucleus of the mallard duck, where they form a somewhat compact group (Bons et al. 1977, 1978a; Oksche 1978); the medioseptal region, POA and MBH of the chicken and pheasant (Hoffman et al. 1978b); the POA of the Japanese quail (Oksche 1978); the SPOA and AHA of the domestic hen (Sterling and Sharp 1982), where they are more diffuse than in the mallard duck. The reports of reactive perikarya in the dorsolateral part of the AN (McNeill et al. 1976), the infundibular area of the mallard duck (Bons et al. 1978b) and the periventricular area of the MBH in pheasant and chicken (Hoffman et al. 1978b) seem doubtful to Sterling and Sharp (1982) because of the use of the Sorrentino 'F' antiserum which contains an ACTH antibody (Clayton and Hoffman 1979a) and the inability to verify this pattern in the domestic hen with Arimura's 743 antiserum.

Reptiles

In reptiles, perikarya have been observed only in the snake *Elaphe climacophora* (Nozaki and Kobayashi 1979) where they are chiefly in the SPOA (median septal nucleus and adjacent MPO).

Amphibians

In amphibians, reactive perikarya were first observed in a paired nucleus of the caudal diencephalon, in castrated *Bufo vulgaris* (Doerr-Scott and Dubois 1975); in an unpaired nucleus, in front of the optic recess, in *Rana pipiens* and *Rana temporaria* (Alpert et al. 1976) and in *Rana esculenta* (Goos et al. 1976); chiefly in the median septal nucleus but also in the adjacent MPO nucleus and the bed nucleus of the hippocampal commissure of *Rana catesbeiana* and *Cynopus pyrrhogaster ensicauda* (Nozaki and Kobayashi 1979) and in the newt (Kubo et al. 1979).

Fishes

In fishes, small faintly reactive perikarya have been found in the area dorsalis pars medialis of the telencephalon, on both sides of the ventriculis communis in *Salmo gairdneri* (Goos and Murathanoglu 1977); in the platyfish (Schreibman et al. 1979) and in the agnatha *Entosphenus japonica* (Nozaki and Kobayashi 1979); in the POA of adult pacific lampreys, *Entosphenus tridentata* (Crim et al. 1979a); in the nucleus preopticus pars magnocellularis and periventricularis posterior of *Gasterosteus aculeatus* (Borg et al. 1982); and in the posterior preoptic nucleus of *Lampetra richardsoni* (Crim et al. 1979b).

4. LHRH PATHWAYS

4.1. HYPOTHALAMIC REACTIVE LHRH PATHWAYS

For the reasons previously discussed (section 1.), reactive LHRH axons have been identified by nearly all groups engaged in the immunocytochemical study of LHRH systems.
They are generally more numerous and easily seen in the ME than elsewhere in the
brain. Projections to brain areas other than the ME utilize diffuse pathways rather than
condensed tracts. We will nevertheless retain the word 'tract' which is of common use
(Table 2).

Infundibular tracts

The LHRH septo/preoptico-infundibular tract (SPIT) and the LHRH tubero-infundibular tract (TIT) are the two major components of the LHRH infundibular tract. These
two tracts terminate mainly in the ME but some of their axons may reach the hypophysial stalk or, rarely, the hilus of the neural lobe; for this reason we will use the expression
'infundibular tract', instead of 'median eminence tract'. The SPIT is the major LHRH
hypothalamic tract in the rat. Its overall origin is well known since the characterization
of LHRH perikarya topography but its fascicular components and their respective origins have been only recently specified by various groups: Ibata et al. (1979a) have described a main basolateral paired pathway innervating most of the ME and an accessory
descending pathway innervating the rostral and most caudal part of the ME.
Merchenthaler et al. (1980a) and Réthelyi et al. (1981) distinguish a median, two medial
and two lateral fascicles, with a certain percentage of crossed axons (particularly in the
inner plexiform layer of the ME), the TIT being devoid of LHRH axons. Kawano and
Daikoku (1981), in addition to mediobasal and lateral LHRH fibers, point out that a
minor portion of infundibular LHRH is produced by cells located in the basal tuberal
hypothalamus. Bennett-Clarke and Joseph (1982) describe a first pathway originating
from cell bodies of the ventrolateral group and following a lateral course; a medial
somewhat dorsal pathway following a periventricular route and a thin medial and ventral pathway. Hoffman and Gibbs (1982) using deafferentation experiments describe
four tracts (Fig. 3). Three of these tracts originate from most rostral perikarya (caudal
septum and MPO): (1) a ventral suboptic tract (which is sufficient to assume gonado-
trophic function); (2) a tract running along the floor of the third ventricle; and (3) a
tract coursing along its walls; the 4th tract, originating from the more laterocaudal perikarya, courses with the MFB and enters the more caudal ME. The modifications of the
LHRH SPIT have been studied in rat during ontogenesis (Gross and Baker 1979;
Kawano et al. 1980; Paull 1978); post-natal period (Daikoku et al. 1982; Elkind-Hirsch

TABLE 2. *Hypothalamic reactive LHRH pathways*

Main origin	List of tracts	Sites of ending
SPOA	LHRH septo/preoptico-infundibular tract	Infundibulum
MBH	LHRH tubero-infundibular tract	Infundibulum
POA/AHA	LHRH preoptico-terminal tract	OVLT
POA/AHA	LHRH preoptico-supraoptic tract	Supraoptic area
Hypothalamus	LHRH ventricular tract	Third ventricle
Hypothalamus	LHRH hypothalamo-hypothalamic networks	Hypothalamus

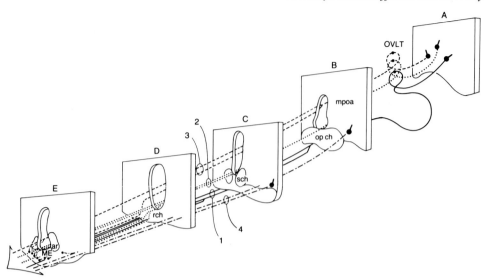

Fig. 3. Tracts of LHRH axons to the median eminence (ME) arise from a triangular field of cells whose apex lies in the caudal septum just rostral to the OVLT within the preoptic periventricular area, level *A*. The rostral-most group of cells initiates 3 tracts: (1) a tract which traverses under the optic chiasm; (2) a tract which traverses along the floor of the third venticle; and (3) a tract which traverses along the lateral walls of the third ventricle. The more lateral and caudal LHRH cells seen in levels *B* and *C* give rise to a 4th tract that courses with the fibers of the medial forebrain bundle and enters the more caudal ME. Fibers from all the tracts branch as they course to the ME and begin to merge at the retrochiasmatic area (rch), level *D*. Then they continue to the ME, level *E*. Since terminals en passant may be found in the OVLT as the LHRH fibers loop around the vessels, loops with dots are indicated. ar: arcuate nucleus; sch: suprachiasmatic nucleus: mpoa: medial preoptic area; op ch: optic chiasm. (Reproduced from Hoffman (1983), by courtesy of the Publisher.)

et al. 1981; Ibata et al. 1981); circadian rhythm (Kerdelhué et al. 1973); estrous cycle (Ibata et al. 1978; Kobayashi et al. 1978; Polkowska and Jutisz 1979); in aged animals (Hoffman and Sladek 1980; Merchenthaler et al. 1980b) and after deafferentation (Hoffman and Gibbs 1982; Scott and Knigge 1981; Taketani et al. 1980). The LHRH SPIT of the hamster (Hoffman 1983; Jennes and Stumpf 1980b) and mouse (Hoffman 1983) are similar to that of the rat. In the guinea pig, the LHRH SPIT was thought to be the major component of the LHRH infundibular tract (Barry and Dubois 1976; Barry et al. 1973a, 1974, 1975) but work from Silverman's laboratory (Krey and Silverman 1978, 1981; Silverman 1976; Silverman and Krey 1978a; Silverman et al. 1979) has emphasized the role of LHRH TIT in lesioned animals, where it maintains preovulatory LH release and ovulation. They now think that axons coming from the SPOA terminate mainly in the ventral and lateral parts and in the zona interna of ME and that axons from cells of the MBH terminate in the mediodorsal portion of the stalk and the post infundibular ME. In dog (Barry and Dubois 1975) and rabbit (Barry 1976a) the SPIT is well developed; in the cat (Barry and Dubois 1976) it seems to be the most important (or even the unique) component of the LHRH infundibular tract, as in prosimians (Barry 1980a) where Galago shows in addition a suboptic tract similar to the subchiasmatic tract later described in rat by Hoffman and Gibbs (1982).

In birds, the axons of the LHRH infundibular tract are distributed vertically to the capillaries of the intercalar plexus, at the level of the rostral and caudal ME (Calas et al. 1973; McNeill et al. 1976; De Reviers and Dubois 1974; Sharp et al. 1975) and come from reactive perikarya of the SPOA (Bons et al. 1978b; Oksche 1978; Sterling and Sharp 1982) (Fig. 4).

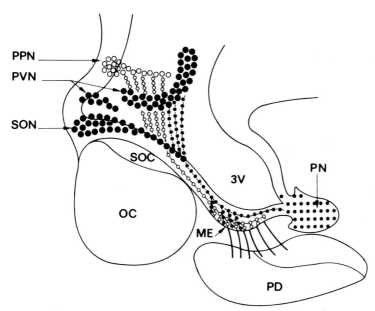

Fig. 4. Diagrammatic representation of neurosecretory systems in the hypothalamus of the duck; sagittal view. Nuclear areas containing LHRH (○) and vasotocin (●) perikarya. LHRH (○—○) and vasotocin (●—●) pathways. ME, median eminence; OC, optic chiasma; PD and PN, pars distalis and pars nervosa of the pituitary; PPN periventricular preoptic nucleus; PVN, paraventricular nucleus; SOC supraoptic commissure; SON, supraoptic nucleus; 3V, third ventricle. (Reproduced from Bons et al. (1978a), by courtesy of The Editors of *Cell and Tissue Research*.)

In reptiles, reactive axons of the SPIT have been observed in the ME of a few genera: Thamnophis, Elaphe, Geoclemys, Gekko, but have been followed from their origin up to the ME only in *Elaphe climacophora* (Nozaki and Kobayashi 1979) (Fig. 5).

In amphibians, the SPIT is also the major projection to the ME in Bufo (Doerr-Scott and Dubois 1975); various species of Rana (Goos et al. 1976; Nozaki and Kobayashi 1979); Xenopus (Doerr-Scott and Dubois 1976; Nozaki and Kobayashi 1979) (Fig. 6) and *Cynopus pyrrhogaster ensicauda* (Nozaki and Kobayashi 1979).

In fish, *Salmo gairdneri* (Goos and Murathanoglu 1977), *Anguilla japonica* (eel), *Fuga niphobles* (puffer) and *Entosphenus japonica* (lamprey) (Nozaki and Kobayashi 1979), most of the reactive axons of rostral origin terminated in the proximal portion of the neurohypophysis, contiguous with the rostral pituitary.

The LHRH tubero-infundibular tract has been difficult to characterize in the guinea pig (see 'Mammals' under section 3.1.). In dog (Barry and Dubois 1975) and rabbit (Barry 1976a) this tract is clearly visible. In monkeys (Barry and Carette 1975a,b; Barry et al. 1975; Hoffman et al. 1978b; Marshall and Goldsmith 1980; Silverman et al. 1977; Zimmerman and Antunés 1976) and in human (Barry 1976b, 1977; Bloch 1977; Bugnon et al. 1976, 1977b; Paulin et al. 1977), the TIT seems to be the principal component of the LHRH infundibular tract. In birds its existence remains in doubt (see 'Birds' under section 3.2.) and it seems to be absent in lower vertebrates, except in Xenopus, which contains some reactive perikarya near the floor of the infundibulum (Doerr-Scott and Dubois 1976).

The LHRH infundibular tract (LHRH 'hypothalamo-infundibular' or 'hypothalamo-median eminence' tract) has been the subject of numerous studies because it comprises

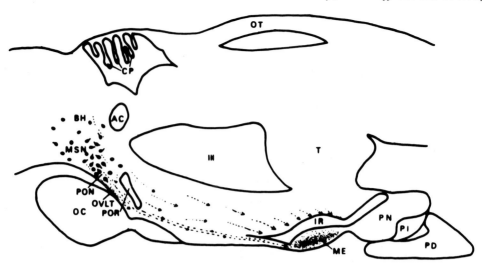

Fig. 5. Topographic distribution of immunoreactive perikarya (black circles) in the brain of the snake *Elaphe climacophora*. They are projected on a nearly midsagittal plane. Only one half of the perikarya is shown. Small dots show immunoreactive fiber terminals. Broken lines indicate the immunoreactive fiber pathways to the median eminence. (Reproduced from Nozaki and Kobayashi (1979), by courtesy of the Editors of *Archivum Histologicum Japonicum*.)

the preterminal and terminal portions of axons which were first to be characterized (Baker et al. 1974; Barry 1980a; Barry et al. 1973a; Calas et al. 1973; King et al. 1974; Kordon et al. 1974; Léonardelli et al. 1973b; Mazzuca and Dubois 1974; Pelletier et al. 1974; Zimmerman et al. 1974). This tract consists of various components (ventral or anterior; lateral; dorsolateral; dorsal or posterior; axial or periaxial) lengthening the various fascicles which come from perikarya of the SPOA and/or MBH, it may be partly crossed. The quantity of reactive material is generally greater in the dorsal and dorsolateral parts of the ME (Fig. 7). With the exception of a usually minor axial bundle, most of the axons of the LHRH infundibular tract run outside of the zona fibrillaris of the ME, through the zona externa, and give rise to radiating collaterals, with dilated endings situated close to the pericapillary basement membrane of the primary portal plexus of the pituitary (intercalar plexus and intra-infundibular loops). Electron microscopic studies of LHRH infundibular axons and pericapillary endings have been performed in rat (Ibata and Watanabe 1977; Krisch 1978; Nozaki et al. 1979; Pelletier et al. 1976), guinea pig (Silverman and Desnoyers 1976), man (Bugnon et al. 1977c, 1978), baboon (Marshall and Goldsmith 1980), mallard duck (Calas et al. 1974) and Xenopus (Doerr-Scott et al. 1978). The axons contain numerous specific granules, ranging from 60–130 nm and terminate in close contact with the basement membrane surrounding the pericapillary spaces.

The LHRH infundibular tract (or some of its components) show modifications under various conditions in rat (see 'Mammals' under section 3.1.); in guinea pig during the fetal and perinatal life (Barry and Dubois 1974d), estrous cycle (Barry and Dubois 1974a,b), gestation (Barry and Dubois 1974b), late pregnancy and parturition (Jennes and Croix 1980a); in sheep during various reproductive states (Polkowska et al. 1980) or after anterior deafferentation (Polkowska 1981); in ovariectomized rat after suckling (Culler et al. 1982); in fetal and early post-natal mouse (Gross and Baker 1977).

188

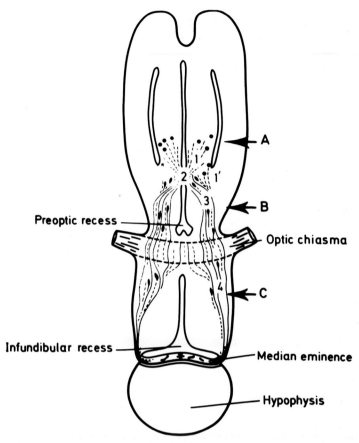

Fig. 6. Diagrammatic horizontal section through the forebrain of *Xenopus laevis* indicating the positions of the perikarya and the LHRH-like neurosecretory fiber pathways. A. Two groups of LHRH-like cells in the septal zone of the telencephalon. (These more dorsal cells are superimposed.) B. LHRH-like cells on either side of the preoptic recess among the neurosecretory fibers. C. LHRH-like cells in the infundibulum. (1) Paired neurosecretory bundles running dorsoventrally through the telencephalon and forming a single bundle (2) between the posterior edge of the telencephalic furrow and the anterior edge of the preoptic recess. The bundle divides into two (3) and the two resulting bundles fan out on either side of the preoptic recess running above the optic chiasma along the ventral edge of the infundibulum; (4) the fibers terminate in the external zone of ME. (Reproduced from Doerr-Scott and Dubois (1976), by courtesy of the Editors of *Cell and Tissue Research.*)

Preoptico-terminal tract

The LHRH preoptico-terminal tract (PTT) has been well characterized in guinea pig (Barry et al. 1973a); monkeys (Barry and Carette 1975a,b: Mazzuca 1977; Silverman et al. 1977; Zimmerman and Antunés 1976); rabbit (Barry 1976a; Flerkó et al. 1978); man (Barry 1977; Bugnon et al. 1977a) and Tupia (Barry 1980a). Reactive LHRH axons were also described in the OVLT of rat (Barry et al. 1973a; King et al. 1974; Kordon et al. 1974; Krause 1979; Pelletier 1976; Pelletier et al. 1977), but the perikarya giving rise to these axons were difficult to demonstrate (see section 1.). In primates, on the contrary, the PTT is clearly visible, with its perikarya and axons (or axon collaterals) and constitutes, after the LHRH infundibular tract, the major efferent hypothalamic

189

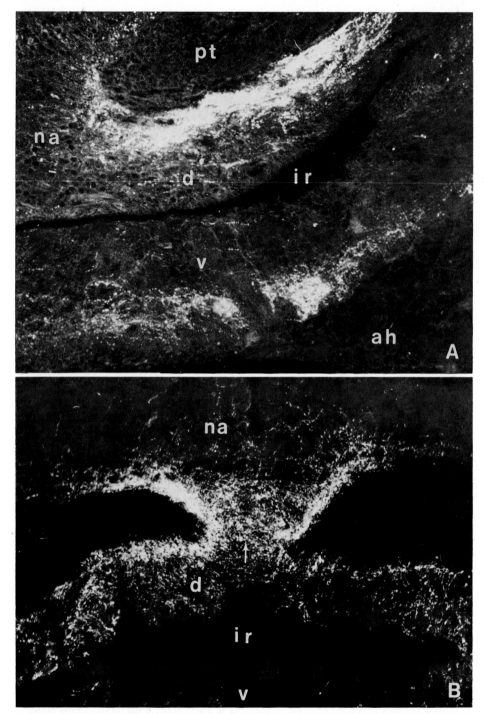

Fig. 7. LHRH infundibular tract. A. sagittal section in the guinea pig at the level of the ME (Barry, personal document). B. Coronal cryostat section in the rat at the level of the ME (Bugnon, personal document). ah: adenohypophysis; d: dorsal lip of median eminence; ir: infundibular recess; na: nucleus arcuatus; pt: pars tuberalis; v: ventral lip of ME; white arrow: crossed fibers of the dorsal component of the LHRH infundibular tract. × 210.

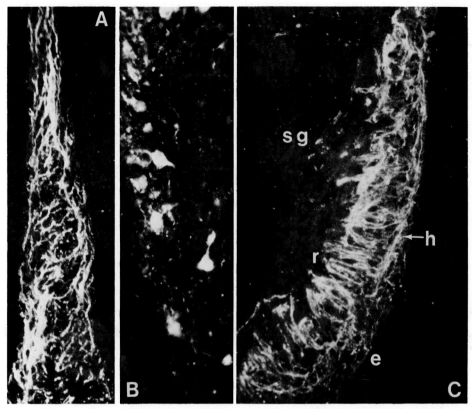

Fig. 8. LHRH preoptico-terminal tract in the squirrel monkey. A. Middle coronal section of the LT; two upper thirds. B. Sagittal section of the LT; reactive perikarya. C. Sagittal section of the two lower thirds of the LT. A–C × 300. e: ependyma; h: hypendymal plexus; r: radiating collaterals; sg: subglial rostral layer. (From Barry, personal documents.)

pathway for LHRH cell bodies (Fig. 8). The reactive axons form an important hypendymal plexus, giving rise to radiating collaterals with pericapillary endings along the short external and long internal vascular loops of the OVLT; some of these axons may reach the subglial rostral layer or the ventricular recess. In non-primates, particularly in rodents, some cells of the POA/AHA contribute simultaneously to the OVLT and to the ME projections (Bennett-Clarke and Joseph 1982), some axons from the SPIT passing through the OVLT (Hoffman and Gibbs 1982; Samson and McCann 1979), and even forming terminals en passant (Hoffman and Gibbs 1982). Conspicuous changes of the PTT have been observed in rat during the estrous cycle (Sétáló et al. 1976b; Wenger 1976; Wenger and Léonardelli 1980), after hypothalamic deafferentation (Weiner et al. 1975), or hypophysectomy (Wenger et al. 1978); in guinea pig during late pregnancy and parturition (Jennes and Croix 1980a); in squirrel monkey during the estrous cycle (Barry 1979a). It seems therefore that this tract has a functional role in mammals, even if the destination of the venous blood from the OVLT remains debatable. In birds (Oksche 1978; Sterling and Sharp 1982) reactive (possibly terminal) axons are present in the OVLT but Nozaki and Kobayashi (1979) think that in amphibians, the reaction product concentrated in the ventral surface of the preoptic recess is not in nerve terminals.

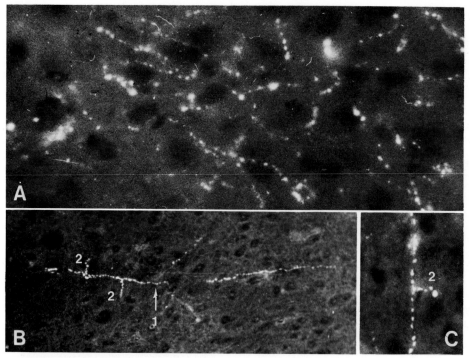

Fig. 9. A. Pericellular axonic endings of the LHRH preoptico-supraoptic tract, AHA; ×900. B. LHRH axon of the SPIT, 1: axonic branching, 2: short collaterals, AHA; ×400. C. LHRH axon in the premammillary area; ×900. A–C: gestating guinea pig. (From Barry, personal documents.)

Preoptico-supraoptic tract

The LHRH preoptico-supraoptic tract (PSOT), observed in the guinea pig (Barry et al. 1973a; Jennes and Croix 1980a; Silverman 1976), originates from perikarya of the POA/ AHA and terminates mainly in the supraoptic crest (Fig. 9,A) and suprachiasmatic region. It is interesting to note that these areas are implicated in the control of sexual behavior in rat, for references see Rodriguez-Sierra and Komisaruk (1982).

Ventricular tract

The LHRH ventricular tract may be formed by numerous and obvious projections of LHRH axons (or other cell body processes) into the third ventricle. These LHRH 'hypothalamo-ventricular' projections (Knigge et al. 1980) have been observed mainly in rat (Bennett-Clarke and Joseph 1982; Burchanowski et al. 1979; Hoffman and Gibbs 1982; Jennes and Stumpf 1980c; Joseph et al. 1981; Piekut and Knigge 1981). Yet, as depicted in Figure 3, these may be axons coursing along the ventricular surface rather than into the ventricular lumen.

Electron microscopic studies (Kawano et al. 1980) indicate that these axons do not extend through the ependyma. Similar fibers were previously observed in the OVLT of primates, accompanied by a few supraependymal perikarya (Barry and Carette 1975a, b) reminiscent of the liquor-contacting neurons of Vigh-Tichman and Vigh (1974).

Intrahypothalamic tracts

LHRH hypothalamo-hypothalamic networks originate from LHRH cell bodies or processes, axons particularly, forming (by means of short or medium collaterals) true synapses, terminals en passant or synaptoid contacts (Fig. 9, A–C). Reactive LHRH terminals are seen in various hypothalamic areas: AHA, supraoptic crest, AN, medial mammillary nucleus (Barry et al. 1973a, 1974; Clayton and Hoffman 1979a; Jennes and Croix 1980a; Silverman 1976), and paraventricular nucleus (Hoffman 1983). Dendritic or somal bridges have also been observed between a certain percentage of LHRH cells (Marshall and Goldsmith 1980) as well as axo-somatic LHRH juxtaposition or closely entwined dendrites (Hoffman 1983). Synaptic contacts between reactive LHRH processes (or sometimes reactive LHRH perikarya) and reactive fibers (Kozlowski et al. 1980; Hisano et al. 1981; Krisch 1980b) were observed with the electron microscope.

4.2. EXTRAHYPOTHALAMIC LHRH PROJECTIONS

The central nervous system distribution of LHRH fibers to areas other than the ME has been extensively studied in mammals such as guinea pigs (Barry and Dubois 1976; Barry et al. 1973a; Silverman 1976), primate (Barry and Carette 1975a; Silverman et al. 1977), hamster (Jennes and Stumpf 1980b; Phillips et al. 1980, 1982), mouse (Clayton and Hoffman 1979a; Hoffman 1983), and rat (Hoffman 1983; Krey and Silverman 1978; Liposits and Sétáló 1980; Witkin et al. 1982). To date, only one non-mammalian species has been fully examined (Múnz et al. 1981). Due to the paucity of information on the non-mammalian species this discussion will focus on mammals; primarily rodent species. Three primary targets of the LHRH system have been noted: (1) *olfactory system;* (2) other projections of the *limbic system;* and (3) areas involved in *reproductive behavior* which do not fall into the first two categories. A diagrammatic representation of all the LHRH projections (both hypothalamic and extrahypothalamic) in the rat is shown in Figures 10 and 11.

Olfactory projections

That LHRH axons might project to the olfactory brain centers was first suggested by Barry et al. (1973a) and later verified (Hoffman et al. 1979; Jennes and Stumpf 1980b; Phillips et al. 1980, 1982; Silverman and Krey 1978a). In certain species such as the hamster (Figs 12 and 13) the olfactory bulb receives two projections: a superficial one which extends into the olfactory bulb along the blood vessels at the medial surface of the olfactory peduncle, and a deep projection which enters the main olfactory bulb from a tract that runs along the subependymal zone of the lateral ventricle. The superficial projection terminates predominantly in the periglomerular and external plexiform layers of the caudal main and accessory olfactory bulb. The mouse and rat have only the superficial projection (Fig. 14).

LHRH connections in the olfactory bulb are altered by urine odors (Dluzen et al. 1981), suggesting a physiological role for the peptide. Since the sites in which the LHRH fibers are found correspond closely to areas of the olfactory bulb which are activated during maternal pup-retrieving behavior, the LHRH projections may be participating in this and other reproductive olfactory functions as well.

In addition to olfactory bulb projections, LHRH axons extend to other olfactory brain centers. LHRH axons are found within the islands of Calleja, in the piriform cor-

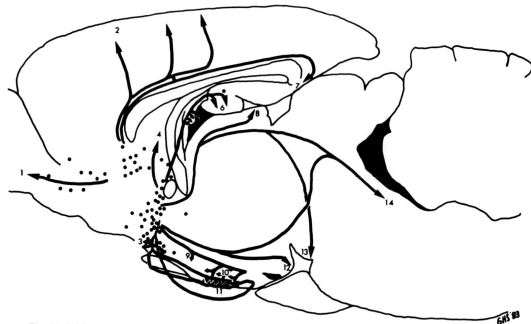

Fig. 10. Midline projections of the rat LHRH system. This figure of a rat brain in parasagittal section illustrates the hypothalamic and extrahypothalamic LHRH projections that are located close to midline. They include projections to: (1) the olfactory bulb (main and accessory); (2) anterior cingulate cortex; (3) organum vasculosum of the lamina terminalis; (4) medial septum; (5) subfornical organ; (6) dorsal hippocampus; (7) subiculum of the dorsal hippocampal region; (8) habenula; (9) paraventricular nucleus of the hypothalamus; (10) arcuate nucleus of the hypothalamus; (11) median eminence; (12) medial mammillary nucleus; (13) interpeduncular nucleus; and (14) central gray of the mesencephalon.

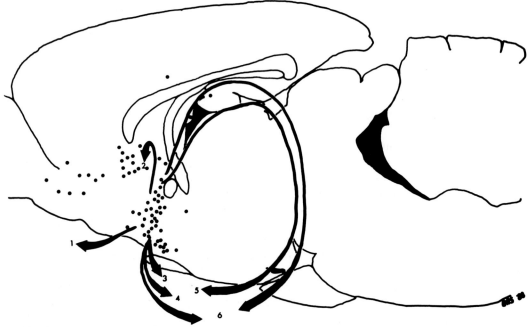

Fig. 11. Lateral projections of the rat LHRH system. This figure illustrates the more lateral projections of LHRH axons. These include projections to: (1) piriform cortex; (2) lateral septum; (3) supraoptic nucleus; (4) cortical nucleus of the amygdala; (5) medial nucleus of the amygdala; (6) ventral subiculum.

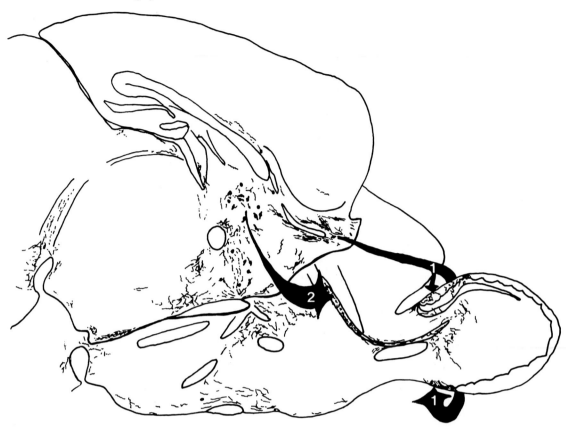

Fig. 12. LHRH pathways to the olfactory bulb of the hamster. LHRH cells that are found in association with the medial olfactory tract give rise to a superficial LHRH projection (1) to the periglomerular regions of the main and accessory olfactory bulbs. A deep LHRH projection (2) arises from the LHRH cells in the medial septum, courses along the subependymal surface of the lateral ventricle and extends to the ependymal region of the main olfactory bulb. This deep projection is absent in the rat and mouse.

tex and within the nucleus of the lateral olfactory tract. As in other projection fields, occasional LHRH neurons can be found in these areas as well (Fig. 15).

Other limbic system projections

In addition to the olfactory system, LHRH axons extend to a number of limbic areas. Projections to the medial (Fig. 16) and cortical amygdaloid (Fig. 17) nuclei were among the first extrahypothalamic projections observed (Barry et al. 1973a; Clayton and Hoffman 1979a; Jennes and Stumpf 1980b; Marshall and Goldsmith 1980; Silverman and Krey 1978a; Sternberger and Hoffman 1978). LHRH fibers present in this area enter from the stria terminalis (Fig. 16) or via the amygdalo-fugal pathway. Some of the fibers within the latter pathway may continue through to the hippocampus (Fig. 12). It is of interest that the medial and cortical amygdala nuclei send projections back to the regions in which the LHRH neurons lie (Kevetter and Winans 1981) and that lesions in the medial amygdala produce disruption of the estrous cycle as well as alterations in reproductive and maternal behavior.

A second limbic system projection extends into the hippocampus from LHRH fibers

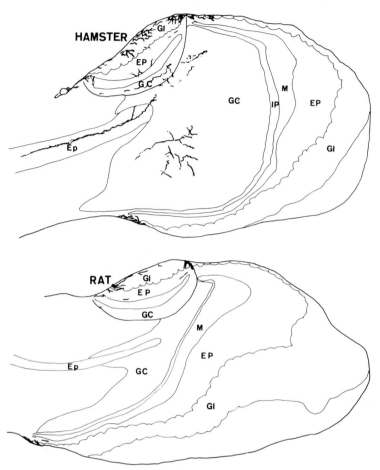

Figs 13 and 14. Comparison of LHRH distribution in the olfactory bulb of the hamster (13) and rat (14). Parasagittal sections of the olfactory bulb close to the mid-sagittal plane illustrate the presence of the deep and superficial LHRH projections in the hamster and superficial projection in the rat. In both species, projections to the main olfactory bulb are confined to the caudal regions of the bulb.

which pass through the subfornical organ (Figs 10, 18 and 19). These fibers generally terminate in the stratum radiatum (Fig. 20) or lacunosum/moleculaire (Fig. 21) but can be found in other dorsal hippocampal regions as well. LHRH cell bodies extend into the hippocampus along with these fibers (Fig. 21). 'Stray' cells can also be found within the subfornical organ (Fig. 22). A second LHRH projection to the hippocampus is found in the lacunosum/molecularis of the ventral subiculum. Although not completely characterized, this projection probably originates in part from cells in the septum which sends axons through the fimbria of the fornix (Fig. 23) as well as receiving some contribution from the amygdalo-fugal pathway.

The cingulate cortex is another component of the limbic system that receives LHRH axons. This projection was first noted in the hamster (Jennes and Stumpf 1980b). The LHRH fibers are oriented in a rostral to caudal plane and extend for long distances within the superficial layers of the cingulate close to the anterior hippocampus (Fig. 24) or travel within the corpus callosum (Fig. 19) and then radiate to layer I of cingulate (Fig. 25). Although not of high density the arrangement of these projections allows for

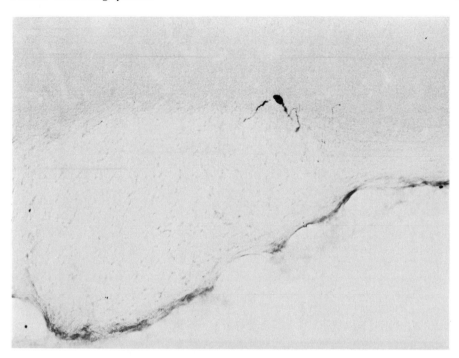

Fig. 15. Cells in the piriform cortex. Occasionally stray LHRH neurons are found in association with LHRH axonal projections to the olfactory regions. In the case illustrated, one such neurons is located just above the lateral olfactory tract in the piriform cortex.

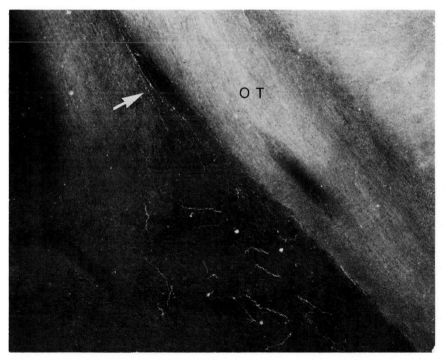

Fig. 16. Axons in the medial amygdaloid nucleus. LHRH axons traverse through the stria terminalis (arrow) to the medial amygdala, as is depicted in this frontal section. OT, optic tract.

197

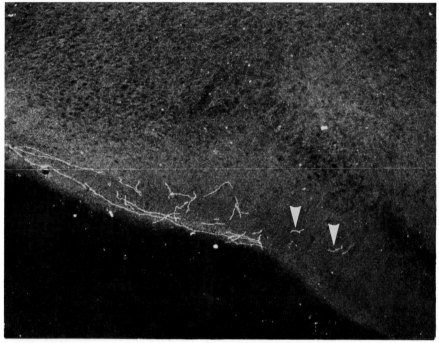

Fig. 17. LHRH axons of the cortical amygdala. LHRH axons are found in the superficial layers of the cortical amygdala. A few axons are observed in the adjacent piriform cortex (arrowheads).

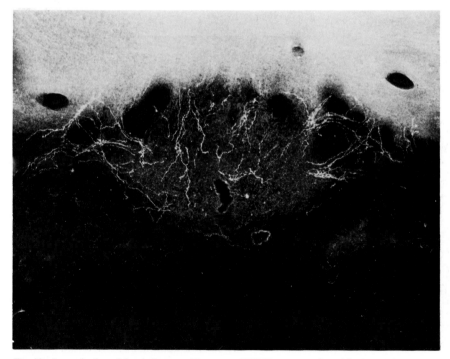

Fig. 18. Axons in the subfornical organ. Numerous LHRH axons are found in the subfornical organ particularly in association with the vessels of its lateral borders.

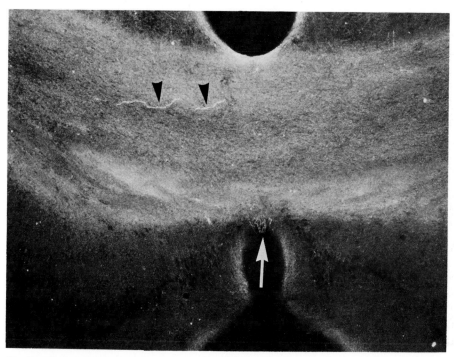

Fig. 19. Fibers coursing to the hippocampus. Some of the LHRH fibers (arrow) continue caudalward from the subfornical organ, and course toward the hippocampus. At this level, a few fibers are found in the corpus callosum (arrowheads).

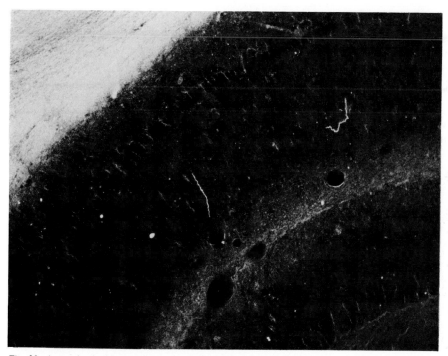

Fig. 20. Axons in the hippocampus. Scattered LHRH axons are present in various regions of the hippocampus. Two fibers can be seen extending in the stratum radiatum of the dorsal hippocampal CA1 region.

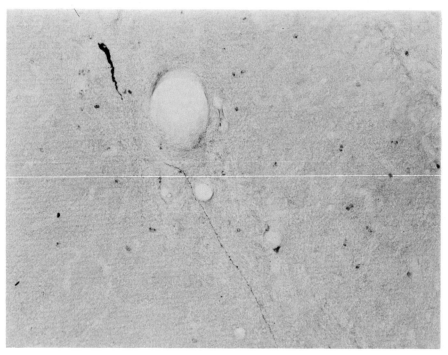

Fig. 21. Fiber and cell in the hippocampus. Occasionally, LHRH cell bodies are found within the dorsal hippocampus. Although the example depicts a cell in the stratum molecularis, the cells can be found in any of the layers where LHRH axons are present. An axon coursing within the stratum lacunosum is also shown.

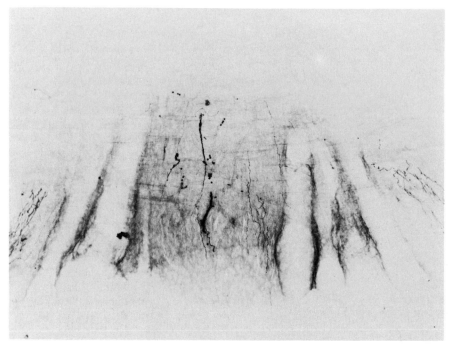

Fig. 22. Cells in the subfornical organ. 'Stray' LHRH cell bodies can be associated with any of the regions where axonal projections are found. Frequently these cells are seen in and around the subfornical organ.

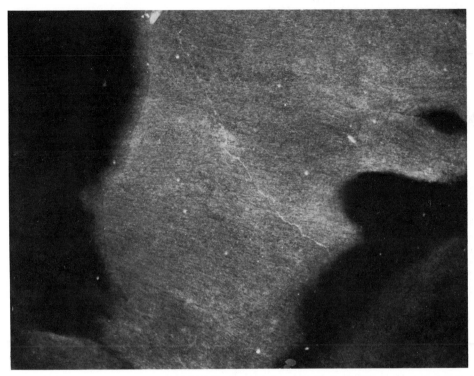

Fig. 23. Axons in the fornix. Scattered LHRH axons are found in the fornix. These appear to terminate in the ventral hippocampus.

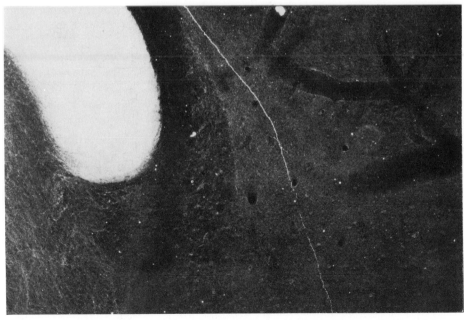

Fig. 24. Axons in the cingulate cortex. Sparse LHRH fibers extend for long distances in the cingulate cortex close to the anterior hippocampus, as is seen in this parasagittal section (rostral is to the right).

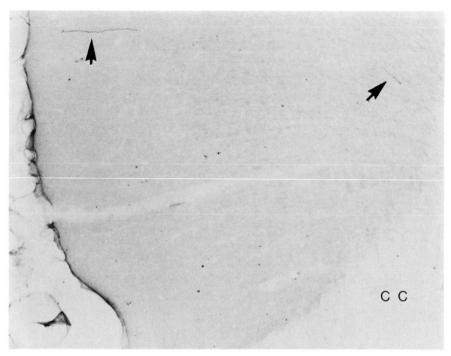

Fig. 25. Axons in the cingulate cortex. Some of the LHRH fibers extend radially from the corpus callosum (CC) in the lateral cingulate cortex toward layer I of this structure (arrows).

a maximization of the effect of these fibers on the cingulate neurons. In the hamster, a small population of LHRH cell bodies focused in the anterior cingulate (mainly within layer II) was observed. In rat or mouse an occasional cell is observed close to the induseum griseum (Fig. 26).

Within the lateral septum, another sparse LHRH projection is observed (Fig. 27). The ventral portion of the lateral septum close to the lateral ventricle appears to be the target of this projection in the rat and mouse. In the hamster, as was discussed under the olfactory projections, the LHRH fibers of the lateral septum continue along the subependymal zone of the lateral ventricle and extend anteriorly into the olfactory bulb.

Scattered LHRH fibers were also observed in the medial septal nucleus. In the hamster, some differences in this projection in males versus females was noted. The female appeared to possess a denser innervation of the medial septum than the male.

The epithalamic centers also constitute part of the limbic system. Of these the medial habenula receives LHRH fibers (Hoffman 1983) (Fig. 28) from either the stria medullaris or midline thalamus. The association of this nucleus with reproductive behavior further suggests that LHRH regulates non-endocrine reproductive function.

Centers controlling reproductive behavior

Besides the various regions of the limbic system and olfactory centers a number of brain areas influence reproductive behavior. Of these the central gray of the mesencephalon has received a great deal of attention since stimulation of that area produces reproductive postures (Moss and Dudley 1980), and application of gonadal steroids or LHRH

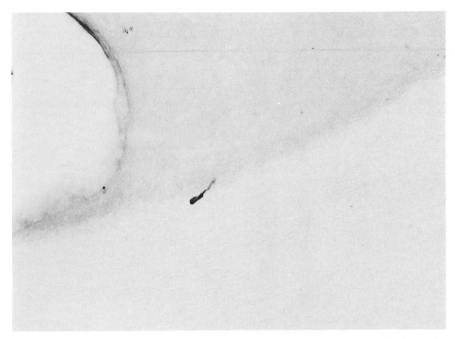

Fig. 26. Cell in the cingulate cortex. A 'stray' LHRH cell is sometimes observed in the deepest layers of the cingulate cortex.

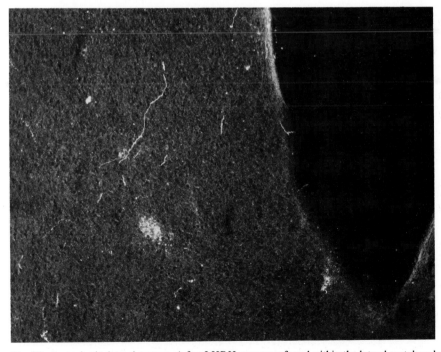

Fig. 27. Axons in the lateral septum. A few LHRH axons are found within the lateral septal nucleus, particularly within the ventral portion of anterior half of the nucleus.

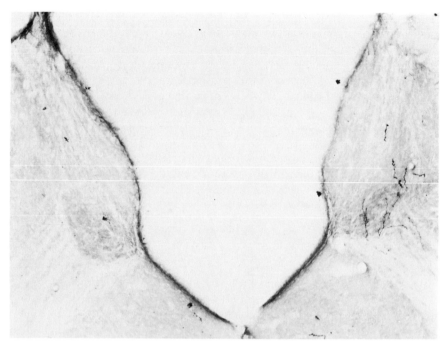

Fig. 28. Fibers of the habenula. LHRH axons are found in the ventrolateral portion of the medial habenula. Although most animals possess a bilateral projection, some animals appear to have a unilateral projection.

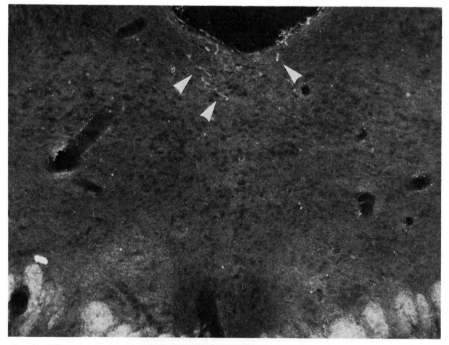

Fig. 29. Fibers in the mesencephalic central gray. LHRH axons course along the ventricular surface from the preoptic area and hypothalamus to the mesencephalon where the axons enter the central gray (arrowheads). The axons appear to terminate within the central gray as well as the dorsal raphe.

mimicks that effect. It was thus not surprising that in that region LHRH fibers are present (Liposits and Sétáló 1980). This projection (Fig. 29), in the rat, arises in the preoptic/medial septal junction and courses with the ventricle around the borders of the thalamus to the mesencephalon. In the hamster it extends along the ventricle only at the ventral border of the thalamus. The fibers then ascend to the central gray and the dorsal nucleus. The projection to the central gray is absent in the mouse.

Other projections

In addition to the projections discussed above sparse LHRH fibers have been noted in the interpeduncular nucleus (Silverman 1976; Witkin et al. 1982) and in the superior colliculus (Silverman 1976). The function of these projections remains unknown.

5. CONCLUDING REMARKS

The topography of LHRH systems is in good agreement with biological, biochemical and radioimmunoassays (see Barry 1979b). Their differential modifications under various circumstances suggest that, in addition to its major prehypophysiotropic action, LHRH may also be distributed by the blood from the OVLT and by the cerebrospinal fluid or act through what I had formerly called 'neurosecretory synapses' (Barry et al. 1973b), as a neuroregulator in numerous neuroendocrine, neurovegetative or behavioral integrated processes. LHRH endings may also have a mediator role in the effects of steroids (Hoffman 1983), probably in association with GABAergic or histaminergic neurons and steroid concentrating cells (SCC). The partial overlapping between SCC cells (Pfaff and Keiner 1973; Stumpf 1970; Warembourg 1977a,b) and LHRH neurons, the interrelationship between LHRH cells or processes and aminergic neurons (Agnati et al. 1977; Ajika 1979; Hoffman et al. 1982; Ibata et al. 1979b; McNeill et al. 1980; Wilkes et al. 1979); the hypothalamic topography of neurotransmitter receptors (Biegon et al. 1982; Block and Billar 1981; Leibovitz et al. 1982; Meibach 1982; Young and Kuhar 1980) and the results of microiontophoretic experiments with LHRH and neurotransmitters (Carette 1976, 1978; Dyer and Dyball 1974; Felix and Phillips 1979; Kelly and Moss 1976; Moss et al. 1976; Poulain 1974; Poulain and Carette 1974, 1976; Sawakami et al. 1976) suggest various hypotheses concerning the possible mechanisms of control of LHRH neurons, as highly simplified in Figure 30 (Barry 1980b, 1982; Hoffman et al. 1982).

It must be noted that the neural control of LHRH perikarya and LHRH endings varies according to their locations (SPOA, MBH, OVLT, ME, etc.) and that if no axo-axonal synapses have been found by electron microscopy in the ME or OVLT, this fact does not preclude the existence of 'functional' contacts between monoaminergic or enkephalinergic fibers and LHRH endings, for example at the level of ME (Fig. 30). On the other hand, specific contacts may also exist between LHRH axons and tanycytes or tanycyte processes in the median eminence but their role is not known; it is also the case for the special surface covering made by tanycyte processes in the zones of termination of LHRH fibers described by Réthelyi et al. (1981).

The experimental study of the control of LHRH hypothalamic systems can be carried out on LHRH nerve terminals (De Paolo et al. 1982; Negro-Vilar et al. 1979; Samson et al. 1981), MBH or ME explants (Ojeda et al. 1982; Rotsztejn et al. 1978), superfused hypothalamic tissue (Kim and Ramirez 1982); LHRH neurons in primary cultures

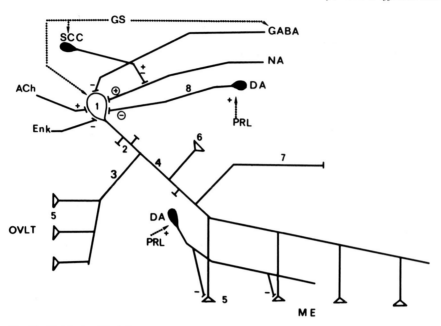

Fig. 30. Highly simplified diagram of the main presumed neuro-hormonal afferents and the main axonic effer-
ences of LHRH-producing neurons of hypothalamic systems. 1: LHRH perikaryon; 2: short collaterals; 3:
axonic projection to the OVLT; 4: axonic projection to the ME; 5: radiating collaterals with dilated pericapillary endings; 6: supraependymal (intraventricular) endings; 7: long collateral, forming 'neurosecretory' synapses, as short collaterals; 8: dopaminergic axons of the incerto-hypothalamic tract. DA: dopaminergic cells;
GABA: GABAergic axons; NA: noradrenergic axons; PRL: prolactin; GS: gonadal steroids; SCC: steroid
concentrating cells. Only the main actions of some neurotransmitters have been indicated. LHRH-producing
neurons of the SPIT may have projections of type 3 or 4, or of both types; LHRH-producing neurons of
the TIT seem to be devoid of type 3 projections. (From Barry, personal drawing.)

(Feldman et al. 1977; Knigge et al. 1977) as well as 'organotypic' cultures of selected
hypothalamic areas (Toran-Allerand 1978).

Although LHRH neurons seem to be distinct from cells which produce other neuropeptides (Dubois 1976; Hökfelt et al. 1978), an ACTH(17–39)-like substance as well as
β-endorphin (Léonardelli and Tramu 1979) have been detected in human hypothalamic
LHRH neurons (Tramu and Pillez 1977), and lastly LHRH-like immunoreactivity has
been observed in some CRF_{41}-positive neurons of rodents (Tramu and Pillez 1981). In
a separate study LHRH and CRF_{41} were found in distinctly different cells (Bugnon et
al. 1982).

Several LHRH hypothalamic systems need further studies but two basic problems remain to be solved.
– the accurate synaptic organization of these systems, namely: the distribution of their
  various types of axonal endings, round specific (OVLT and ME) or 'local' capillaries;
  neural projections to the ventricular or outer surface of the brain; short or long collaterals giving rise to 'neurosecretory' or better 'liberinergic' synapses, with interneurons
  or specific (dopaminergic, neuroendocrine, comportmental, etc.) effector neurons; or
  extra-hypothalamic projections to various target sites.
– the chemical nature and functions of the various neural afferents to the somato-den-
  dritic field and axonal processes of each subpopulation of LHRH neurons, as well
  as the identification of their specific membrane receptors. It seems that this last prob-

lem has to be *at first* approached by means of ultrastructural immunocytochemistry (and later hybridization histochemistry), in spite of all its difficulties, because it is one of the most significant challenges of chemical neuroanatomy for the next years.

6. ACKNOWLEDGMENTS

The authors would like to acknowledge the technical assistance of Ms Judy VanLare.

7. REFERENCES

Agnati LF, Fuxe K, Hökfelt T, Goldstein M, Jeffcoate S (1977): A method to measure the distribution pattern of specific nerve terminals in sampled regions. Studies on tyrosine hydroxylase, LHRH, TRH and GIH immunofluorescence. *J. Histochem. Cytochem., 25,* 1222–1236.
Ajika K (1979): Simultaneous localization of LHRH and catecholamines in rat hypothalamus. *J. Anat., 128,* 331–347.
Alpert LC, Brawer JR, Jackson MD, Patel Y (1975): Somatostatin and LHRH: immunohistochemical evidence for distinct hypothalamic distribution. *Fed. Proc., 34,* 239.
Alpert LC, Brawer JR, Jackson MD, Reichlin R (1976): Localization of LH-RH in frog brain *(Rana pipiens* and *Rana catesbeiana). Endocrinology, 98,* 910–921.
Amos M, Burgus R, Blackwell R, Vale W, Fellows R, Guillemin R (1971): Purification, aminoacid composition and N-terminus of the hypothalamic luteinizing hormone-releasing factor (LRF) of bovine origin. *Biochem. Biophys. Res. Commun., 44,* 205–210.
Arimura A, Sato H, Coy DH, Worobec RB, Schally AV, Yanaihara N, Hashimoto T, Sukura N (1975): The antigenic determinant of the LH-releasing hormone for three different antisera. *Acta Endocrinol. (Copenhagen), 78,* 222–231.
Baker BL, Dermody WC (1976): Effect of hypophysectomy on immunocytochemically demonstrated gonadotropin releasing hormone in the rat brain. *Endocrinology, 98,* 1116–1122.
Baker BL, Dermody WC, Reel JR (1974): Localization of luteinizing hormone-releasing hormone in the rat brain as observed with immunocytochemistry. *Am. J. Anat., 139,* 129–134.
Baker BL, Dermody WC, Reel JR (1975): Distribution of gonadotropin releasing hormone in the rat brain as observed with immunocytochemistry. *Endocrinology, 97,* 125–135.
Barry J (1976a): Characterization and topography of LH-RH neurons in the rabbit. *Neurosci. Lett., 2,* 201–205.
Barry J (1976b): Characterization and topography of LH-RH neurons in the human brain. *Neurosci. Lett., 3,* 287–291.
Barry J (1977): Immunofluorescence study of LH-RH neurons in man. *Cell Tissue Res., 181,* 1–14.
Barry J (1979a): Immunofluorescence study of the preoptico-terminal LHRH tract in the female squirrel monkey during the oestrous cycle. *Cell Tissue Res., 198,* 1–13.
Barry J (1979b): Immunohistochemistry of luteinizing hormone-releasing hormone producing neurons of the vertebrates. *Int. Rev. Cytol., 60,* 179–221.
Barry J (1980a): Immunofluorescence study of LRH-producing neurons in Prosimians *(Tupaia* and *Galago). Cell Tissue Res., 206,* 355–365.
Barry J (1980b): Convergence et articulation réciproque des neurones aminergiques et peptidergiques dans l'hypothalamus. *Ann. Endocrinol., 41,* 457–465.
Barry J (1982): Systèmes neurohormonaux contrôlant les fonctions gonadotropes et prolactiniques. *Contracept. Fertil. Sex., 10,* 711–718.
Barry J, Carette B (1975a): Immunofluorescence study of LRF neurons in primates. *Cell Tissue Res., 164,* 163–178.
Barry J, Carette B (1975b): Etude en immunofluorescence des neurones élaborateurs de LRF chez les Cébidés. *C. R. Acad. Sci., 281,* 735–738.
Barry J, Croix D (1978): Immunofluorescence study of the hypothalamo-infundibular LRH tract and serum gonadotropin levels in the female squirrel monkey during the oestrous cycle. *Cell Tissue Res., 192,* 215–226.
Barry J, Dubois MP (1974a) Immunofluorescence study of the preoptico-infundibular LHRH neurosecretory pathway of the guinea pig during the estrous cycle. *Neuroendocrinology, 15,* 200–208.

Barry J, Dubois MP (1974b): Study of the preoptico-infundibular LH-RH neurosecretory pathway in female guinea pig during gestation and the oestrous cycle. In: Knowles F, Vollrath G (Eds), *Neurosecretion. The Final Neuroendocrine Pathway, 1st Ed.*, pp. 148–153. Springer, Berlin/Heidelberg/New York

Barry J, Dubois MP (1974c) Etude comparée en immunofluorescence des neurones élaborateurs de LRF chez les Mammifères. *Arch. Anat. Microsc. Morphol. Exp., 63*, 363–374.

Barry J, Dubois MP (1974d) Etude en immunofluorescence de la différenciation prénatale des cellules élaboratrices de LH-RF et de la maturation de la voie neurosécrétrice préoptico-infundibulaire chez le cobaye. *Brain Res., 67*, 103–113.

Barry J, Dubois MP (1975): Immunofluorescence study of LRF producing neurons in the cat and the dog. *Neuroendocrinology, 18*, 290–298.

Barry J, Dubois MP (1976): Immunoreactive LRF neurosecretory pathways in mammals. *Acta Anat., 94*, 497–503.

Barry J, Dubois MP, Poulain P (1973a): LRF producing cells of the mammalian hypothalamus. *Z. Zellforsch. Mikrosk. Anat., 146*, 351–366.

Barry J, Dubois MP, Poulain P, Léonardelli J (1973b): Charactérisation et topographie des neurones hypothalamiques immunoréactifs avec des anticorps anti LRF de synthèse. *C. R. Acad. Sci., 276*, 3191–3193.

Barry J, Dubois MP, Carette B (1974): Immunofluorescence study of the preoptico-infundibular LRF neurosecretory pathway in normal, castrated and testosterone treated male guinea pig. *Endocrinology, 95*, 1416–1423.

Barry J, Girod C, Dubois MP (1975): Topographie des neurones élaborateurs de LRF chez les Primates. *Bull. Assoc. Anat., 59*, 103–110.

Bennett-Clarke C, Joseph SA (1982): Immunocytochemical distribution of LHRH neurons and processes in the rat: hypothalamic and extrahypothalamic locations. *Cell Tissue Res., 221*, 493–504.

Biegon A, Rainbow TC, McEwen BS (1982): Quantitative autoradiography of serotonin receptors in the rat brain. *Brain Res., 242*, 197–204.

Bloch B (1977): Les neurones producteurs de LH-RH chez l'Homme au cours de la vie foetale. *Ann. Sci. Univ. Besançon, 5*, 1–213.

Block BA, Billar RB (1981): Properties and regional distribution of cholinergic receptors in the rat hypothalamus. *Brain Res., 212*, 152–158.

Bons N, Kerdelhué B, Assenmacher I (1977): Présence de neurones élaborateurs de LH-RH dans l'hypothalamus antérieur du canard *(Anas platyrhynchos)*. *C. R. Acad. Sci., 285*, 1327–1330.

Bons N, Kerdelhué B, Assenmacher I (1978a): Immunocytochemical identification of an LHRH producing system originating in the preoptic nucleus of the duck. *Cell Tissue Res., 188*, 99–106.

Bons N, Kerdelhué B, Assenmacher I (1978b): Mise en évidence d'un deuxième systeme neurosécreteur à LHRH dans l'hypothalamus du canard. *C. R. Acad. Sci., 287*, 145–148.

Borg B, Goos HJT, Terlou M (1982): LHRH-immunoreactive cells in the brain of the three-spined stickleback, *Gasterosteus aculeatus* (Gasterosteidae). *Cell Tissue Res., 226*, 695–699.

Bugnon C, Bloch B, Fellmann D (1976): Mise en évidence cytoimmunologique des neurones à LH-RH chez le foetus humain. *C. R. Acad. Sci., 282*, 1625–1628.

Bugnon C, Bloch B, Fellmann D (1977a): Cytoimmunological study of gonadotroph hypothalamo-hypophyseal axis in human fetus. *J. Steroid Biochem., 8*, 565–575.

Bugnon C, Bloch B, Lenys D, Fellmann D (1977b): Etude cytoimmunologique des neurones hypothalamiques à LH-RH chez le foetus humain. *Brain Res., 128*, 249–262.

Bugnon C, Bloch B, Lenys D, Fellmann D (1977c): Ultrastructural study of the LH-RH containing neurons in the human fetus. *Brain Res., 137*, 175–180.

Bugnon C, Bloch B, Lenys D, Fellmann D (1978): Cytoimmunological study of the LH-RH neurons in human fetal life. In: Scott DE, Kozlowski GP, Weindl A (Eds), *Brain-Endocrine Interaction, 1st Ed., Vol. 3*, pp. 183–196. Karger, Basel.

Bugnon C, Fellmann D, Gougeot A, Cardot J (1982): Ontogeny of the corticoliberin neuroglandular system in rat brain. *Nature (London), 298*, 159–161.

Burchanowski BT, Sternberger AL (1980): Improved visualization of luteinizing hormone-releasing hormone by immunocytochemical staining of thick vibratome sections. *J. Histochem. Cytochem., 28*, 361–363.

Burchanowski BT, Knigge KM, Sternberger LA (1979): Rich ependymal investment of luliberin (LHRH) fibers revealed immunocytochemically in an image like that from Golgi stain. *Proc. Natl Acad. Sci. USA, 76*, 6671–6674.

Calas A, Kerdelhué B, Assenmacher I, Jutisz M (1973): Les axones à LH-RH de l'éminence médiane. Mise en évidence chez le canard par une technique immunocytochimique. *C. R. Acad. Sci., 277*, 2765–2767.

Calas A, Kerdelhué B, Assenmacher I, Jutisz M (1974): Les axones à LH-RH de l'éminence médiane. Etude ultrastructurale chez le canard par une technique immunocytochimique. *C. R. Acad. Sci., 278*, 2557–2559.

Carette B (1976): Iontophorèse de noradrénaline sur des neurones des aires septale, préoptique et hypothalamique antérieure. *C. R. Acad. Sci., 282*, 1877–1880.

Carette B (1978): Responses of preoptic-septal neurons to iontophoretically applied histamine. *Brain Res., 145*, 391–395.

Clarke C (1977): Immunocytochemical localization of LHRH and SRIF in the rat CNS. *Anat. Rec., 187*, 356.

Clayton CH, Hoffman GE (1979a): Immunocytochemical evidence for anti-LHRH and anti-ACTH activity in the 'F' antiserum. *Am. J. Anat., 155*, 139–143.

Clayton CJ, Hoffman GE (1979b): Immunocytochemical visualization of luteinizing hormone-releasing hormone (LHRH) in vibratome sectioned murine brain. *Soc. Neurosci. Abstracts*, 119.1.

Crim JW, Urano A, Gorbman A (1979a): Immunocytochemical studies of luteinizing hormone-releasing hormone in brains of agnathan fishes. I. Comparisons of adult Pacific lamprey *(Entosphenus tridentata)* and the Pacific hagfish *(Eptatretus stouti)*. *Gen. Comp. Endocrinol., 37*, 294–305.

Crim JW, Urano A, Gorbman A (1979b): Immunocytochemical studies of luteinizing hormone-releasing hormone in brain of agnathan fishes. II. Patterns of immunoreactivity in larval and maturing western brook lamprey *(Lampetra richardsoni)*. *Gen. Comp. Endocrinol. 38*, 290–299.

Culler D, McArthur WH, Dees WL, Oweris RE, Harms PG (1982): Immunocytochemical evidence that suckling inhibits the postovariectomy depletion of median eminence luteinizing hormone releasing hormone. *Neuroendocrinology, 34*, 258–264.

Daikoku S, Hisano S, Maki Y (1982): Immunocytochemical demonstration of LHRH-neurons in young rat hypothalamus. *Arch. Histol. Jpn., 45*, 69–82.

Dees WL, Sorensen AM Jr, Kemp WM, McArthur NH (1981a): GnRH localization in the equine brain and infundibulum: an immunohistochemical study. *Brain Res., 208*, 123–134.

Dees WL, Sorensen AM Jr, Kemp WM, McArthur NH (1981b): Immunocytochemical localization of gonadotropin-releasing hormone (GnRH) in the brain and infundibulum of the sheep. *Cell Tissue Res., 215*, 181–191.

De Paolo LV, Ojeda SR, Negro-Vilar A, McCann SM (1982): Alterations in the responsiveness of median eminence luteinizing hormone-releasing hormone nerve terminals to norepinephrine and prostaglandin E_2 in vitro during the rat estrous cycle. *Endocrinology, 110*, 1999–2005.

De Reviers M, Dubois MP (1974): Binding of synthetic-LRF antibodies in the ME of the cockerel. *Hormone Metab. Res., 6*, 94.

Dluzen DE, Ramirez VD, Carter CS, Getz LL (1981): Male vole urine changes luteinizing hormone releasing hormone and norepinephrine in female olfactory bulb. *Science, 212*, 573–575.

Doerr-Scott J, Clauss RO, Dubois MP (1978): Localisation histochimique au microscope électronique d'une hormone GnRH dans l'éminence médiane de *Xenopus laevis* Daud. *C. R. Acad. Sci., 286*, 477–479.

Doerr-Scott J, Dubois MP (1975): Localisation et identification d'un centre LH-RF dans l'encéphale du carpaud *Bufo vulgaris. C. R. Acad. Sc., 180*, 285–289.

Doerr-Scott J, Dubois MP (1976): LH-RH like system in the brain of *Xenopus laevis* Daud. Immunohistochemical identification. *Cell Tissue Res., 172*, 477–486.

Dubois MP (1976): Immunocytological evidence of LH-RH in hypothalamus and median eminence: a review. *Ann. Biol. Anim. Biochim. Biophys., 16*, 177–194.

Dyer RG, Dyball REJ (1974): Evidence for a direct effect of LRF and TRF on single unit activity in rostral hypothalamus. *Nature (London), 252*, 486–488.

Elkind-Hirsch K, King JC, Gerall AA, Arimura A (1981): The luteinizing hormone-releasing hormone (LHRH) system in normal and estrogenized neonatal rat. *Brain Res. Bull., 7*, 645–654.

Feldman SC, Johnson AB, Bornstein MB, Campbell CT (1977): Luteinizing hormone releasing hormone (LHRH) neurons in cultures of fetal rat hypothalamus. *Neuroendocrinology, 28*, 131–137.

Felix D, Phillips I (1979): Inhibitory effects of luteinizing hormone releasing hormone (LH-RH) on neurons in the organum vasculosum laminae terminalis (OVLT). *Brain Res., 169*, 204–208.

Flerkó B, Sétáló G, Vigh A, Arimura A, Schally AV (1978): The luteinizing hormone-releasing hormone (LH-RH) neuron system in the rat and rabbit. In: Scott DE, Kozlowski GP, Weindl A (Eds), *Brain-Endocrine Interactions, 1st Ed., Vol. 3*, pp. 108–116. Karger, Basel.

Goldsmith PC, Ganong WF (1975): Ultrastructural localization of luteinizing hormone releasing hormone in the median eminence of the rat. *Brain Res., 97*, 181–193.

Goos HJT, Murathanoglu O (1977): Localization of gonadotropin releasing hormone (GnRH) in the forebrain neurohypophysis of the trout *(Salmo gairdneri)*. *Cell Tissue Res., 181*, 163–168.

Goos HJT, Lichtenberg PJM, Van Oordt PGW (1976): Immunofluorescence studies on gonadotropin releasing hormone (GnRH) in the forebrain and the neurohypophysis of the green frog *Rana esculenta*. *Cell Tissue Res., 168*, 325–334.

Gross DS, Baker BL (1977): Immunohistochemical localization of gonadotrophin releasing hormone (GnRH) in the fetal and early post natal mouse brain. *Am. J. Anat., 148*, 195–216.

209

Gross DS, Baker BL (1979): Developmental correlation between hypothalamic gonadotropin-releasing hormone and hypophysial luteinizing hormone. *Am. J. Anat., 154*, 1–10.

Hattori M, Wakabayashi K, Nozaki M (1980): Differences of Japanese quail LH-RF from mammalian LH-RF revealed by biological and immunocytochemical study. *Gen. Comp. Endocrinol., 41*, 217–224.

Hisano H, Kawano H, Maki Y, Daikoku S (1981): Electromicroscopic study of immunoreactive LHRH perikarya with special reference to neuronal regulation. *Cell Tissue Res., 220*, 511–518.

Hoffman GE (1976): Immunocytochemical localization of luteinizing hormone-releasing hormone (LHRH) in murine and primate brain. *Anat. Rec., 184*, 429.

Hoffman GE (1983): LHRH neurons and their projections. In: Sano Y, Ibata Y, Zimmerman EA (Eds), *Structure and Function of Peptidergic and Aminergic Neurons*, Ch. 12, pp. 183–201. Japan Scientific Societies Press, Tokyo.

Hoffman GE, Gibbs FP (1982) LHRH pathways in rat brain: deafferentation spares a sub-chiasmatic LHRH projection to the median eminence. *Neuroscience, 7*, 179–193.

Hoffman GE, Sladek JR Jr (1980): Age-related changes in dopamine, LHRH and somatostatin in rat hypothalamus. *Neurobiol. Aging, 1*, 27–37.

Hoffman GE, Knigge KM, Moynihan JA, Melnyk A, Arimura A (1978a): Neuronal fields containing luteinizing hormone-releasing hormone (LHRH) in mouse brain. *Neuroscience, 3*, 219–231.

Hoffman GE, Melnyk V, Hayes T, Bennett-Clarke C, Fowler E (1978b): Immunocytology of LHRH neurons. In: Scott DE, Kozlowski GP, Weindl A (Eds), *Brain-Endocrine Interactions, Vol. 3*, pp. 67–82. Karger, Basel.

Hoffman GE, Davis B, Macrides F (1979): LHRH neurons send axons to the olfactory bulb in the hamster. *Soc. Neurosci. Abstracts*, 177.3.

Hoffman GE, Wray S, Goldstein M (1982): Relationship of catecholamines and LHRH: light microscopic study. *Brain Res. Bull., 8*, 417–430.

Hökfelt T, Elde R, Fuxe K, Johansson O, Ljungdahl A, Goldstein M, Luft R, Efendic S, Nilsson G, Ganten D, Jeffcoate SL, Said S, Perez de la Mora M, Possani L, Tapia R, Teran L, Palacios R (1978): Aminergic and peptidergic pathways in the nervous system with special reference to the hypothalamus. *Ass. Res. Nervous Mental Dis., 56*, 69–136.

Ibata Y, Watanabe K (1977): A morphological survey of the median eminence: fluorescence histochemistry and electron microscopy and immunohistochemistry. *Arch. Histol. Jpn., 40*, 303–315.

Ibata Y, Watanabe K, Kimura H, Sano Y, Sin S, Hashimura E, Imagawa K (1978): Distribution of LH-RH nerve endings in the median eminence of proestrus female rat: fluorescence and peroxidase anti-peroxidase (PAP) immunohistochemistry. *Endocrinol. Jpn., 25*, 141–148.

Ibata Y, Watanabe K, Kinoshita H, Kubo S, Sano Y, Sin S, Hashimura E, Imagawa K (1979a): The location of LHRH neurons in the rat hypothalamus and their pathways to the median eminence. *Cell Tissue Res., 198*, 381–395.

Ibata Y, Watanabe K, Kinoshita H, Kubo S, Sano Y, Sin S, Hashimura E, Imagawa K (1979b): Detection of catecholamine and luteinizing hormone-releasing hormone (LHRH) containing nerve endings in the median eminence and the organon vasculosum laminae terminalis by fluorescence histochemistry and immunocytochemistry on the same microscopic sections. *Neurosci. Lett., 11*, 181–186.

Ibata T, Tani N, Obata HL, Tanaka M, Kubo S, Fukui K, Fujimoto N, Kinoshita H, Watanabe K, Sano Y, Hashimura E, Sin S, Imagawa K (1981): Correlative ontogenetic development of catecholamine- and LHRH-containing nerve ending in the median eminence of the rat. *Cell Tissue Res., 216*, 31–38.

Jackson GL (1971): Comparison of rat and chicken luteinizing hormone-releasing factors. *Endocrinology, 89*, 1460–1463.

Jennes L, Croix D (1980a): Changes in the LH-RH immunoreactivity of hypothalamic structures during late pregnancy and after parturition in the guinea pig. *Cell Tissue Res., 205*, 121.

Jennes L, Stumpf WE (1980b): LHRH-systems in the brain of the golden hamster. *Cell Tissue Res., 209*, 239–256.

Jennes LJ, Stumpf WE (1980c): LHRH-neuronal projections to the inner and outer surface of the brain. *Neuroendocrinol. Lett., 2*, 241–247.

Joseph SA, Piekut DT, Knigge KM (1981): Immunocytochemical localization of luteinizing hormone-releasing hormone (LHRH) in vibratome sectioned brain. *J. Histochem., Cytochem., 29*, 247–254.

Kawano H, Daikoku S (1981): Immunohistochemical demonstration of LHRH neurons and their pathways in the rat hypothalamus. *Neuroendocrinology, 32*, 179–186.

Kawano H, Watanabe YG, Daikoku S (1980): Light and electron microscopic observations on the appearance of immunoreactive LHRH in perinatal rat hypothalamus. *Cell Tissue Res., 213*, 465–474.

Kelly MJ, Moss RL (1976): Quantitative evaluation and determination of the biological potency of iontophoretically applied luteinizing hormone-releasing hormone (LRF). *Neuropharmacology, 15*, 325–328.

Kerdelhué B, Jutisz M, Gillessen D, Studer RD (1973): Obtention of antisera against the decapeptide which

210

stimulates the release of pituitary gonadotropins and development of its radioimmunoassay. *Biochim. Biophys. Acta, 297,* 540–548.

Kerdelhué B, Palkovits M, Karteszi M, Reinberg A (1981): Circadian variation in substance P, luliberin (LHRH) and thyroliberin (TRH) in hypothalamic and extrahypothalamic brain nuclei of adult male rats. *Brain Res., 206,* 405–413.

Kevetter GA, Winans SS (1981): Connections of the corticomedial amygdala in the golden hamster. I. Efferents of the 'vomeronasal amygdala'. *J. Comp. Neuroendocrinol., 197,* 81–98.

Kim K, Ramirez VD (1982): In vitro progesterone stimulates the release of luteinizing hormone-releasing hormone from superfused hypothalamic tissue from ovariectomized estradiol-primed prepuberal rats. *Endocrinology, 111,* 750–757.

King JC, Gerall AA (1976): Localization of luteinizing hormone-releasing hormone. *J. Histochem. Cytochem., 24,* 829–845.

King JC, Millar P (1979): Heterogeneity of vertebrate luteinizing hormone-releasing hormone. *Science, 206,* 67–69.

King JC, Parson JA, Erlanden SL, Williams TH (1974): Luteinizing hormone-releasing hormone (LHRH) pathway of the rat hypothalamus revealed by the unlabeled antibody peroxidase-antiperoxidase method. *Cell Tissue Res., 153,* 211–217.

King JC, Elkind KE, Gerall AA, Millar RP (1978): Investigation of the LH-RH system in the normal and neonatally steroid treated male and female rat. In: Scott DE, Kozlowski GP, Weindel A (Eds), *Brain-Endocrine Interactions, 1st Ed., Vol. 3,* pp. 97–107. Karger, Basel.

King JC, Tobet SA, Snavely SL, Arimura A (1980): The LHRH system in normal and androgenized female rat. *Peptides, 1, Suppl. 1,* 85–100.

Knigge KM, Hoffman GE, Scott DE, Sladek JR (1977): Identification of catecholamine and LH-RH containing neurons in primary cultures of dispersed cells of the basal hypothalamus. *Brain Res., 120,* 395–405.

Knigge KM, Joseph SA, Hoffman GE (1978): Organization of LRF- and SRIF neurons in the endocrine hypothalamus. In: Reichlin S, Baldessarini RJ, Martin JB (Eds), *The Hypothalamus, 1st Ed.,* Ch. 2, pp. 49–67. Raven Press, New York.

Knigge KM, Hoffman GE, Joseph SA, Scott DE, Sladek CD, Sladek JR Jr (1980): Recent advances in structure and function of the endocrine hypothalamus. In: Morgane PJ, Panksepp J (Eds), *Handbook of the Hypothalamus, Vol. 2,* Ch. 2, pp. 63–164. Marcel Dekker, Inc., New York/Basel.

Kobayashi MR, Lu KH, Moore RY, Yen SSC (1978): Regional distribution of hypothalamic luteinizing hormone-releasing hormone in proestrus rats: effects of ovariectomy and estrogen replacement. *Endocrinology, 102,* 98–105.

Kordon C, Kerdelhué B, Pattou E, Jutisz M (1974): Immunohistochemical localization of LH-RH in axons and nerve terminals of the rat median eminence. *Proc. Soc. Exp. Biol. Med. 147,* 122–127.

Kozlowski GP, Hostetter G (1978): Cellular and subcellular localization and behavioral effects of gonadotrophin-releasing hormone (Gn-RH) in the rat. In: Scott DE, Kozlowski GP, Weindl A (Eds), *Brain-Endocrine Interactions, Vol. 3,* pp. 138–153. Karger, Basel.

Kozlowski GP, Chu L, Hostetter G, Kerdelhué B (1980): Cellular characteristics of immunolabeled luteinizing hormone release hormone (LHRH) neurons. *Peptides, 1,* 37–46.

Krause K (1979): Comparative distribution of LH-RH and somatostatin in the supraoptic crest (OVLT) of the rat. *Neurosci. Lett., 11,* 177–180.

Krey LC, Silverman AJ (1981): The luteinizing hormone-releasing hormone (LH-RH) neuronal networks of the guinea pig brain. III. The regulation of cyclic gonadotropin secretion. *Brain Res., 229,* 429–444.

Krey LC, Silverman AJ (1978): The luteinizing hormone-releasing hormone (LH-RH) neuronal networks of the guinea pig brain. II. The regulation of gonadotropin secretion and the origin of terminals in median eminence. *Brain Res., 157,* 247–255.

Krisch B (1978): The distribution of LHRH in the hypothalamus of the thirsting rat. A light and electromicroscopical study. *Cell Tissue Res., 186,* 135–148.

Krisch B (1980a): Immunocyochemistry of neuroendocrine systems: vasopressin, somatostatin, luliberin. *Prog. Histochem. Cytochem., 13,* 1–163.

Krisch B (1980b): Two types of luliberin-immunoreactive perikarya in the preoptic area of the rat. *Cell Tissue Res., 212,* 443–455.

Kubo S, Watanabe K, Ibata Y, Sano Y (1979): LH-RH neuron system of the newt by immunocytochemical study. *Arch. Histol. Jpn., 42,* 235–242.

Leibovitz SF, Jahnwar-Uniyal M, Dworkin B, Makman HM (1982): Distribution of α-adrenergic, β-adrenergic and dopaminergic receptors in discrete hypothalamic areas of rat. *Brain Res., 233,* 97–114.

Léonardelli J, Dubois MP (1974): Commandes aminergiques et cholinergiques des cellules élaboratices de LH-RH chez le cobaye. *Ann. Endocrinol., 35,* 639–645.

Léonardelli J, Tramu G (1979): Immunoreactivity for β-endorphin in LH-RH neurons of the fetal human hypothalamus. *Cell Tissue Res., 203,* 201–207.

211

Léonardelli J, Hermand E, Tramu G (1973a): Action du sulpiride sur les neurones élaborateurs de LH-RH. *C. R. Soc. Biol. Filiales, 167*, 1815–1819.

Léonardelli J, Barry J, Dubois MP (1973b): Mise en évidence par immunofluorescence d'un constituant immunologiquement apparenté au LH-RF dans l'hypothalamus et l'éminence médiane des Mammifères. *C. R. Acad. Sci., 276*, 2043–2046.

Léonardelli J, Dubois MP, Poulain P (1974): Effect of exogenous serotonin on LH-RH secreting neurons in the guinea pig hypothalamus as revealed by immunofluorescence. *Neuroendocrinology, 15*, 69–72.

Léonardelli J, Tramu G, Hermand E (1978): Mélatonine et cellules à gonadolibérine (LH-RH) de l'hypothalamus du rat. *C. R. Soc. Biol. Filiales, 172*, 481–484.

Liposits ZS, Sétáló G (1980): Descending luteinizing hormone-releasing hormone (LH-RH) nerve fibers to the midbrain of the rat. *Neurosci. Lett., 20*, 1–4.

Marshall PE, Goldsmith PC (1980): Neuroregulatory and neuroendocrine GnRH pathways in the hypothalamus and forebrain of the baboon. *Brain Res., 193*, 353–372.

Matsuo H, Arimura A, Nair RMG, Schally AV (1971): Synthesis of the porcine LH and FSH releasing hormone by the solid phase method. *Biochem. Biophys. Res. Commun., 45*, 822–827.

Mazzuca M (1977): Immunocytochemical and ultrastructural identification of luteinizing hormone-releasing hormone (LH-RH) containing neurons in the vascular organ of the lamina terminalis of the squirrel monkey. *Neurosci. Lett., 5*, 123.

Mazzuca M, Dubois MP (1974): Detection of luteinizing hormone releasing hormone in the guinea pig median eminence with an immunoenzymatic technique. *J. Histochem. Cytochem., 22*, 993–996.

McNeill TH, Kozlowski GP, Abel JH Jr, Zimmerman EA (1976): Neurosecretory pathways in the Mallard duck *(Anas platyrhynchos)* brain: localization by aldehyde fuchsin and immunoperoxidase techniques for neurophysin (NP) and gonadotrophin releasing hormone (GnRH). *Endocrinology, 95*, 1323–1332.

McNeill TH, Scott DE, Sladek JR Jr (1980): Simultaneous monamine histofluorescence and neuropeptides immunocytochemistry. I. Localization of catecholamines and gonadotropin-releasing hormone in the rat median eminence. *Peptides, 1*, 59–68.

Meibach RC (1982): A detailed protocol for the in vitro radioautographic visualization of serotoninergic receptors. *J. Histochem. Cytochem. 30*, 831.

Merchenthaler I, Kovács G, Lovász JG, Sétáló G (1980a): The preoptico-infundibular LH-RH tract of the rat. *Brain Res., 198*, 63–74.

Merchenthaler I, Lengvari J, Horváth J, Sétáló G (1980b): Immunohistochemical study of LHRH-synthetisizing neuron system of aged female rats. *Cell Tissue Res., 209*, 499–503.

Millar RP, Aehnelt C, Rossier G (1977): Higher molecular weight immunoreactive species of luteinizing hormone releasing hormone: possible precursors of the hormone. *Biochem. Biophys. Res. Commun., 74*, 720–731.

Monahan M, Rivier J, Burgus R, Amoss M, Blackwell R, Vale W, Guillemin R (1971): Synthèse totale par phase solide d'un décapeptide qui stimule la sécrétion des gonadotropines hypophysaires LH et FSH. *C. R. Acad. Sci., 273*, 508–510.

Moss RL, Dudley C (1980): Luteinizing hormone-releasing hormone: a role in extrapituitary function. In: Barker JL, Smith TG Jr (Eds), *The Role of Peptides in Neuronal Function*, pp. 455–478. Marcel Dekker, Inc., New York.

Moss RL, Kelly MJ, Dudley C (1976): Responsiveness of medial preoptic neurons to releasing hormones and neurohumoral agents. *Fed. Proc., 34*, 219.

Münz H, Stumpf WE, Jennes L (1981): LHRH systems in the brain of the platyfish. *Brain Res., 221*, 1–13.

Negro-Vilar A, Ojeda SR, McCann SM (1979): Catecholaminergic modulation of luteinizing hormone-releasing hormone release by median eminence terminals in vitro. *Endocrinology, 104*, 1749–1757.

Nett TM, Akbar A, Niswender GD, Hedlund M, White WF (1973): A radioimmunoassay for gonadotropin releasing hormone (GnRH) in serum. *J. Clin. Endocrinol., 36*, 880–885.

Nozaki M, Kobayashi H (1979): Distribution of LHRH-like substances in the vertebrate brains as revealed by immunocytochemistry. *Arch. Histol. Jpn., 42*, 201–219.

Nozaki M, Taketani Y, Minaguchi H, Kigawa T, Kobayashi H (1979): Distribution of LHRH in rat and mouse brain with special reference to tanycytes. *Cell Tissue Res., 197*, 195–212.

Ojeda SR, Negro-Vilar A, McCann SM (1982): Evidence for involvement of alpha-adrenergic receptors in norepinephrine-induced prostaglandin E_2 and luteinizing hormone-releasing hormone release from the median eminence. *Endocrinology, 110*, 409–412.

Oksche A (1978): Evolution, differentiation and organization of hypothalamic systems controlling reproduction. In: Scott DE, Kozlowski GP, Weindl A (Eds), *Brain Endocrine Interactions, Vol. 3*, pp. 1–15. Karger, Basel.

Paull WK (1978): Perinatal neuroendocrine morphology and the localization of LHRH in neonatal rats. In: Scott DE, Kozlowski GP, Weindl A (Eds), *Brain Endocrine Interaction, Vol. 3*, pp. 16–32. Karger, Basel.

Paulin C, Dubois MP, Barry J, Dubois PM (1977): Immunofluorescence study of LH-RH producing cells in the human fetal hypothalamus. *Cell Tissue Res., 182*, 341–345.

Pelletier G (1976): Immunohistochemical localization of hypothalamic hormones at the electron microscope level. In: Labrie F, Meites J, Pelletier G (Eds), *Hypothalamus and Endocrine Functions, Vol. 3*, pp. 433–450. Plenum Press, New York.

Pelletier G, Labrie F, Puviani R, Arimura A, Schally AV (1974): Immunohistochemical localization of luteinizing hormone-releasing hormone in the rat median eminence. *Endocrinology, 95*, 314–317.

Pelletier G, Leclerc R, Dubé D (1976): Immunohistochemical localization of hypothalamic hormones. *J. Histochem. Cytochem., 24*, 864–871.

Pelletier G, Leclerc R, Dubé D, Arimura A, Schally AV (1977): Immunohistochemical localization of luteinizing hormone-releasing hormone (LH-RH) and somatostatin in the organum vasculosum of the lamina terminalis of the rat. *Neurosci. Lett., 4*, 27–31.

Pfaff D, Keiner M (1973): Atlas of estradiol concentrating cells in the central nervous system of the female rat. *J. Comp. Neurol., 151*, 121–158.

Phillips HS, Hostetter G, Kerdelhué B, Kozlowski GP (1980): Immunocytochemical localization of LHRH in central olfactory pathways of hamster. *Brain Res., 193*, 574–579.

Phillips HS, Ho BT, Linner JG (1982): Ultrastructural localization of LHRH-immunoreactive synapses in the hamster accessory olfactory bulb. *Brain Res., 246*, 193–204.

Piekut DT, Knigge KM (1981): immunocytochemical analysis of the rat pineal gland using antisera generated against analogs of luteinizing hormone releasing hormone (LHRH). *J. Histochem. Cytochem., 29*, 616–622.

Polkowska J (1981): Immunocytochemistry of luteinizing hormone releasing hormone (LHRH) and gonadotropic hormones in the sheep after anterior deafferentation of the hypothalamus. *Cell Tissue Res., 220*, 637–649.

Polkowska J, Jutisz M (1979): Local changes in immunoreactive gonadotrophin releasing hormone in the rat median eminence during the estrus cycle. Correlation with the pituitary luteinizing hormone. *Neuroendocrinology, 28*, 281–288.

Polkowska J, Dubois MP, Domanski E (1980): Immunocytochemistry of luteinizing hormone releasing hormone (LHRH) in the sheep hypothalamus during various reproductive stages. Correlation with the gonadotropic hormones of the pituitary. *Cell Tissue Res., 208*, 327–341.

Poulain P (1974): Excitation des neurones de la région préoptico-septale par application iontophorétique d'acétylcholine. *C. R. Acad. Sci., 279*, 1773–1775.

Poulain P, Carette B (1974): Iontophoresis of prostaglandins on hypothalamic neurons. *Brain Res., 79*, 311–314.

Poulain P, Carette B (1976): Actions of iontophoretically applied prolactin on septal and preoptic neurons in the guinea pig. *Brain Res., 116*, 172–176.

Réthelyi M, Vigh S, Sétáló G, Merchenthaler I, Flérko B, Petrusz P (1981): The luteinizing hormone-releasing hormone containing pathways and their co-termination with tanycyte processes in and around the median eminence and in the pituitary stalk of the rat. *Acta Morphol. Acad. Sci. Hung., 29*, 259–283.

Richoux JP, Dubois MP (1976): Détection immunocytologique de peptides immunologiquement apparentés au LRH et au SRIF chez le lérot dans différentes conditions. *C. R. Soc. Biol. Filiales, 170*, 860–867.

Rodriguez-Sierra JF, Komisaruk BR (1982): Common hypothalamic sites of sexual receptivity in female rats by LHRH, PGE$_2$ and progesterone. *Neuroendocrinology, 35*, 363–369.

Rotsztejn WH, Drouva SV, Pattou C, Kordon C (1978): Met-enkephalin inhibits in vitro dopamine-induced release from mediobasal hypothalamus of male rats. *Nature (London), 274*, 281–282.

Samson WK, McCann SM (1979): Effects of lesions in the organum vasculosum lamina terminalis on the hypothalamic distribution of luteinizing hormone-releasing hormone and gonadotropin secretion in the ovariectomized rat. *Endocrinology, 105*, 939–946.

Samson WK, Snyder G, Fawcett C, McCann SM (1980): Chromatographic and biologic analysis of ME and OVLT LHRH. *Peptides, 1*, 97–102.

Samson WK, Burton KP, Reeves JP, McCann SM (1981): Vasoactive intestinal peptides stimulates luteinizing hormone-releasing hormone from median eminence synaptosomes. *Regul. Peptides, 2*, 253–264.

Sawakami M, Sakuma Y, Kawakami M (1976): Electrophysiological evidences for possible participation of periventricular neurons in anterior pituitary regulation. *Brain Res., 101*, 79–94.

Schally AV, Arimura A, Baba Y, Nair RMG, Matsuo J, Redding TW, Debeljuk L, White WF (1971): Isolation and properties of the FSH- and LH-releasing hormone. *Biochem. Biophys. Res. Commun., 43*, 393–399.

Schreibman MP, Halpern RL, Goos HJT, Margolis-Kazan H (1979): Identification of luteinizing hormone-releasing hormone (LHRH) in the brain and pituitary gland of a fish by immunocytochemistry. *J. Exp. Zool., 210*, 153–159.

213

Scott PM, Knigge KM (1981): Immunocytochemistry of luteinizing hormone-releasing hormone, vasopressin and corticotropin following deafferentation of the basal hypothalamus of the male rat brain. *Cell Tissue Res., 21*, 393–402.

Sétáló G, Vigh S, Schally AV, Arimura A, Flerkó B (1975): LH-RH containing neural elements in the rat hypothalamus. *Endocrinology, 96*, 135–142.

Sétáló G, Vigh S, Schally AV, Arimura A, Flerkó B (1976a): Immunohistological study of the origin of LH-RH containing nerve fibers of the rat hypothalamus. *Brain Res., 103*, 597–602.

Sétáló G, Vigh S, Schally AV, Arimura A, Flerkó B (1976b): Changing immunoreactivity of the LH-RH containing nerve terminals in the organum vasculosum lamina terminalis. *Acta Biol. Acad. Sci. Hung., 27*, 75–77.

Sharp PJ, Haase E, Fraser HM (1975): Immunofluorescent localization of sites binding anti-synthetic LH-RH serum in the medium eminence of the green finch *(Chloris chloris L)*. *Cell Tissue Res., 162*, 83–91.

Shin SH, Howitt C (1977): Evidence for the existence of LHRH binding protein. *Neuroendocrinology, 24*, 14–23.

Sievertsson H, Chang JK, Bogentoft C, Currie BL, Folkers K, Bowers CY (1971): Synthesis of the luteinizing hormone releasing hormone of the hypothalamus and its hormonal activity. *Biochem. Biophys. Res. Commun., 44*, 1566–1571.

Silverman AJ (1976): Distribution of luteinizing hormone-releasing hormone (LHRH) in the guinea pig brain. *Endocrinology, 99*, 30–41.

Silverman AJ, Desnoyers P (1976): Ultrastructural immunocytochemical localization of luteinizing hormone-releasing hormone (LH-RH) in the median eminence of the guinea pig. *Cell Tissue Res., 169*, 157–166.

Silverman AJ, Krey LC (1978a): The luteinizing hormone releasing hormone (LH-RH) neuronal networks of the guinea pig brain. I. Intra- and extrahypothalamic projections. *Brain Res., 157*, 233–246.

Silverman AJ, Zimmerman EA (1978b): Pathways containing luteinizing hormone-releasing hormone (LH-RH) in the mammalian brain. In: Scott DE, Kozlowski GP, Weindl A (Eds), *Brain-Endocrine Interactions, Vol. 3*, pp. 83-96. Karger, Basel.

Silverman AJ, Antunés JL, Ferin M, Zimmerman EA (1977): The distribution of luteinizing hormone-releasing hormone (LH-RH) in the hypothalamus of the rhesus monkey; light microscopic study using immunoperoxidase technique. *Endocrinology, 101*, 134–142.

Silverman AJ, Krey LC, Zimmerman EA (1979): A comparative study of the luteinizing hormone-releasing hormone (LH-RH) neuronal networks in mammals. *Biol. Reprod., 20*, 98–110.

Sterling RJ, Sharp PJ (1982): The localization of LH-RH neurons in the diencephalon of the domestic hen. *Cell Tissue Res., 222*, 283–298.

Sternberger LA, Hoffman GE (1978): Immunocytology of luteinizing hormone-releasing hormone. *Neuroendocrinology, 25*, 111–128.

Stumpf WE (1970): Estrogen neurons and estrogen neuron system in the periventricular brain. *Am. J. Anat., 129*, 207–218.

Taketani Y, Nozaki M, Taga M, Minaguchi H, Kigawa T, Sakamoto S, Kobayashi H (1980): Effect of hypothalamic deafferentation on the distribution of luteinizing hormone-releasing hormone (LHRH) in the rat brain. *Endocrinol. Jpn., 27*, 297–305.

Toran-Allerand CD (1978): The luteinizing hormone-releasing hormone (LH-RH) neurons in cultures of the newborn mouse hypothalamus/preoptic area: ontogenetic aspects and response to steroids. *Brain Res., 149*, 257–265.

Tramu G, Pillez A (1981): Localization immunocytochimique des terminaisons à corticolibérine dans l'éminence médiane du cobaye et du rat. *C. R. Acad. Sci., 294*, 107–114.

Tramu G, Léonardelli J, Dubois MP (1977): Immunohistochemical evidence for an ACTH-like substance in hypothalamic LH-RH neurons. *Neurosci. Lett., 6*, 305–309.

Vigh-Teichman I, Vigh B (1974): The infundibular cerebrospinal fluid contacting neurons. *Adv. Anat. Embryol. Cell Biol., 50*, 7–91.

Warembourg MY (1977a): Radioautographic localization of estrogen-concentrating cells in the brain and pituitary of the guinea pig. *Brain Res., 123*, 357–362.

Warembourg MY (1977b): Topographical distribution of estrogen-concentrating cells in the brain and pituitary of the squirrel monkey. *Neurosci. Lett., 5*, 315–319.

Weindl A, Sofroniew MV (1978): Neurohormones and circumventricular organs. An immunohistochemical investigation. In: Scott DE, Kozlowski GP, Weindl A (Eds), *Brain-Endocrine Interactions, Vol. 3*, pp. 117–137. Karger, Basel.

Weiner RI, Pattou E, Kerdelhué B, Lordon C (1975): Differential effects of hypothalamic deafferentation upon luteinizing hormone-releasing hormone in the median eminence and organum vasculosum of the lamina terminalis. *Endocrinology, 97*, 1597–1600.

214

Wenger T (1976): Ultrastructural changes in the nerve terminals of the vascular organ of the lamina terminalis in the rat during the estrous cycle. *Neurosci. Lett., 3*, 29–32.

Wenger T, Léonardelli J (1980): Circadian and cyclic LHRH variations in the organum vasculosum of the lamina terminalis of female and male rats. *Neuroendocrinology, 31*, 331–337.

Wenger T, Gerendai I, Halasz B (1978): Effect of hypophysectomy on the luteinizing hormone-releasing hormone content of the organum vasculosum of the lamina terminalis in the female rat. *Brain Res., 157*, 157–160.

Wilkes MM, Kobayashi RM, Yen SSC, Moore RY (1979): Monoamine neuron regulation of LRF neurons innervating the organum vasculosum laminae terminalis and median eminence. *Neurosci. Lett., 13*, 41–46.

Witkin JW, Paden CM, Silverman A (1982): The luteinizing hormone-releasing hormone (LHRH) system in the rat brain. *Neuroendocrinology, 35*, 429–438.

Wray S, Hoffman GE (1982): LHRH cells: a variation with maturation. *Soc. Neurosci. Abstracts*, 29.2.

Wray S, Hoffman GE (1983): Postnatal maturation of the LHRH system. *Soc. Neurosci. Abstracts*, 294.1.

Young WC III, Kuhar MJ (1980): Noradrenergic α_1 and α_2 receptors: light microscopic autoradiographic localization. *Proc. Ntl Acad. Sci. USA, 77*, 1696–1700.

Zimmerman EA, Antunés JL (1976): Organization of the hypothalamic pituitary system: current concepts from immunocytochemical studies. *J. Histochem. Cytochem., 24*, 807–815.

Zimmerman EA, Hsu KC, Ferin M, Kozlowski GP (1974): Localization of gonadotropin releasing hormone (Gn-RH) in the hypothalamus of the mouse by immunoperoxidase technique. *Endocrinology, 95*, 1–8.

CHAPTER V

β-Endorphin, α-MSH, ACTH, and related peptides*

HENRY KHACHATURIAN, MICHAEL E. LEWIS, KANG TSOU AND
STANLEY J. WATSON

1. INTRODUCTION

β-Endorphin, α-MSH, ACTH, and related substances belong to a distinct family of peptides derived from a single precursor molecule, proopiomelanocortin (POMC) (Fig. 1). To date, this precursor, POMC, has been localized to both the pituitary gland and the brain (for review, see Akil and Watson 1983; Akil et al. 1984; Chrétien and Seidah 1981; Eipper and Mains 1980; Herbert et al. 1980; Krieger et al. 1980; O'Donohue and Dorsa 1982; Watson et al. 1984; Khachaturian et al. 1985).

Since β-endorphin has known opiate characteristics, it also belongs to one of three opioid peptide families, the most studied other members of which are Met-enkephalin and Leu-enkephalin, derived from proenkephalin (see Comb et al. 1982; Gubler et al. 1982; Noda et al. 1982), and dynorphin A, dynorphin B, and α-neo-endorphin, derived from prodynorphin (see Kakidani et al. 1982). All these peptides share the common opioid core amino acid sequence Tyr-Gly-Gly-Phe-Leu or Tyr-Gly-Gly-Phe-Met, the latter of which is incorporated into β-endorphin.

Since POMC peptides are present in both the pituitary and the brain, they must be regarded as potential hormones or neuromodulators/neurotransmitters. The co-localization of these substances in the same pituitary cells or brain neurons raises many questions regarding the regulation of their synthesis, storage, release, and possible coordinate action. For example, the regulation of synthesis and storage could occur at several levels: (1) transcription of the POMC gene to messenger RNA, (2) translation of the

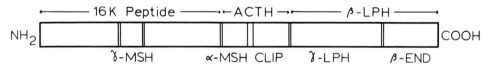

Fig. 1. Schematic model of proopiomelanocortin molecule indicating the position of several peptide products. Double bars indicate dibasic cleavage sites. β-END = β-endorphin. β-LPH = β-lipotropin. CLIP = corticotropin-like intermediate lobe peptide.

---

*This work was supported by NIDA grant DA00265 and NIDA Center grant DA00154 to SJW; NIMH training grant MH15794 to HK.

Handbook of Chemical Neuroanatomy, Vol. 4: GABA and Neuropeptides in the CNS, Part I.
A. Björklund and T. Hökfelt, editors.
© Elsevier Science Publishers B.V., 1985.

mRNA to precursor, (3) proteolytic processing of precursor to peptide, or (4) post-translational processing (such as acetylation) which may alter the biological properties of the final products. Furthermore, although the several POMC peptides have the same general distribution within the central nervous system, the regulation of release and co-ordinate action might involve: (1) differential processing of the precursor and products which may result in quantitative differences in the regional distribution of stored peptides in the neuron, (2) possible differential distribution of receptors for each individual peptide, or (3) agonistic, antagonistic, or synergistic effects of the several peptides on a given target cell.

In this chapter, we present a detailed description of the anatomical distribution of the POMC peptides in the rat central nervous system, along with brief reviews of the biochemical nature of these substances, and their possible physiological roles in pain, stress, cardiovascular control, respiration, neuroendocrine control, thermoregulation, consummatory and sexual behavior, aggression, locomotion, and reinforcement and learning processes.

2. BACKGROUND

The first of the POMC-derived peptides to be recognized for their biological activities were the melanocyte-stimulating hormones (MSH's) for their effects on the melanotrophs and ACTH for its effect on the adrenal gland (see Baker 1979). The structure of ACTH was elucidated by Li et al. (1955), and that of α- and β-MSH by Lee and Lerner (1956). Later, in the process of purifying corticotropin from sheep pituitary glands, Li (1964) discovered a lipolytic peptide with some biological activity similar to that of ACTH. The functional significance of this peptide, β-lipotropin, remained obscure until it was proposed to be the precursor of β-MSH (Chrétien and Li 1967). These latter investigators had identified another lipolytic peptide, γ-lipotropin, and had shown it to be contained within the bovine β-lipotropin molecule (β-LPH(1–58)), with β-MSH constituting β-LPH(41–58).

In the early 1970's, the demonstration of high affinity stereospecific opiate receptor sites in the central nervous system (Pert and Snyder 1973; Simon et al. 1973; Terenius 1973) prompted the search for endogenous ligands. In 1975, Hughes and co-workers described the first two endogenous opioid peptides in mammalian brain, namely Met- and Leu-enkephalin, and noted the existence of the Met-enkephalin amino acid sequence within that of β-lipotropin (β-LPH(61–65)). A year later, Li and Chung (1976), Bradbury et al. (1976), and Chrétien et al. (1976) independently isolated and characterized a third opioid peptide, β-endorphin, from the pituitary, and showed its amino acid sequence also to exist within that of β-lipotropin (β-LPH(61–91)). Simultaneously, β-endorphin was shown to be a potent substance in a wide variety of opiate test systems (Bradbury et al. 1976; Chrétien et al. 1976; Cox et al. 1975; De Wied 1977; Guillemin et al. 1976; Li and Chung 1976; Loh et al. 1976; Rubinstein et al. 1977; Tseng et al. 1976a,b). Subsequently, it became known that β-lipotropin and β-endorphin shared a common precursor with α-MSH and ACTH (hence the name proopiomelanocortin) and several other peptides (Mains et al. 1977; Roberts and Herbert 1977). Shortly thereafter, with the application of cDNA cloning techniques, several investigators were able to determine the full structure of the POMC precursor (Drouin and Goodman 1980; Nakanishi et al. 1979; Roberts et al. 1979; Whitfeld et al. 1982) (Fig. 1).

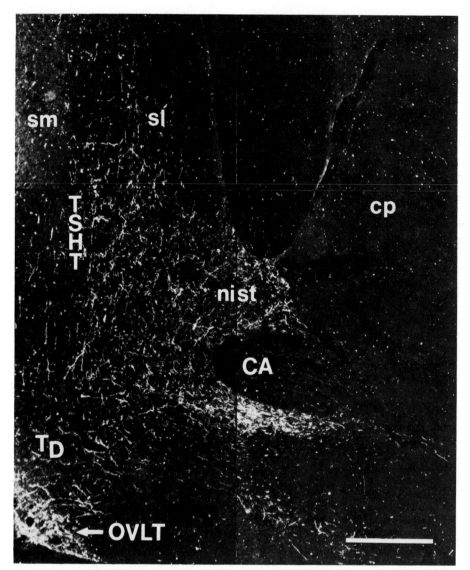

Fig. 2. Montage at frontal plane *A 7.5*: note fiber flow into the nucleus interstitialis stria terminalis (nist); and ventral lateral septum (sl) via tractus septohypothalamicus (TSHT) (or hypothalamoseptalis). Note also fibers in the tractus diagonalis (TD); and the organum vasculosum lamina terminalis (OVLT). *16K* immunoreactivity. Bar = 400 μm.

2.1. PITUITARY GLAND

In the anterior lobe of the pituitary, the corticotrophs process the POMC molecule into ACTH and β-lipotropin as major products, whereas in the intermediate lobe melanotrophs, β-lipotropin and ACTH are cleaved into β-endorphin, γ-lipotropin, and α-MSH and corticotropin-like intermediate lobe peptide (CLIP), respectively (Benjannet et al. 1980; Eipper and Mains 1978; Gianoulakis et al. 1979; Zakarian and Smyth 1979). In

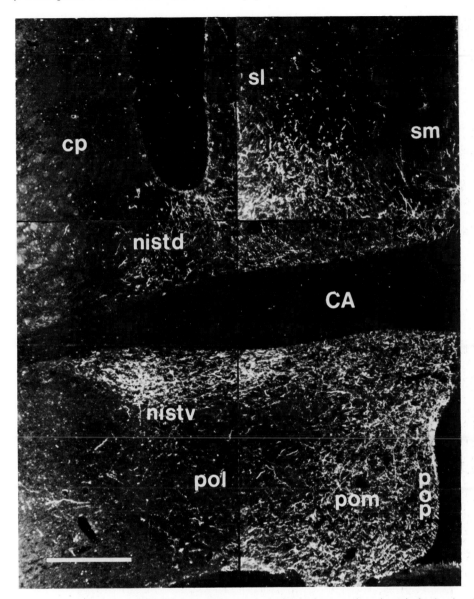

Fig. 3. Montage at frontal plane *A 7.2*: note fiber concentration in the preoptic periventricular (pop) and pre-optic medial (pom) nuclei; nucleus interstitialis stria terminalis, pars ventralis (nistv) and pars dorsalis (nistd); and ventral lateral septum (sl). *16K* immunoreactivity. Bar = 400 μm.

the *brain*, the proteolytic processing of the POMC precursor appears to be similar to that found in the intermediate lobe (see Watson et al. 1980).

The pituitary is the major site of POMC biosynthesis. The first immunocytochemical study of β-lipotropin showed this peptide to be localized to anterior lobe corticotrophs and all cells of the intermediate lobe (Moon et al. 1973). This observation made it apparent that a relationship must exist between β-lipotropin and ACTH in the anterior lobe, and β-lipotropin and α-MSH in the intermediate lobe. The work of several laboratories

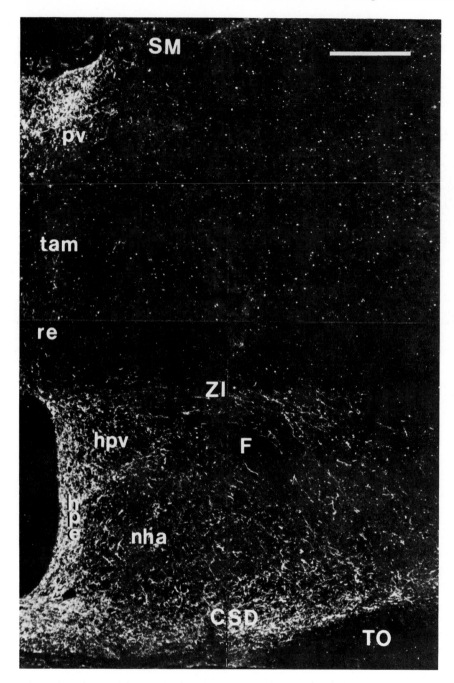

Fig. 4. Montage at frontal plane *A 5.3*: note fiber concentration in the hypothalamic periventricular (hpe), paraventricular (hpv) and anterior (nha) nuclei; and the periventricular nucleus of thalamus (pv). Note also fiber flow in the zona incerta (ZI) and the supraoptic decussation (CSD). *16K* immunoreactivity. Bar = 400 μm.

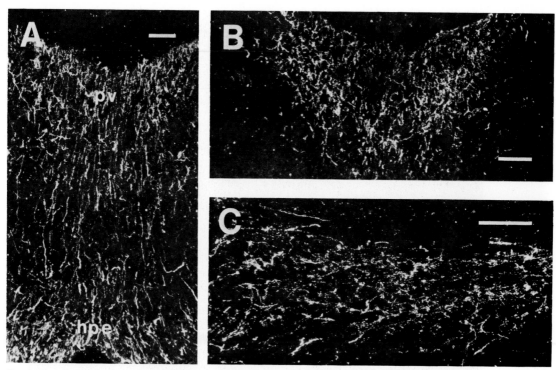

Fig. 5. The periventricular nucleus of the thalamus is depicted at 3 different levels. *A* (frontal plane *A 6.3*) shows a rostral level where *16K* immunoreactive fibers flow from periventricular hypothalamic nucleus (hpe) into the periventricular thalamic nucleus (pv). *B* (frontal plane *A 4.1*): *16K* immunoreactive fibers at a more caudal level of the nucleus. *C* (parasagittal plane *Lat. 0.1*): note fiber flow in the rostral-caudal (left-right) areas of the nucleus; *β*-endorphin immunoreactivity. Bar = 100 μm.

led to the impression of a more direct link between *β*-lipotropin, *β*-endorphin, ACTH and *α*-MSH (Bloom et al. 1977; Pelletier et al. 1977; Weber et al. 1978). They showed *β*-lipotropin, ACTH, and *β*-endorphin immunoreactivities to be localized in the corticotrophs, and likewise that *β*-endorphin, *β*-lipotropin, and *α*-MSH immunoreactivities were localized in the melanotrophs, thus raising the possibility that these peptides are biosynthetically related. As already mentioned, the biochemical studies of Mains et al. (1977) and Roberts and Herbert (1977) elucidated the structure of the common prohormone (with an apparent molecular weight of 31 kilodaltons) which gave rise to all of these peptides. The discovery of the '31K' precursor (i.e., POMC) thus explained the findings of the preceding anatomical co-localization studies (Bloom et al. 1977; Pelletier et al. 1977; Weber et al. 1978). The '31K' precursor contains *β*-lipotropin at its COOH-terminus, ACTH in the middle, and a '16K fragment' (16K) piece at the NH$_2$-terminus. 16K immunoreactivity has also been shown to be localized to the same pituitary cells that store ACTH, *β*-lipotropin and *β*-endorphin (Pelletier 1980, and our own observations). From both biochemical and anatomical studies, it is apparent that precursor biosynthesis and subsequent processing and packaging of final products occur in the same granules of anterior lobe corticotrophs and intermediate lobe melanotrophs.

2.2. CENTRAL NERVOUS SYSTEM

In the central nervous system, POMC-producing neurons are located in the arcuate nu-

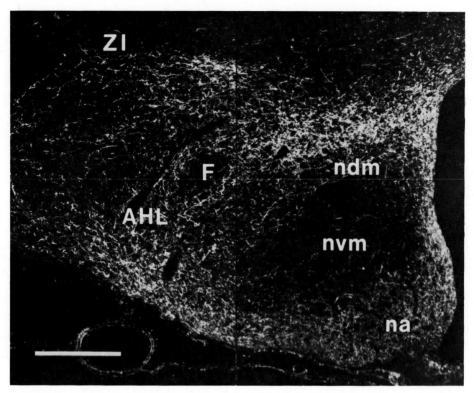

Fig. 6. Montage at frontal plane *A 4.1*: note immunoreactivity in the arcuate nucleus (na), and also fiber flow in the dorsomedial nucleus (ndm), zona incerta (ZI) and lateral hypothalamic area (AHL). *16K* immunoreactivity. Bar = 400 μm.

cleus and periarcuate regions of the medial-basal hypothalamus, with projections throughout the brain. Recently, a second, less extensive group of POMC neurons has been described in caudal medulla in the nucleus tractus solitarius (Schwartzberg and Nakane 1981,1983). Our own observations (Khachaturian et al. 1983a) place these latter neuronal perikarya in the caudal part of the nucleus tractus solitarius and nucleus commissuralis among the perikarya of the A2 noradrenergic cell group.

Numerous immunocytochemical studies have dealt with the distribution of POMC products, viz. β-lipotropin, β-endorphin, ACTH, α-MSH and γ-MSH, in neuronal perikarya, projections, and terminals in the brain of several species (Bloch et al. 1978, 1979; Bloom et al. 1978a,b, 1980; Finley et al. 1981a; Jacobowitz and O'Donohue 1978; Khachaturian et al. 1981, 1984a,b; Nilaver et al. 1979; Pelletier et al. 1978; Sofroniew 1979; Watson and Akil 1981; Watson et al. 1977b, 1978a,b; Zimmerman et al. 1978). Watson et al. (1977b) and Bloom et al. (1978a) demonstrated β-lipotropin and β-endorphin immunoreactivities to occur in hypothalamic neurons, and further showed that these neurons were separate from those which contain the enkephalins (Elde et al. 1976; Watson et al. 1977a). Additional evidence for the separateness of the β-endorphin/β-lipotropin neuronal system and the enkephalin neuronal systems was provided by lesion experiments (Akil et al. 1978b; Watson et al. 1978a). Electrolytic lesions placed in the hypothalamus resulted in a decrease in brain β-endorphin/β-lipotropin levels without affecting enkephalin levels. On the other hand, midbrain lesions caused a depletion of enkephalins rostral to the lesion site, but failed to influence the levels of β-endorphin and β-

222

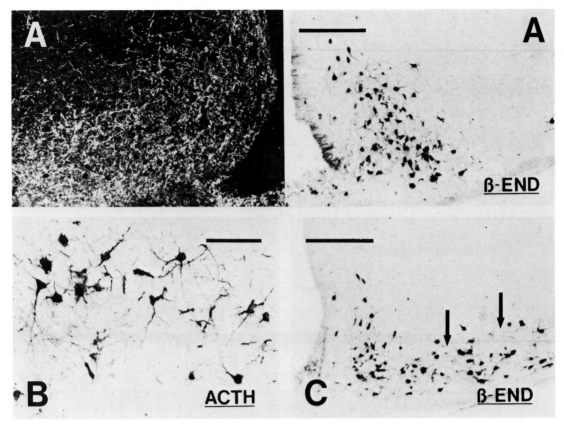

Fig. 7. A (frontal plane *A 3.8*): arcuate nucleus at caudal level showing *16K* immunoreactive fibers and *β*-endorphin (*β*-END) perikarya. *B* (frontal plane *A 4.9*): *ACTH* immunoreactive arcuate perikarya demonstrating processes. *C* (frontal plane *A 4.9*): arcuate nucleus at a more rostral level showing immunoreactive *β*-endorphin (*β*-END) perikarya also in the peri-arcuate region (arrows). Bar (A, C) = 200 μm. Bar (B) = 100 μm.

lipotropin (Akil et al. 1978b). It is now clear that *β*-endorphin-producing neurons are anatomically distinct from those producing either the enkephalins (Elde et al. 1976; Finley et al. 1981b; Hökfelt et al. 1977; Khachaturian et al. 1983b,c; Sar et al. 1978; Simantov et al. 1977; Uhl et al. 1979; Watson et al. 1977a) or dynorphin (Khachaturian et al. 1982; Vincent et al. 1982; Watson et al. 1981, 1982a,b; Weber and Barchas 1983).

After the demonstration of *β*-lipotropin and *β*-endorphin in brain, several investigators began to search for neuronally synthesized ACTH and α-MSH. Krieger et al. (1977) had shown the presence of ACTH immunoreactivity in the central nervous system of normal as well as hypophysectomized rats, lending support for its *de novo* synthesis in the brain. Soon thereafter, Watson et al. (1978a) were able to demonstrate the presence of *β*-endorphin, *β*-lipotropin and ACTH, immunoreactivities in the same arcuate neuronal perikarya. Numerous other light and electron microscopic immunocytochemical studies confirmed the co-localization of several POMC peptides in the same arcuate neurons (Bloch et al. 1978; Nilaver et al. 1979; Pelletier 1979; Sofroniew 1979). The ACTH antiserum used by Watson et al. (1978a) 'stained' the anterior lobe corticotrophs much more readily than either intermediate lobe or brain. Since the antigenic determinant of that antibody was directed against ACTH(11–24), the possibility that the brain processed ACTH into α-MSH (N-acetyl-ACTH(1–13)-NH$_2$), much like that which occurred in the intermediate lobe melanotrophs, became increasingly apparent. Support for this idea was provided by light and electron microscopic demonstrations of α-MSH immunoreactivity in brain, showing its distribution to be identical to that of ACTH, β-endorphin and β-lipotropin immunoreactivities (Dube and Pelletier 1979; Jacobowitz and O'Donohue 1978; Pelletier 1979; Pelletier and Dube 1977; Van Leeuwen et al. 1979; Watson 1980; Watson and Akil 1979, 1980a,b). Watson and Akil (1980a,b) further showed that the arcuate perikarya which contained β-endorphin also contained α-MSH and other POMC peptides, concluding that the processing of brain POMC indeed resembled that of the intermediate lobe, resulting in the production of β-endorphin-like and α-MSH-like peptides. Apparently, the brain POMC neurons cleaved β-lipotropin into β-endorphin, and ACTH into α-MSH and CLIP. In support of this hypothesis, Barnea et al. (1979) showed that ACTH concentrations decreased gradually as the brain region dissected was further removed from the POMC-producing neuronal perikarya in the hypothalamus, thus arguing that as POMC is transported away from the perikaryon it is gradually processed into final peptide products.

3. IMMUNOCYTOCHEMISTRY OF POMC PEPTIDES (*Table 1*)

3.1. ANATOMICAL DISTRIBUTION OF NEURONAL PERIKARYA

The major site of immunoreactive β-endorphin/α-MSH/ACTH/16K perikarya is the arcuate nucleus of the medial-basal hypothalamus in its rostral-caudal extent (Atlas, A 3.2–4.9; L 0.1–0.9 and Figs 7, 9). Other scattered perikarya exist in the peri-arcuate region in an area ventral to the ventromedial nucleus (Atlas, A 4.1–4.9; Lat. 0.9 and Fig. 7C). These POMC-containing perikarya are parvocellular and in 20-μm thick tissue sections exhibit numerous dendritic processes and occasionally a rather thin axonal projection which appears beaded a short distance from the perikaryon (Fig. 7B). These perikarya are immunoreactive to all POMC peptide products. A second group of perikarya, the majority of which reside in the dorsolateral hypothalamus, exhibit immunoreactivity to α-MSH antisera but not to any other POMC peptide antisera (Fig. 22) (see section on α-MSH, p. 242). A third group of neuronal perikarya, also immunoreactive to all POMC peptides, reside in the caudal regions of the nucleus tractus solitarius pars commissuralis, in the caudal medulla (Atlas, P 7.4; Lat 0.4 and Figs 17A, 20B). This latter group, as well as neurons of the arcuate nucleus, are more easily identifiable in embryonic stages, without colchicine pre-treatment (Fig. 20) (Khachaturian et al. 1983a). It is interesting to note that in the arcuate nucleus of the hypothalamus, and in the nucleus tractus solitarius, POMC perikarya reside in close proximity to both enkephalin-containing and dynorphin-containing perikarya. The latter nuclei are the only regions in the brain where all three opioid-containing neuronal perikarya are so closely clustered. Furthermore, many dopaminergic perikarya also are localized within the arcuate nucleus, with projections to the median eminence. Likewise, a major noradrenergic cell group, A2 (Dahlström and Fuxe 1964), resides in the caudal nucleus tractus solitarius (Fig. 17C). The co-existence of the two POMC neuronal groups with other opioid and catecholaminergic perikarya may have interesting functional implications for a coordinate role of these neurons in hormone and cardiovascular regulation.

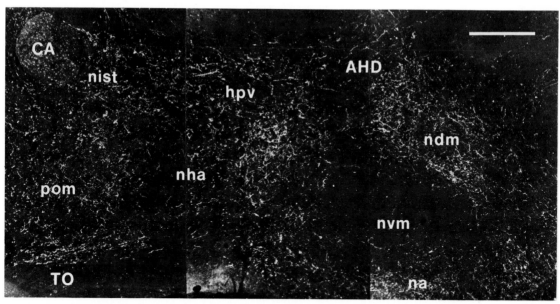

Fig. 8. Montage at parasagittal plane *Lat. 0.4*: distribution of β-endorphin immunoreactive fibers throughout the hypothalamus and preoptic area. Note fiber density in the dorsomedial (ndm) *vs* ventromedial (nvm) nuclei. Note flow of fibers from anterior hypothalamic nucleus (nha) into the medial preoptic nucleus (pom). Also note immunoreactivity in the arcuate nucleus (na), paraventricular nucleus (hpv) and dorsal hypothalamic area (AHD). Bar = 500 μm.

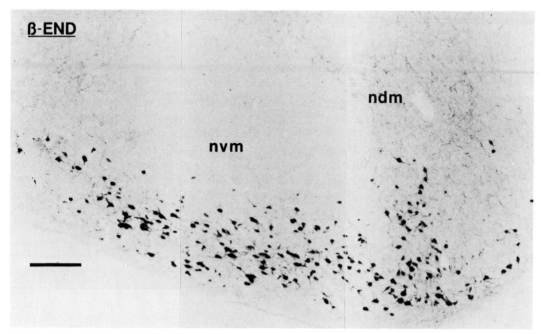

Fig. 9. Montage at parasagittal plane *Lat. 0.4*: arcuate nucleus in its rostral-caudal (left-right) extent showing the distribution of immunoreactive β-endorphin (β-END) perikarya. Bar = 200 μm.

TABLE 1. *List of antisera*

Antibody	Source	Specificity	Key cross-reactivities
β-End (affinity purified)	Watson/Akil	β-LPH(77–91)	6–8% XR with β-LPH, not XR with Met-Enk, ACTH, or α-MSH
ACTH(X3)	Watson/Akil	ACTH(20–24)	Not XR with β-LPH, β-End, α-MSH, β-MSH, or Met-Enk
α-MSH(X2)	Watson/Akil	COOH-terminus	Not XR with ACTH(1–24), ACTH(17–39), ACTH(1–39), β-End, or β-LPH
α-MSH(X2)	Pelletier	COOH-terminus	Not XR with ACTH
α-MSH	Weber/Voigt	COOH-terminus	≪ 1% XR with ACTH
α-MSH	Vaudry	COOH-terminus	≪ 0.1% XR with ACTH
α-MSH(X3)	Immunonuclear Corp.	COOH-terminus	Not XR with ACTH(1–24), ACTH(1–39)
16K fragment (affinity purified)(X3)	Mains/Eipper	NH₂-terminus of 31K precursor	≪ 1% XR with β-End, β-LPH, ACTH

β-End = β-endorphin. β-LPH = β-lipotropin. Met-Enk = Met-enkephalin. Leu-Enk = Leu-enkephalin. X = Number of different sera. XR = Cross-reactive.

3.2. PROJECTIONAL SYSTEMS

Immunoreactive β-endorphin/α-MSH/ACTH/16K processes are distributed widely throughout the neuraxis. The only brain areas that are for the most part devoid of immunoreactive β-endorphin, ACTH, or 16K fibers are the cerebral cortex, striatum, hippocampus, cerebellum, and olfactory bulb, at least within the limitations of immunocytochemistry. These same areas appear to contain an α-MSH-like immunoreactive material localized to neuronal processes and terminals (Fig. 23). These latter fibers presumably originate from the non-arcuate (i.e., non-POMC) hypothalamic neuronal perikarya which also exhibit α-MSH-like immunoreactivity (see section on α-MSH, p. 242). From the POMC perikarya of the arcuate region, three major fiber projectional systems can be described. For the most part, these projections do not follow 'classical' anatomical pathways, and when they do, it does not appear that they form a major component of that pathway.

Rostral projections

Rostral projections of arcuate POMC neurons can be traced through periventricular regions of the hypothalamus and preoptic area (Atlas, A 5.7–7.2; Lat. 0.1–0.9 and Figs

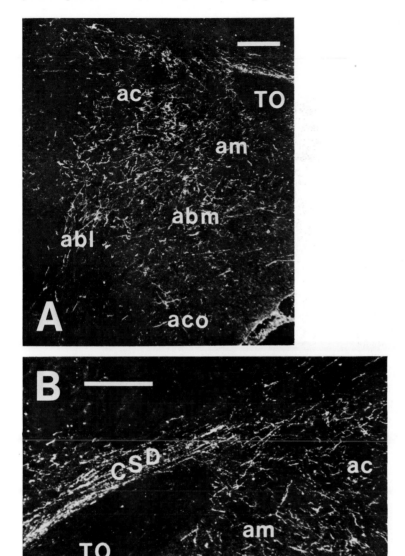

Fig. 10. Amygdala. *A, B* (frontal plane *A 4.9*): note flow of *16K* immunoreactive fibers into the amygdala via the dorsal supraoptic commissure (CSD) innervating the central (ac), medial (am), basomedial (abm), basolateral (abl), and cortical (aco) amygdaloid nuclei. Bar = 200 μm.

3,4,8). These midline fibers continue into the telencephalon, some coursing further rostrally into the olfactory-associated areas, while others turn dorsally to innervate septal and other limbic structures. Some of these fibers course through the diagonal band (of Broca) and septohypothalamic (or hypothalamoseptal) tract (Atlas, A 7.5–8.9; Lat. 0.1–0.9 and Fig. 2). Others enter the stria terminalis which exhibits immunoreactivity throughout its entire course to the amygdala (Atlas, A 3.4–6.7; Lat. 1.4–3.9). Another group of rostrally projecting periventricular hypothalamic fibers follow a more dorsal

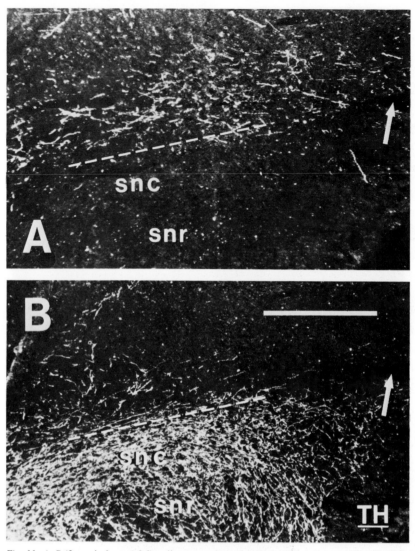

Fig. 11. A, B (frontal plane *A 2.2*): adjacent sections showing *16K* immunoreactive fibers (A) coursing dorsal to the substantia nigra pars compacta (snc). For comparison, tyrosine hydroxylase (TH) immunoreactivity is shown in *B*. (TH antiserum was a kind gift of Dr T. Joh, Cornell University.) Note dorsal boundry of snc marked by dashed line. Also note position of common capillary marked by the arrows. Bar = 400 μm.

course just caudal to the anterior commissure and enter the thalamus (Atlas, A 6.3; Lat. 0.1–0.4 and Fig. 5A). Here again they run in the periventricular regions, gradually changing course to flow in a caudal direction (Atlas, A 3.4–6.3; Lat. 0.1 and Figs 4,5). Some are seen to enter the stria medullaris thalami. Others innervate various thalamic and habenular (epithalamic) regions. A continuation of the periventricular thalamic projection enters the mesencephalon dorsally and continues in a periaqueductal and periventricular (fourth ventricle) course, innervating many structures in the midline raphe and reticular formation (Atlas A 0.2–2.6; P 0.1–2.8; Lat. 0.1–0.9 and Figs 12, 13, 15).

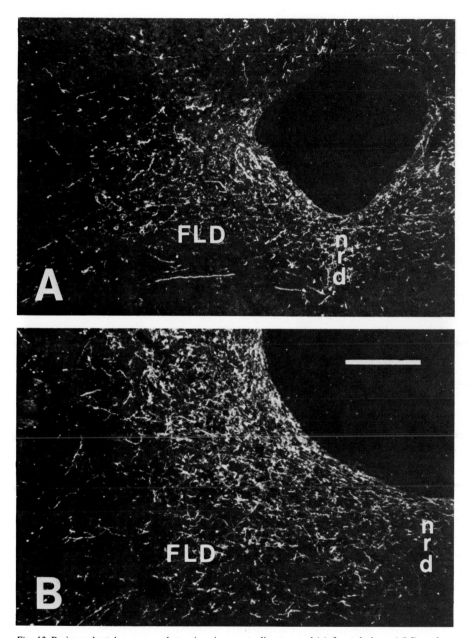

Fig. 12. Periaqueductal gray, or substantia grisea centralis at rostral (*A*, frontal plane *A 0.2*), and more caudal (*B*, frontal plane *P 0.5*) levels. Note also position of dorsal longitudinal fasciculus (FLD) and nucleus raphe dorsalis (nrd). *16K* immunoreactivity. Bar = 200 μm.

Lateral projections

Lateral projections from arcuate POMC perikarya are distributed broadly throughout the hypothalamus, especially in its ventral aspects (Atlas, A 3.2–6.3; Lat. 0.1–1.9 and Figs 4, 6). Generally speaking, the distributional density of these fibers diminishes from

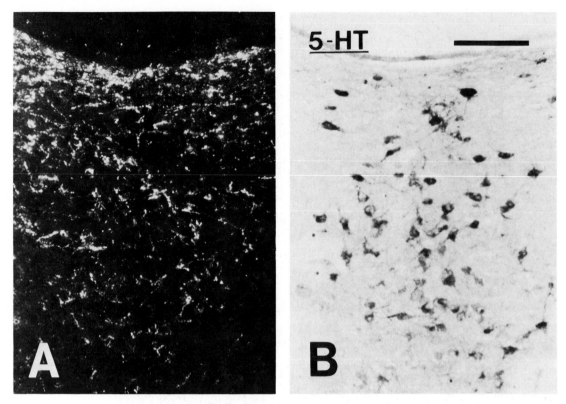

Fig. 13. Nucleus raphe dorsalis. *A*, *B* (frontal plane *P 0.5*): adjacent sections showing distribution of immuno-reactive *16K* fibers in the dorsal raphe nucleus (A). For comparison, serotonin (5-HT) immunoreactive peri-karya are shown in *B*. Bar = 100 μm.

midline to more laterally located structures. Rostrally, these fibers innervate lateral pre-optic, anterior hypothalamic and anterior amygdaloid areas (Atlas, A 5.7–6.7; Lat. 0.4–1.4 and Figs 3,4). Most other hypothalamic regions also appear to be directly innervated by fibers coursing rostro-laterally, dorso-laterally or caudo-laterally from the arcuate nucleus in its entire rostral-caudal extent (Figs 4, 6, 8). Some of these fibers are organized into distinct projectional systems as described above and which are detailed below. Other scattered fibers can be traced in almost all directions, and do not seem to belong to any distinct projectional system. Many such fibers are seen within the medial fore-brain bundle as it courses through the lateral hypothalamic area. However, a distinct laterally projecting system is situated in the floor of the diencephalon, coursing within the supraoptic decussation, dorsal to the optic tracts (Atlas, A 3.4–5.7 and Figs 4, 10). These fibers can be traced laterally from the arcuate POMC perikarya into the amygda-loid region. Caudally and laterally, these fibers appear to be sandwiched between the optic tract and the cerebral peduncle. In the temporal region, they innervate the amyg-daloid nuclear complex (Atlas, A 2.6–5.7; Lat. 2.4–3.9 and Fig. 10). As already men-tioned, another possible source of amygdaloid innervation is fibers travelling in the stria terminalis. These latter fibers might originate from the rostrally projecting POMC fibers in the telencephalon. Conversely, fibers from medial amygdaloid areas might enter the stria terminalis to innervate rostral limbic structures.

230

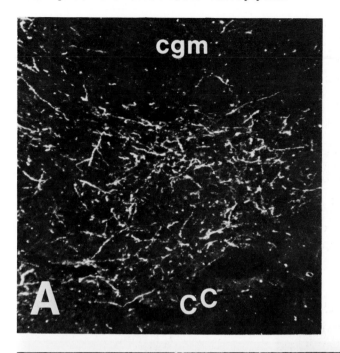

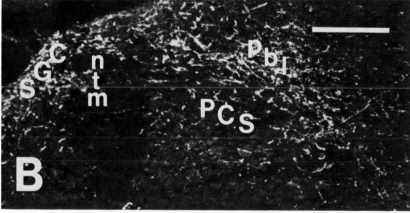

Fig. 14. A (frontal plane *A 1.6*): *16K* immunoreactive fibers in the lateral reticular formation of mesencephalon sandwiched between the medial geniculate nucleus (cgm) and the crus cerebri (OC). This laterally-caudally projecting system contributes to the innervation of the parabrachial nucleus (pbl) shown in *B* (frontal plane *P 1.5*), situated near the superior cerebellar peduncle (PCS). *16K* immunoreactivity. Bar = 200 μm.

Caudal projections

Caudal projections of the arcuate POMC neurons are rather complex and run in multiple directions. Within the hypothalamus, these fibers course through posterior hypothalamic and supramammillary regions (Atlas, A 2.6–3.8; Lat. 0.2–0.9). Periventricular posterior hypothalamic projections enter the periventricular central gray substance of the thalamus (Atlas, A 2.8–3.2; Lat. 0.1). Here they course in a more dorsal direction and appear to continue their periventricular course into the mesencephalic periaqueduc-

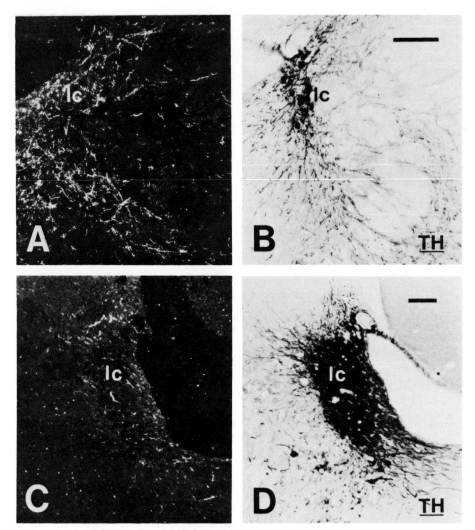

Fig. 15. A, B (frontal plane *P 1.5*): adjacent sections at rostral pole of locus ceruleus (lc). *C, D* (frontal plane *P 2.8*): adjacent sections at a more middle level of locus ceruleus. Note denser concentration of *16K* immuno-reactive fibers at the rostral pole (A) versus the middle level of lc (C). For comparison, tyrosine hydroxylase (TH) immunoreactivity is shown in *B* and *D*. Bar = 100 μm.

tal gray (Atlas, A 0.2–2.6; P 0.1; Lat. 0.1–1.4 and Fig. 12). Some of these fibers course through the dorsal longitudinal fasciculus (of Schutz) (Fig. 12). This latter projection appears to join the periventricular thalamic projections (described above) in the dorsal mesencephalon to innervate primarily the periaqueductal and collicular areas.

Besides this periventricular system, a major component of the caudal projectional system enters the mesencephalon ventrally from the supramammillary hypothalamic region (Atlas, A 2.6–3.2; Lat. 0.1–1.4). These fibers course through the ventral tegmental area dorsal to the interpeduncular nuclear complex, and continue in either a midline dorsal and caudal direction or a more lateral and caudal direction (Atlas, A 0.2–2.8; Lat. 0.1–2.9 and Fig. 11). The midline dorsal-caudal fibers project through the ventral and dorsal tegmental areas, sandwiched between the decussations of the ventral and dorsal tegmen-

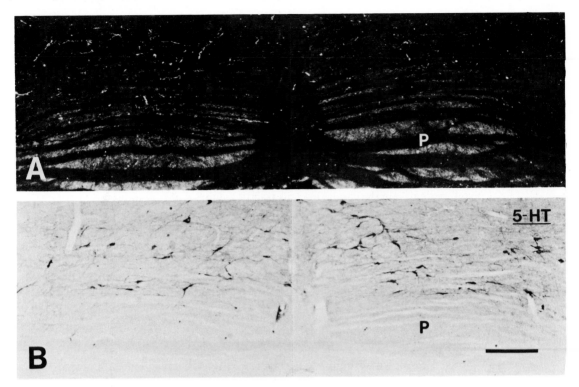

Fig. 16. Nucleus raphe magnus, *A, B* (frontal plane *P 4.5*): adjacent sections showing scattered *16K* immuno-reactive fibers in raphe magnus region (A) dorsal to the pyramidal tract (P). For comparison, serotonin (*5-HT*) immunoreactive perikarya are shown in *B*. Bar = 200 μm.

tum rostrally and the decussation of the brachium conjunctivum (superior cerebellar pe-duncle) caudally (Atlas, Lat. 0.1–0.9). Before entering the dorsal raphe and periaque-ductal regions, they also course in between (and through) the fibers of medial longitudinal fasciculus on either side. These fibers contribute to the innervation of peri-aqueductal and other dorsal reticular sites in the brainstem. The more lateral-caudal projecting fibers course through the ventral tegmental area and continue laterally sand-wiched between the medial lemniscus dorsally and the substantia nigra and cerebral pe-duncle ventrally (Atlas, A 1.6–2.6; Lat. 1.4–2.9 and Fig. 11). In the lateral-most regions of the mesencephalon, in an area just dorsal to the cerebral peduncle, these latter fibers enter the pons (Atlas, A 0.2; Lat. 2.4 and Fig. 14A). Also, in the area stretching between the periaqueductal regions and dorsolateral mesencephalon, the lateral-caudal project-ing fibers appear to be continuous with the periaqueductal-periventricular projection system (Atlas, A 0.2–1.6). This latter region of immunoreactive POMC fibers is situated ventral to the pretectal area and superior colliculus and dorsal to the red nucleus and decussation of the brachium conjunctivum (Atlas, A 0.2–1.6). Once within the pons, the distinction between the periaqueductal and the lateral-dorsal projecting systems is less clear. Both systems appear to contribute to the innervation of dorsolateral pontine structures around the brachium conjunctivum and continue caudally into the pontine and medullary reticular formation (Atlas, A 0.2; P 0.1–2.3; Lat. 0.1–2.4 and Figs 12, 13, 14, 15). Together, the latter systems appear to innervate the dorsal and lateral re-gions of both pons and medulla. In the caudal medulla, the dorsally projecting fibers become sparse; however, in the region of the vago-solitary complex, a sharp increase in fiber density can perhaps be attributed to the intrinsic POMC perikarya of the nucleus tractus solitarius region (Atlas, P 7.4; Lat. 0.4 and Fig. 17A) (see ahead).

Yet another component of the caudal projection system enters the mesencephalon and pons from more ventral aspects (Atlas, A 0.2; Lat. 0.4–1.9). In the ventral pontine region, scattered POMC immunoreactive fibers can be traced through midline raphe areas as well as more laterally situated reticular sites (Atlas, P 3.9–8.0; Lat. 0.1–2.4 and Figs 16, 18). No prominent fiber bundle can be depicted in the ventral pons or medulla; however, some reticular areas appear to contain a denser distribution of fibers than others, especially in the raphe and lateral reticular sites. Again in the caudal medulla, a general concentration of fibers can be noted in the ventral reticular regions, which can perhaps be attributed to the neurons located in the solitary complex.

From perikarya in the caudal nucleus tractus solitarius pars commissuralis (Fig. 17A), which demonstrate immunoreactivity to β-endorphin, α-MSH, ACTH, and 16K (Khachaturian et al. 1983a), laterally and ventrally projecting fibers appear to innervate caudal medullary reticular formation (Atlas, P 7.4; Lat. 0.4). Further tract-tracing studies are needed to determine which areas are innervated by the arcuate POMC projections, and which from the solitary complex POMC fibers. By the same token, POMC fibers detected in the spinal cord (Fig. 19), could conceivably have risen from either of the two POMC neuronal groups.

3.3. DISTRIBUTION OF FIBERS AND TERMINALS

From the foregoing description of POMC fiber projectional systems, it is apparent that a wide array of central nervous system structures are innervated by the arcuate and solitary complex POMC neurons. However, it is not always easy to distinguish between a terminal innervation area and an area through which immunoreactive fibers course *en route* to other regions. This is also true for immunoreactivity seen within the classical (i.e., myelinated) bundles that interconnect virtually the entire central nervous system. Thus, the occasional single immunoreactive fibers seen within the intermediate olfactory tract, genu of the corpus callosum, anterior commissure, fornix, stria medullaris thalami, lateral optic tract, mammillothalamic tract, fasciculus retroflexus (habenulo-interpeduncular tract), medial lemniscus, posterior commissure, lateral regions of the cerebral peduncle, collicular commissures, decussation of the brachium conjunctivum as well as brachium conjunctivum (superior cerebellar peduncle), medial longitudinal fasciculus, tractus solitarius, and spinal trigeminal tract, most probably represent fibers that are merely coursing through, rather than within, these myelinated bundles. On the other hand, several other 'classical' bundles do contain sufficient concentrations of immunoreactive fibers which course in the general direction (either anterograde or retrograde) of the myelinated fibers, such that one must at least consider the possibility that these represent real projections. Among these are the septohypothalamic (or in this case, more appropriately, hypothalamoseptal) tract (Fig. 2), tractus diagonalis (diagonal band of Broca) (Fig. 2), stria terminalis, supraoptic commissure (Figs 4, 10), and dorsal longitudinal fasciculus (of Schutz) (Fig. 12) coursing through the periventricular and periaqueductal gray substance.

On the opposite page is a listing of central nervous system regions that contain immunoreactive fibers and terminals. For simplicity, the density of immunoreactive structures within each region or nucleus has been categorized as *dense*, *medium*, *light*, or *scattered*. Specific brain areas are listed from rostral to caudal, followed by subnuclei, subdivisions, or regions in parentheses.

Dense

Lateral septum (ventrolateral) (Figs 2, 3)
Interstitial (bed) nucleus of stria terminalis (ventral) (Figs 2, 3, 8)
Preoptic nucleus (median, periventricular, suprachiasmatic, medial) (Figs 3, 8)
Central nucleus of amygdala (Fig. 10)
Organum vasculosum of the lamina terminalis (Fig. 2)
Periventricular nucleus of hypothalamus (Fig. 4)
Paraventricular nucleus (pars parvocellularis) (Figs 4, 8)
Arcuate nucleus of hypothalamus and peri-arcuate regions (Figs 6, 7, 8)
Dorsomedial nucleus of hypothalamus (dorsal) (Figs 6, 8)
Periventricular nucleus of thalamus (Figs 4, 5)
Substantia grisea periventricularis, at the junction of thalamus and midbrain
Substantia grisea centralis or periaqueductal gray (medial, lateral) (Fig. 12)
Lateral (dorsal) parabrachial nucleus (Fig. 14)

Medium

Medial septum (ventral) (Figs 2, 3)
Interstitial (bed) nucleus of stria terminalis (dorsal) (Figs 2, 3)
Lateral preoptic nucleus, or area (medial) (Fig. 3)
Medial nucleus of amygdala (dorsal) (Fig. 10)
Anterior hypothalamic nucleus or area (Figs 4, 8)
Paraventricular nucleus (pars magnocellularis) (Figs 4, 8)
Posterior hypothalamic nucleus or area
Lateral hypothalamic area (medial) (Fig. 6)
Zona incerta (Figs 4, 6)
Supramammillary region
Periaqueductal gray (dorsal) (Fig. 12)
Area cuneiformis
Lateral mesencephalic reticular formation (lateral to periaqueductal gray)
Mesencephalic nucleus of trigeminal (rostral) (Fig. 14)
Substantia grisea periventricularis (just rostral to locus ceruleus) (Fig. 15)
Mesencephalic nucleus of trigeminal (caudal)
Nucleus tractus solitarius (caudal, area of A2 noradrenergic cells) (Fig. 17)
Nucleus commissuralis (area of A2 noradrenergic cells) (Fig. 17)
Lateral reticular nucleus (area of A1 noradrenergic cells) (Fig. 18)

Light

Nucleus accumbens (extreme medial)
Lateral septum (dorsomedial) (Figs 2, 3)
Medial septum (dorsal) (Figs 2, 3)
Nucleus of the diagonal band (of Broca) (Fig. 2)
Lateral preoptic area (lateral) (Fig. 3)
Anterior amygdaloid area (medial)
Medial nucleus of amygdala (ventral) (Fig. 10)
Other amygdaloid nuclei (basomedial, basolateral) (Fig. 10)
Dorsomedial nucleus of hypothalamus (ventral) (Figs 6, 8)
Lateral hypothalamic area (lateral) (Fig. 6)
Ventral tegmental area
Pretectal area (medial, lateral)

Dorsal raphe nucleus (Fig. 13)
Inferior colliculus (medial and ventral regions near periaqueductal gray)
Main sensory nucleus of trigeminal
Medial (ventral) parabrachial nucleus
Nucleus raphe magnus (medial, ventral) (Fig. 16)
Nucleus reticularis paragigantocellularis
Area of A5 noradrenergic cells
Nucleus tractus solitarius (rostral)

Scattered

Anterior olfactory nucleus (pars posterior)
Anterior cingulate cortex (occasional single fibers in deeper layers)
Nucleus accumbens (medial, ventral)
Medial and lateral septum (extreme dorsal)
Anterior amygdaloid area (lateral)
Other amydaloid nuclei (intercalated, cortical) (Fig. 10)
Transitional zone between periamygdaloid and piriform cortices (occasional single fibers)
Suprachiasmatic nucleus
Supraoptic nucleus (occasional single fibers)
Ventromedial nucleus of hypothalamus (Figs 6, 8)
Premammillary nuclei (ventral, dorsal)
Paratenialis nucleus of thalamus (occasional midline)
Anterior nucleus of thalamus (occasional midline) (Fig. 4)
Rhomboideus nucleus of thalamus (occasional midline)
Reuniens nucleus of thalamus (occasional midline) (Fig. 4)
Medial nucleus of thalamus, pars medialis (occasional midline)
Posterior nucleus of thalamus, pars medialis (occasional midline)
Habenula, or epithalamus (medial, lateral)
Nucleus linearis of mesencephalon (pars rostralis and caudalis)
Substantia nigra (pars compacta) (Fig. 11)
Oculomotor nucleus (Edinger-Westphal)
Superior colliculus (deeper strata)
Inferior colliculus (lateral, superficial)
Nucleus centralis superior (occasional single fibers in raphe medianus)
Dorsal nucleus of the lateral lemniscus
Nucleus locus ceruleus (Fig. 15)
Dorsal tegmental nucleus
Nucleus raphe pontis (occasional single fibers)
Motor nucleus of trigeminal (occasional single fibers)
Nucleus reticularis pontis oralis
Nucleus reticularis pontis caudalis
Nucleus raphe magnus (dorsal)
Nucleus raphe obscurus (occasional single fibers)
Nucleus reticularis gigantocellularis
Nucleus reticularis parvocellularis
Nucleus raphe pallidus (occasional single fibers)
Nucleus ambiguus
Nucleus of spinal tract of trigeminal (caudal, occasional single fibers)
Dorsal motor nucleus of vagus (Fig. 17)
Nucleus reticularis medulla oblongata
Dorsal gray horn of spinal cord (all laminae)
Dorsolateral fasciculus of spinal cord (Lissauer's tract) (Fig. 19)
Area dorsal to the central canal of spinal cord (dorsal lamina X) (Fig. 19)

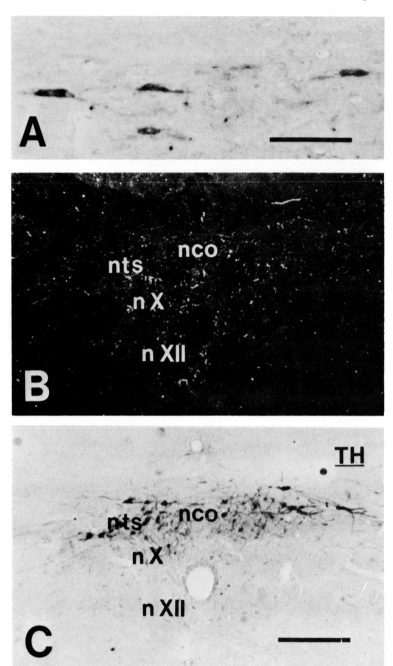

Fig. 17. A, B, C (frontal plane P 7.4). A shows immunoreactive β-endorphin perikarya in the caudal nucleus tractus solitarius. *B* and *C* are adjacent sections showing the distribution of *16K* immunoreactive fibers (B) in the region of the nucleus tractus solitarius (nts), nucleus commissuralis (nco), dorsal motor nucleus of the vagus (nX), and the hypoglossal nucleus (nXII). For comparison, tyrosine hydroxylase (TH) immunoreactive perikarya belonging to the noradrenergic cell group A2 (Dahlström and Fuxe 1964) are shown in *C*. Bar (A) = 50 μm. Bar (B, C) = 200 μm.

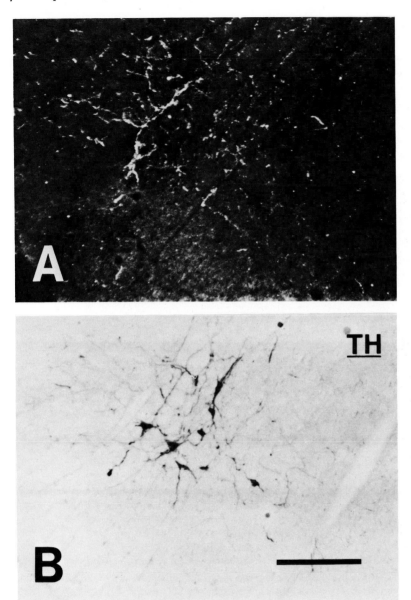

Fig. 18. A, B (frontal plane *P 7.4*): adjacent sections showing immunoreactive *16K* fibers (A) concentrated in the vicinity of tyrosine hydroxylase (TH) immunoreactive perikarya in the lateral reticular nucleus. These perikarya (B) belong to the noradrenergic group A1 (Dahlström and Fuxe 1964). Bar = 200 μm.

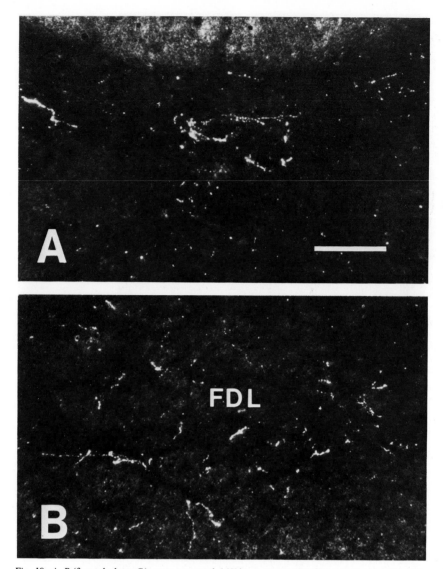

Fig. 19. A, B (frontal plane C_l): note scattered *16K* immunoreactive fibers in the vicinity of the spinal central canal (A), as well as the dorsal lateral fasciculus (FDL) of the spinal cord (B). Bar = 100 μm.

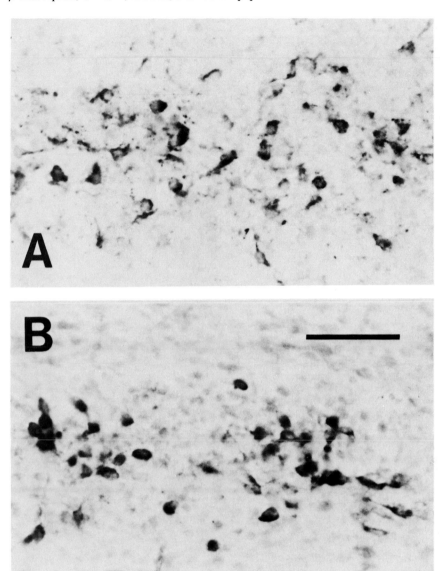

Fig. 20. 21-day-old rat embryo. *16K* immunoreactive perikarya in the arcuate nucleus (A) and the nucleus tractus solitarius (B) are easily demonstrable *without* colchicine pre-treatment. Bar = 50 μm.

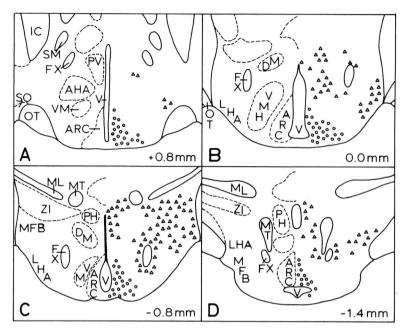

Fig. 21. Comparative distribution of arcuate β-endorphin/α-MSH perikarya (circles) and α-2 (α-MSH) perikarya (triangles) in the rat hypothalamus at selected frontal planes redrawn from the stereotaxic atlas of the rat brain (Pellegrino et al. 1979). AHA: anterior hypothalamic area. ARC: arcuate nucleus. DM: dorsomedial nucleus. FX: fornix. IC: internal capsule. LHA: lateral hypothalamic area. MFB: medial forebrain bundle. ML: medial lemniscus. MT: mammillothalamic tract. OT: optic tract. PH: posterior hypothalamus. PV: paraventricular nucleus. SM: stria medullaris. SO: supraoptic nucleus. V: third ventricle. VM/VMH: ventromedial nucleus. ZI: zona incerta.

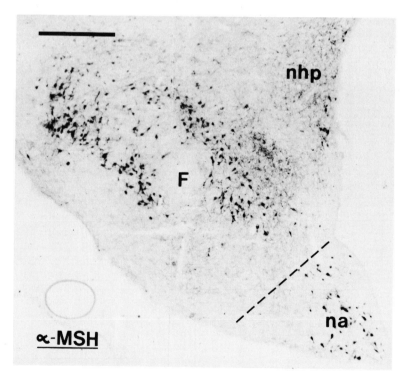

Fig. 22. Montage at frontal plane *A 3.8*: note distribution of α-2 neuronal perikarya in the lateral hypothalamic area surrounding the fornix (F). The α-MSH perikarya of the arcuate nucleus (na) are seen medial to the dashed line. Bar = 400 μm.

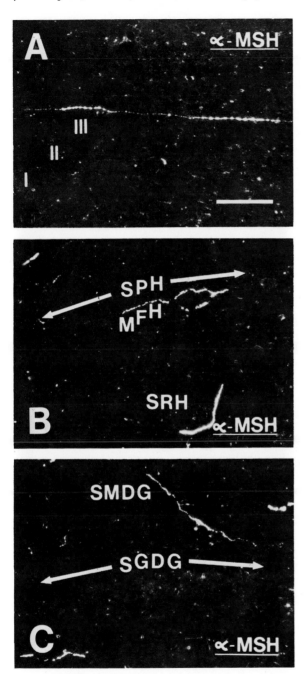

Fig. 23. α-MSH immunoreactive fibers in several cerebral cortical laminae (A); hippocampal mossy fibers (MFH) near stratum pyramidale (SPH), and in stratum radiatum (SRH) (B); and in the dentate gyrus stratum moleculare (SMDG) near stratum granulosum (SGDG) (C). These fibers presumably originate from the α-2 neurons of the hypothalamus. Bar = 100 μm.

4. THE NON-POMC α-MSH-LIKE IMMUNOREACTIVE SYSTEM IN BRAIN

In the process of studying the brain distribution of α-MSH-like material, Watson and Akil (1979) discovered a widespread group of hypothalamic neurons located outside of the arcuate region which were immunoreactive to several α-MSH antisera, but not to antisera of any other POMC peptide. That initial observation has been confirmed in both the rat (Guy et al. 1980, 1981; Watson 1980; Watson and Akil 1980a) and cat (Micevych and Elde 1982) hypothalamus. This second set of α-MSH immunoreactive neurons (termed 'α-2' to distinguish them from the arcuate α-MSH neurons) are detectable only after colchicine pretreatment. These neurons appear to project exclusively to the striatum, hippocampus, cerebral cortex and olfactory bulb, regions which appear to be virtually devoid of projections immunoreactive for other POMC peptides. The immunoreactive material in these cells is likely to be α-MSH-like since the immunoreactivity in the perikaryal region (Jegou et al. 1983) and in cortex and hippocampus (unpublished observation in O'Donohue and Dorsa 1982) has been reported to behave similarly to α-MSH on high-performance liquid chromatography (HPLC). Furthermore, immunocytochemical studies with 8 different α-MSH antisera (Table 1) have yielded no significant differences in the immunoreactive signal seen in the α-2 neurons (Watson and Akil 1979, 1980a). The signal obtained from all 8 antisera could be blocked by 20 μM α-MSH (N-acetyl-ACTH(1–13)-NH$_2$), des-acetyl-α-MSH and diacetyl-α-MSH, but not with N-acetyl-ACTH(1–13) or ACTH(1–13). Hence, the COOH-terminus amidation appears to be essential for the antibody recognition site (Watson, in preparation). It can be concluded from these studies that α-MSH-like immunoreactivity (α-MSH-LI) in both the arcuate and α-2 systems must be similar in their COOH-terminal regions.

While it is possible, in the absence of sequence data, to argue that the material in α-2 neurons may not be authentic α-MSH, there is presently no specific evidence to that effect. Using coupled HPLC and radioimmunoassay, several laboratories have investigated the nature of the α-MSH-LI in hypothalamus versus pituitary (Loh et al. 1980; O'Donohue et al. 1979, 1982; Akil and Watson, in preparation). It is generally agreed that the major product in rat intermediate lobe is α-MSH, with some evidence of des-acetyl-α-MSH (Loh et al. 1980) and some diacetyl-α-MSH (Akil and Watson, in preparation). The hypothalamus appears to contain a large amount of des-acetyl-α-MSH and some α-MSH (Loh et al. 1980; O'Donohue 1982). However, there is presently no evidence of other immunoreactive species which may derive from α-2 and are not seen in arcuate or pituitary cells containing POMC. If the α-2 neurons do contain authentic α-MSH, it is either synthesized from POMC which is processed very differently from POMC in arcuate neurons, or is synthesized from a non-POMC precursor.

4.1. DISTRIBUTION OF α-2 PERIKARYA

Anatomically, the COOH-terminal α-MSH-LI is localized to the α-2 perikarya which are distributed from middle to posterior hypothalamus in the rat (Figs 21, 22). The regions which contain α-2 perikarya are, from medial to lateral: periventricular nucleus, dorsal region of the ventromedial nucleus, perikarya surrounding the fornix, ventral zona incerta, and a large number of perikarya in the lateral hypothalamic area. These perikarya number in the range of 6,000–10,000 on one side of the brain, almost twice the number of arcuate POMC perikarya on the same side (Khachaturian et al. in preparation). The α-2 group can be separated from the arcuate POMC group by both chemical and physical means, for further characterization studies. Rats can be treated neonatally with monosodium glutamate (MSG) to induce neuron damage in the medial-basal hypothalamus (see Olney 1979). This results in the destruction of approximately 75% of arcuate POMC perikarya without any effect on the α-2 neurons. Furthermore, the medial-basal hypothalamus can be surgically isolated with a Halasz knife, resulting in the complete differentiation of the arcuate nucleus (see Halasz 1969). No arcuate POMC perikarya survive this procedure, while the α-2 neurons remain apparently unaffected (Khachaturian et al. in preparation).

4.2. THE α-2 PROJECTIONS

α-MSH-LI fibers are scattered throughout the caudate-putamen nuclear complex. In the hippocampal formation, α-MSH-LI fibers are seen in the dentate gyrus stratum moleculare (the dendritic field of the granule cells) (Fig. 23C), and in the hilus, where axons of the granule cells converge into the mossy fiber projection to the hippocampal fields CA3 and CA2. Within the hippocampus, α-MSH-LI fibers appear in the stratum oriens (the dendritic field of pyramidal cells) in fields CA1, CA2 and CA3, within the mossy fiber layer, as well as throughout stratum radiatum (Fig. 23B). Moreover, immunoreactive fibers are often seen to traverse several strata, coursing through stratum granulosum (granule cell layer of dentate gyrus), and stratum pyramidale (pyramidal cell layer of hippocampus). Fibers are also seen in the hippocampal fimbriae. In the cerebral cortex, α-MSH-LI fibers are scattered throughout most cortical laminae in the frontal, parietal, occipital, cingulate, entorhinal, and piriform regions (Fig. 23A). Fibers were often seen traversing several laminae and finally ending in lamina I where they are often oriented horizontal to the pial surface. Also in the cingulum bundle, many α-MSH-LI fibers are seen oriented in parallel with the corpus callosum, presumably projecting within this bundle. In the olfactory bulb, scattered α-MSH-LI fibers are seen in the anterior olfactory nucleus, within the intermediate olfactory tract (presumably projecting rostrally), and the glomerular external plexiform, mitral cell, and internal plexiform layers of the olfactory bulb.

There appear to exist several possible pathways which might carry α-MSH-LI axons from the α-2 neurons to their innervation fields. In particular, α-MSH-LI fibers were detected in the following regions: (1) The medial forebrain bundle (MFB) and its rostral extension, the cingulum bundle, contain α-MSH-LI fibers. Many α-2 neurons are located in the lateral hypothalamic area, through which the MFB projects, connecting brainstem structures with more rostral cortical and limbic areas of the brain. Thus, α-MSH-LI fibers might project via the MFB to the neocortex and hippocampus (through the cingulum bundle). (2) The fornix, through which fibers from the hippocampal formation project to the hypothalamus and other limbic areas, also contains α-MSH-LI fibers. Many α-2 perikarya are seen surrounding the columns of the fornix, some of which could project to the hippocampus via this route. (3) Many α-MSH-LI fibers are also seen projecting directly laterally from the hypothalamus, coursing over the optic tracts and entering into the amygdala region, thereby possibly gaining access to both the amygdaloid complex and the hippocampus. However, it is not clear whether these fibers represent the arcuate β-endorphin/α-MSH projections or the α-2 projections. (4) α-MSH-LI fibers are also seen in the intermediate olfactory tract, through which they might gain access to the olfactory bulb. Conversely, these α-MSH-LI fibers might originate from the bulb itself, since perikarya containing α-MSH immunoreactivity have been described in the mitral cell layer (O'Donohue and Jacobowitz 1980).

In MSG-lesioned rats (without colchicine pre-treatment), the fiber projections of the arcuate β-endorphin/α-MSH system appear to be diminished, as indicated by a decrease in intensity of the immunoreactivity in the periventricular thalamus, amygdala and periaqueductal gray, all areas which normally receive innervation from the arcuate POMC neurons. In contrast, no loss of immunoreactivity was noted in the hippocampal and cortical fiber systems in the MSG-treated rats, indicating the possible origin of these fibers from the hypothalamic α-2 neurons. Thus, it seems possible to separate, albeit not completely, the arcuate and α-2 neuronal systems by means of neonatal MSG-induced lesions.

In rats with knife-cut isolations of the medial-basal hypothalamus, also without colchicine pre-treatment, the fiber projections of the arcuate β-endorphin/α-MSH neurons were completely abolished. And, as expected, no loss of α-MSH-LI fibers was noted in the projection systems of the α-2 neurons. Apparently, surgical isolation of the arcuate nucleus results in a more complete depletion of immunoreactivity in the β-endorphin/α-MSH neuronal projection system arising from this nucleus, perhaps due to retrograde and anterograde degeneration of the neurons from the point of severance of the axons by the knife-cut. Further, the procedure leaves the α-2 neurons intact, thereby providing a method for the complete isolation of the arcuate and α-2 neuronal systems.

5. PHYSIOLOGY AND PATHOPHYSIOLOGY OF POMC PEPTIDES

The dramatic behavioral and physiological effects of POMC peptides, as well as their possible involvement in psychiatric states, have been extensively reviewed elsewhere (Akil and Watson 1983; Beckwith and Sandman 1982; Berger et al. 1982; Bolles and Fanselow 1982; Holaday and Loh 1981; Koob and Bloom 1982; O'Donohue and Dorsa 1982; Watson et al. 1985). In general, it has been difficult to extrapolate from the effects of POMC peptide administration (i.e., pharmacology) to likely physiological roles of these peptides. While it is clear that these peptides can exert potent effects following intracerebral, intracerebroventricular, or even peripheral administration, such evidence, by itself, is not adequate to demonstrate a particular physiological role. To provide only a single example, it is known that β-endorphin can act at both μ and δ opioid receptor subtypes (Lord et al. 1977), but that the distribution of these receptors is much more extensive than that of β-endorphin-containing neuronal systems (cf. Goodman et al. 1980; Lewis et al. 1983a,b, 1984, 1985 to the maps presented here); it is clear that intraventricular administration of β-endorphin would result in activation of opiate receptors which are anatomically unrelated to endogenous β-endorphin systems, producing effects which have no physiological significance. The most persuasive arguments for physiological significance arise from the convergence of multiple lines of evidence (e.g., when pharmacological studies provide results consistent with independent studies of changes in response to physiological challenges). Below, we briefly summarize various studies pointing to some possible physiological and pathophysiological roles of POMC peptides. We have not reviewed the possible role of these peptides in human psychopathology since this subject has been considered elsewhere (Akil and Watson 1983; Watson et al. 1984, 1985) and is not amenable to anatomically based analyses in non-human subjects.

5.1. ANALGESIA

When β-endorphin is administered centrally, it is a very potent opiate, producing long-lasting analgesia, tolerance, and naloxone-precipitable withdrawal (Loh et al. 1976; Tseng et al. 1976a,b). The possible physiological significance of the opiate analgesic action is supported by findings that electrical stimulation of the periaqueductal gray and other brain regions where *β*-endorphin-immunoreactive fibers are present, results in analgesia (Mayer et al. 1971; Richardson and Akil 1977) which is naloxone-reversible (Akil et al. 1979; Hosobuchi et al. 1977), and in increased levels of *β*-endorphin immunoreactivity in cerebrospinal fluid (Akil et al. 1978a; Hosobuchi et al. 1979). Naloxone-reversible analgesia is also induced by stressors such as footshock (Akil et al. 1976; Lewis et al. 1980; Madden et al. 1972), which appear to activate both the pituitary and brain POMC systems (Guillemin et al. 1977; Lewis et al. 1981; Rossier et al. 1977; Shiomi and Akil 1982). Nevertheless, the role of *β*-endorphin in mediating stress-induced analgesia remains controversial (Lewis et al. 1981; Lim et al. 1982; Millan et al. 1980, 1981; Shiomi and Akil 1982), so that while stress is a clear physiological stimulus to *β*-endorphin release, the subsequent physiological role of the peptide in this situation is less clear. A possible physiological role for the non-opioid POMC peptides in analgesia should also be considered, since ACTH produces analgesia via a non-opioid receptor and is additive with *β*-endorphin in producing analgesia, and *γ*-MSH, while inactive alone, potentiates the analgesia produced by ACTH peptides (Walker et al. 1980).

5.2. CARDIOVASCULAR REGULATION

The cardiovascular actions of *β*-endorphin and other opioids have been fully reviewed by Holaday (1983) and will be mentioned only briefly here. Intracisternal administration of *β*-endorphin has been reported to induce an initial transient elevation of heart rate and arterial pressure followed by delayed hypotension and bradycardia (Laubie et al. 1977). These actions are not unique to *β*-endorphin; similar effects were also observed with D-Ala^2-Met-enkephalinamide and morphine (Bolme et al. 1978). The cardiovascular pharmacology of the opioids has proven to be very complex, with actions depending upon the central (or peripheral) locus and opioid receptor subtypes involved (Feuerstein and Faden 1982; Hassen et al. 1982; Holaday and Faden 1982). Uncovering a selective physiological role of *β*-endorphin is difficult, since it can act at both *μ* and *δ* receptor subtypes; for example, in nucleus tractus solitarius, which is critically involved in the baroreceptor and chemoreceptor reflex arcs, both receptor subtypes are present (Goodman et al. 1980) as well as all three opioid peptide systems (Khachaturian et al. 1982, 1983b,c, 1985). Although there is compelling evidence for a role of endogenous opioids in some pathophysiological states, including shock, spinal injury, and hypotension (Holaday 1983), the specific role of *β*-endorphin in these non-homeostatic conditions remains to be clarified. A possible role of α-MSH in cardiovascular regulation should be considered, since microinjection of this peptide into the dorsomedial hypothalamic nucleus, but not elsewhere within hypothalamus, resulted in an increase in heart rate (Diz and Jacobowitz 1983).

5.3. RESPIRATORY REGULATION

Central administration of *β*-endorphin produces the same marked depression of respiration (Moss and Friedman 1978) which is classically observed with opiate alkaloids. Since both *μ* and *δ* agonists produce similar respiratory depressive effects (Florez et al. 1982), *β*-endorphin could be acting at either site. Although endogenous opioids have been implicated in respiratory pathophysiology (Holaday and Loh 1981), a specific role of β-endorphin has not yet been demonstrated.

5.4. NEUROENDOCRINE REGULATION

As might have been predicted from the complex and often contradictory literature on opiate alkaloid effects on neuroendocrine function (Holaday and Loh 1981), the actions of β-endorphin on hormone responses have often proven difficult to evaluate. Some of the clearest results, however, have been obtained in studies of the anterior pituitary hormones, prolactin and growth hormone. Numerous investigators have shown that β-endorphin is a very effective releaser of both hormones (for review, see Holaday and Loh 1981), apparently at the hypothalamic level. A physiological role of endogenous opioids in their regulation was suggested by the finding that naloxone decreases basal plasma prolactin and growth hormone levels (Bruni et al. 1977; Shaar et al. 1977), although this effect was not observed in all subsequent studies (e.g., Martin et al. 1979); in any case, there is no clear evidence yet for a specific physiological role of β-endorphin in the regulation of these hormones. Although a role in the regulation of vasopressin has been proposed, the experimental findings fail to demonstrate much consistency: β-endorphin has been reported to stimulate (Van Vugt and Meites 1980; Weitzman et al. 1977), inhibit (Iversen et al. 1980; Van Wimersma Greidanus et al. 1979, 1981), or have no effect at all (Reid et al. 1981) upon vasopressin release. An inhibitory effect of β-endorphin upon oxytocin release has been reported (Clarke et al. 1979), but its physiological significance requires further study. In one of the very few anatomically oriented investigations of opioid effects on hormones, Parvizi and Ellendorff (1980) reported that β-endorphin inhibited luteinizing hormone release following administration into amygdala but not hypothalamus. However, other investigators (Shultz et al. 1981) have found that injection of anti-β-endorphin antibodies into the arcuate nucleus of hypothalamus caused an increase in luteinizing hormone release, implicating β-endorphin in this region in the physiological control of the hormone.

One particularly interesting endocrine target of β-endorphin may be the POMC-synthesizing cells themselves (Holaday and Loh 1981). The potential interactions seem to be complex, since β-endorphin can stimulate α-MSH release (Van Wimersma Greidanus et al. 1979), an effect which is attenuated by γ-MSH (Van Ree et al. 1981). Other POMC peptides also have potent endocrine actions: α-MSH has complex effects on growth hormone release (O'Donohue and Dorsa 1982), and ACTH can inhibit opiate alkaloid or peptide-stimulated prolactin release (Ferri et al. 1982; Kanyicska et al. 1983).

5.5. THERMOREGULATION

Determining the physiological role of β-endorphin in thermoregulation has been complicated by the complex relationship between opiate actions on body temperature and a host of variables, including species, dose, ambient temperature, route of administration, degree of tolerance, endocrine status, and degree of stress (Clark 1979; Holaday and Loh 1981). Attempting to account for a diversity of reported findings, Holaday and Loh (1981) have proposed that endorphins may be hyperthermic regulators in states of perceived cold, and hypothermic regulators at normal ambient temperatures and in conditions of heat stress. The hyperthermic and hypothermic effects of β-endorphin are differentially sensitive to naloxone (Bloom and Tseng 1981; Holaday and Loh 1981), indicating a possible involvement of different receptors. The proposed physiological role of β-endorphin in hypothermia-mediated heat adaptation (Holaday and Loh 1981) is intriguing and deserves further investigation. The reported hypothermic actions of the POMC-related peptides, ACTH(1–24) and α-MSH (Glyn and Lipton 1981), as well as the reversal of β-endorphin effects by γ-MSH (Van Ree et al. 1981), require further consideration from the viewpoint of the heat adaptation hypothesis. A physiological role of septal α-MSH in control of fever has also been proposed (Glyn-Bollinger et al. 1983; Murphy et al. 1983); since the septum receives a rich innervation by POMC fibers, the interaction of α-MSH with other POMC peptides in this region should be considered.

5.6. CONSUMMATORY BEHAVIOR

Several investigators have suggested a role for β-endorphin in the regulation of food intake. Feeding can be increased by central administration of β-endorphin (Grandison and Guidotti 1977; McKay et al. 1981) and decreased by peripheral or central administration of naloxone (Holtzman 1974; see for later references Olson et al. 1979, 1980, 1981, 1982). Genetically obese mice (ob/ob) and rats (fa/fa), which have elevated concentrations of pituitary and plasma β-endorphin immunoreactivity, stop overeating in response to opiate antagonists (Margulis et al. 1978; Recant et al. 1980). However, the role of β-endorphin has been questioned since the onset of obesity in ob/ob mice precedes the appearance of increased pituitary β-endorphin immunoreactivity (Rossier et al. 1979; but see Garthwaite et al. 1980). Other investigators have also suggested that the elevated levels of peptide may be a consequence rather than a cause of the hyperphagia and resultant obesity (Deutch and Martin 1983). A role for endogenous opiates in stress-induced eating has been proposed on the basis of naloxone studies (Lowy et al. 1980; Morley and Levine 1980) although a specific role for β-endorphin has not yet been demonstrated. The proposed endorphin–obesity link has also been questioned on the basis of findings that pituitary β-endorphin levels were unrelated to weight gains resulting from several obesity-inducing treatments (Gunion and Peters 1981). The role of β-endorphin, in particular, in the regulation of food intake has been questioned on the basis of the finding that adrenalectomy increases β-endorphin levels but not eating or naloxone inhibition of eating (see Olson et al. 1982).

A physiological role for β-endorphin in the regulation of water intake is also controversial. A large number of investigations have demonstrated that opiate antagonists inhibit drinking in water-deprived and undeprived animals (see Olson et al. 1981, 1982 for references); such findings raised the possibility that endogenous opioids facilitate drinking behavior, a view consistent with reports that opiate agonists usually stimulate fluid intake (Olson et al. 1982). However, β-endorphin, as well as other opioids, have been reported to inhibit drinking stimulated by angiotensin II (Summy-Long et al. 1981a), as well as drinking associated with relative cellular dehydration, hypovolemia, or eating (Summy-Long et al. 1981c). Although the inhibitory actions are naloxone-reversible and not due to a general sensory-motor dysfunction, naloxone itself was also found to inhibit drinking stimulated by angiotensin II (Summy-Long et al. 1981b). Resolution of these seemingly paradoxical findings is necessary for a further understanding of the role of endorphins in thirst. However, since hypophysectomy does not attenuate the suppressant effect of naloxone on water intake (Brown et al. 1980), it appears that pituitary β-endorphin, at least, does not have a significant role in naloxone-suppressable drinking.

5.7. SEXUAL BEHAVIOR

A physiological role of endogenous opioids in regulating sexual behavior has been proposed since naloxone was found to stimulate copulatory responses in male rats (Hetta 1977; McIntosh et al. 1980) and lordosis behavior in female rats (Sirinathsinghji et al. 1983). Conversely, β-endorphin potently inhibits copulatory behavior in male rats (McIntosh et al. 1980; Meyerson 1981; Meyerson and Terenius 1977) and lordosis behavior in female rats (Sirinathsinghji et al. 1983). The release of endogenous opioids, including β-endorphin, during sexual behavior has been suggested by several investigators (Murphy et al. 1979; Szechtman et al. 1981; but see Goldstein and Hansteen 1977), although a specific role of β-endorphin in regulating (e.g., terminating or reinforcing) such behavior has not yet been demonstrated. A role for α-MSH and/or ACTH in regulating sexual behavior has also been proposed since central administration of ACTH in males results in penile erection, copulatory movements, and ejaculation (Bertolini et al. 1969; Ferrari et al. 1963), and in females, α-MSH stimulates lordosis behavior (Thody et al. 1981).

5.8. AGGRESSIVE AND DEFENSIVE BEHAVIOR

Endogenous opioids have been proposed to have a role in regulating agonistic behaviors. Shock-elicited aggression was enhanced by naloxone in 2 studies (Fanselow et al. 1980; Gorelick et al. 1981), but reduced in another investigation using different procedures (McGivern et al. 1981). The relationship of these effects to β-endorphin systems is presently unknown. ACTH has been more extensively investigated for a role in agonistic behavior. The acute effect of ACTH in enhancing fighting behavior, which appears to be mediated through adrenal as well as extra-adrenal influences (Brain and Evans 1977), contrasts with the chronic effect of the peptide in suppressing fighting behavior (Brain and Poole 1974). α-MSH has been reported to promote the secretion of an aggression-eliciting pheromone (Nowell and Wouters 1975) as well as to inhibit aggressive behavior (Paterson et al. 1978); however, it would be remarkable if both effects occurred together under physiological conditions, since attack would be elicited toward an animal simultaneously rendered unable to defend itself.

5.9. LOCOMOTION AND GROOMING

Intraventricular administration of β-endorphin can result in a catatonic-like immobilization (Bloom et al. 1976; Jacquet and Marks 1976) which is followed by or preceded by hyperactivity, depending upon the dose (Segal et al. 1977). An anatomical dissection of this effect was begun by Stinus et al. (1980) who reported only locomotor activation following β-endorphin administration into the ventral tegmental area. ACTH can also exert biphasic effects upon motor activity; the inhibitory effect of high doses, but not the stimulatory effect of low doses, could be blocked with naltrexone (Amir et al. 1980), indicating opioid mediation. Intraventricular injection of ACTH/α-MSH-related peptides also induces prolonged grooming behavior (Gispen and Isaacson 1981) which can also be elicited by β-endorphin (Gispen et al. 1976) and suppressed by opiate antagonists (Gispen and Wiegant 1976) and γ-MSH (Van Ree et al. 1981). These findings are consistent with evidence for low affinity interactions of ACTH with opioid receptors (Akil et al. 1980; Terenius et al. 1975), the physiological significance of which is yet undetermined. A physiological role for ACTH has been suggested on the basis of findings that

intraventricular administration of ACTH antiserum decreases novelty-induced grooming (Dunn et al. 1979).

5.10. MEDIATION OF ENDOGENOUS REWARD

Belluzzi and Stein (1977) have suggested a role for endogenous opioids in mediating
drive-reduction reward, partly on the basis of findings that naloxone reduces brain self-
stimulation rates. Although this result was not obtained by some investigators (e.g., Van
der Kooy et al. 1977), others have defined procedural conditions for demonstrating the
effect (Schaefer and Michael 1981). ACTH(4–10) was found to facilitate self-stimulation
at low response rates, which the investigators suggested was due to enhancement of the
rewarding properties of the stimulation (Nyakas et al. 1980). However, there are difficulties in using self-stimulation rates as a measure of reinforcement value (Valenstein
1964). A role for endogenous opioids in reinforcement may be indicated by the finding
that naloxone itself can act as a negative reinforcer, generating and maintaining escape
responding in non-dependent monkeys (Downs and Woods 1976). The rewarding properties of β-endorphin (Van Ree et al. 1979) and ACTH (Jouhaneau-Bowers and Le
Magnen 1979) have been demonstrated in self-administration studies, although such
findings are not direct evidence for a physiological role of these peptides in reward.

5.11. LEARNING AND MEMORY

The study of the role of POMC-related peptides in learning and memory is intrinsically
difficult; these processes cannot be measured directly, but only inferred from task performance, which itself is sensitive to changes in sensory or motor function, or motivatio-
nal and affective states. Thus, changes in the performance of a 'memory task' following
some treatment are not necessarily due to an effect on 'memory' *per se*. For example,
β-endorphin and related peptides were found to delay extinction of a pole-jump avoidance task (De Wied et al. 1978b); while this effect could be interpreted as a stabilization
of memory, there are alternate interpretations, including enhanced arousal, attention,
or fear motivation, or a decreased ability to shift or stop an established behavioral response. In one-trial passive avoidance tests, post-trial administration of β-endorphin
(during the 'consolidation phase') was reported to impair retention performance
(Martinez and Rigter 1980); however, other investigators have reported enhanced retention performance (De Wied et al. 1978a; Kovacs et al. 1983). Post-trial administration
of vasopressin has also been reported to produce bimodal effects (Sahgal et al. 1982),
which may indicate an effect of the peptide on processes other than memory (e.g., on
arousal; see Koob and Bloom 1982). Although Izquierdo (1982) has proposed the existence of an 'endogenous amnestic mechanism' mediated by β-endorphin, the evidence
at present is not unequivocal.

ACTH and α-MSH peptides have frequently been shown to exert potent effects
(usually facilitatory) on learning and memory task performance (see for review Eipper
and Mains 1980). There appears to be a consensus that these effects are not upon memory consolidation *per se*, but occur through increasing arousal, attention, or the motiva-
tional significance of environmental stimuli. The effect of α-MSH on performance is sen-
sory-selective in that visual, but not auditory, discrimination performance is enhanced
(Handelmann et al. 1983). In contrast to α-MSH, γ-MSH impairs reversal performance
on a visual discrimination task (O'Donohue et al. 1981b). The performance-enhancing
effect of α-MSH depends upon N-acetylation (O'Donohue et al. 1981a, 1982), indicating
a possible regulatory process for modulating the functional activity of the peptide.

5.12. TOWARD AN INTEGRATIVE PHYSIOLOGY OF BRAIN POMC SYSTEMS

The previous sections discussed separately a variety of potential physiological actions of POMC-related peptides; however, it is likely that these actions do not occur in isolation from one another, but in some cases may reflect components of integrated physiological responses. This is particularly likely in cases where the POMC systems appear to be activated by potent psychobiological challenges (e.g., certain stressors) which elicit complex physiological and behavioral responses. It is possible that 'defense-motivational' theories (Bolles and Fanselow 1980; Masterson and Crawford 1982) may help in the formulation of a useful integrative framework for future studies.

In reviewing the foregoing sections, it appears that a major difficulty in interpreting the physiological significance of many studies has been a lack of anatomical orientation; i.e., can the proposed actions of the peptides be related to their anatomical distribution? We hope that our presentation of coronal and parasagittal stereotaxic maps of pathways containing POMC-related peptides will assist investigators who wish to explore the diverse actions of these peptides in a more anatomical context.

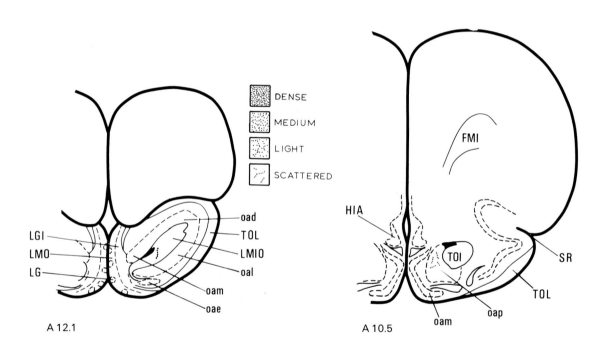

Frontal Atlas. These schematic frontal sections through the rat CNS demonstrate the distribution of POMC-containing neuronal perikarya (solid circles), processes (dotted lines) and terminals (dotted accumulations of various densities) in the right side of the brain and cervical spinal cord. *For abbreviations*, consult the General Abbreviations List, p. 609 and the text for details.
Parasagittal Atlas. These schematic parasagittal sections, redrawn from the stereotaxic atlas of the rat brain (Paxinos and Watson 1982), show the distribution of POMC-containing perikarya (solid circles), processes (dotted lines) and terminals (dotted accumulations of various densities) in the CNS. These drawings better demonstrate the rostral and caudal projections of the POMC neurons. Consult the General Abbreviations List, p. 609 and the text for details.

250

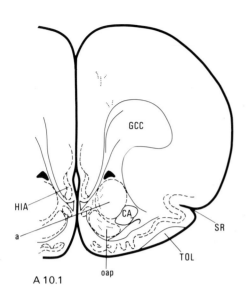

A 10.1

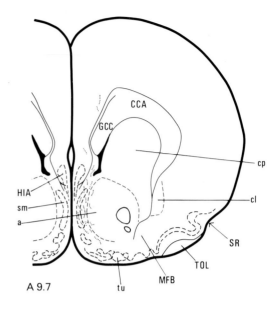

A 9.7

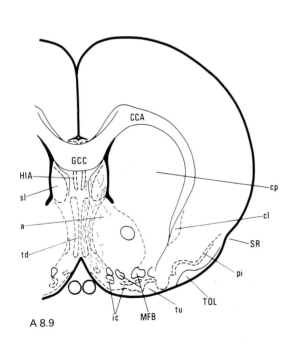

A 8.9

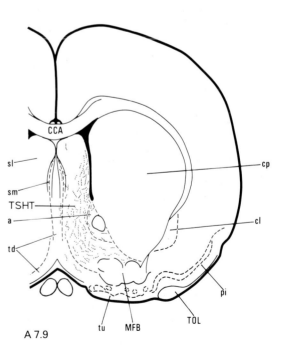

A 7.9

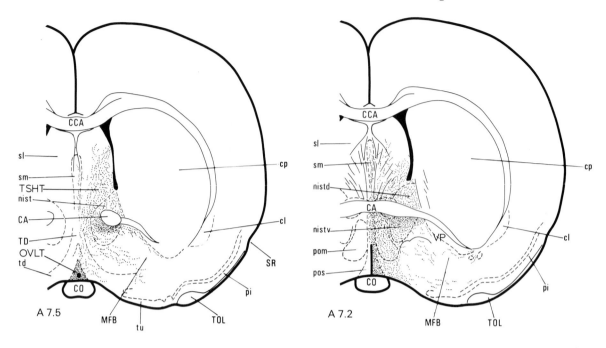

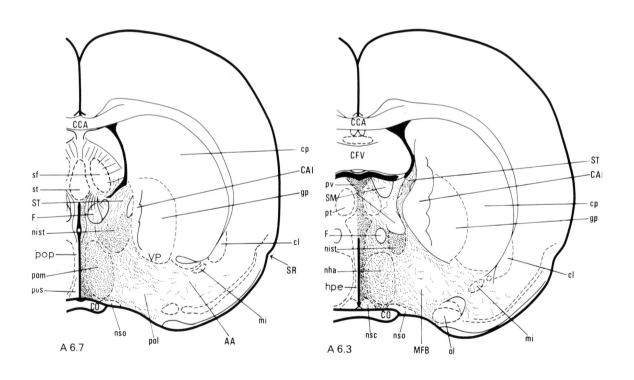

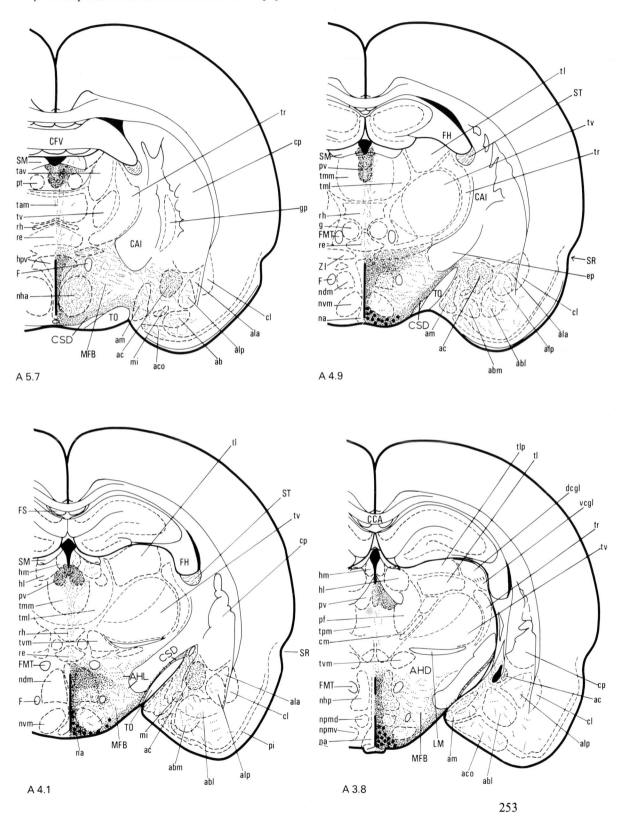

A 5.7

A 4.9

A 4.1

A 3.8

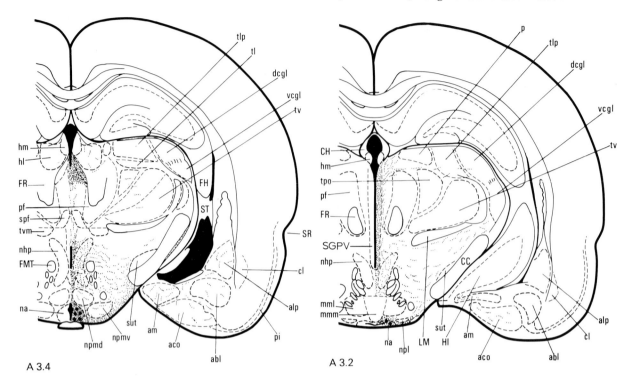

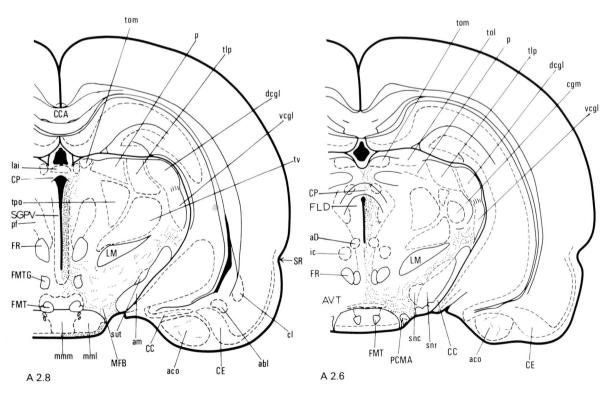

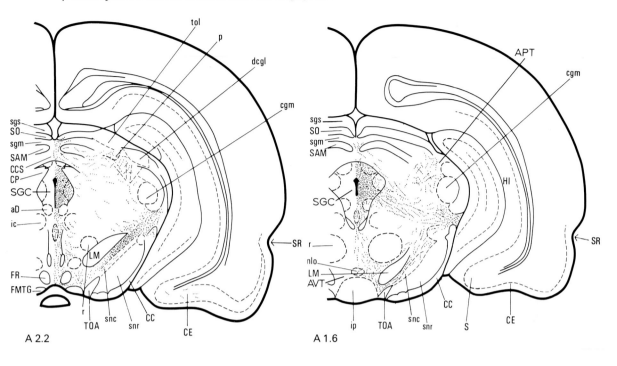

A 2.2

A 1.6

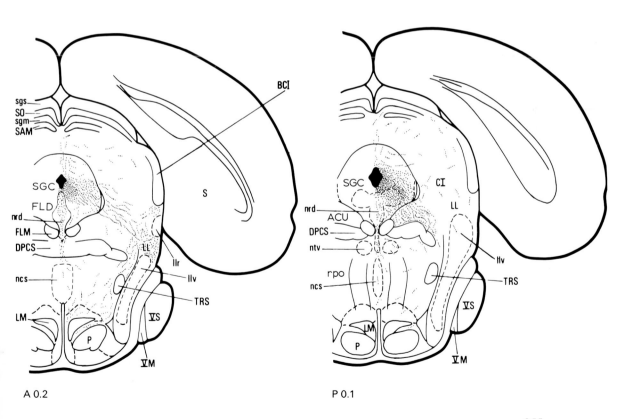

A 0.2

P 0.1

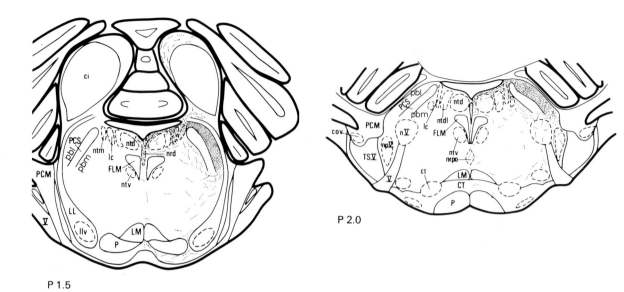

P 1.5

P 2.0

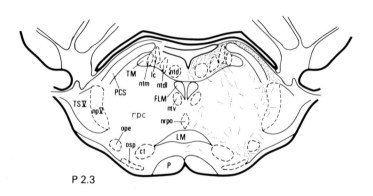

P 2.3

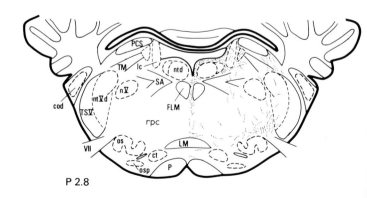

P 2.8

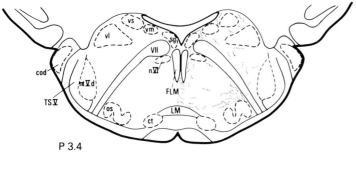

P 3.4

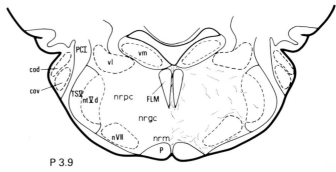

P 3.9

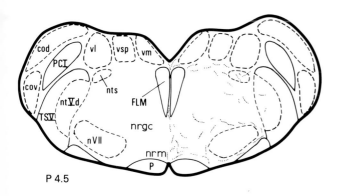

P 4.5

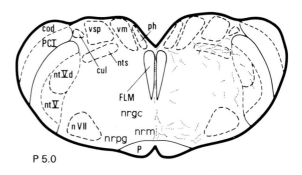

P 5.0

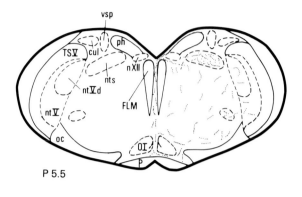

P 5.5

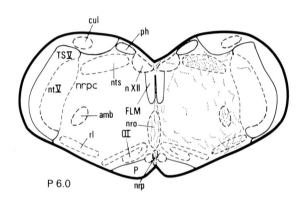

P 6.0

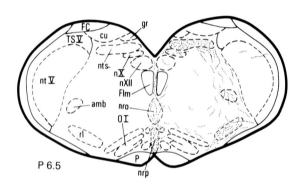

P 6.5

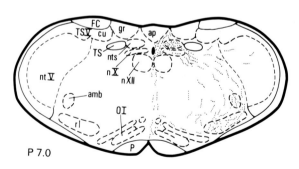

P 7.0

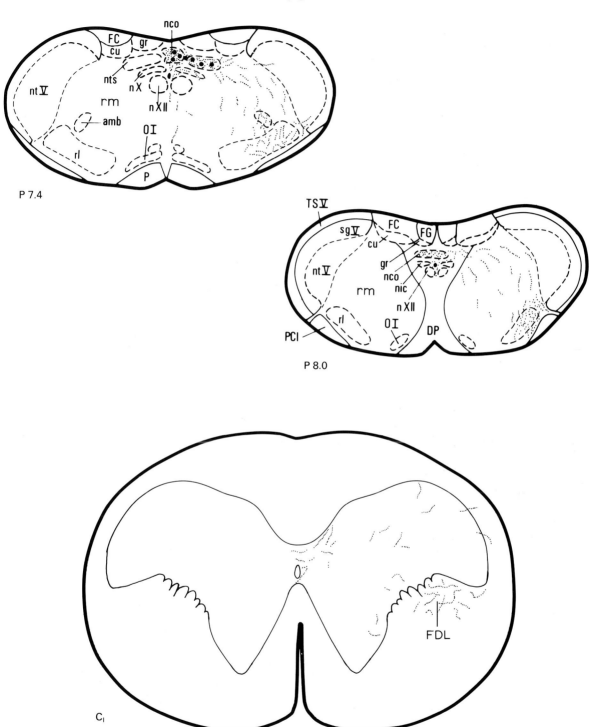

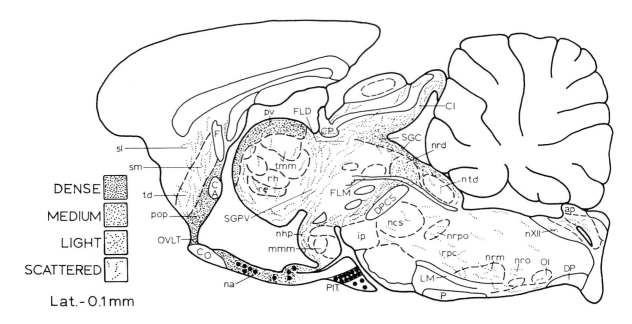

DENSE

MEDIUM

LIGHT

SCATTERED

Lat.-0.1mm

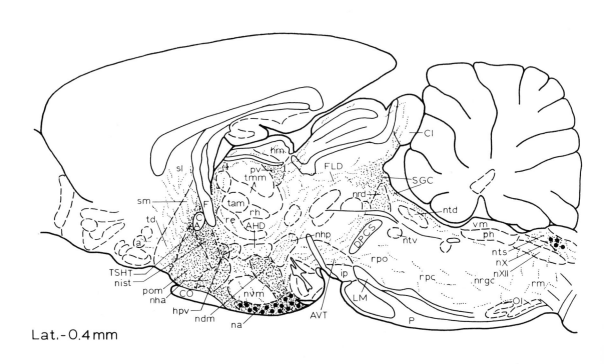

Lat.-0.4mm

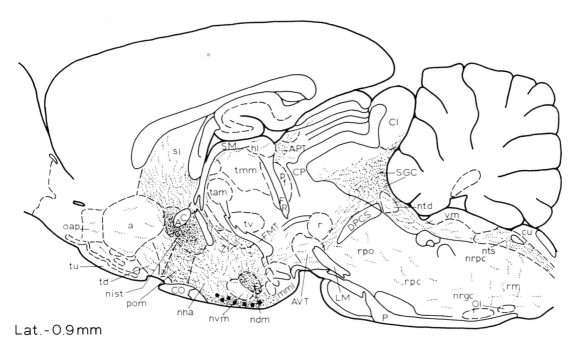

Lat.-0.9 mm

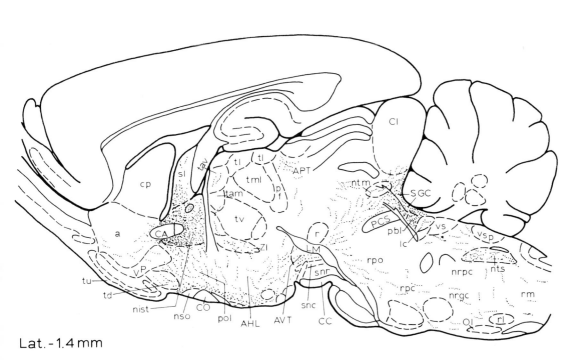

Lat.-1.4 mm

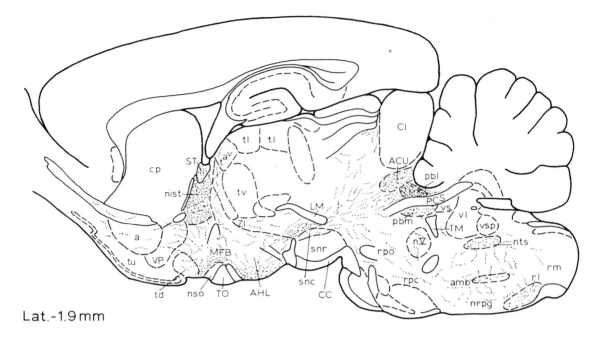

Lat.-1.9mm

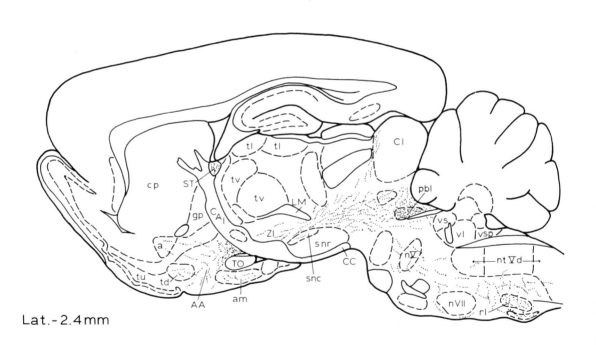

Lat.-2.4mm

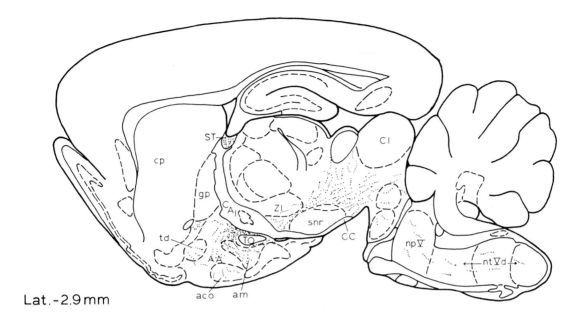

Lat.-2.9mm

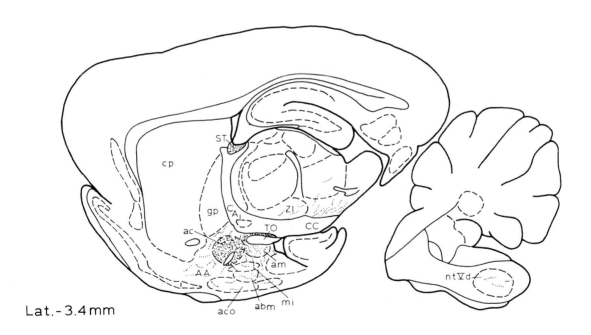

Lat.-3.4mm

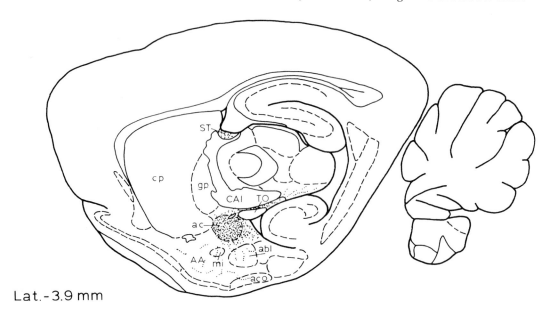

Lat.-3.9 mm

6. ACKNOWLEDGMENTS

The authors are indebted to Mr Per H. Kjeldsen of the University of Michigan, School of Dentistry, for expert photographic assistance, and Mrs Marcia Ritchie for manuscript preparation.

7. REFERENCES

Akil H, Watson SJ (1983): Beta-endorphin and biosynthetically related peptides in the central nervous system. In: Iversen, L, Iversen SD, Snyder, SH (Eds), *Handbook of Psychopharmacology, Vol. 16*, pp. 209–253. Plenum, New York.

Akil H, Madden J, Patrick RL, Barchas JD (1976): Stress-induced increase in endogenous opiate peptides: concurrent analgesia and its partial reversal by naloxone. In: Kosterlitz H (Ed.), *Opiates and Endogenous Opioid Peptides*, pp. 63–70. Elsevier, Amsterdam.

Akil H, Richardson DE, Barchas JD, Li CH (1978a): Appearance of beta-endorphin-like immunoreactivity in human ventricular cerebrospinal fluid upon analgesic electrical stimulation. *Proc. Natl Acad. Sci. USA, 75*, 5170–5172.

Akil H, Watson SJ, Berger PA, Barchas JD (1978b): Endorphins, beta-lipotropin and ACTH: biochemical, pharmacological and anatomical studies. In: Trabucchi M, Costa E (Eds), *The Endorphins: Advances in Biochemistry and Psychopharmacology, Vol. 18*, pp. 125–139. Raven Press, New York.

Akil H, Watson SJ, Barchas JD, Li CH (1979): Beta-endorphin immunoreactivity in rat and human blood: radioimmunoassay, comparative levels and physiological alterations. *Life Sci., 24*, 1659–1666.

Akil H, Hewlett W, Barchas JD, Li CH (1980): Binding of [³H]beta-endorphin to rat brain membranes: characterization and opiate properties. *Eur. J. Pharmacol., 64*, 1–8.

Akil H, Watson SJ, Young E, Lewis ME, Khachaturian H, Walker JM (1984): Endogenous opioids: biology and function. In: Cowan WM (Ed.), *Annual Review of Neuroscience, 7*, 223–255.

Amir S, Galina H, Blair R, Brown ZW, Amit Z (1980): Opiate receptors may mediate the suppressive but not the excitatory action of ACTH on motor activity in rats. *Eur. J. Pharmacol., 66*, 307–313.

Baker B (1979): The evolution of ACTH, MSH and LPH – structure, function and development. In: Barrington EJW (Ed.), *Hormones and Evolution, Vol. 20*, pp. 643–722. Academic Press, New York.

Barnea A, Cho G, Porter JC (1979): Intracellular processing of alpha-MSH and ACTH in hypothalamic neurons: a preliminary study. *Soc. Neurosci. Abstracts, 5*, 523.

Beckwith BE, Sandman CA (1982): Central nervous system and peripheral effects of ACTH, MSH and related neuropeptides. *Peptides, 3*, 411–420.

Belluzzi JD, Stein L (1977): Enkephalin may mediate euphoria and drive-reduction reward. *Nature (London), 266*, 556–558.

Benjannet S, Seidah NG, Routhier R, Chretien M (1980): A novel human pituitary peptide containing the gamma-MSH sequence. *Nature (London)*, *285*, 415–416.

Berger PA, Akil H, Watson SJ, Barchas JD (1982): Behavioral pharmacology of the endorphins. *Annu. Rev. Med.*, *33*, 397–415.

Bertolini A, Vergoni W, Gessa GL, Ferrari W (1969): Induction of sexual excitement by the action of adreno-corticotrophic hormone in brain. *Nature (London)*, *221*, 667–669.

Bloch B, Bugnon C, Fellman D, Lenys D (1978): Immunocytochemical evidence that the same neurons in the human infundibular nucleus are stained with anti-endorphins and antisera of other related peptides. *Neurosci. Lett.*, *10*, 147–152.

Bloch B, Bugnon C, Fellman D, Lenys D, Gouget A (1979): Neurons of the rat hypothalamus reactive with antisera against endorphins, ACTH, MSH and beta-lipotropin. *Cell Tissue Res.*, *204*, 1–15.

Bloom AS, Tseng L-F (1981): Effects of beta-endorphin on body temperature in mice at different ambient temperatures. *Peptides*, *2*, 293–297.

Bloom F, Segal D, Ling N, Guillemin R (1976): Endorphins: profound behavioral effects in rats suggest new etiological factors in mental illness. *Science*, *194*, 630–632.

Bloom F, Battenberg E, Rossier J, Ling N, Guillemin R (1978a): Neurons containing beta-endorphin in rat brain exist separately from those containing enkephalin: immunocytochemical studies. *Proc. Natl Acad. Sci. USA*, *75*, 1591–1595.

Bloom F, Rossier J, Battenberg E, Bayon A, French E, Henricksen SJ, Siggins GR, Segal D, Browne R, Ling N, Guillemin R (1978b); Beta-endorphin: cellular localization, electrophysiological and behavioral effects. In: Costa E, Trabucchi M (Eds), *Advances in Biochemical Psychopharmacology: The Endorphins*, Vol. 18, 89–109. Raven Press, New York.

Bloom F, Battenberg E, Shibasaki T, Benoit R, Ling N, Guillemin R (1980): Localization of gamma-melano-cyte stimulating hormone (gamma-MSH) immunoreactivity in rat brain and pituitary. *Regul. Peptides*, *1*, 205–222.

Bloom FE, Battenberg E, Rossier J, Ling N, Leppaluoto J, Vargo TM, Guillemin R (1977): Endorphins are located in the intermediate and anterior lobes of the pituitary gland, not in the neurohypophysis. *Life Sci.*, *20*, 43–48.

Bolles RC, Fanselow MS (1980): A perceptual-defensive-recuperative model of fear and pain. *Behav. Brain Sci.*, *3*, 291–323.

Bolles RC, Fanselow MS (1982): Endorphins and behavior. *Annu. Rev. Psychol.*, *33*, 87–101.

Bolme P, Fuxe K, Agnati LF, Bradley R, Smythies J (1978): Cardiovascular effects of morphine and opioid peptides following intracisternal administration in chloralose-anesthetized rats. *Eur. J. Pharmacol.*, *48*, 319–324.

Bradbury AF, Feldberg WF, Smyth DG, Snell C (1976): Lipotropin C-fragment: an endogenous peptide with potent analgesic activity. In: Kosterlitz HW (Ed.), *Opiates and Endogenous Opioid Peptides*, pp. 9–17. Elsevier, Amsterdam.

Brain PR, Evans AE (1977): Acute influences of some ACTH-related peptides on fighting and adrenocortical activity in male laboratory mice. *Pharmacol. Biochem. Behav.*, *7*, 425–433.

Brain PR, Poole AE (1974): The role of endocrines in isolation-induced intermale fighting in albino laboratory mice. 1. Pituitary adrenocortical influences. *Aggress. Behav.*, *1*, 39–69.

Brown DR, Blank MS, Holtzman SG (1980): Suppression by naloxone of water intake induced by deprivation and hypertonic saline in intact and hypophysectomized rats. *Life Sci.*, *26*, 1535–1542.

Bruni JF, Van Vugt D, Marshall S, Meites J (1977): Effects of naloxone, morphine and methionine enkephalin on serum prolactin, luteinizing hormone, follicle stimulating hormone, thyroid stimulating hormone and growth hormone. *Life Sci.*, *21*, 461–466.

Chrétien M, Li CH (1967): Isolation, purification and characterization of gamma-lipotropic hormone from sheep pituitary glands. *Can. J. Biochem.*, *45*, 1163–1174.

Chrétien M, Benjannet S, Dragon N, Seidah NG, Lis M (1976): Isolation of peptides with opiate activity from sheep and human pituitaries: relationship to beta-lipotropin. *Biochem. Biophys. Res. Commun.*, *72*, 472–478.

Chrétien M, Seidah NG (1981): Chemistry and biosynthesis of pro-opiomelanocortin: ACTH, MSH's, endorphins and their related peptides. *Mol. Cell. Endocrinol.*, *21*, 101–127.

Clarke G, Wood P, Merrick L, Lincoln DW (1979): Opiate inhibition of peptide release from the neurohumoral terminals of hypothalamic neurons. *Nature (London)*, *282*, 746–748.

Clark WG (1979): Influence of opioids on central thermoregulatory mechanisms. *Pharmacol. Biochem. Behav.*, *10*, 609–613.

Comb J, Seeburg PH, Adelman J, Eiden L, Herbert E (1982): Primary structure of the human Met- and Leu-enkephalin precursor and its mRNA. *Nature (London)*, *295*, 663–666.

Cox BM, Ophiem KE, Teschemacher H, Goldstein A (1975): A peptide-like substance from pituitary that acts like morphine. 2. Purification and properties. *Life Sci., 16*, 1777–1782.

Dahlström A, Fuxe K (1964): Evidence for the existence of monoamine-containing neurons in the central nervous system. I. Demonstration of monoamines in the cell bodies of brain stem neurons. *Acta Physiol. Scand., 62 (Suppl. 232)*, 1–36.

De Wied D (1977): Behavioral effects of neuropeptides related to ACTH, MSH, and beta-lipotropin. *Ann. NY Acad. Sci., 297*, 263–274.

De Wied D, Kovacs GL, Bohus B, Van Ree JM, Greven JM (1978a): Neuroleptic activity of the neuropeptide beta-lipotropin (62–77) ([des-tyr²]gamma-endorphin; (DTgammaE). *Eur. J. Pharmacol., 49*, 427–436.

De Wied D, Bohus B, Van Ree JM, Urban I (1978b): Behavioral and electrophysiological effects of peptides related to lipotropin (B-LPH). *J. Pharmacol. Exp. Therap., 204*, 570–580.

Deutch AY, Martin RJ (1983): Mesencephalic dopamine modulation of pituitary and central beta-endorphin: relation to food intake regulation. *Life Sci., 33*, 281–287.

Diz DI, Jacobowitz DM (1983): Cardiovascular effects of intrahypothalamic injection of alpha-melanocyte stimulating hormone. *Brain Res., 270*, 265–272.

Downs DA, Woods JH (1976): Naloxone as a negative reinforcer in rhesus monkeys: effects of dose, schedule, and narcotic regimen. *Pharmacol. Rev., 27*, 397–406.

Drouin J, Goodman MH (1980): Most of the coding region of rat ACTH beta-lipotropin precursor gene lacks intervening sequences. *Nature (London), 288*, 610–613.

Dube D, Pelletier G (1979): Further studies on the immunohistochemical localization of alpha-MSH in the rat brain. *Neurosci. Lett., 12*, 171–176.

Dunn AJ, Green EJ, Isaacson RL (1979): Intracerebral adrenocorticotropic hormone mediates novelty-induced grooming in the rat. *Science, 203*, 283.

Eipper BA, Mains R (1978): Existence of a common precursor to ACTH and endorphin in the anterior and intermediate lobes of the rat pituitary. *J. Supramol. Struct., 8*, 247–262.

Eipper BA, Mains RE (1980): Structure and biosynthesis of pro-adrenocorticotropin/endorphin and related peptides. *Endocrine Rev., 1*, 1–27.

Elde R, Hökfelt T, Johansson O, Terenius L (1976): Immunohistochemical studies using antibodies to leucine-enkephalin: initial observations on the nervous system of the rat. *Neuroscience, 1*, 349–351.

Fanselow MS, Sigmundi RA, Bolles RC (1980): Naloxone pretreatment enhances shock-elicited aggression. *Physiol. Psychol., 8*, 369–371.

Ferrari W, Gessa GL, Vargil L (1963): Behavioral effects induced by intracisternally injected ACTH and MSH. *Ann. NY Acad. Sci., 104*, 330–345.

Ferri S, Cocchi D, Locatelli V, Spampinato S, Miller E (1982): ACTH-(1–24) counteracts the prolactin-releasing effect of an opioid. *Eur. J. Pharmacol., 77*, 143–145.

Feuerstein G, Faden AI (1982): Hypothalamic sites for cardiovascular regulation by mu, delta or kappa opioid agonists. *Life Sci., 31*, 2197–2200.

Finley JCW, Lindström P, Petrusz P (1981a): Immunocytochemical localization of beta-endorphin-containing neurons in the rat brain. *Neuroendocrinology, 33*, 28–42.

Finley JCW, Maderdrut JL, Petrusz P (1981b): The immunocytochemical localization of enkephalin in the central nervous system of the rat. *J. Comp. Neurol., 198*, 541–565.

Florez J, Hurle MA, Mediavilla A (1982): Respiratory responses to opiates applied to the medullary ventral surface. *Life Sci., 31*, 2189–2197.

Garthwaite TL, Martinson DR, Tsing LF, Hagen TC, Menachan LA (1980): A longitudinal hormonal profile of the genetically obese mouse. *Endocrinology, 107*, 671–676.

Gianoulakis C, Seidah NG, Chrétien M (1979): In vitro biosynthesis and chemical characterization of ACTH and ACTH fragments by the rat pars intermedia. International Narcotic Research Conference. In: Way WL (Ed.), *Endogenous and Exogenous Opiate Agonists and Antagonists*, pp. 289–292. Pergamon Press, New York.

Gispen WH, Isaacson RL (1981): ACTH-induced excessive grooming in the rat. *Pharmacol. Therap., 12*, 209–246.

Gispen WH, Wiegant VM (1976): Opiate antagonists suppress ACTH-(1–24) induced excessive grooming in the rat. *Neurosci. Lett., 2*, 159–164.

Gispen WH, Wiegant VM, Bradbury AF, Hulme EC, Smyth DG, Snell CR, De Wied D (1976): Induction of excessive grooming in the rat by fragments of lipotropin. *Nature (London), 264*, 794–795.

Glyn JR, Lipton JM (1981): Hypothermic and antipyretic effects of centrally administered ACTH(1–24) and alpha-melanotropin. *Peptides, 2*, 177–187.

Glyn-Bollinger JR, Bernardini GL, Lipton JM (1983): Alpha-MSH injected into the septal region reduces fever in rabbits. *Peptides, 4*, 199–203.

266

Goldstein A, Hansteen RW (1977): Evidence against involvement of endorphins in sexual arousal and orgasm in man. *Arch. Gen. Psychiatry, 34*, 1179–1180.

Goodman RR, Snyder SH, Kuhar MJ, Young III WS (1980): Differentiation of delta and mu opiate receptor localizations by light microscopic autoradiography. *Proc. Natl Acad. Sci. USA, 77*, 6239–6243.

Gorelick DA, Elliott ML, Sbordone RJ (1981): Naloxone increases shock-elicited aggression in rats. *Res. Commun. Substance Abuse, 2*, 419–422.

Grandison L, Guidotti A (1977): Stimulation of food intake by muscimol and beta-endorphin. *Neuropharmacology, 16*, 533–536.

Gubler U, Seeburg P, Hoffman BJ, Gage LP, Udenfriend S (1982): Molecular clonig establishes proenkephalin as precursor of enkephalin-containing peptides. *Nature (London), 295*, 206–208.

Guillemin R, Ling N, Burgus R (1976): Endorphins, peptides d'origine hypothalamique et neurohypophysaire d'activité morphinomimétique. Isolement et structure moléculaire d'alpha-endorphin. *C. R. Acad. Sci., Ser. D, 282*, 783–785.

Guillemin R, Vargo T, Rossier J, Minick S, Ling N, Rivier C, Vale W, Bloom F (1977): Beta-endorphin and adenocorticotropin are secreted concomitantly by the pituitary gland. *Science, 197*, 1367–1369.

Gunion MW, Peters RH (1981): Pituitary beta-endorphin, naloxone and feeding in several experimental obesities. *Am. J. Physiol., 241*, R173–R184.

Guy J, Leclerc R, Vaudry H, Pelletier G (1980): Identification of a second category of alpha-melanocyte-stimulating hormone neurons in the rat hypothalamus. *Brain Res., 199*, 135–146.

Guy J, Vaudry H, Pelletier G (1981): Differential projections of two immunoreactive alpha-melanocyte stimulating hormone neurons in the rat brain. *Brain Res., 220*, 119–202.

Halasz B (1969): The endocrine effects of isolation of the hypothalamus from the rest of the brain. In: Ganong WF, Martini L (Eds), *Frontiers in Neuroendocrinology*, pp. 307–342. Oxford University Press, New York.

Handelmann GE, O'Donohue TL, Forrester D, Cook W (1983): Alpha-melanocyte stimulating hormone facilitates learning of visual but not auditory discriminations. *Peptides, 4*, 145–148.

Hassen AH, Feuerstein GZ, Faden AI (1982): Cardiovascular responses to opioid agonists injected into the nucleus of tractus solitarius of anesthetized cats. *Life Sci., 31*, 2193–2196.

Herbert E, Budarf M, Phillips M, Rosa P, Policastro P, Oates E, Roberts JL, Seidah NG, Chrétien M (1980): The presence of a presequence in the common precursor to ACTH and endorphin and the role of glycosylation in processing of the precursor and secretion of ACTH and endorphin. *Ann. NY Acad. Sci., 343*, 79–93.

Hetta J (1977): Effects of morphine and naltrexone on sexual behavior in the male rat. *Acta Pharmacol. Toxicol., 41 (Suppl. IV)*, 53.

Hökfelt T, Elde R, Johansson O, Terenius L, Stein L (1977): The distribution of enkephalin-immunoreactive cell bodies in the rat central nervous system. *Neurosci. Lett., 5*, 25–31.

Holaday J (1983): Cardiovascular effects of endogenous opiate systems. *Annu. Rev. Pharmacol. Toxicol., 23*, 541–594.

Holaday JW, Faden AI (1982): Selective cardiorespiratory differences between third and fourth ventricular injections of 'mu' and 'delta' opiate agonists. *Fed. Proc., 41*, 1468.

Holaday JW, Loh HH (1981): Neurobiology of beta-endorphin and related peptides. In: Li CH (Ed.), *Hormonal Proteins and Peptides, Vol. 10*, pp. 202–291. Academic Press, New York.

Holtzman SG (1974): Behavioral effects of separate and combined administration of naloxone and d-amphetamine. *J. Pharmacol. Exp. Therap., 189*, 51–60.

Hosobuchi Y, Adams JE, Linchitz R (1977): Pain relief by electrical stimulation of the central gray matter in humans and its reversal by naloxone. *Science, 197*, 183–186.

Hosobuchi Y, Rossier J, Bloom FE, Guillemin R (1979): Stimulation of human periaqueductal gray for pain relief increases immunoreactive beta-endorphin in ventricular fluid. *Science, 203*, 279–281.

Hughes J, Smith TW, Kosterlitz HW, Fothergill LA, Morgan BA, Morris HR (1975): Identification of two related pentapeptides from the brain with potent opiate agonist activity. *Nature (London), 258*, 577–579.

Iversen LL, Iversen SD, Bloom FE (1980): Opiate receptors influence vasopressin release from nerve terminals in rat neurohypophysis. *Nature (London), 284*, 350–351.

Izquierdo I (1982): Beta-endorphin and forgetting. *Trends Pharmacol. Sci., 3*, 455–457.

Jacobowitz DM, O'Donohue TL (1978): Alpha-melanocyte-stimulating hormone: immunohistochemical identification and mapping in neurons of rat brain. *Proc. Natl Acad. Sci., 75*, 6300–6304.

Jacquet YF, Marks N (1976): The C-fragment of beta-lipotropin: an endogenous neuroleptic or antipsychotogen? *Science, 194*, 632–635.

Jegou S, Tonon MC, Guy J, Vaudry H, Pelletier G (1983): Biological and immunological characterization of alpha-melanocyte-stimulating hormone in two neuronal systems of the rat brain. *Brain Res., 260*, 91–98.

Jouhaneau-Bowers M, Le Magnen J (1979): ACTH self-administration in rats. *Pharmacol. Biochem. Behav.*, *10*, 325–328.

Kakidani H, Furutani Y, Takahashi H, Noda M, Morimoto Y, Hirose T, Asai M, Inayama S, Nakanishi S, Numa S (1982): Cloning and sequence analysis of cDNA for porcine beta-neo-endorphin/dynorphin precursor. *Nature (London)*, *298*, 245–249.

Kanyicska B, Stark E, Horvath G, Simonyi A, Fekete MIK (1983): Long term ACTH induced diminished responsiveness of prolactin secretion to morphine. *Life Sci.*, *33*, 55–63.

Khachaturian H, Tsou K, Watson SJ (1981): Beta-endorphin and alpha-MSH in the rat brain: a comparative immunocytochemical analysis. *Soc. Neurosci. Abstracts*, 7, 93.

Khachaturian H, Watson SJ, Lewis ME, Coy D, Goldstein A, Akil H (1982): Dynorphin immunocytochemistry in the rat central nervous system. *Peptides*, *3*, 941–954.

Khachaturian H, Alessi NE, Munfakh N, Watson SJ (1983a): Ontogeny of opioid and related peptides in the rat CNS and pituitary: an immunocytochemical study. *Life Sci.*, *33 (Suppl. I)*, 61–64.

Khachaturian H, Lewis ME, Hollt V, Watson SJ (1983b): Telencephalic enkephalinergic systems in the rat brain. *J. Neurosci.*, *3*, 844–855.

Khachaturian H, Lewis ME, Watson SJ (1983c): Enkephalin systems in diencephalon and brain stem of the rat. *J. Comp. Neurol.*, *220*, 310–320.

Khachaturian H, Dores RM, Watson SJ, Akil H (1984a): Beta-endorphin/ACTH immunocytochemistry in the CNS of the lizard *Anolis carolinensis*: evidence for a major mesencephalic cell group. *J. Comp. Neurol.*, *229*, 576–584

Khachaturian H, Lewis ME, Haber SN, Akil H, Watson SJ (1984b): Proopiomelanocortin peptide immunocytochemistry in rhesus monkey brain. *Brain Res. Bull.*, *13*, 785–800.

Khachaturian H, Lewis ME, Schäfer MK-H, Watson SJ (1985): Anatomy of CNS opioid systems. *Trends Neurosci.*, *8*, 111–119

Koob GF, Bloom FE (1982): Behavioral effects of neuropeptides: endorphins and vasopressin. *Annu. Rev. Physiol.*, *44*, 571–582.

Kovacs GL, Bohus B, De Wied D (1983): Effects of beta-endorphin and its fragments on inhibitory avoidance behavior in rats. *Psychoneuroendocrinology*, *8*, 411–420

Krieger DT, Liotta A, Brownstein MJ (1977): Presence of corticotropin in brain of normal and hypophysectomized rats. *Proc. Natl Acad. Sci. USA*, *74*, 648–652.

Krieger DT, Liotta AS, Brownstein MJ, Zimmerman EA (1980): ACTH, beta-lipotropin and related peptides in brain, pituitary and blood. *Recent Prog. Hormone Res.*, *36*, 277–344.

Laubie M, Schmitt H, Vincent M, Remond G (1977): Central cardiovascular effects of morphinomimeticpeptides in dogs. *Eur. J. Pharmacol.*, *46*, 67–71.

Lee TH, Lerner AB (1956): Isolation of melanocyte-stimulating hormone from hog pituitary gland. *J. Biol. Chem.*, *221*, 943–959.

Lewis JW, Cannon JT, Liebeskind JC (1980): Opioid and non-opioid mechanisms of stress analgesia. *Science*, *208*, 623–625.

Lewis JW, Cannon JT, Liebeskind JC, Akil H (1981): Alterations in brain beta-endorphin immunoreactivity following acute and chronic stress. *Pain, Suppl. 1*, S263.

Lewis ME, Khachaturian H, Watson SJ (1983a): Comparative distribution of opiate receptors and three opioid peptide systems in rhesus monkey central nervous system. *Life Sci.*, *33 (Suppl I)*, 239–242.

Lewis ME, Pert A, Pert CB, Herkenham M (1983b): Opiate receptor localization in rat cerebral cortex. *J. Comp. Neurol.*, *216*, 339–358.

Lewis ME, Khachaturian H, Akil H, Watson SJ (1984): Anatomical relationship between opioid peptides and receptors in rhesus monkey brain. *Brain Res. Bull.*, *13*, 801–802

Lewis ME, Khachaturian H, Watson SJ (1985): Combined autoradiographic-immunocytochemical analysis of opiate receptors and opioid peptide neuronal systems in brain. *Peptides, 6, Suppl. 1*, 37–47

Li CH (1964): Lipotropin, a new active peptide from pituitary glands. *Nature (London)*, *201*, 924.

Li CH, Chung D (1976): Isolation and structure of an untriakontapeptide with opiate activity from camel pituitary glands. *Proc. Natl Acad. Sci. USA*, *73*, 1145–1148.

Li CH, Geschwind II, Cole RD, Raake ID, Harris JI, Dixon JS (1955): Amino-acid sequence of alpha-corticotropin. *Nature (London)*, *176*, 687–689.

Lim AT, Wallace M, Oei TP, Gibson S, Romas N, Pappas W, Clements J, Funder JW (1982): Footshock analgesia. Lack of correlation with pituitary and plasma immunoreactive-beta-endorphin. *Neuroendocrinology*, *35*, 236–241.

Loh HH, Tseng LF, Wei E, Li CH (1976): Beta-endorphin as a potent analgesic agent. *Proc. Natl Acad. Sci. USA*, *73*, 2895–2899.

Loh, PY, Eskay RL, Brownstein M (1980): Alpha-MSH-like peptides in rat brain: identification and changes in level during development. *Biochem. Biophys. Res. Commun.*, *94*, 916–923.

Lord JAH, Waterfield AA, Hughes J, Kosterlitz HW (1977): Endogenous opioid peptides: multiple agonists and receptors. *Nature (London)*, *267*, 495–499.

Lowy MT, Maickal RP, Yim GK (1980): Naloxone reduction of stress-related feeding. *Life Sci.*, *26*, 2113–2118.

Madden J, Akil H, Patrick RL, Barchas JD (1977): Stress-induced parallel changes in central opioid levels and pain responsiveness in the rat. *Nature (London)*, *265*, 358–360.

Mains RE, Eipper BA, Ling N (1977): Common precursor to corticotropins and endorphins. *Proc. Natl Acad. Sci. USA*, *74*, 3014–3018.

Margules DL, Moisset B, Lewis MJ, Shibuya H, Pert CB (1978): Beta-endorphin is associated with overeating in genetically obese mice (ob/ob) and rats (fa/fa). *Science*, *202*, 988–991.

Martin JP, Tolis G, Woops I, Guyla H (1979): Failure of naloxone to influence physiological growth hormone and prolactin secretion. *Brain Res.*, *168*, 210–215.

Martinez Jr JL, Rigter H (1980): Endorphins alter acquisition and consolidation of an inhibitory avoidance response in rats. *Neurosci. Lett.*, *19*, 197–201.

Masterson FA, Crawford M (1982): The defense motivation system: a theory of avoidance behavior. *Behav. Brain Sci.*, *5*, 661–696.

Mayer DJ, Wolfle TL, Akil H, Carder B, Liebeskind JC (1971): Analgesia from electricial stimulation in the brainstem of the rat. *Science*, *174*, 1351–1354.

McGivern RF, Lobaugh NJ, Collier AC (1981): Effect of naloxone and housing conditions on shock-elicited reflexive fighting: influence of immediate prior stress. *Physiol. Psychol.*, *9*, 251–256.

McIntosh TK, Vallano ML, Barfield RJ (1980): Effects of morphine, beta-endorphin and naloxone on catecholamine levels and sexual behavior in the male rat. *Pharmacol. Biochem. Behav.*, *13*, 435–441.

McKay LD, Kenney NJ, Edens NK, Williams RH, Woods SC (1981): Intracerebroventricular beta-endorphin increases food intake of rats. *Life Sci.*, *29*, 1429–1434.

Meyerson BJ (1981): Comparison of the effects of beta-endorphin and morphine on exploratory and socio-sexual behavior in the male rat. *Eur. J. Pharmacol.*, *69*, 453–463.

Meyerson BJ, Terenius L (1977): Beta-endorphin and male sexual behavior. *Eur. J. Pharmacol.*, *42*, 191–192.

Micevych PE, Elde RD (1982): Neurons containing alpha-melanocyte stimulating hormone and beta-endorphin immunoreactivity in the rat hypothalamus. *Peptides*, *3*, 655–662.

Millan MJ, Przewlocki R, Herz A (1980): A non-beta-endorphinergic adenohypophyseal mechanism is essential for an analgetic response to stress. *Pain*, *8*, 343–353.

Millan MJ, Przewlocki R, Kerlicz M, Gramsch C, Hollt V, Herz A (1981): Stress-induced release of brain and pituitary beta-endorphin: major role of endorphins in generation of hyperthemia, not analgesia. *Brain Res.*, *208*, 325–338.

Moon HD, Li CH, Jennings BM (1973): Immunohistochemical and histochemical studies of pituitary beta-lipotropin. *Anat. Rec.*, *175*, 524–538.

Morley JE, Levine AS (1980): Stress-induced eating is mediated through endogenous opiates. *Science*, *209*, 1259–1261.

Moss IR, Friedman E (1978): Beta-endorphin: effects on respiratory regulation. *Life Sci.*, *23*, 1271–1276.

Murphy MR, Bowie DL, Pert CB (1979): Copulation elevates plasma beta-endorphin in the male hamster. *Soc. Neurosci. Abstracts*, *5*, 470.

Murphy MT, Richards DB, Lipton JM (1983): Antipyretic potency of centrally administered alpha-melanocyte stimulating hormone. *Science*, *221*, 192–193.

Nakanishi S, Inoue A, Kita T, Nakamura M, Chang ACY, Cohen SN, Numa S (1979): Nucleotide sequence of cloned cDNA for bovine corticotropin-beta-lipotropin precursor. *Nature (London)*, *278*, 423–427.

Nilaver G, Zimmerman EA, Defendini R, Liotta A, Krieger DA, Brownstein M (1979): Adrenocorticotropin and beta-lipotropin in hypothalamus. *J. Cell Biol.*, *81*, 50–58.

Noda M, Furutani Y, Takahashi H, Toyosato M, Hirose T, Inayama S, Nakanishi S, Numa S (1982): Cloning and sequence analysis of cDNA for bovine adrenal preproenkephalin. *Nature (London)*, *295*, 202–206.

Nowell NW, Wouters A (1975): Release of aggression-promoting pheromone by male mice treated with alpha-melanocyte-stimulating hormone. *J. Endocrinol.*, *65*, 36P–37P.

Nyakas C, Bohus B, De Wied D (1980): Effects of ACTH-(4–10) on self-stimulation behavior in the rat. *Physiol. Behav.*, *24*, 759–764.

O'Donohue TL, Jacobowitz DM (1980): Studies on alpha-melanotropin in the central nervous system. In: Beers Jr RF, Bassett EG (Eds), *Polypeptide Hormones*, pp. 203–222. Raven Press, New York.

O'Donohue TL, Dorsa DM (1982): The opiomelanotropinergic neuronal and endocrine systems. *Peptides*, *3*, 353–395.

O'Donohue TL, Miller RL, Jacobowitz PM (1979): Identification, characterization and stereotaxic mapping of intraneuronal alpha-melanocyte-stimulating hormone-like immunoreactive peptides in discrete regions of the rat brain. *Brain Res.*, *176*, 101–123.

O'Donohue TL, Handelmann GE, Chaconas T, Miller RL, Jacobowitz DM (1981a): Evidence that N-acetylation regulates the behavioral activity of alpha-MSH in the rat and human central nervous system. *Peptides, 2*, 333–344.

O'Donohue TL, Handelmann GE, Loh YP, Olton DS, Leibowitz J, Jacobowitz DM (1981b): Comparison of biological and behavioral activities of alpha- and gamma-melanocyte stimulating hormones. *Peptides, 2*, 101–104.

O'Donohue TL, Handelmann GE, Miller RL, Jacobowitz DM (1982): N-acetylation regulates the behavioral activity of alpha-melanotropin in a multineurotransmitter neuron. *Science, 215*, 1125–1127.

Olney JW (1979): Excitotoxic amino acids: research application and safety implications. In: Filer LF (Ed.), *Glutamic Acid: Advances in Biochemistry and Physiology*, pp. 287–319. Raven Press, New York.

Olson GA, Olson RD, Kastin AJ, Coy DH (1979): Endogenous opiates: through 1978. *Neurosci. Biobehav. Rev., 3*, 285–299.

Olson GA, Olson RD, Kastin AJ, Coy DH (1980): Endogenous opiates: 1979. *Peptides, 1*, 365–379.

Olson GA, Olson RD, Kastin AJ, Coy DH (1981): Endogenous opiates: 1980. *Peptides, 2*, 349–369.

Olson GA, Olson RD, Kastin AJ, Coy DH (1982): Endogenous opiates: 1981. *Peptides, 3*, 1039–1072.

Parvizi N, Ellendorff F (1980): Beta-endorphin alters luteinizing hormone secretion via the amygdala but not the hypothalamus. *Nature (London), 286*, 812–813.

Paterson AT, Rickerby J, Simpson J, Vickers C (1978): Melanocyte-stimulating hormone and the pineal in the control of territorial aggression (proceedings). *J. Physiol., 285*, 45P.

Paxinos G, Watson C (1982): *The Rat Brain in Stereotaxic Coordinates*. Academic Press, Sydney.

Pellegrino LJ, Pellegrino AS, Cushman AJ (1979): *A Stereotaxic Atlas of the Rat Brain, Second Edition*. Plenum Press, New York.

Pelletier G (1979): Ultrastructural immunohistochemical localization of adrenocorticotropin and beta-lipotropin in the rat brain. *J. Histochem. Cytochem., 27*, 1046–1048.

Pelletier G (1980): Ultrastructural localization of a fragment (16K) of the common precursor for adrenocorticotropin (ACTH) and beta-lipotropin (B-LPH) in the rat hypothalamus. *Neurosci. Lett., 16*, 85–90.

Pelletier G, Dube D (1977): Electron microscopic immunohistochemical localization of alpha-MSH in the rat brain. *Am. J. Anat., 150*, 201–206.

Pelletier G, Leclerc R, LaBrie F, Cote J, Chrétien M, Lis M (1977): Immunohistochemical localization of beta-lipotropin hormone in the pituitary gland. *Endocrinology, 100*, 770–776.

Pelletier G, Desy L, Lissitszky J-C, Labrie F, Li CH (1978): Immunohistochemical localization of beta-lipotropin in the human hypothalamus. *Life Sci., 22*, 1799–1804.

Pert CB, Snyder SH (1973): Opiate receptor: demonstration in nervous tissue. *Science, 179*, 1011–1014.

Recant L, Voyles NR, Luciano M, Pert CB (1980): Naltrexone reduces weight gain, alters 'beta-endorphin', and reduces insulin output from pancreatic islets of genetically obese mice. *Peptides, 1*, 309–313.

Reid RL, Yen SSC, Artmon H, Fisher DA (1981): Effects of synthetic beta-endorphin on release of neurohypophyseal hormones. *Lancet, 2*, 1169–1170.

Richardson DE, Akil H (1977): Pain reduction by electrical stimulation in man. Part 1: Acute administration in periaqueductal and periventricular sites. *J. Neurosurg., 47*, 178–183.

Roberts JL, Herbert E (1977): Characterization of a common precursor to corticotropin and beta-lipotropin: identification of beta-lipotropin peptides and their arrangement relative to corticotropin in the precursor synthesized in a cell-free system. *Proc. Natl Acad. Sci. USA, 74*, 5300–5304.

Roberts JL, Seeburg PH, Shine J, Herbert E, Baxter JD, Goodman HM (1979): Corticotropin and beta-endorphin: construction and analysis of recombinant DNA complementary to mRNA for the common precursor. *Proc. Natl Acad. Sci. USA, 76*, 2153–2157.

Rossier J, French ED, Rivier C, Ling N, Guillemin R, Bloom FE (1977): Footshock induced stress increases beta-endorphin levels in blood but not brain. *Nature (London), 270*, 618–620.

Rossier J, Rogers J, Shibasaki T, Guillemin R, Bloom FE (1979): Opioid peptides and alpha-melanocyte-stimulating hormone in genetically obese (ob/ob) mice during development. *Proc. Natl Acad. Sci. USA, 76*, 2077–2080.

Rubinstein M, Stein S, Gerber LD, Udenfriend S (1977): Isolation and characterization of the opioid peptides from rat pituitary: beta-lipotropin. *Proc. Natl Acad. Sci. USA, 74*, 3052–3055.

Sahgal A, Keith AB, Wright C, Edwardson JA (1982): Failure of vasopressin to enhance memory in a passive avoidance task in rats. *Neurosci. Lett., 28*, 87–92.

Sar M, Stumpf WE, Miller RJ, Chang K-J, Cuatrecasas P (1978): Immunohistochemical localization of enkephalin in rat brain and spinal cord. *J. Comp. Neurol., 182*, 460–482.

Schaefer GH, Michael RP (1981): Threshold differences for naloxone and naltrexone in the hypothalamus and midbrain using fixed ratio brain self-stimulation in rats. *Psychopharmacology, 74*, 17–22.

Schwartzberg DG, Nakane PK (1981): Pro-ACTH/endorphin antigenicities in medullary neurons of the rat. *Soc. Neurosci. Abstracts, 7*, 224.

Schwartzberg DG, Nakane PK (1983): ACTH-related peptide containing neurons within the medulla oblongata of the rat. *Brain Res., 276*, 351–356.

Segal DS, Browne RG, Bloom F, Ling N, Guillemin R (1977): Beta-endorphin: endogenous opiate or neuroleptic? *Science, 198*, 411–413.

Shaar CJ, Frederickson RCA, Dininger NB, Jackson L (1977): Enkephalin analogues and naloxone modulate the release of growth hormone and prolactin – evidence for regulation by an endogenous opioid peptide in brain. *Life Sci., 21*, 853–860.

Shiomi H, Akil H (1982): Pulse-chase studies of the POMC/beta-endorphin system in the pituitary of acutely and chronically stressed rats. *Life Sci., 31*, 2271–2273.

Shultz R, Wilhelm A, Pirke KM, Gramsch C, Herz A (1981): Beta-endorphin and dynorphin control serum luteinizing hormone level in immature female rats. *Nature (London), 294*, 757–759.

Simantov R, Kuhar MJ, Uhl GR, Snyder SH (1977): Opioid peptide enkephalin: immunohistochemical mapping in rat central nervous system. *Proc. Natl Acad. Sci. USA, 74*, 2167–2171.

Simon EJ, Hiller JM, Edelman I (1973): Stereospecific binding of the potent narcotic analgesic [³H]etorphine to rat-brain homogenate. *Proc. Natl Acad. Sci. USA, 70*, 1947–1949.

Sirinathsinghji DJS, Whittington PE, Audsley A, Fracer HM (1983): Beta-endorphin regulates lordosis in female rats by modulating LH-RH release. *Nature (London), 301*, 62–64.

Sofroniew MV (1979): Immunoreactive beta-endorphin and ACTH in the same neurons of the hypothalamic arcuate nucleus in the rat. *Am. J. Anat., 154*, 283–289.

Stinus L, Koob GF, Ling N, Bloom FE, Le Moal M (1980): Locomotor activation induced by infusion of endorphins into the ventral tegmental area: evidence for opiate-dopamine interactions. *Proc. Natl Acad. Sci. USA, 77*, 2323–2327.

Summy-Long JY, Keil LC, Deen K, Rosella L, Severs WB (1981a): Endogenous opioid peptide inhibition of the central actions of angiotensin. *J. Pharmacol. Exp. Ther., 217*, 619–629.

Summy-long JY, Keil LC, Deen K, Severs WB (1981b): Opiate regulation of angiotensin-induced drinking and vasopressin release. *J. Pharmacol. Exp. Ther., 217*, 630–637.

Summy-Long JY, Rosella LM, Keil LC (1981c): Effects of centrally administered endogenous opioid peptides on drinking behavior, increased plasma vasopressin concentrations and pressor response to hypertonic sodium chloride. *Brain Res., 221*, 343–357.

Szechtman H, Herskhowitz M, Simantov R (1981): Sexual behavior decreases pain sensitivity and stimulates endogenous opioids in male rats. *Eur. J. Pharmacol., 70*, 279–285.

Terenius L (1973): Characteristics of the 'receptor' for narcotic analgesics in synaptic plasma membrane fraction from rat brain. *Acta Pharmacol. Toxicol., 33*, 377–384.

Terenius L, Gispen WH, De Wied D (1975): ACTH-like peptides and opiate receptors in the rat brain: structure-activity studies. *Eur. J. Pharmacol., 33*, 395–399.

Thody AJ, Wilson CA, Everard D (1981): Alpha-melanocyte stimulating hormone stimulates sexual behavior in the female rat. *Psychopharmacology, 74*, 153–156.

Tseng LF, Loh HH, Li CH (1976a): Beta-endorphin as a potent analgesic by intravenous injection. *Nature (London), 263*, 239–240.

Tseng LF, Loh HH, Li CH (1976b): Beta-endorphin: cross tolerance to and cross-physical dependence on morphine. *Proc. Natl Acad. Sci. USA, 73*, 4187–4189.

Uhl GR, Goodman RR, Kuhar MJ, Childers SR, Snyder SH (1979): Immunocytochemical mapping of enkephalin containing cell bodies, fibers and nerve terminals in the brain stem of the rat. *Brain Res., 116*, 75–94.

Valenstein ES (1964): Problems of measurement and interpretation with reinforcing brain stimulation. *Psychol. Rev., 71*, 415–437.

Van der Kooy D, Le Piane FG, Phillips AG (1977): Apparent independence of opiate reinforcement and electrical self-stimulation systems in the rat. *Life Sci., 20*, 981–986.

Van Leeuwen FW, Swaab DF, De Raay C, Fisser B (1979): Immunoelectron-microscopical demonstration of alpha-melanocyte-stimulating hormone-like compound in the rat brain. *J. Endocrinol., 80*, 59P–60P.

Van Ree JM, Smyth DG, Colpaert FC (1979): Dependence-creating properties of lipotropin C-fragment (beta-endorphin): evidence for its internal control of behavior. *Life Sci., 24*, 495–502.

Van Ree JM, Bohus B, Csontos M, Gispen WH, Greven HM, Nijkamp FP, Opmeer FA, De Rotte GA, Van Wimersma Greidanus TB, Witter A, De Wied D (1981): Behavioral profile of gamma-MSH: relationship with ACTH and beta-endorphin action. *Life Sci., 28*, 2875–2888.

Van Vugt DA, Meites J (1980): Influence of endogenous opiates on anterior pituitary function. *Fed. Proc., 39*, 2533–2538.

Van Wimersma Greidanus TB, Thody TJ, Verspaget H, De Rotte GA, Goedemans HJH, Croset G, Van Ree JM (1979): Effects of morphine and beta-endorphin on basal and elevated plasma levels of alpha-MSH and vasopressin. *Life Sci., 24*, 579–586.

271

Van Wimersma Greidanus TB, Van Ree JM, Goedemans HJH, Van Dam AF, Andringa-Bakker EAD, De Wied D (1981): Effects of beta-endorphin fragments on plasma levels of vasospressin. *Life Sci., 29*, 783–788.

Vincent SR, Hökfelt T, Christensson I, Terenius L (1982): Dynorphin-immunoreactive neurons in the central nervous system of the rat. *Neurosci. Lett., 33*, 185–190.

Walker JM, Akil H, Watson SJ (1980): Evidence for homologous actions of pro-opiocortin products. *Science, 210*, 1247–1249.

Watson SJ (1980): Alpha-MSH in brain beta-endorphin neurons, and other neurons as well. In: Way EL (Ed.), *Endogenous and Exogenous Opiate Agonists and Antagonists*, pp. 127–130. Pergamon Press, New York.

Watson SJ, Akil H (1979): Presence of two alpha-MSH positive cell groups in rat hypothalamus. *Eur. J. Pharmacol., 58*, 101–103.

Watson SJ, Akil H (1980a): Alpha-MSH in rat brain: occurrence within and outside brain beta-endorphin neurons. *Brain Res., 182*, 217–223.

Watson SJ, Akil H (1980b): On the multiplicity of active substances in single neurons: beta-endorphin and alpha-MSH as a model system. In: De Wied D, Van Keep PA (Eds), *Hormones and the Brain*, pp. 73–86. MTP Press, Lancaster.

Watson SJ, Akil H (1981): Anatomy of beta-endorphin-containing structures in pituitary and brain. In: Li CH (Ed.), *Hormonal Proteins and Peptides, Vol. 10*, pp. 171–201. Academic Press, New York.

Watson SJ, Akil H, Sullivan SO, Barchas JD (1977a): Immunocytochemical localization of methionine-enkephalin: preliminary observations. *Life Sci., 25*, 733–738.

Watson SJ, Barchas JD, Li CH (1977b): Beta-lipotropin: localization in cells and axons in rat brain by immunocytochemistry. *Proc. Natl Acad. Sci. USA, 74*, 5155–5158.

Watson SJ, Akil H, Richard CW, Barchas JD (1978a): Evidence for two separate opiate peptide neuronal systems and the coexistence of beta-lipotropin, beta-endorphin and ACTH immunoreactivities in the same hypothalamic neurons. *Nature (London), 275*, 226–228.

Watson SJ, Richard CW, Barchas JD (1978b): Adrenocorticotropin in rat brain: immunocytochemical localization in the cells and axons. *Science, 200*, 1180–1182.

Watson SJ, Akil H, Walker JM (1980): Anatomical and biochemical studies of the opioid peptides and related substances in the brain. *Peptides, 1 (Suppl. 1)*, 11–20.

Watson SJ, Akil H, Ghazarossian V, Goldstein A (1981): Dynorphin immunocytochemical localization in brain and peripheral nervous system: preliminary studies. *Proc. Natl Acad. Sci. USA, 78*, 1260–1263.

Watson SJ, Akil H, Fischli A, Goldstein A, Zimmerman E, Nilaver G, Van Wimersma Greidanus TB (1982a): Dynorphin and vasopressin: common localization in magnocellular neurons. *Science, 216*, 85–87.

Watson SJ, Khachaturian H, Akil H, Coy D, Goldstein A (1982b): Comparison of the distribution of dynorphin systems and enkephalin systems in brain. *Science, 218*, 1134–1136.

Watson SJ, Akil H, Khachaturian H, Young E, Lewis ME (1984): Opioid systems: anatomical, physiological and clinical perspectives. In: Collier HOJ, Hughes J, Rance MJ, Tyers MB (Eds), *Opioids: Past, Present and Future*, pp. 145–178. Taylor and Francis Ltd., London.

Watson SJ, Khachaturian H, Lewis ME, Akil H (1985): Chemical neuroanatomy as a basis for biological psychiatry. In: Berger PA, Brodie HKH (Eds), *American Handbook of Psychiatry, Vol. 8*. Basic Books, Inc., New York. In press.

Weber E, Barchas JD (1983): Immunohistochemical distribution of dynorphin B in rat brain: relation to dynorphin A and alpha-neo-endorphin system. *Proc. Natl Acad. Sci. USA, 80*, 1125–1129.

Weber E, Voigt R, Martin R (1978): Concomitant storage of ACTH and endorphin-like immunoreactivity in the secretory granule of anterior pituitary corticotrophs. *Brain Res., 157*, 385–390.

Weitzman RE, Fisher DA, Minick S, Ling N, Guillemin R (1977): Beta-endorphin stimulates secretion of arginine vasopressin in vivo. *Endocrinology, 101*, 1643–1646.

Whitfeld PL, Seeburg PH, Shine J (1982): The human pro-opiomelanocortin gene: organization, sequence and interspersion with repetitive DNA. *DNA, 1*, 133–136.

Zakarian S, Smyth D (1979): Distribution of active and inactive forms of endorphins in rat pituitary and brain. *Proc. Natl Acad. Sci. USA, 76*, 5972–5976.

Zimmerman EA, Liotta A, Krieger DT (1978): Beta-lipotropin in brain: localization in hypothalamic neurons by immunoperoxidase technique. *Cell Tissue Res., 186*, 393–398.

CHAPTER VI

Distribution of enkephalin-containing neurons in the central nervous system*

PETER PETRUSZ, ISTVAN MERCHENTHALER AND
JEROME L. MADERDRUT

1. INTRODUCTION

Recombinant DNA** technology has revealed the presence of at least 3 distinct genes that code for precursor proteins containing the sequences of one or more opioid peptides (Nakanishi et al. 1979; Comb et al. 1982; Gubler et al. 1982; Noda et al. 1982; Kakidani et al. 1982). The principal goal of this chapter is to describe the anatomical distribution of the perikarya, fibers and nerve terminals that contain either the precursor protein, preproenkephalin (preproenkephalin A), or smaller peptide fragments derived from this precursor by proteolytic processing (Fig. 1). This goal requires unique markers that discriminate the products derived from the preproenkephalin gene from both the products of the preproopiomelanocortin (PPOMC) and the preprodynorphin (preproenkephalin B) genes (Fig. 1).

Although DNA complementary to messenger RNA coding for mammalian preproenkephalin has only been cloned and sequenced from bovine adrenal medulla (Gubler et al. 1982; Noda et al. 1982) and human pheochromocytoma (Comb et al. 1982), compelling indirect evidence suggests the presence of a similar (or identical) precursor protein in the bovine and human brain, respectively (Rossier et al. 1980; Baird et al. 1982; Dandekar and Sabol 1982; Höllt et al. 1982; Liston et al. 1983; Pittius et al. 1983; Liston and Rossier 1984). Compelling indirect evidence also suggests the presence of a similar precursor protein in the brain and spinal cord of the rat (Rossier et al. 1980a; Boarder et al. 1982; Ikeda et al. 1982; Legon et al. 1982; Majane et al. 1983; Sabol et al. 1983; Tang et al. 1983; Yang et al. 1983; Lindberg and Yang 1984; Yoshikawa et al. 1985;

*Parts of our studies were supported by Grants Number NS 14904 and NS 20402 from the United States Public Health Service.
**Abbreviations used in this Chapter: APP, avian pancreatic polypeptide; BAM 12P, bovine adrenal medullary opioid dodecapeptide; BAM 22P, bovine adrenal medullary opioid docosapeptide; CNS, central nervous system; CRF, corticotropin releasing factor; DAB, 3,3'-diaminobenzidine; DNA, deoxyribonucleic acid; ENK-7, (Met^5)-enkephalin-Arg^6-Phe^7; ENK-8, (Met^5)-enkephalin-Arg^6-Gly^7-Leu^8; FMRF, phenylalanine-methionine-arginine-phenylalanine; GABA, γ-amino-N-butyric acid; HPLC, high pressure liquid chromatography; HRP, horseradish peroxidase; Leu-ENK, (Leu^5)-enkephalin; -LI, -like immunoreactivity; Met-ENK, (Met^5)-enkephalin; PAP, peroxidase-antiperoxidase; PPOMC, preproopiomelanocortin; RIA, radioimmunoassay; RNA, ribonucleic acid; SP, substance P. *For all other abbreviations*, see the General Abbreviations List, p. 609.

Handbook of Chemical Neuroanatomy. Vol. 4: GABA and Neuropeptides in the CNS, Part I.
A. Björklund and T. Hökfelt, editors.
© Elsevier Science Publishers B.V., 1985.

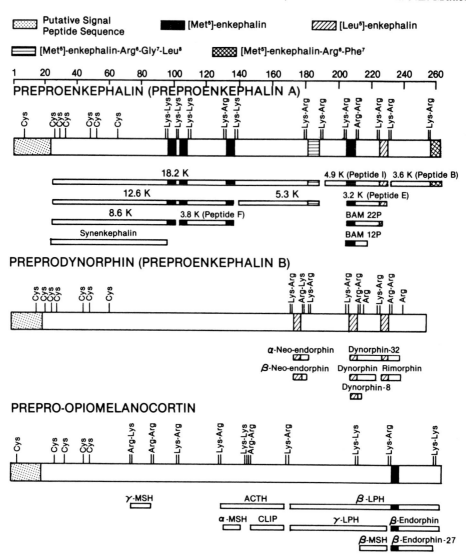

Fig. 1. Schematic representation of the proteolytic processing of the 3 opioid peptide-containing prohormones. The paired and single basic amino acids that serve as processing sites are indicated. Only peptides that have been isolated from one or more mammalian tissues and characterized by biochemical methods are illustrated. This figure is a modification of schematics previously published by Nakanishi et al. (1979), Udenfriend and Kilpatrick (1983), and Rossier et al. (1983). These 3 papers should be consulted for further information about the structure and processing of the 3 polyhormonal precursors.

cf. Kojima et al. 1982). The proenkephalin precursors in the bovine adrenal medulla and human pheochromocytoma each contain 4 copies of (Met^5)-enkephalin (Met-ENK) and a single copy of (Leu^5)-enkephalin (Leu-ENK), the opioid heptapeptide (Met^5)-enkephalin-Arg^6-Phe^7 (ENK-7), and the opioid octapeptide (Met^5)-enkephalin-Arg^6-Gly^7-Leu^8 (ENK-8); each internal opioid peptide sequence is flanked by pairs of basic amino acids (Fig. 1) that are the usual processing signals in polyhormonal precursors (Docherty and Steiner 1982; Douglass et al. 1984; Loh et al. 1984). The opioid heptapeptide ENK-7 which forms the carboxyl terminus of preproenkephalin, has a pair of basic amino acids only preceding its amino terminus. All 4 distinct opioid peptides predicted from the amino acid sequence of preproenkephalin to be end products of sequential processing by a trypsin-like enzyme followed by a carboxypeptidase B-like enzyme had previously been isolated and sequenced from extracts of the bovine adrenal medulla (Stern et al. 1979; Kilpatrick et al. 1981). An opioid docosapeptide (BAM 22P) and an opioid dodecapeptide (BAM 12P) that contain the Met-ENK sequence at their amino termini have been isolated from the bovine adrenal medulla and sequenced (Mizuno et al. 1980a,b). Antisera directed against either the carboxyl terminus of either ENK-7 or ENK-8 (e.g., Williams and Dockray 1982), or the non-enkephalin-containing sequences of preproenkephalin (e.g., Bloch et al. 1983; Liston et al. 1983) are potentially candidates for the required unique markers for the preproenkephalin gene.*

Most of the early systematic studies of the immunohistochemical distribution of enkephalin pentapeptide-like immunoreactivity (pentapeptide-LI) in the mammalian brain and spinal cord (Elde et al. 1976; Hökfelt et al. 1977a; Simantov et al. 1977; Watson et al. 1977; Sar et al. 1978; Uhl et al. 1979) were completed before the isolation and sequencing of dynorphin (dynorphin A) (Goldstein et al. 1979) and α-neo-endorphin (Kangawa et al. 1979) from porcine pituitary and hypothalamic extracts, respectively. Although the authors of these pioneering studies were conscious to varying degrees of the need to discriminate between neuronal systems expressing some of the 'end-products' of the PPOMC (β-lipotropin and β-endorphin) and the preproenkephalin (Leu- and Met-ENK) gene (cf. Bloom et al. 1978), they used antisera that in most (and perhaps all) cases did not discriminate between the expression of the preprodynorphin gene and the preproenkephalin gene. Thus, an unknown number of neuronal systems labeled as enkephalin-containing by these authors were, in fact, dynorphin-containing neuronal systems.

Although the preproenkephalin precursor is apparently identical in the adrenal medulla, the pituitary and the central nervous system (CNS), proteolytic processing appears to vary (at least quantitatively) between different tissues (Baird et al. 1982; Weber et al. 1983a; Lindberg and Yang 1984). The PPOMC and the preprodynorphin precursors also show differential processing by different tissues (Gramsch et al. 1980; Eipper and Mains 1981; Weber et al. 1982; Seizinger et al. 1984). Immunocytochemical techniques can be used to examine either proteolytic precursor processing during axonal transport from perikarya to nerve terminals or differential precursor processing at the level of individual perikarya and between specific terminal fields (e.g., McGinty and Bloom 1983; Williams and Dockray 1983a).

A technique for the selective deposition of silver crystals on the 3,3'-diaminobenzidine (DAB) polymer used to localize horseradish peroxidase (HRP) in immunocytochemical bridge methods (Ordronneau et al. 1981) substantially increases the intensity of dendritic and axonal staining (Merchenthaler et al. 1982a,b). This technique in combination

---

*Although antisera directed toward the free C-terminus of either Leu-ENK (e.g. Khachaturian et al. 1983a,b) or Met-ENK (e.g. Altschuler et al. 1982) can have a high degree of specificity for the free enkephalin pentapeptides as opposed to dynorphin, rimorphin, α-neo-endorphin, and β-endorphin, they are intrinsically incapable of discriminating either between Leu-ENK derived from proenkephalin or prodynorphin, or between Met-ENK derived from proenkephalin or PPOMC. Since the Leu-ENK sequences in dynorphin, rimorphin and α-neo-endorphin are immediately followed by pairs of basic amino acids (Fig. 1), the possibility that Leu-ENK can be cleaved from these peptides in some tissues is quite real (cf. Udenfriend and Kilpatrick 1983). The further processing of dynorphin, rimorphin and/or α-neo-endorphin in some regions of the CNS to yield Leu-ENK has recently been suggested (Zamir et al. 1983a; Kilpatrick et al. 1983b; Zamir et al. 1984). Therefore, antisera directed toward the free C-terminus of Leu-ENK cannot be used to discriminate between neurons expressing the preproenkephalin and the preprodynorphin genes.

with thick Vibratome sections should permit a more complete description of enkephalin-containing pathways and a better correlation of the morphology of immunocytochemically stained perikarya with cell types defined by classical Golgi methods (cf. Grzanna et al. 1978; Sofroniew and Glassman 1981; see also the chapter by A. Björklund in *Vol. 1* of This Series) than previously possible (e.g., Maley et al. 1983). A secondary goal of this chapter is to supply a better definition of the morphology of enkephalin-containing neurons than previous investigators.

A variety of double-labeling techniques using either adjacent sections or the simultaneous localization of two markers in the same section have provided evidence for the co-localization of enkephalin-LI with each of the classical neurotransmitters as well as several structurally unrelated peptide transmitter candidates (see 4.3.). In some of these cases the evidence is, however, indirect; many possible cases of co-localization suggested by comparisons between studies on the localization of enkephalin-LI and the localization of other putative neurotransmitters have yet to be examined using double-labeling techniques (cf. Stengaard-Pedersen and Larsson 1981). The final goal of this chapter is to examine some additional potential cases of co-localization of enkephalin-LI with immunoreactivity for other peptide transmitter candidates.

2. MATERIALS AND METHODS

2.1. SOURCES OF TISSUES

Twenty-four adult Sprague-Dawley rats were purchased from ARS/Sprague-Dawley (Madison, WI). Some of the rats were sacrificed 24 hours following a bilateral stereotaxic injection of colchicine (100 μg dissolved in 10 μl of saline) into the lateral ventricles. Three human brains were gifts from Drs R.V. Randall and S. Ikazaki (Departments of Internal Medicine and Pathology, Mayo Clinic, Rochester, MN). One 4-month-old lamb was a gift from Dr J.C. Rose (Department of Physiology and Pharmacology, Bowman Gray School of Medicine, Winston-Salem, NC). Three adult cats and one 8-day-old White Leghorn (*Gallus domesticus*) chicken were also used. One cat had 1 mg of colchicine injected into the lateral ventricles 24 hours prior to sacrifice; the other cat had 1 mg of colchicine injected into the lumbar subarachnoid space 24 hours prior to sacrifice (Maderdrut et al. 1982).

2.2. PREPARATION OF TISSUES

The rats were anesthetized with ether and were perfused through the ascending aorta with 50 ml of 1% paraformaldehyde followed by 250 ml of 4% paraformaldehyde in 0.1 M phosphate buffer (pH 7.4). The 4-month-old lamb and the 8-day-old chicken were perfused with corresponding larger and smaller volumes of the same fixatives, respectively. The 3 cats were perfused as described by Ordronneau and Petrusz (1980); the 3 humans were perfused within 4 hours of death with 4% paraformaldehyde. Thirty minutes after completion of the perfusion, the brain and spinal cord were carefully removed, cut into smaller pieces, and immersed in the same fixative overnight. The tissues were then either embedded in paraffin or cut at 50 μm using a Lancer Vibratome. Paraffin-embedded tissues were sectioned serially at 5 or 8 μm.

2.3. PRIMARY ANTISERA

All primary antisera were raised in rabbits. The anti-Leu-ENK serum was a gift from Dr R.J. Miller (Department of Pharmacological and Physiological Science, University of Chicago, Chicago, IL). The preparation, RIA specificity and immunohistochemical specificity of the antiserum have been described (Miller et al. 1978; Finley et al. 1981a). The antiserum shows about 4% cross-reactivity with dynorphin by RIA (A. Goldstein, personal communication). The BAM 22P antiserum was purchased from Peninsula Laboratories, Inc. (Belmont, CA). The antiserum shows no cross-reactivity with either Met-ENK or Leu-ENK by RIA. The anti-ENK-7 serum (L150) was a gift from Dr D.J. Dockray (Department of Physiology, University of Liverpool, Liverpool, United Kingdom). The antigen was made by coupling ENK-7 to thyroglobulin with glutaraldehyde. The antiserum is directed toward the C-terminus of ENK-7 and requires a free terminal carboxyl group for recognition (Williams and Dockray 1983a). The molluscan peptide, FMRF-amide (Greenberg and Price 1983) is not recognized by antiserum L150 (Williams and Dockray 1983a); the distribution of FMRF-amide-LI in the rat CNS is distinct from the distribution of ENK-7-LI (Williams and Dockray 1983b). The anti-dynorphin(1–17) serum (R3-121481) was a gift from Dr A. Goldstein (Addiction Research Center, Palo Alto, CA). The antigen was made by coupling dynorphin to thyroglobulin with glutaraldehyde. The antiserum shows no cross-reactivity with Leu-ENK by RIA. The antiserum recognizes both N-terminally and C-terminally extended variants of dynorphin. The anti-rimorphin (dynorphin B) serum (13S) was also a gift from Dr A. Goldstein. The antigen was made by coupling rimorphin to thyroglobulin with glutaraldehyde. The antiserum shows no cross-reactivity with Leu-ENK, dynorphin or α-neo-endorphin by RIA. The antiserum recognizes both N-terminally and C-terminally extended variants of rimorphin (Cone and Goldstein 1982a). The β-endorphin antiserum (222-1) was raised in our laboratory. The preparation, RIA specificity and immunohistochemical specificity of the antiserum have been described (Finley et al. 1981b). The corticotropin-releasing factor (CRF) antiserum (SV-22) was a gift from Drs S. Vigh and A.V. Schally (Department of Medicine, Tulane University, New Orleans, LA). The preparation, RIA specificity and immunohistochemical specificity of the antiserum have been described (Vigh et al. 1982; Merchenthaler et al. 1982b). The anti-oxytocin serum was a gift from Dr L.W. Swanson (Salk Institute, La Jolla, CA). The preparation, RIA specificity and immunohistochemical specificity of the antiserum have been described (Vandesande and Dierickx 1975).

2.4. IMMUNOCYTOCHEMICAL METHODS

The Vibratome sections were pretreated with a graded series of ethanol to enhance the penetration of antibodies (Merchenthaler et al. 1982b). All Vibratome sections were stained by the unlabeled-antibody peroxidase-antiperoxidase (PAP) method (Sternberger 1979); all paraffin sections were stained by the 'double PAP' method (Ordronneau et al. 1981).

After completion of the DAB reaction step, some of the Vibratome sections were processed for the selective deposition of silver crystals onto the DAB polymer (Gallyas et al. 1982; Merchenthaler et al. 1982a,b). The selective deposition of silver is based on the ability of the DAB polymer to catalyze the reaction between silver ions (from $AgNO_3$) and a reducing agent (formaldehyde). Nonspecific deposition of silver is prevented by suppression of the catalytic activity of the tissue by prior oxidation with perchloric acid. In the resulting Golgi-like images, contrast is markedly enhanced, neuronal morphology is displayed with greater fidelity, and fibers can be traced for longer distances than in conventionally stained preparations (Merchenthaler et al. 1982a,b). By augmenting even the weakest sites of DAB deposition, the silver method increases the sensitivity (detection limit) of immunocytochemistry by about two orders of magnitude (Gallyas et al. 1982).

The distribution of proenkephalin-derived peptides was compared to that of PPOMC- and prodynorphin-derived peptides by localizing antigens in the same section with contrasting chromogens (Joseph and Sternberger 1979).

2.5. CONTROLS AND DEFINITIONS

Method specificity was tested by a series of increasing dilutions of the primary antiserum resulting in a gradual decrease and eventual disappearance of the immunological staining (Petrusz et al. 1980). Possible interference by endogenous peroxidase(s) was either ruled out by staining some sections beginning with the DAB step or prevented by preincubating the sections in absolute methanol containing 1% H_2O_2 (Burns 1978). Antiserum specificity was tested by absorption with either the peptide used for immunization or other structurally related and structurally unrelated peptides (Petrusz et al. 1980). Sections stained for the simultaneous localization of two antigens, and adjacent sections stained alternately for two structurally unrelated peptides provided additional controls of antiserum specificity. These double-staining techniques were also used to determine whether two proenkephalin-derived peptides occurred in the same perikarya and whether processes containing proenkephalin-derived peptides formed apparent contacts with perikarya containing PPOMC- and/or prodynorphin-derived peptides.

The term 'enkephalin pentapeptide-LI' is used in this chapter to encompass all tissue antigenic sites which bind antibodies that are *specific* for either Leu- or Met-ENK, the major criterion for specificity being competitive inhibition of the binding (as tested in simultaneous immunohistochemical staining) by either Leu- or Met-ENK, respectively (cf. Petrusz et al. 1976, 1980). This definition clearly includes not only authentic Leu- or Met-ENK but also other structurally related molecules containing either the complete Leu- or Met-ENK sequences (e.g., peptide E and peptide F) or an antigenic fragment of the Leu- or Met-ENK sequences (e.g., BAM 22P) as well as structurally unrelated molecules containing either the complete Leu- or Met-ENK sequences (e.g., dynorphin and β-endorphin) or an antigenic fragment of the Leu- or Met-ENK sequences (e.g., FMRF-amide). Absorption tests for possible cross-reacting molecules are valid only for the molecules that have actually been tested with the antiserum in simultaneous immunohistochemical staining and cannot be extrapolated to similar molecules that have not been tested. The results of RIA specificity tests, while suggestive, cannot provide definitive information about the recognition of the corresponding antigens following fixation. It should be re-emphasized that RIA specificity tests of polyclonal antisera only define the recognition properties of those antibody populations in the serum that bind the labeled tracer (Petrusz et al. 1976). The analogous terms 'ENK-7-LI', 'BAM 22P-LI', etc., are used with the same reservations. These reservations are implicit when terms such as 'enkephalin-containing' are used to describe the distribution of an antigen seen with immunohistochemical techniques. This does not necessarily imply any definable non-specificity of the particular antiserum but simply represents an inherent limitation in the accuracy with which antigens localized by immunohistochemical techniques with either poly- or monoclonal antisera can be specified.

3. RESULTS

3.1. GENERAL

The detection of enkephalin-containing neuronal cell bodies, processes and terminals was enhanced in this study by several technical improvements. These include the use of colchicine pretreatment, thick Vibratome sections, silver-gold intensification of the DAB polymer and, most importantly, antisera with unique specificity for products of the preproenkephalin gene (see 1. and 2.).

Immunocytochemical staining with the Leu-ENK antiserum was always more intense than with the ENK-7 antiserum in tissues from both normal and colchicine-treated animals (cf. Williams and Dockray 1983a). Although the ENK-7 antiserum was substantially more effective than the BAM 22P antiserum in staining cell bodies and nerve processes in the rat and cat CNS, the BAM 22P antiserum was substantially more effective than the ENK-7 antiserum in staining chromaffin cells in the adrenal medulla of both rat and cat (cf. Baird et al. 1982; Höllt et al. 1982). The distribution of BAM 22P immunoreactive perikarya and neuronal processes in the brain and spinal cord of the rat was apparently identical to the distribution of ENK-7 immunoreactive perikarya and neuronal processes (cf. Khachaturian et al. 1983a,b).

Although immunoreactive perikarya could be detected in normal rats with the ENK-7 antiserum, the staining intensity was dramatically enhanced following intracerebroventricular injection of colchicine without any significant decrement in the staining intensity of immunoreactive fibers and nerve terminals. Therefore, the description of enkephalin-LI and the distributional maps of ENK-7-LI presented in this chapter are based almost completely (with only a few exceptions that are clearly indicated) on the results obtained from colchicine-treated rats.

Based on specificity tests conducted either by us or by Williams and Dockray (1982, 1983a), and on theoretical grounds (see 1. and Fig. 1), we assume that the ENK-7 antiserum labels specifically neurons that contain at least one product of the preproenkephalin gene and does not label neurons that contain only opioid peptides that are products of either the PPOMC or the preprodynorphin gene. The distribution of 'enkephalin' reported in this chapter is based on our unpublished results with the ENK-7 antiserum (L150). With a few exceptions (e.g., the hypothalamic magnocellular nuclei or the hippocampal mossy fiber system), the distribution of ENK-7-LI overlaps as least in broad outline with the distribution of enkephalin pentapeptide-LI described by earlier investigators who used antisera to Leu- or Met-ENK which could potentially also recognize peptides derived from prodynorphin (e.g., Elde et al. 1976; Hökfelt et al. 1977a; Simantov et al. 1977; Watson et al. 1977; Sar et al. 1978; Uhl et al. 1979; Finley et al. 1981a). Apparent discrepancies between our results and those reported in earlier publications will be discussed in Section 4.1.

The vast majority of ENK-7 immunoreactive cells were small to medium-size bipolar or multipolar neurons with perikarya having diameters of 7–30 μm. However, staining was also observed within some of the largest perikarya of the rat CNS (e.g., gigantocellular reticular neurons in the brainstem raphe). In addition, abundant immunoreactivity was observed in neuronal processes and terminal-like structures throughout the CNS. Here, the staining was characterized by punctate accumulations of the reaction product along the extent of the processes. Although light microscopy alone is not sufficient to decide whether these varicosities represent *en passant* synaptic contacts, data from the literature strongly suggest that at least a portion of them do serve that purpose (e.g., about 25% of the varicosities in the striatum, according to Pickel et al. 1980a,b). Several pericellular basket-like terminals were also observed in the rat CNS, e.g., in the lateral septal nucleus. In addition, many individual varicose fibers seemed to occur in close apposition to neuronal cell bodies, suggesting axosomatic synaptic contacts (e.g., around motoneurons in the spinal cord). The general ultrastructural features of peptidergic neurons are discussed by Pickel (Chapter II) and will not be explicitly reviewed here.

The detailed localization of the structures labeled by antiserum L150 in the rat CNS is described in the following sections and is illustrated in the Atlas.

3.2. TELENCEPHALON

Perikarya were labeled with the antiserum to ENK-7 in the olfactory bulb, olfactory tubercle, nucleus accumbens, septal nuclei, bed nucleus of the stria terminalis, diagonal band of Broca, basal ganglia, amygdala, hippocampal formation, and in several paleocortical and neocortical regions. In the olfactory bulb, small immunoreactive perikarya were observed in the periglomerular regions as well as in the internal granular layer (Fig. 2), and in the anterior olfactory nuclei. The former group contained small round cells while the two latter groups also included fusiform cell bodies. Occasionally the processes of the fusiform perikarya in the internal granular layer could be seen running radially through the internal plexiform layer and disappearing in the external plexiform layer. A population of cells extended into the olfactory tubercle and continued laterally in the piriform cortex, mainly in layer II. Only scattered and weakly stained perikarya were seen in the cingulate cortex and in regions of the frontal, parietal and occipital neocortex, where they were located mainly in layers II and III. Small perikarya were also labeled in the nucleus accumbens (Fig. 3), the lateral septal nucleus, and the lateral part of the bed nucleus of the stria terminalis. In the lateral septum, many unlabeled multipolar perikarya were surrounded very densely by labeled terminals, giving the impression of perikaryal staining (Fig. 4; cf. Stengaard-Pedersen and Larsson 1983). However, several clearly labeled perikarya were also present in the medial regions of the lateral septum. Enkephalin-immunoreactive cells were seen in the medial septal nucleus (Fig. 4). Numerous perikarya were stained in the vertical and horizontal limbs of the diagonal band of Broca (Fig. 5). Small, dispersed enkephalin-containing cells were found in the caudate-putamen (Fig. 6). The areas that contained the cells and fibers throughout the striatum were interspersed in a mosaic-like manner (cf. Graybiel et al. 1981) with round or oval areas devoid of immunostaining (Fig. 6). A similar pattern of ENK-7-immunoreactive fibers was seen in the human globus pallidus. The immunoreactive cell bodies in the striatum were uniformly distributed both rostrally and caudally, but tended to aggregate in the medial and ventral regions at the level of the preoptic-anterior hypothalamic area (Fig. 6).

All of the amygdaloid nuclei contained scattered cells stained by the antiserum to ENK-7, with the greatest number of cells in the lateral and central nuclei (Fig. 7; see also Fig. 6). In the hippocampal region, a few scattered and weakly stained cells were seen in the pyramidal layer (the majority in the CA1 field and, less frequently, in other regions). Labeled perikarya were also seen in the granular layer of the dentate gyrus and in the subiculum. Most of the perikarya in the pyramidal layer were fusiform, and

---

Atlas. Schematic representation of ENK-7 immunoreactive cell bodies and fibers in the rat brain, as represented in 20 coronal planes. Fiber densities are represented in a 4-graded scale, from scattered (widely spaced thin lines) to very dense (thick lines). *For abbreviations,* see the General Abbreviations List, p. 609.

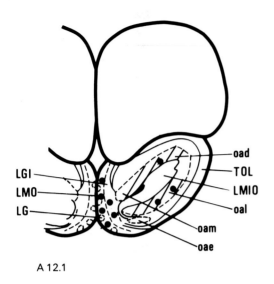

A 12.1

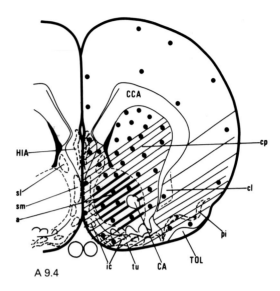

A 9.4

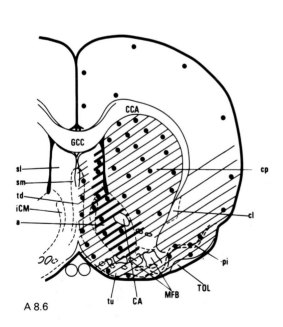

A 8.6

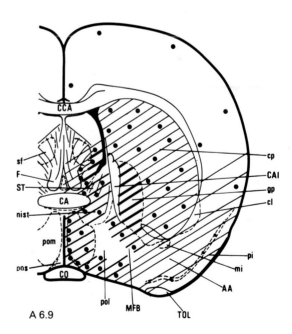

A 6.9

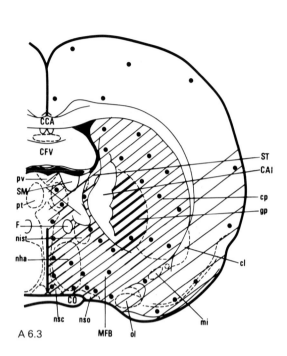

A 6.3

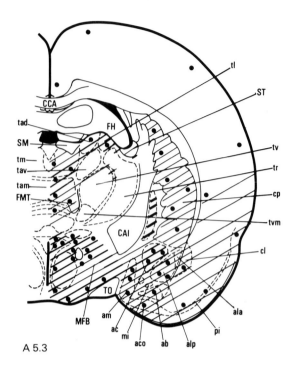

A 5.3

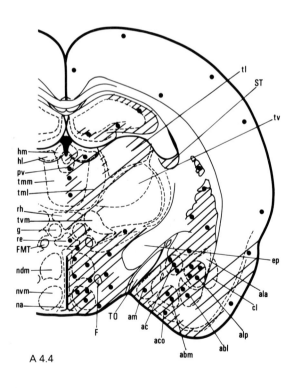

A 4.4

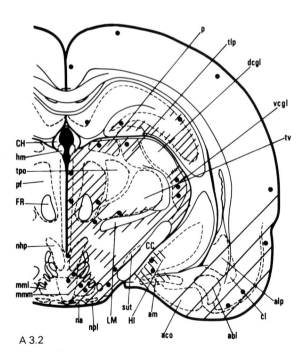

A 3.2

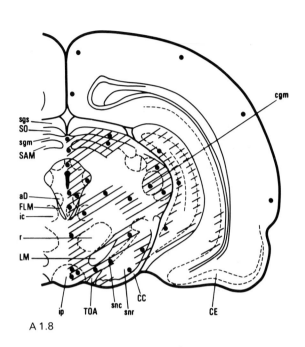

A 1.8

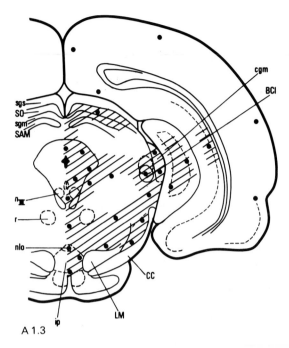

A 1.3

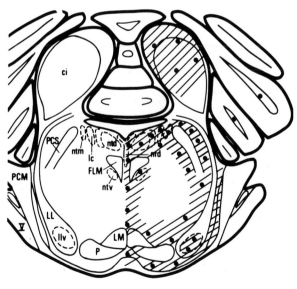

P 1.5

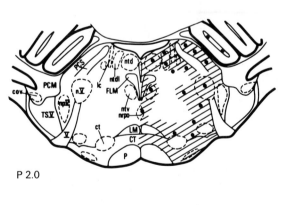

P 2.0

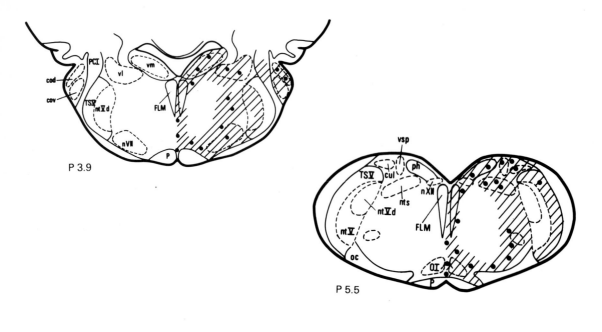

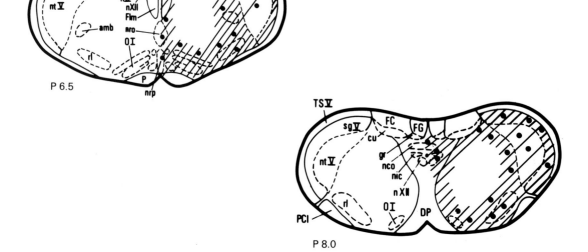

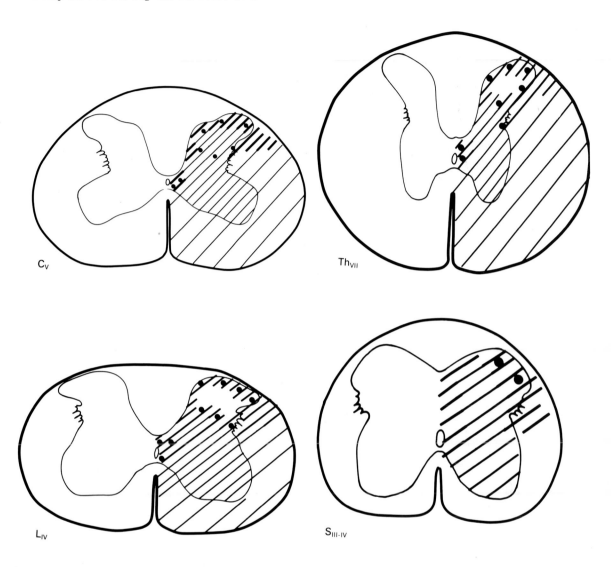

their processes were extended parallel to the dendritic tree of the pyramidal cells.

Neuronal processes were stained with the antiserum to ENK-7 in all of the above areas. However, the density and the distribution of these processes was different and characteristic for each region. The processes of the neurons in the cerebral cortex and olfactory bulb extended for only a short distance from their perikarya. Cells in the internal granular layer of the olfactory bulb sent their processes toward the outer layers as far as the external plexiform layer (Fig. 2). A dense accumulation of stained fibers was seen in the nucleus accumbens, especially in its ventromedial portion (Fig. 3), and in the horizontal and vertical limbs of the diagonal band of Broca. The densest accumulation of enkephalin-containing processes in the entire CNS was seen in the globus pallidus, the ansa lenticularis and the amygdaloid complex, forming a continuous field extending over these areas (Fig. 6).

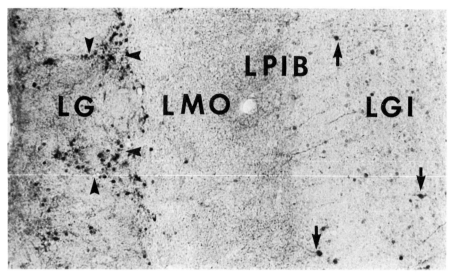

Fig. 2. Enkephalin-containing perikarya and neuronal processes in the olfactory bulb of the rat. Small, round perikarya surround the olfactory glomeruli (arrowheads). Scattered enkephalin-containing cell bodies are seen in the lamina granularis interna (arrows). Some of these cells are fusiform with processes that run through the lamina plexiformis interna. LG: lamina glomerulosa; LGI: lamina granulosa interna; LMO: lamina molecularis; LPIB: lamina plexiformis interna bulbi olfactorii. Colchicine treated; Vibratome section; Leu-ENK antiserum; silver intensification. × 210.

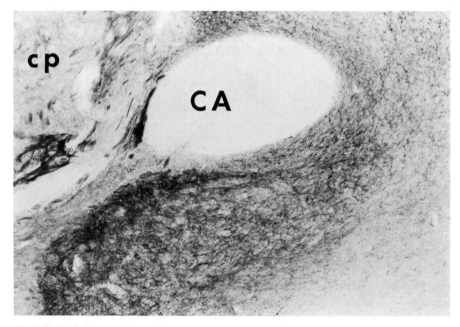

Fig. 3. Enkephalin-containing perikarya and neuronal processes in the nucleus accumbens of the rat. Dense accumulations of immunoreactive fibers are seen in the ventral portion of the nucleus. CA: commissura anterior; cp: caudatus putamen. Colchicine treated; Vibratome section; Leu-ENK antiserum; silver intensification. × 80.

286

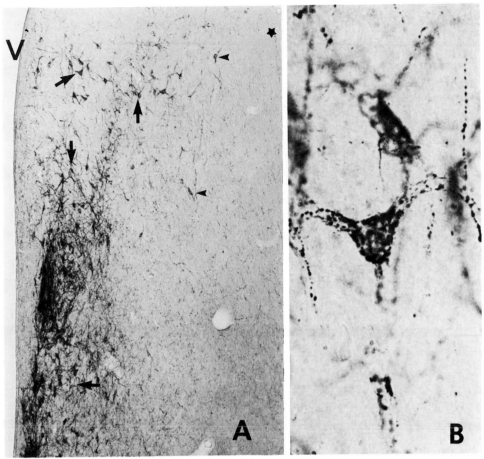

Fig. 4. A. Enkephalin-containing perikarya and neuronal processes in the lateral septal nucleus of the rat. Many of the unlabeled perikarya are multipolar and are surrounded by a dense network of labeled terminals (arrows). Only a few enkephalin-containing perikarya are seen in the medial septal nucleus (arrowheads). The midline is indicated by an asterisk. Dense accumulations of immunoreactive fibers are seen in the basal portion of the lateral septal nucleus. V: lateral ventricle. Colchicine treated; Vibratome section; Leu-ENK antiserum; silver intensification. × 80. *B.* High power view from the same field as Figure 4A (see upper arrow) of an unstained perikaryon surrounded by bouton-like processes. × 800.

3.3. DIENCEPHALON

Thalamus

In the thalamus, scattered perikarya were recognized by the antiserum to ENK-7 in the paraventricular, paratenial, and anterior basal medial, ventral and lateral nuclei (Fig. 8). Enkephalin-containing neuronal processes in the thalamus were less abundant than in other regions of the diencephalon. In the anterior region of the thalamus (Fig. 8), ENK-7-immunoreactive fibers were observed laterally in the anterior ventral thalamic nucleus. More medially, a dense aggregate of immunoreactive neuronal processes was seen between the paratenial nucleus, the anterior medial thalamic nucleus, and the paraventricular nucleus. Enkephalin-positive fibers were also observed in the stellatocellular

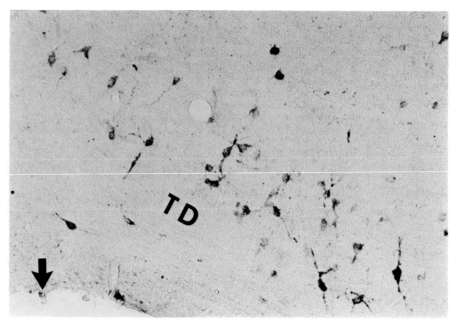

Fig. 5. Enkephalin-containing perikarya in the horizontal limb of the diagonal band of Broca (TD) of the rat. The basal surface is indicated by an arrow in the midline. Colchicine treated; Vibratome section; ENK-7 antiserum; silver intensification. × 210.

and rotundocellular periventricular nuclei, the rhomboid nucleus, the nucleus reuniens, the medial thalamic nucleus (the lateral region of the lateral part of this nucleus and the medial region of the medial part of this nucleus), the medial area of the posteromedial thalamic nucleus, the medial portion of the parafascicular nucleus, and the ventral portion of the ventral thalamic nucleus (dorsal to the medial lemniscus). Scattered fibers were also seen in the lateral and medial habenula.

Hypothalamus

Numerous small perikarya were stained with the ENK-7 antiserum in the medial preoptic nucleus, the ventromedial region of the lateral preoptic nucleus, and the periventricular preoptic nucleus (Fig. 9). A few scattered cell bodies were also found in the lateral region of the lateral preoptic nucleus. In the mid-hypothalamic region, strongly stained immunoreactive perikarya were observed in the perifornical region (Fig. 10A). In the paraventricular nucleus, immunoreactive perikarya, stained with medium intensity (Fig. 10A), were found only in the parvocellular subdivisions (cf. Swanson and Kuypers 1980), while somewhat larger but weakly stained cell bodies were seen in the lateral peripheral zone of the nucleus (Figs 10A and B). This difference in staining intensity (observed within the same section) was also seen with the BAM 22P antiserum. Dual staining with contrasting chromogens in the same Vibratome section revealed that the majority of the ENK-7-immunoreactive perikarya in the paraventricular nucleus did not contain CRF-LI (cf. Merchenthaler et al. 1982b). Antisera to both dynorphin and rimorphin produced intense staining in the magnocellular cell bodies of the paraventricular nucleus, the supraoptic nucleus, and the accessory magnocellular nuclei, but gave

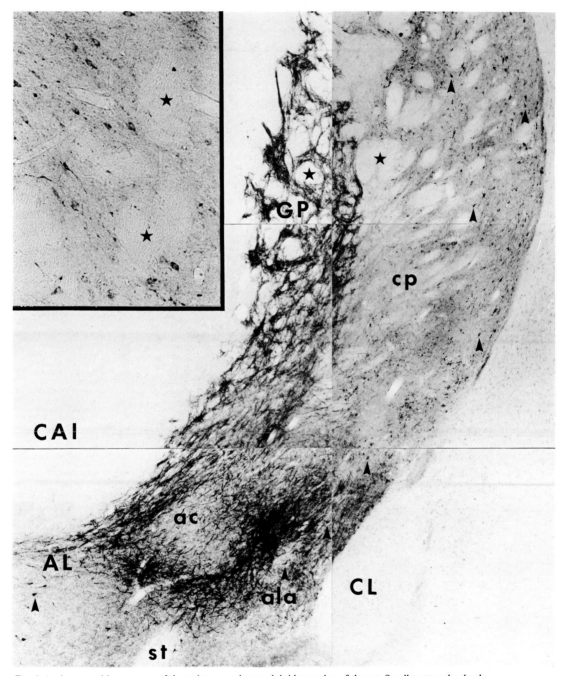

Fig. 6. A photographic montage of the striatum and amygdaloid complex of the rat. Small scattered enkepha-lin-containing cells are seen in the putamen and among immunoreactive neuronal processes in the amygdaloid complex (arrowheads). Dense accumulations of immunoreactive fibers are seen in the globus pallidus (GP), ansa lenticularis (AL), and the lateral and central amygdaloid nuclei. Both enkephalin-containing perikarya in the putamen and enkephalin-containing fibers in the globus pallidus are distributed in a mosaic-like pattern with round or oval areas that are devoid of staining (stars) interspersed between the stained areas. ac: nucleus amygdaloideus centralis; ala: nucleus amygdaloideus lateralis; cp: nucleus caudatus putamen; CAI: capsula interna; CL: claustrum; st: stria terminalis. Colchicine treated; Vibratome section; ENK-7 antiserum; silver intensification. × 64. *Inset:* High power view of enkephalin-containing perikarya in the putamen. × 168.

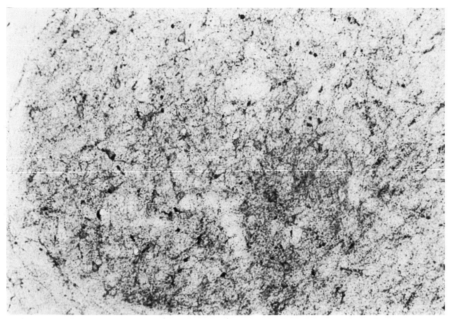

Fig. 7. Enkephalin-containing perikarya and neuronal processes in the central amygdaloid nucleus of the rat. Enkephalin-containing cell bodies are masked by numerous intensely stained immunoreactive neuronal processes. Colchicine treated; Vibratome section; ENK-7 antiserum; silver intensification. × 210.

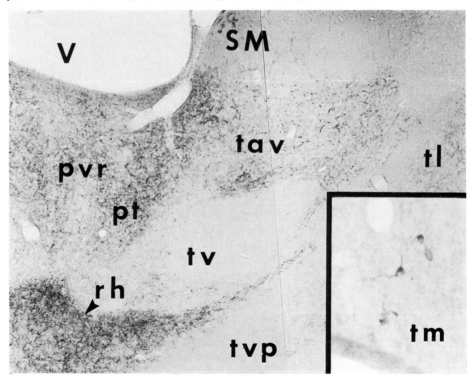

Fig. 8. Enkephalin-containing neuronal processes in the thalamus of the rat. Most of the immunoreactive fibers are in the paraventricular (pvr), paratenial (pt), rhomboid (rh), anterior medial (tm), and lateral (tl) thalamic nuclei. The ventral thalamic nucleus (tv) has very few immunoreactive neuronal processes. *Inset:* Multi-

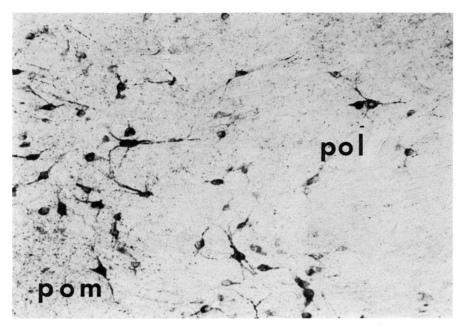

Fig. 9. Enkephalin-containing perikarya in the medial (pom) and lateral (pol) preoptic nuclei of the rat. The majority of the immunoreactive perikarya are in the medial preoptic nucleus with far fewer immunoreactive perikarya in the lateral preoptic nucleus. Colchicine treated; Vibratome section; ENK-7 antiserum; silver intensification. × 210.

very weak staining of some additional small cell bodies located between the paraventricular nucleus and the fornix (Fig. 10C). The dynorphin and rimorphin antisera also stained numerous thick varicose fiber profiles in the internal zone of the median eminence. Dual stainings with contrasting chromogens in the same paraffin or Vibratome sections revealed that the vast majority of the oxytocin-immunoreactive perikarya did not contain ENK-7-LI. Medium-size, often fusiform ENK-7-positive cell bodies were seen in a region immediately dorsal to the supraoptic nuclei. In the human hypothalamus, the ENK-7 antiserum stained perikarya in the lateral hypothalamus (including the perifornical area) and in the arcuate nucleus.

Scattered but still quite numerous and intensely stained cells were seen throughout the hypothalamus. Distinct groups of cells were present in the suprachiasmatic, ventromedial (Fig. 11), dorsomedial and arcuate nuclei (Fig. 12) and in the substantia innominata. Enkephalin-containing cells in the arcuate nucleus were small, round or fusiform, and few in number (Fig. 12B); in contrast, the arcuate nucleus contained numerous larger, stellate cell bodies which stained with the β-endorphin antiserum (Fig. 12A). These latter cell bodies extended beyond the boundaries of the arcuate nucleus throughout the medial-basal hypothalamus, and laterally along the base of the brain into the lateral hypothalamus. In the posterior hypothalamus, ENK-7-positive cell bodies were found in the caudal part of the arcuate nucleus and in the dorsomedial, premammillary (Fig. 13), and medial, lateral and posterior mammillary nuclei.

----

polar enkephalin-containing cell bodies in the medial thalamic nucleus. SM: stria medullaris thalami; tav: nucleus anterior ventralis; tvp: nucleus ventralis thalami, pars parvocellularis; V: third ventricle. Colchicine treated; Vibratome section; ENK-7 antiserum; silver intensification. × 80.

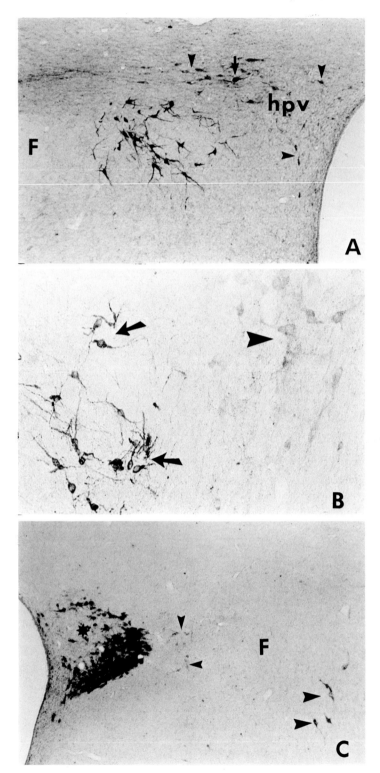

Immunoreactive neuronal processes were uniformly distributed throughout the entire hypothalamus and in the ventral amygdalofugal tract, coursing from the vicinity of the amygdala into the hypothalamic region. The external zone of the median eminence contained a moderate number of immunoreactive fibers and terminals; only a few fibers were seen in the internal zone. The infundibulum and the neural stalk also contained immunoreactive fibers. Although the supraoptic nucleus did not contain either ENK-7 or BAM-22P-immunoreactive cell bodies, many immunoreactive varicose fibers were observed among the unstained magnocellular perikarya within this nucleus. A moderate density of ENK-7 immunoreactive processes was seen in the external zone of both the human and the lamb median eminence, with a few scattered fibers in the internal zone.

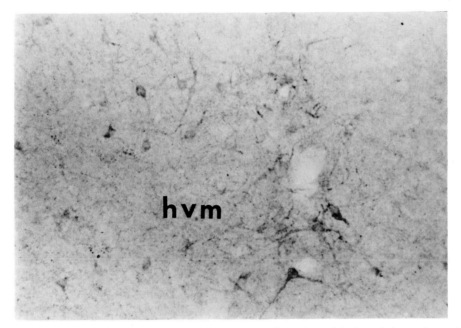

Fig. 11. Enkephalin-containing perikarya in the ventromedial nucleus of the hypothalamus (hvm) of the rat. Colchicine treated; Vibratome section; ENK-7 antiserum; unintensified. × 210.

Fig. 10. A. Enkephalin-containing perikarya in the perifornical region of the hypothalamus of the rat at the level of the paraventricular nucleus (hpv). Intensely stained perikarya are seen between the fornix (F) and the paraventricular nucleus. Small scattered perikarya are seen in the lateral and periventricular subdivisions (arrowheads) of the paraventricular nucleus (Swanson and Kuypers 1980). An intensely stained magnocellular perikaryon (arrow) is situated among the less intensely stained parvocellular perikarya (arrowheads). Colchicine treated; Vibratome section; ENK-7 antiserum; silver intensification. × 96. *B.* Enkephalin-containing perikarya in the paraventricular nucleus and the perifornical region of the rat. This high power illustration is from a Vibratome section adjacent to the section used for *A*. Two populations of immunoreactive perikarya can be seen. One group of cells located in the perifornical region (arrows) is stained far more intensely than the other group of cells located in the magnocellular subdivision of the posteromedial paraventricular nucleus (arrowhead). ENK-7 antiserum; silver intensification. × 168. *C.* Dynorphin-containing perikarya in the magnocellular subdivision of the posterior paraventricular nucleus of the rat. This illustration is from a Vibratome section adjacent to the section used for *B*. The dynorphin-containing perikarya are arranged in a circular pattern within the paraventricular nucleus (asterisk) and display few processes. Immunoreactive perikarya in the lateral hypothalamus (large arrowheads) are fusiform in shape. Small weakly stained perikarya can be seen between the paraventricular nucleus and the fornix (small arrowheads). Dynorphin antiserum; silver intensification. × 64.

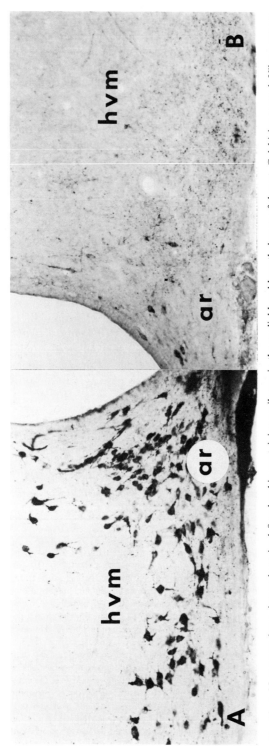

Fig. 12. A. Numerous, large, intensely stained β-endorphin-containing perikarya in the medial basal hypothalamus of the rat. Colchicine treated; Vibratome section; β-endorphin antiserum; silver intensification. × 190. *B.* Enkephalin-containing perikarya in the medial basal hypothalamus of the rat. Only a few small immunoreactive perikarya are seen in the arcuate nucleus (ar). hvm: nucleus ventromedialis. Colchicine treated; Vibratome section; ENK-7 antiserum; silver intensification. × 190.

Posterior pituitary

Fine beaded ENK-7 immunoreactive fibers were present in the posterior lobe (infundibular process). They were located close to the surface of the posterior lobe, along its anterior border, near the pars intermedia. In contrast, dynorphin antisera stained large (often several micrometers in diameter), round, oval or irregular structures throughout the extent of the posterior lobe.

Subthalamus and metathalamus

In the subthalamic region, immunoreactive cell bodies were observed in the entopeduncular nucleus, the zona incerta, the H_2 field of Forel, and in the ventral nucleus of the lateral geniculate body (Fig. 14).

Enkephalin-immunoreactive fibers were observed in all of the aforementioned regions and in the marginal layer of the medial geniculate body. A larger group of horizontally running fibers was seen just below, and a smaller bundle just above, the medial lemniscus.

3.4. MESENCEPHALON

Figure 15 is a photographic montage demonstrating a large area of the caudal mesencephalic tegmentum stained with the antiserum to ENK-7. Immunoreactive perikarya were present in the ventral portion of the periaqueductal gray (including cell bodies in the dorsal raphe, the dorsal tegmental nucleus, and the third and fifth cranial nerve motor nuclei), the cuneiform nucleus (Fig. 16), the ventromedial portion of the ventral teg-

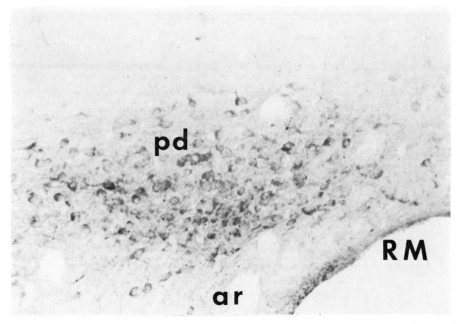

Fig. 13. Enkephalin-containing round perikarya with few processes in the dorsal premammillary nucleus (pd) of the rat. ar: arcuate nucleus; RM: recessus mamillaris. Colchicine treated; Vibratome section; ENK-7 antiserum; unintensified. × 210.

mental nucleus, the median raphe nuclei, the interpeduncular nucleus, and scattered in the midbrain reticular formation. This latter group of cells formed a continuous band between the crus cerebri and the central gray. Immunoreactive cell bodies were also seen in the substantia nigra, pars compacta (Fig. 17). In the tectum, the ENK-7 antiserum labeled cell bodies in the superior and inferior colliculi and in the dorsal part of the central gray. Enkephalin-containing neuronal processes were observed in all of the above regions. In addition, fibers were seen in the substantia nigra, pars reticularis. Dense accumulations of fibers were observed in the supramammillary and dorsal tegmental decussations.

3.5. METENCEPHALON

The antiserum to ENK-7 revealed a large number of cell bodies in the lateral and medial parabrachial nuclei. Immunoreactive cell bodies were also seen in the medial and lateral vestibular nuclei, in the central gray matter (most of them close to the midline in the dorsal raphe), and in the region of the dorsal tegmental nucleus. Enkephalin-containing cells were also demonstrated in the locus ceruleus, the subcerulear region, the nucleus raphes pontis, the ventral and dorsal cochlear nuclei, and the nucleus reticularis pontis. Scattered cells were also seen in the lateral trapezoid nucleus, in the nucleus of the lateral lemniscus, and throughout the reticular formation of the pons. In the cerebellum, medium-size, round perikarya were seen throughout the granular layer of the cortex, but were most numerous near the layer of the Purkinje cells (Fig. 18). Scattered small immunoreactive cells were also seen in the cerebellar prepositus and fastigial nuclei.

The distribution of ENK-7-immunoreactive neuronal processes in the pons was similar to that of the perikarya. Scattered fibers were observed in the central gray, extending in the midline ventrally into the region of the raphe nuclei and laterally into the mesencephalic trigeminal nucleus and the lateral aspect of the nucleus reticularis pontis. Larger concentrations of fibers were present in the dorsal and ventral parabrachial nuclei, and on both sides of the superior cerebellar peduncle. Ventrally, scattered fibers were seen in the lateral trapezoid nucleus, the facial and raphe nuclei, and the parvocellular and

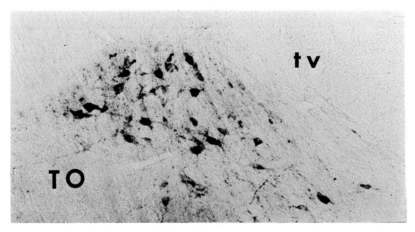

Fig. 14. Several enkephalin-containing perikarya in the ventral geniculate nucleus of the rat. TO: tractus opticus; tv: ventral thalamic nucleus. Colchicine treated; Vibratome section; ENK-7 antiserum; silver intensification. × 189.

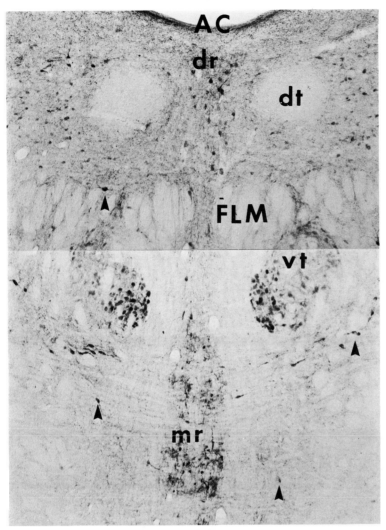

Fig. 15. A photographic montage of a large region of the caudal mesencephalic tegmentum of the rat. Enkephalin-containing perikarya are seen in the ventral portion of the periaqueductal gray including perikarya in the dorsal raphe (dr), the dorsal tegmental nucleus (dt) and the area just lateral to the nucleus, the ventromedial portion of the ventral nucleus (vt), and the median raphe nucleus (mr). Scattered immunoreactive perikarya are also seen in the reticular formation (arrowheads). AC: aqueductus cerebri; FLM: fasciculus longitudinalis medialis. Colchicine treated; Vibratome section; ENK-7 antiserum; silver intensification. × 72.

gigantocellular reticular nuclei. In the cerebellum, immunoreactive fibers were seen occasionally in the molecular layer, the white matter, and the cerebellar peduncles.

3.6. MYELENCEPHALON

Figure 19 is a photographic montage demonstrating the distribution of ENK-7-LI in a coronal section at the mid-level of the medulla oblongata. Immunoreactive perikarya are present in the prepositus hypoglossal nucleus, the reticular formation, the nucleus

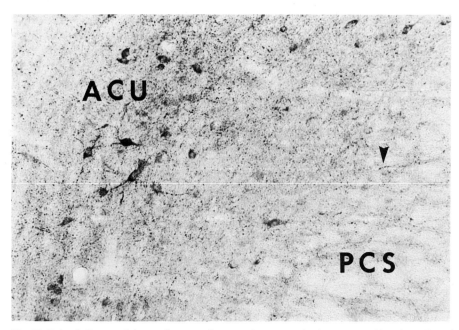

Fig. 16. Enkephalin-containing perikarya and neuronal processes in the area cuneiformis (ACU) of the rat. Multipolar immunoreactive cells are seen lateral to the pedunculus cerebellaris superior (PCS). The peduncle contained scattered enkephalin-immunoreactive neuronal processes (arrowhead). Colchicine treated; Vibratome section; ENK-7 antiserum; silver intensification. × 210.

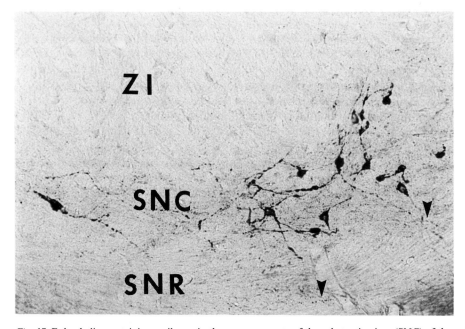

Fig. 17. Enkephalin-containing perikarya in the pars compacta of the substantia nigra (SNC) of the rat. Scattered immunoreactive fibers can be seen in the pars reticularis of the substantia nigra (SNR) in the same section (arrowheads). ZI: zona incerta. Colchicine treated; Vibratome section; ENK-7 antiserum; silver intensification. × 210.

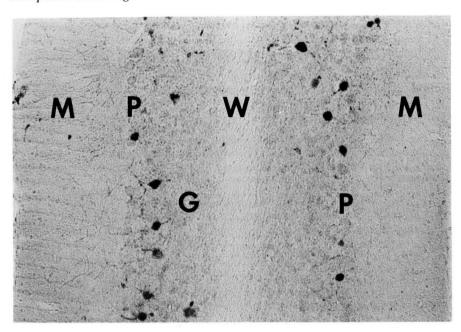

Fig. 18. Enkephalin-containing presumptive Golgi cells in the cerebellar cortex of the rat. The medium-size, round perikarya are located in the granular layer (G) of the cortex with the greatest concentration of immuno-reactive perikarya occurring near the border with the Purkinje cell layer (P). Only a few immunoreactive fibers can be seen in the molecular layer (M). W: white matter. Colchicine treated; Vibratome section; ENK-7 antiserum; silver intensification. × 210.

raphes obscurus, the nucleus raphes magnus, the nucleus raphes pallidus, the lateral part of the inferior olive, the paragigantocellular nucleus, the nucleus ambiguus, the nucleus of the solitary tract (see also Fig. 20), and scattered throughout the reticular formation. In addition, ENK-7-immunoreactive cell bodies were seen in the lateral reticular nucleus (Fig. 21), the area postrema, the commissural nucleus, and the substantia gelatinosa as well as the deeper laminae of the spinal trigeminal nucleus (Fig. 22A,B).

Most regions of the medulla contained a continuous network of immunoreactive fibers (Fig. 19). A denser plexus of fibers was seen in the vicinity of the fourth ventricle, in the region of the prepositus hypoglossal nucleus, and the solitary nucleus and tract, extending laterally, within the medial and spinal vestibular nuclei, into the peripheral regions of the spinal trigeminal nucleus (Fig. 22). The spinal trigeminal complex contained ENK-7-LI throughout its rostro-caudal extent. The density of the immunoreactivity increased continuously in a rostro-caudal direction, with by far the densest accumulation in the caudal third of the medulla. The fiber network also extended throughout the lateral region of the parvocellular reticular nucleus, the lateral part of the gigantocellular reticular nucleus, the dorsal reticular nucleus, the nucleus ambiguus, the inferior olivary complex, and the raphe nuclei. Fibers were also observed in the midline area of the reticular formation coursing from the region of the periaqueductal gray to more ventral structures.

3.7. SPINAL CORD

Immunoreactive perikarya were found in the marginal zone (lamina I) and the substan-

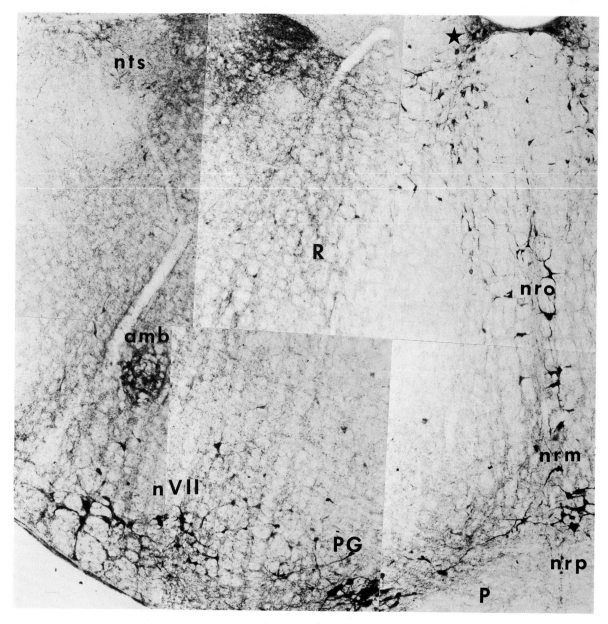

Fig. 19. A photographic montage of the middle level of the medulla oblongata of the rat. Enkephalin-containing perikarya are present in the prepositus hypoglossal nucleus (star), the nucleus raphes obscurus (nro), the nucleus raphes magnus (nrm), the nucleus raphes pallidus (nrp), the paragigantocellular nucleus of the medulla (PG), among the motoneurons in the facial nucleus (nVII), the nucleus ambiguus (amb), the nucleus of the solitary tract (nts), and scattered throughout the reticular formation (R). A continuous network of immunoreactive fibers extends throughout the medulla. P: pyramis. Colchicine treated; Vibratome section; Leu-ENK antiserum; silver intensification. × 60.

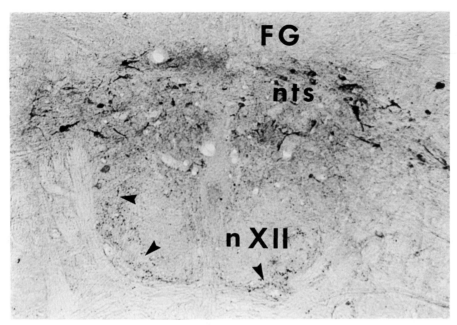

Fig. 20. Enkephalin-containing perikarya in the nucleus of the solitary tract (nts) of the rat. Small, fusiform or multipolar cells are extended in the horizontal plane within the borders of the nucleus. Immunoreactive processes are seen in the nucleus of the hypoglossal nerve (nXII) in the same section (arrowheads). FG: fasciculus gracilis. Colchicine treated; Vibratome section; ENK-7 antiserum; silver intensification. × 210.

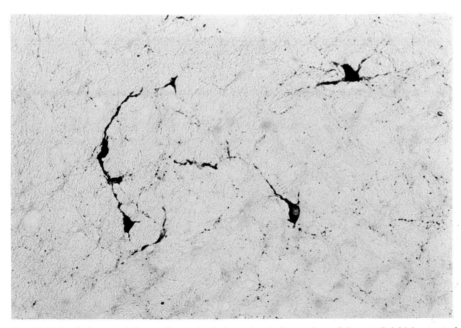

Fig. 21. Enkephalin-containing perikarya in the lateral reticular nucleus of the rat. Colchicine treated; Vibratome section; ENK-7 antiserum; silver intensification. × 210.

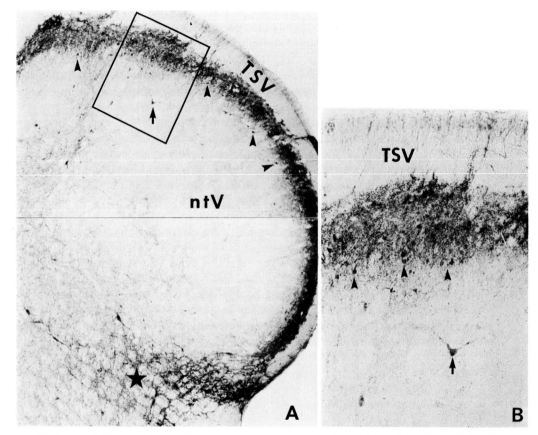

Fig. 22. A. Enkephalin-containing perikarya and neuronal processes in the caudal medulla of the rat. Small enkephalin-containing perikarya are seen in the substantia gelatinosa (arrowheads) and deeper laminae (arrow) of the nucleus tractus spinalis nervi trigemini (ntV). Large immunoreactive perikarya are seen in the lateral reticular nucleus in the same section (star). A dense plexus of immunoreactive fibers is seen in the substantia gelatinosa and a less dense plexus of immunoreactive fibers covers the lateral reticular nucleus. TSV: tractus spinalis nervi trigemini. Colchicine treated; Vibratome section; ENK-7 antiserum; silver intensification. × 56. *B.* A high power view of the rectangular area outlined in *A.* Small enkephalin-containing perikarya in the substantia gelatinosa (arrowheads) and a large cell body in deeper lamina of the spinal trigeminal nucleus (arrows). TSV: tractus spinalis nervi trigemini. × 147.

tia gelatinosa (lamina II) of the dorsal horn of the spinal gray matter. Most cell bodies were located in the deeper region of the substantia gelatinosa. Scattered cells were also seen in the medial portion of lamina IV, in laminae V–VII, and in lamina X, around the central canal (Fig. 23). A dense accumulation of immunoreactive fibers was present in the marginal zone (Fig. 24) and continued ventrally along the lateral edge of the dorsal horn to the level of lamina V. (This fiber distribution is particularly clear in Fig. 26.) Another area with dense fiber staining was the dorsomedial portion of the lateral funiculus (Fig. 24). Fibers in laminae VIII and IX were located close to motoneurons, suggesting the possibility of axosomatic synaptic contacts (Fig. 25). The cervical, thoracic and lumbar segments of the spinal cord appeared to contain comparable levels of ENK-7-LI, with the exception of the intermediolateral column which, when present, always contained a heavy concentration of immunoreactive fibers. A diminished number of immunoreactive cell bodies and fibers was seen in the sacral cord, especially in its

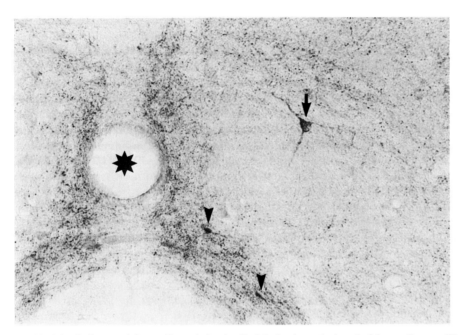

Fig. 23. Enkephalin-containing perikarya in lamina X of the lumbar spinal cord of the rat. Two small immuno-reactive perikarya are seen in the medial surface of the dorsal horn (arrowheads). A larger cell body (arrow) is seen in lamina X near the central canal (asterisk). Colchicine treated; Vibratome section; ENK-7 antiserum; silver intensification. × 210.

caudal portions. The distribution of ENK-7-immunoreactive fibers in the sheep spinal cord (Fig. 26) was similar to the distribution seen in the rat.

Leu-ENK-LI was seen at all levels of the chicken spinal cord. A dense accumulation of immunoreactive processes was seen in the superficial laminae of the dorsal horn (Fig. 27A) and surrounding the central canal (Fig. 27B). A dense accumulation of immuno-reactive processes was also seen in the ventral horn at the brachial and lumbar levels. It is noteworthy that immunoreactive perikarya in the chicken spinal cord were readily demonstrated without pretreatment with colchicine (Fig. 27C; cf. Bayon et al. 1980a; De Lanerolle et al. 1981).

3.8. COMPARISON OF THE DISTRIBUTION OF PROENKEPHALIN-, PRODYNORPHIN- AND PROOPIOMELANOCORTIN-DERIVED PEPTIDES

The antiserum to β-endorphin stained a population of neurons in the medial-basal hy-pothalamic region that was clearly distinct from neurons stained with the antiserum to ENK-7 (or to Leu-ENK; cf. Finley et al. 1981a). The existence of separate populations of proenkephalin and PPOMC-containing perikarya is already obvious on the basis of the morphological features of the two cell populations (Fig. 11A and B): the cells stained with the anti-β-endorphin serum are numerous, large, stellate or polygonal, with fairly long processes, and occupy a large area within the medial-basal hypothalamus, extend-ing beyond the boundaries of the arcuate nucleus, especially laterally along the basal surface; the cells stained with the anti-ENK-7 serum are much fewer, small, round cells with short or no visible processes, and are found (in this region) only within the arcuate

303

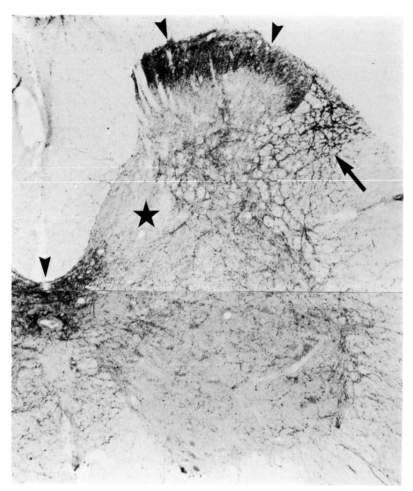

Fig. 24. Enkephalin-containing neuronal processes in the rostral lumbar spinal cord of the rat. Dense accumulations of immunoreactive fibers (arrowheads) are seen in laminae I and II and in lamina X posterior to the central canal. A dense network of enkephalin-containing fibers can also be seen in the dorsomedial portion of the lateral funiculus (arrow). Scattered fibers are seen throughout the gray matter and in the lateral and anterior funiculi of the white matter. Clarke's column is almost completely devoid of immunoreactive fibers (star). Colchicine treated; Vibratome section; ENK-7 antiserum; silver intensification. × 72.

nucleus. The projecting axons of β-endorphin neurons appear as long, thick varicose processes, while those of enkephalin neurons are fine, thin, beaded fibers which are difficult to trace continuously for longer distances (cf. Finley et al. 1981b). In addition to these morphological differences, dual immunocytochemical stainings, demonstrating two antigens in the same section, have also established that the antigens recognized by these two antisera reside in two distinct neuronal populations. In similar dual-stained preparations we observed close apposition between β-endorphin-containing cell bodies and enkephalin-containing fibers in the arcuate nucleus, suggesting axosomatic synaptic contacts. In addition, in 'single-stained' sections, β-endorphin-immunoreactive fibers appeared to surround unstained medium-size perikarya in the arcuate nucleus (cf. Kiss and Williams 1983).

The situation is somewhat less clear with regard to the comparative distribution of

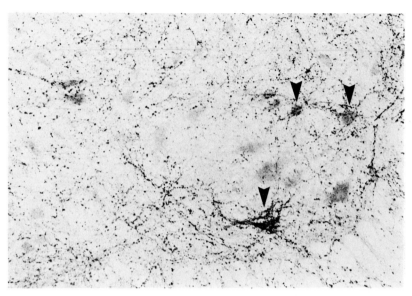

Fig. 25. Motoneurons in lamina IX of the lumbar ventral horn of the rat surrounded by enkephalin-containing neuronal processes (arrowheads). Colchichine treated; Vibratome section; ENK-7 antiserum; silver intensification. × 189.

ENK-7 versus dynorphin immunoreactive perikarya, although our results seem to suggest that the antigens recognized by these antisera are also localized in separate neuronal systems. However, our current studies on the comparative distribution of these two systems in the forebrain have been restricted to the hypothalamus (Fig. 9) and the posterior pituitary; furthermore, our observations (see 3.2. and 4.3.) are in apparent conflict with some of the results reported from other laboratories. The antiserum to dynorphin stained intensely many large cell bodies in the paraventricular, supraoptic and accessory magnocellular nuclei, and large (often several μm in diameter) fibers and terminals throughout the posterior pituitary. In contrast, the antiserum to ENK-7 did not stain any cells in the supraoptic nucleus, stained very weakly a few magnocellular cell bodies only in the lateral periphery of the paraventricular nucleus, and only scattered small beaded fibers around the periphery of the posterior pituitary.

The highest density of both ENK-7 and dynorphin immunoreactive fibers in the lumbar spinal cord of the cat was in the superficial laminae of the dorsal horn (cf. Przewlocki et al. 1983) and the area surrounding the central canal (lamina X). The highest density of both ENK-7 and dynorphin immunoreactive fibers in the caudal medulla of the cat was in the superficial laminae of the nucleus caudalis (cf. Maderdrut et al. 1982). Both ENK-7- and dynorphin-containing perikarya were concentrated in the superficial laminae of the dorsal horn, the lateral portion of laminae IV-V and the area surrounding the central canal of the cat lumbar spinal cord. Both ENK-7- and dynorphin-containing perikarya were concentrated in the superficial laminae of nucleus caudalis and the lateral reticular nucleus of the cat caudal medulla. Although both ENK-7- and dynorphin-containing perikarya had a similar morphology and a similar distribution in both the lumbar spinal cord and the caudal medulla, separate populations of perikarya appeared to be labeled by the two antisera.

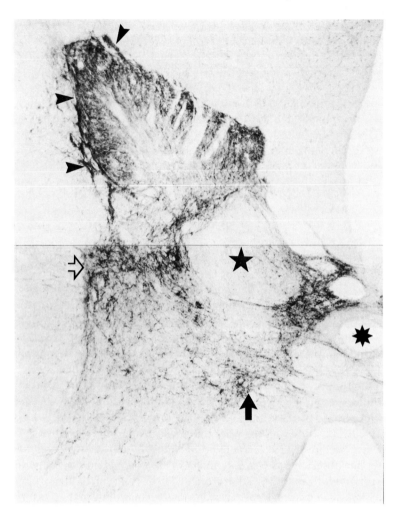

Fig. 26. Enkephalin-containing neuronal processes in the rostral lumbar spinal cord of the lamb. The gross distribution of immunoreactive fibers is similar to the distribution in the rat (see Fig. 25). Dense accumulations of immunoreactive processes are seen in laminae I and II which continue ventrally along the lateral edge of the dorsal horn (arrowheads), in lamina X around the central canal (asterisk), and in the lateral edge of lamina V (open arrow). Scattered fibers are seen in the anterior column with a higher concentration of fibers in the medial portion bordering lamina VIII (arrow). Clarke's column is almost completely devoid of immunoreactive fibers (star). Normal lamb; Vibratome section; ENK-7 antiserum; silver intensification. × 67.

Fig. 27. A. Enkephalin-containing perikarya and neuronal processes in the lumbar spinal cord of a young chicken. Dense accumulations of immunoreactive fibers are seen in laminae I and II, in lamina X around the central canal (star), and in the dorsal intermediate gray matter. PF: posterior funiculus. Normal chicken; Vibratome section; Leu-ENK antiserum; silver intensification. × 80. *B.* High power view of immunoreactive processes in lamina X from the same Vibratome section as *A.* The midline is indicated by a star. × 210. *C.* High power view of the rectangular area outlined in *A.* A dense aggregation of enkephalin-containing perikarya is indicated by arrows. A few weakly stained perikarya are seen in the medial region of the dorsal horn (large arrowhead). The lateral margin of the dorsal horn is surrounded by small arrowheads. LF: lateral funiculus. × 210.

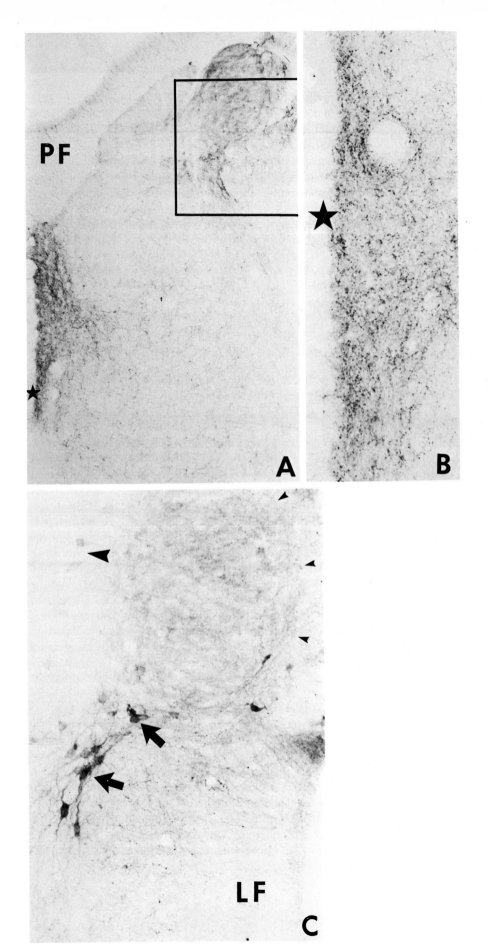

PF

A

B

C

LF

4. DISCUSSION

4.1. COMPARISON WITH EARLIER IMMUNOCYTOCHEMICAL STUDIES

The distribution of enkephalin in the mammalian CNS has been studied extensively by both RIA and immunocytochemical methods. Since the pertinent RIA studies are reviewed by Palkovits and Brownstein (Chapter 1), only immunocytochemical studies will be considered in depth in this chapter.

The general distribution of immunocytochemically identifiable enkephalin in the mammalian CNS has been described and/or mapped by Elde et al. (1976), Hökfelt et al. (1977a), Simantov et al. (1977), Watson et al. (1977), Johansson et al. (1978), Sar et al. (1978), Uhl et al. (1979), Wamsley et al. (1980), Finley et al. (1981a), Stengaard-Pedersen and Larsson (1981), Weber et al. (1981a), Haber and Elde (1982a,b), Khachaturian et al. (1983a,b), Williams and Dockray (1983a), and Bouras et al. (1984). In addition, numerous publications have dealt with the detailed immunocytochemical or experimental-immunocytochemical analysis of enkephalin-containing perikarya, fibers and terminals in selected areas of the mammalian CNS, such as the cerebral cortex (McGinty et al. 1984), the olfactory bulb and tubercle (Bogan et al. 1982; Davis et al. 1982), the retina (Altschuler et al. 1982), the amygdala (Wray et al. 1981; Roberts et al. 1982; Wray and Hoffman 1983; Veening et al. 1984), the septum and the stria terminalis (Uhl et al. 1978; Sakanaka et al. 1982; Beauvillain et al. 1983; Stengaard-Pedersen and Larsson 1983; Woodhams et al. 1983; Gall and Moore 1984), the hippocampus (Gall et al. 1981; Fitzpatrick and Johnson 1981; Hoffman et al. 1983; McGinty et al. 1983; Gall et al. 1984; Roberts et al. 1984; Tielen et al. 1984), the striatum (Pickel et al. 1980a; Graybiel et al. 1981; Haber and Elde 1981; DiFiglia et al. 1982; Williams and Dockray 1982; Somogyi et al. 1982; Haber and Nauta 1983; Bouyer et al. 1984), the hypothalamus and the pituitary (Weber et al. 1978; Tramu and Leonardelli 1979; Beauvillain et al. 1980, 1982, 1984; Rossier et al. 1980b; Tramu et al. 1981; Romagnano et al. 1982; Van Leeuwen et al. 1983; DiFiglia and Aronin 1984), the midbrain and the pons (Pickel et al. 1979, 1980b; Moss et al. 1981; Hunt and Lovick 1982; Léger et al. 1983; Moss and Basbaum 1983; Moss et al. 1983; Graybiel et al. 1984; Kapadia and De Lanerolle 1984; Willard et al. 1984), the cerebellum (Schulman et al. 1981), and the lower brainstem and spinal cord (Hökfelt et al. 1977b; Uhl et al. 1979; Del Fiacco and Cuello 1980; Glazer and Basbaum 1980; Seybold and Elde 1980; Armstrong et al. 1981; Aronin et al. 1981; Gibson et al. 1981; Glazer and Basbaum 1981; Haynes and Zakarian 1981; Hunt et al. 1981b; Jancsó et al. 1981; LaMotte and De Lanerolle 1981; Bennett et al. 1982; Hancock 1982; Holets and Elde 1982; De Lanerolle and LaMotte 1982; Ruda 1982; Sumal et al. 1982; Glazer and Basbaum 1983; Maley et al. 1983; Romagnano and Hamill 1983; Ruda et al. 1983; Charnay et al. 1984; Kalia et al. 1984).

The enkephalinergic system characterized in these publications is one of the most extensive (if not *the* most extensive) defined peptidergic system in the mammalian CNS. Given the vast complexity of this system and the initial uncertainties about the nature of the antigen or antigens recognized by conventional antisera against the enkephalin pentapeptides, it may be considered surprising and rather fortunate that the overall distribution of the 'true' enkephalinergic system, i.e., the system that expresses the preproenkephalin gene, corresponds so well to that outlined in many of the earlier studies. Nevertheless, the results of these earlier studies differ in several specific points from the distribution of ENK-7-LI presented in this chapter. Undoubtedly, part of these differences are due to the unique specificity of our antiserum and our Vibratome-silver intensification technology (see 2.4.). However, a small number of differences remain unexplained even after consideration of these and other technical factors.

Our present data are in nearly total agreement with those reported by Williams and Dockray (1983a) who used the same ENK-7 antiserum (L150) that was used in the present study. The minor differences that do exist are most likely due to either the higher dose of colchicine that we used (100 μg *vs* 60 μg), the amplification in the intensity of the PAP reaction product provided by the silver intensification step (see 2.4.), or other as yet unrecognized methodological factors. Thus, in contrast to the results of Williams and Dockray (1983a) and in agreement with several other studies, we were able to demonstrate scattered enkephalin-containing neurons in the neocortex (cf. Finley et al. 1981a; Khachaturian et al. 1983a; McGinty 1983; McGinty et al. 1984), the granular layer of the olfactory bulb (Fig. 2; cf. Finley et al. 1981a; Bogan et al. 1982; Davis et al. 1982; Khachaturian et al. 1983a), and the substantia nigra, pars compacta (Fig. 17). In addition to presumptive Golgi cells in the cerebellum, we also observed scattered ENK-7-immunoreactive fibers in the cerebellar cortex and white matter (Fig. 18; see also Schulman et al. 1981).

In contrast to the earlier observations of Sar et al. (1978), Micevych and Elde (1980) and Finley et al. (1981a) made with Leu-ENK antisera, the ENK-7 antiserum did not label either magnocellular perikarya in the hypothalamic paraventricular and supraoptic nuclei or a substantial number of coarse varicose fibers in the internal zone of the median eminence. Present evidence indicates that these cells and nerve fibers express the preprodynorphin rather than the preproenkephalin gene (see 4.3.).

Recently, Khachaturian et al. (1983a,b) studied the comparative distribution of Leu-ENK and BAM 22P in the rat brain, the former being based on results obtained with affinity-purified antibodies selected to recognize the free carboxyl terminus of Leu-ENK. Although this resulted in a much improved localization, it must be kept in mind that such an antiserum is incapable of distinguishing between Leu-ENK derived from proenkephalin and Leu-ENK derived from prodynorphin (cf. Udenfriend and Kilpatrick 1983; Zamir et al. 1984; see 1.). Although our present results are largely in agreement with those of Khachaturian et al. (1983a,b), some differences are apparent. In the neocortex (particularly in the deeper layers), the ENK-7 antiserum did not label as extensive a population of cells as seen by Khachaturian et al. (1983a). The ENK-7 antiserum also stained a substantially smaller number of fibers in the hippocampus than the Leu-ENK antiserum used by these authors (see also Williams and Dockray 1983a). On the other hand, the ENK-7 antiserum in our study did label perikarya in several thalamic nuclei, including the paratenial nucleus, and in the granule layer of the cerebellum (Williams and Dockray 1983a; Fig. 18). In further contrast to the results of Khachaturian et al. (1983b), the ENK-7 antiserum stained both perikarya and nerve processes in the dorsal cochlear nucleus. Enkephalin-LI has been localized in several auditory centers such as the dorsal cochlear nucleus, the nucleus of the lateral lemniscus and the medial geniculate body (Johansson et al. 1978; Sar et al. 1978; Uhl et al. 1979; Finley et al. 1981a; Willard et al. 1984). Our results agree with those of Khachaturian et al. (1983a,b) in that the BAM 22P antiserum, although it results in a less intense staining of both perikarya and processes, labels essentially the same neurons as other antisera specific for the products of the preproenkephalin gene. Finally, in contrast to several earlier studies and in agreement with Khachaturian et al. (1983b), we have now recognized ENK-7-immunoreactive perikarya in the motor trigeminal, mesencephalic trigeminal, oculomotor and prepositus hypoglossal nuclei. On the basis of the smaller size of the labeled perikarya and the absence of any detectable enkephalin-containing processes leaving these nuclei, we assume that these cells are interneurons (see also Boone and Aldes 1984). However, further studies are needed to establish the precise nature and role of these enkephalin-containing neurons.

In view of the possibility that Leu-ENK antisera may recognize both proenkephalin- and prodynorphin-derived peptides, it is important to consider the topographical relationship of the neuronal systems that contain these two peptide families (the separate nature of the neurons containing the third family of opiate peptides, the PPOMC family, is well established; see 3.8. and 4.5.). The known products of the prodynorphin gene (dynorphin, rimorphin, dynorphin-8, α-neo-endorphin and β-neo-endorphin) are widely distributed in the CNS and are mutually co-localized within the same neurons (Weber et al. 1981b; Watson et al. 1983). For the most part, the general areas where prodynorphin-derived peptides are found also contain proenkephalin-derived peptides. Such areas include the neocortex, neostriatum, amygdala, hippocampus, periaqueductal gray, several brainstem nuclei (e.g., substantia nigra, locus ceruleus and raphe nuclei), and the spinal cord (for details, see Botticelli et al. 1981; Vincent et al. 1982; Watson et al. 1982; Weber and Barchas 1983; Zamir et al. 1983b). However, closer examination of many of these regions revealed that, with very few exceptions (e.g., the nucleus of the solitary tract: Mulcahy et al. 1983), the two peptide families exist in two distinct neuronal populations (Fig. 10; cf. Vincent et al. 1982; Watson et al. 1982; McGinty and Bloom 1983). In the hippocampus, an extensive system of 'enkephalinergic' cells and fibers has been described (Sar et al. 1978; Fitzpatrick and Johnson 1981; Gall et al. 1981; Finley et al. 1981a). Our current results as well as those of Williams and Dockray (1983a) indicate that only a relatively small part of this system contains proenkephalin-derived peptides. The remaining part, the granule cell-mossy fiber system, appears to contain prodynorphin-derived peptides (McGinty et al. 1983; Weber and Barchas 1983). Similar conclusions can be reached with regard to the hypothalamic magnocellular nuclei (see Fig. 10 and 4.3.), and the arcuate nucleus (cf. McGinty and Bloom 1983). The functional significance of the apparent close association between two (and in some places even three) peptidergic systems, containing different families of endogenous opiate peptides, remains to be elucidated.

4.2. ENKEPHALIN-CONTAINING PATHWAYS

It is apparent from this and from many previous studies that enkephalin-containing neurons constitute a heterogeneous population. The majority appear to be interneurons located in strategic positions to modulate the function of numerous projection pathways and neuronal centers throughout the CNS. However, since a substantial number of enkephalin-containing fibers are found within well-known neuroanatomical pathways, some enkephalinergic neurons are likely to function as projection neurons. The results of the present study and of the study of Williams and Dockray (1983a) confirm that many of the traditional neuroanatomical pathways indeed contain proenkephalin-derived peptides. However, all previous experimental work on 'enkephalinergic' pathways has been carried out with antisera that could potentially cross-react with peptides derived from prodynorphin (cf. Zamir et al. 1984).

Since enkephalin-containing perikarya are apparently absent from the globus pallidus, the exceptionally dense network of enkephalin-immunoreactive fibers and terminals, first recognized by Elde et al. (1976), is likely to be derived from extra-pallidal sources. Experimental studies combining immunocytochemistry with stereotaxic lesions, knife cuts, retrogradely transported markers or neurotoxin administration have established that most of the enkephalin-containing fibers and terminals in the globus pallidus are derived from the neostriatum (Cuello and Paxinos 1978; Brann and Emson 1980; Correa et al. 1981; Del Fiacco et al. 1982). However, the neostriatum may not be the only source of enkephalin-containing afferents to the globus pallidus. Palkovits et al. (1981) noted a significant decrease in the Met-ENK concentration in the globus pallidus after transection of the ansa lenticularis, which carries hypothalamic (from the ventro-medial nucleus) and mesencephalic (from the substantia nigra) afferents to the globus pallidus. Both the ventromedial nucleus and the substantia nigra were found to contain ENK-7-immunoreactive perikarya (see 3.3. and 3.4.), confirming earlier reports based on antisera to Met-ENK or Leu-ENK (e.g., Watson et al. 1977; Johansson et al. 1978; Uhl et al. 1979). Cuello (1983) suggested that neostriatal enkephalin-containing fibers also project to the substantia nigra. However, Zamir et al. (1984) presented experimental evidence to indicate that the high levels of Leu-ENK found in the substantia nigra, although supplied by striatonigral axons, are generated from prodynorphin. The ultra-structural analyses carried out by Pickel et al. (1980a) and Somogyi et al. (1982) are consistent with the concept of a major striatopallidal enkephalin-containing pathway.

Both the nuclear regions and the pathways of the limbic system are rich in enkephalin-like immunoreactivity (see 3.). This includes the olfactory bulb and tubercle, the piri-form, entorhinal and cingulate cortex, the nucleus accumbens, the amygdaloid complex, the lateral septal nucleus, the hippocampus, several thalamic and hypothalamic nuclei, the epithalamus, and parts of the midbrain tegmentum and central gray. Some of the pathways that interconnect these nuclear regions and contain enkephalin-immunoreactive fibers are the entorhinal-hippocampal (perforant) pathway (Gall et al. 1981), the septohypothalamic tract, the ventral amygdalofugal tract, the stria terminalis, and the medial forebrain bundle (see 3.3.). Based on a combined stereotaxic lesioning and immunocytochemical approach, Uhl et al. (1978) were the first to suggest that the stria termi-nalis contained enkephalin-immunoreactive fibers of amygdaloid origin and that these fibers terminated 'almost exclusively' in the bed nucleus of the stria terminalis. Palkovits et al. (1981) approached the same question by measuring the radioimmunoassayable Met-ENK content in several brain regions after stereotaxic transection of the stria ter-minalis at the level where it enters the diencephalon, dorsal to the bed nucleus. They observed a substantial decrease of Met-ENK concentration in the central amygdaloid and suprachiasmatic nuclei, indicating that (1) amygdaloid afferents may also be present in the stria terminalis, and (2) part of the stria terminalis projection to the hypothalamus (to the suprachiasmatic region) may be enkephalinergic. However, the authors point out that their findings may be explained by several alternative mechanisms, such as denerva-tion effects or postoperative ischemia. McLean et al. (1983) found that electrolytic le-sions of the stria terminalis were followed by a significant reduction of the enkephalin content of the habenula, demonstrated by a radioimmunohistochemical method. They suggested that the enkephalin-containing cells of the bed nucleus (Finley et al. 1981a; see 3.2.) may be the source of an enkephalinergic projection to the habenula. This path-way may be part of a proposed multisynaptic opioid peptide-containing limbic pathway extending from the olfactory bulb to the interpeduncular nucleus (cf. Herkenham and Pert 1980).

Our results (see 3.2.) are largely consistent with the view of Stengaard-Pedersen and Larsson (1983) that most of the previously described 'enkephalin-containing perikarya' in the lateral septum are in fact unlabeled neurons surrounded by an exceptionally dense enkephalin-immunoreactive fiber and terminal network. The origin of these enkephalin-containing fibers is most likely the anterior-ventrolateral or perifornical hypothalamic area (Sakanaka et al. 1982; Poulain et al. 1984). In addition, our results (see 3.2.) also indicate that a moderate number of enkephalin-containing perikarya do exist in the medial regions of the lateral septal nucleus (cf. Gall and Moore 1984). Enkephalin-containing fibers were described in the fornix of the rat, monkey and man (Roberts et al. 1983).

The hypothalamus is the source of several pathways that are known to include enkephalin-containing fibers. One of the most important projections, that from the magnocellular nuclei to the posterior pituitary, appears from recent studies to contain predominantly prodynorphin-derived peptides (see 3.3., 4.1. and 4.3.), although the possibility of the existence of proenkephalin-derived peptides in these neurons cannot be discounted (cf. Martin and Voigt 1981; Martin et al. 1983; Vanderhaegen et al. 1983; Van Leeuwen et al. 1983). In fact, BAM 22P (Baird et al. 1982), ENK-7 and ENK-8 (Panula et al. 1983) have all been detected in posterior pituitary extracts. When studied by immunocytochemistry, these proenkephalin-derived peptides are localized in fine varicose fibers located at the periphery of the neurohypophysis (Rossier et al. 1979; Panula et al. 1983; see 3.3.). The origin of these fibers is unknown; their most likely source, at least in the rat, is the parvocellular enkephalin-containing cell population of the paraventricular nucleus (cf. Sawchenko and Swanson 1982; Williams and Dockray 1983a; see 3.3.). This cell population, located primarily in caudal parts of the parvocellular division of the paraventricular nucleus, has also been shown to send long projections to autonomic centers of the brainstem (e.g., dorsal vagal complex) and to the spinal cord (Sawchenko and Swanson 1982). Whether the projections to the brainstem or spinal cord and to the neurohypophysis both arise from a single population of neurons, or whether separate or overlapping populations project to these two major target sites, is not known (cf. Swanson and Kuypers 1980).

Numerous immunocytochemical studies have identified enkephalin-containing fibers and terminals in the external zone of the median eminence, indicating that opioid peptides may be released there in the vicinity of the primary capillary loops of the hypothalamo-hypophyseal portal system (e.g., Hökfelt et al. 1977a; Tramu and Leonardelli 1979; Sar et al. 1978; Beauvillain et al. 1980; Micevych and Elde 1980; Wamsley et al. 1980; Finley et al. 1981a). The perikaryal origin of these enkephalin-containing projections has not been studied systematically. The finding that the administration of the neurotoxin monosodium glutamate to neonatal mice results in nearly total disappearance of enkephalin-containing processes from the median eminence by 60 days of age (Romagnano et al. 1982) suggests that most of these fibers are derived from the medial-basal hypothalamus. However, toxic damage to other brain areas and to fibers passing through the medial-basal hypothalamic area are difficult to exclude in such studies. In a recent report, Hökfelt et al. (1983) suggest that a population of the parvocellular paraventricular neurons that project to the external zone of the median eminence contain immunoreactive enkephalin, PHI-27 and CRF (see also 4.3.). As pointed out by the authors, confirmation of this co-localization within the median eminence (which would implicitly confirm the paraventricular origin of these enkephalin-containing fibers) has to await the application of high-resolution co-localization techniques such as dual immunocytochemical staining at the electron microscopic level.

Several enkephalin-containing pathways and functionally coherent multisynaptic circuits have been recognized in the brainstem and the spinal cord. The presence of immunoreactive enkephalin in the centers and pathways of the vestibulocochlear system has already been discussed (4.1.). In addition, Fex and Altschuler (1981) have demonstrated that some of the cells of the lateral superior olivary complex that project to the cochlea contain Met-ENK (see 4.3.). Brainstem nuclei associated with the regulation of respiratory functions (the parabrachial nuclei, the solitary tract, and the nucleus ambiguus) are also rich in enkephalin-containing cells or processes (Finley et al. 1981a; see 3.5. and 3.6.). Enkephalin-LI has been detected in cranial motor nuclei and thus is likely to play a role in the regulation of motor systems such as the masticatory system (motor nucleus of the trigeminal nerve), eye movements (oculomotor and prepositus hypoglossal nuclei), or facial movements (motor nucleus of the facial nerve) (Khachaturian et al. 1983b; see 3.4.–3.6.). These nuclei appear either to contain enkephalin-immunoreactive interneurons (see 4.1.) or to be innervated by extrinsic enkephalin-containing fibers, probably from the surrounding reticular formation. The reticulo-facial enkephalin-containing pathway identified by Senba and Tohyama (1983) in an experimental immunocytochemical study is an example of such a short pathway. The involvement of enkephalin in the coordination of motor activities is also suggested by its apparent presence in cerebellar mossy fibers in several classes of vertebrates (Schulman et al. 1981). Reports of enkephalin-LI in autonomic preganglionic motoneurons are discussed in Section 4.3.

One of the most extensively studied functional systems which contains abundant enkephalin-immunoreactive perikarya, fibers and terminals is the system involved in pain and analgesia (e.g., Hökfelt et al. 1977b, 1979; Beitz 1982; Ruda 1982; Ruda et al. 1983). The periaqueductal gray, the nucleus raphes magnus, the marginal layer and the substantia gelatinosa of the spinal trigeminal nucleus and the dorsal horn of the spinal cord are all remarkably rich in enkephalin-immunoreactive neuronal structures. Most of these appear to be interneurons (cf. Hökfelt et al. 1977b; Bennett et al. 1982; Maderdrut et al. 1982; Ruda 1982) or propriospinal neurons (Pickel et al. 1983). However, a component of the descending bulbospinal pathways (cf. Basbaum and Fields 1978) has also been demonstrated to be enkephalinergic (Hökfelt et al. 1979; Bowker et al. 1981; Pickel et al. 1983). The perikarya of origin of these fibers appear to be located near the inferior olive, 'presumably in the pars α of the gigantocellular reticular nucleus' (Hökfelt et al. 1979; see Fig. 19). Enkephalin-LI has also been demonstrated in shorter pathways within the brainstem that project to the nucleus raphes magnus (Beitz 1982).

In addition to its occurrence in somatosensory pathways, enkephalin-like immunoreactivity (together with other neuropeptides) has been described in a multisynaptic ascending visceral and taste pathway (Mantyh and Hunt 1984). The system examined by these authors extended from the nodose ganglion to the neocortex via the solitary nucleus, the parabrachial nucleus and the ventral posterior medial nucleus of the thalamus. Enkephalin-LI was present at all central levels examined, and double-labeling with immunocytochemistry and retrograde tracing techniques has demonstrated that some of the peptide-containing neurons in fact form ascending projections between the relay nuclei studied. This work thus provides direct evidence that enkephalin-LI occurs in projection neurons in the rat CNS.

Palmer et al. (1982) detected several enkephalin-containing fiber bundles with immunocytochemistry in the embryonic rat brain that have not been detected with immunocytochemistry in the adult rat brain. These included an apparent pathway between the ventral hypothalamus and the globus pallidus, the mammillothalamic tract, the fasciculus retroflexus, and an apparent mesencephalic projection to (or from) the habenular nuclei. Corroborating evidence for the first pathway has come from experiments on adult rats using stereotaxic lesions and RIA (Palkovits et al. 1981; see above). An enkephalin-containing pathway that is detectable only in the perinatal rat hippocampus has been described by Gall et al. (1984). Enkephalin-containing perikarya and nerve terminals occur in the appropriate locations in the adult rat brain to form all of these transiently detectable pathways (see 3.2., 3.3. and 3.4.). These embryonic and/or perinatal enkephalin-containing pathways may be present (but not detectable) in the adult rat brain. Lowered concentrations or alterations in the processing of proenkephalin in adult axons, interference with the immunohistochemical reactions by myelination or dilution of early appearing enkephalin-containing axons by later appearing non-enkephalin-containing axons could result in spurious negative results in the adult. Since transient anatomical connections (e.g., Innocenti 1981), transient gene expression (e.g., Haynes et al. 1982) and naturally occurring cell death (e.g., Oppenheim et al. 1982) are apparently common developmental processes, it is possible that either these connections no longer exist in the adult or the cells of origin express a different 'transmitter' phenotype in the adult. Therefore, although the transient detection with immunohistochemistry of an enkephalin-containing pathway in the embryonic or perinatal CNS cannot be taken as evidence for the existence of the same pathway in the adult CNS, it should be considered as an important clue to potential enkephalin-containing pathways in the adult which can then be verified by experimental hodological methods.

4.3. CO-LOCALIZATION OF ENKEPHALINS WITH OTHER PUTATIVE TRANSMITTERS

A variety of double-labeling techniques have provided evidence for the localization of enkephalin-LI in neurons within the CNS that also contain either acetylcholine, serotonin, norepinephrine, or GABA. Similar techniques have also provided evidence for the localization of enkephalin-LI in neurons within the CNS that also contain one or more other peptide transmitter candidates.

The preganglionic motoneurons that innervate the mammalian sympathetic (Dalsgaard et al. 1982, 1983) and parasympathetic (Glazer and Basbaum 1980; Kawatani et al. 1983) ganglia as well as those that innervate the avian ciliary ganglion (Erichsen et al. 1981, 1982a,b) have been reported to contain enkephalin-LI. Enkephalin-LI has also been localized in acetylcholinesterase-positive cells in the guinea pig lateral superior olivary complex that project to the cochlea (Altschuler et al. 1983). The evidence for the co-localization of acetylcholine and enkephalin in the same neuron in all these studies is indirect; confirmation of this co-localization can only be attained with antibodies against choline acetyltransferase and a double-labeling technique.

Many of the early systematic studies on the distribution of enkephalin pentapeptide-LI in the mammalian brain described enkephalin-positive perikarya in several of the 'serotonergic' raphe nuclei (e.g., Sar et al. 1978; Uhl et al. 1979; Finley et al. 1981a). Glazer et al. (1981) used antisera against both Leu-ENK and serotonin to double-label perikarya in the same sections through the midbrain nucleus raphes dorsalis and the medullary nucleus paragigantocellularis of the cat. The double-labeled perikarya in both raphe nuclei appeared to be a subpopulation of the serotonin-positive perikarya that had a specific morphology and anatomical distribution within the raphe nuclei. Some perikarya in both raphe nuclei appeared to contain only Leu-ENK-LI. Perikarya containing both serotonin- and substance P-like immunoreactivity (SP-LI) have been described in the nucleus raphes magnus and the nucleus reticularis gigantocellularis (pars α) of the rat (Hökfelt et al. 1978). Enkephalin-containing perikarya have also been described in the same nuclei (Finley et al. 1981a; see 3.5.). Whether enkephalin- and SP-LI occur in identical, separate or overlapping populations of perikarya in the raphe nuclei is unknown (cf. Johansson et al. 1981).

Perikarya containing Leu-ENK-LI in the 'noradrenergic' locus ceruleus and adjacent nuclei were first described in the rat (Finley et al. 1981a) and the lizard (Naik et al. 1981).

314

Antisera against both ENK-7 and BAM 22P also stain perikarya in the locus ceruleus and adjacent nuclei (Khachaturian et al. 1983b; see 3.5.). Charnay et al. (1982) and Léger et al. (1983) used antisera against both enkephalin pentapeptides and tyrosine hydroxylase to double-label the same perikarya in adjacent 8 μm sections through the dorsolateral pontine tegmentum of the cat. Most of the cells containing tyrosine hydroxylase-LI in the locus ceruleus, the subcerulear region, and the medial and lateral parabrachial nuclei also contained enkephalin pentapeptide-LI. Although enkephalin-containing chromaffin cells in the bovine adrenal medulla are predominantly (and perhaps exclusively) epinephrine-containing (as opposed to norepinephrine-containing) chromaffin cells (Livett et al. 1982; Roisin et al. 1983), enkephalins appear to be co-localized with norepinephrine in perikarya in the rostral pons. Whether the 'adrenergic' perikarya in the medulla (Hökfelt et al. 1974) contain both epinephrine and proenkephalin-derived peptides needs to be determined. Perikarya containing both tyrosine hydroxylase- and avian pancreatic polypeptide (APP)-LI have been described in the locus ceruleus of the rat (Hunt et al. 1981a). Whether enkephalin- and APP-LI occur in identical, separate or overlapping populations of noradrenergic perikarya in the locus ceruleus of the rat is unknown (*vide supra*).

Some of the early studies on the distribution of enkephalin pentapeptide-LI in the mammalian brain described Leu-ENK-positive perikarya in the granular layer of the cerebellum with the morphology and distribution previously ascribed to Golgi cells (Sar et al. 1978; Finley et al. 1981; Schulman et al. 1981). The number of Golgi cells containing Leu-ENK-LI comprised a large percentage of the total number of Golgi cells (Finley et al. 1981a; Schulman et al. 1981). Schulman et al. (1981) also reported that Golgi cells in the cerebellum of two species of teleosts contained Leu-ENK-LI. The Golgi cells of the rat cerebellum also contain ENK-7-LI (see 3.5.; Williams and Dockray 1983a). The cerebellar Golgi cells have traditionally been assumed to employ GABA as a transmitter (Eccles et al. 1967). A large percentage of the total number of Golgi cells in the mammalian cerebellum are stained by antisera against the enzyme that synthesizes GABA, L-glutamic acid decarboxylase (Saito et al. 1974; Oertel et al. 1981). These experiments suggest that GABA and enkephalins are co-localized in some cerebellar Golgi cells in mammals. Confirmation of this co-localization with antibodies against both L-glutamic acid decarboxylase (or GABA) and ENK-7, and a double-labeling technique would be useful. Aronin et al. (1984) used antisera against both enkephalin pentapeptides and L-glutamic acid decarboxylase to double-label the same perikarya in adjacent 4 μm sections through the caudate nucleus of the rat. One-half of the perikarya containing enkephalin pentapeptide-LI were estimated to also contain L-glutamic acid decarboxylase-LI using a correction factor derived by staining adjacent sections with the same antiserum. Aronin et al. (1984) suggested that the cells containing only proenkephalin-derived peptides have different striatofugal projections from the cells containing both proenkephalin-derived peptides and GABA.

Some of the early studies on the distribution of enkephalin pentapeptide-LI in the mammalian brain described enkephalin-positive magnocellular neurons in the supraoptic and paraventricular nuclei (e.g., Sar et al. 1978; Micevych and Elde 1980; Finley et al. 1981a) and enkephalin-positive terminals in the pars nervosa of the pituitary (Rossier et al. 1980b; Micevych and Elde 1980). The current concensus appears to be that vasopressin-containing magnocellular neurons in the supraoptic and paraventricular nuclei also contain prodynorphin-derived peptides (see 3.3.; Watson et al. 1982; Weber et al. 1982; Weber and Barchas 1983; Whitnall et al. 1983) and that most of the enkephalin-LI previously described in the hypothalamo-neurohypophyseal pathway is the result of cross-reactivity of the enkephalin pentapeptide antisera with one or more prodynor-phin-derived peptides (see 1. and 4.1.). Vanderhaeghen et al. (1983) used an antiserum against the N-terminal fragment of bovine adrenal proenkephalin which does not con-tain the sequences of either Leu- or Met-ENK (synenkephalin, see Fig. 1) to demon-strate proenkephalin-containing magnocellular neurons in the dorsal part of the bovine supraoptic nucleus and the lateral part of the bovine paraventricular nucleus. Almost all of the synenkephalin-positive perikarya could also be stained in adjacent 5 μm sec-tions by using a specific antiserum against oxytocin; magnocellular neurons visualized by using a specific antiserum against vasopressin were never stained in adjacent sections by using the synenkephalin antiserum (Vanderhaeghen et al. 1983). However, RIA re-sults after discrete bilateral radiofrequency lesions of the supraoptic nuclei have indicat-ed that these nuclei do not contribute to the Met-ENK content of the rat hypothalamus (Millan et al. 1983). Magnocellular neurons containing either ENK-7- or BAM-22P-LI occur only in the lateral part of the paraventricular nucleus in the rat (see 3.3. and 4.1.; Williams and Dockray 1983a). Whether the enkephalin-containing magnocellular neu-rons in the lateral part of the paraventricular nucleus in the rat also contain oxytocin-LI is unknown. Martin and Voigt (1981) and Martin et al. (1983) reported that the distribu-tion of Met-ENK- and oxytocin-LI fibers and terminals in adjacent 0.5 μm sections through the pars nervosa of the rat pituitary was identical. Other investigators have found that the distribution of enkephalin- and oxytocin-containing fibers in the neu-rohypophysis overlaps extensively; however, the morphology and distribution of enke-phalin-containing fibers in the neurohypophyses of the cat (Micevych and Elde 1980) and the rat (see 3.3.) clearly differs from that of the oxytocin-containing fibers (cf. Van Leeuwen et al. 1983).

Hunt et al. (1981a) used antisera against both Met-ENK and APP to double-label perikarya in the intermediolateral column of the sacral spinal cord of the rat. The major-ity of these cells contained both Met-ENK- and APP-LI. Since these spinal visceral mo-toneurons are cholinergic, the coexistence of proenkephalin, APP and acetylcholine in the same neuron seems probable (cf. Glazer and Basbaum 1980). A substantial number of perikarya in the intermediolateral column of the sacral spinal cord of the rat also contain somatostatin-LI (Dalsgaard et al. 1981). Whether perikarya in the sacral inter-mediolateral column contain both proenkephalin and prosomatostatin has not been de-termined. Erichsen et al. (1982a) used antisera against both Leu-ENK and SP to double-label perikarya in several areas of the pigeon CNS, including the avian homologue of the Edinger-Westphal nucleus (accessory oculomotor nucleus). Although many peri-karya contained both Leu-ENK- and SP-LI, some perikarya were immunoreactive for only Leu-ENK or SP. Since these cranial visceral motoneurons are cholinergic (e.g., Landmesser and Pilar 1970), the co-existence of proenkephalin, SP and acetylcholine in the same neuron seems probable. Whether perikarya in the accessory oculomotor nu-cleus also contain APP-LI is unknown (cf. Hunt et al. 1981a).

Hökfelt et al. (1983) used antisera against Leu-ENK and PHI-27 (Tatemoto and Mutt 1981) and the restaining technique of Tramu et al. (1978) to double-label perikarya in the parvocellular subdivision of the paraventricular nucleus of the rat. Some of these double-labeled cells could also be stained by using an antiserum against CRF. Some perikarya in the parvocellular paraventricular nucleus were immunoreactive for only Leu-ENK or PHI-27 (Hökfelt et al. 1983). Only a small fraction of the perikarya in the parvocellular paraventricular nucleus containing CRF-LI also contained ENK-7-LI (see 3.3.).

Tramu et al. (1981) used antisera against both enkephalin pentapeptides and somato-

316

statin and a restaining technique (Tramu et al. 1978) to double-label presumptive nerve terminals in the external zone of the guinea pig median eminence. Most of the somatostatin-immunoreactive nerve terminals surrounding the capillary loops of the portal vessels also appeared to contain enkephalin pentapeptide-LI (see 4.2.). Beauvillain et al. (1984) used both adjacent ultrathin sections and double-labeling of the same ultrathin section with gold particles and DAB polymers for the ultrastructural localization of somatostatin and enkephalin pentapeptides in the external zone of the guinea pig median eminence. All somatostatin-immunoreactive nerve terminals also contained enkephalin pentapeptide-LI granules. More than 70% of the granules containing somatostatin-LI also contained enkephalin-LI. Prodynorphin-derived peptides are concentrated in the *internal* zone of the rat median eminence (see 3.3. *Hypothalamus*). The co-localization of prosomatostatin- and proenkephalin-derived peptides in the same granules is presumptive evidence for the co-release of both peptides (cf. Wilson et al. 1982). However, the results reported by Beauvillain et al. (1984) appear to be in conflict with the observations that most of the somatostatin-containing fibers in the rat median eminence originate from perikarya in the periventricular hypothalamus (e.g., Makara et al. 1983) and that most of the somatostatin-containing perikarya in the periventricular hypothalamus do not contain proenkephalin-derived peptides (e.g., Tramu et al. 1981; see 3.3. *Hypothalamus* and 4.2.).

The co-localization of two or more transmitter candidates within a cell does not constitute, *a priori*, evidence for either co-synthesis within or co-release (*vide supra*) from that cell. However, the increase in the number and intensity of enkephalin-immunoreactive perikarya following blockade of axoplasmic transport (see 3.1.) strongly suggests synthesis in the labeled cell. The recently developed technique of 'hybridization histochemistry' (e.g., Gee et al. 1983) should be able to discriminate between sites of peptide synthesis and sites of secondary peptide uptake and storage. The co-localization of enkephalins with other putative transmitters in some neurons should not be taken to imply that all enkephalin-containing neurons must contain one or more other putative transmitters.

4.4. RELATIONSHIP OF ENKEPHALIN-CONTAINING PATHWAYS TO THE LOCALIZATION OF OPIATE RECEPTORS AND BIOSYNTHETIC ENZYMES

The discovery of opiate receptors in the mammalian brain (Pert and Snyder 1973; Simon et al. 1973; Terenius 1973), unlike the history of most other putative neurotransmitter receptors, preceded and provided the final impetus for the discovery of endogenous opioid ligands in the mammalian brain (Hughes et al. 1975). Consequently, the earliest systematic studies on the distribution of opiate receptors in the mammalian brain and spinal cord with either radioligand binding (e.g., Hiller et al. 1973; Kuhar et al. 1973) or 'dry-mount' autoradiographic (e.g., Pert et al. 1975; Atweh and Kuhar 1977) techniques were completed before the first studies on the immunohistochemical distribution of enkephalin pentapeptides in the mammalian CNS (see 1.).

The initial systematic studies on the immunohistochemical distribution of enkephalin pentapeptide-LI in the brain and spinal cord (e.g., Elde et al. 1976; Simantov et al. 1977) revealed that there was a positive correlation between the density of opiate receptors and the density of enkephalin-containing neuronal processes in different regions. Many areas of the mammalian CNS that had previously been reported to contain high densities of opiate receptors, e.g., laminae I and II of the spinal cord, the nucleus of the solitary tract and the parabrachial nuclei were revealed to also have high densities of enkephalin-containing neuronal processes. However, some regions, previously reported to have high densities of opiate receptors, e.g., the cerebral cortex and the basolateral amygdaloid nucleus, revealed only a few immunoreactive neuronal processes; other regions that had previously been reported to have very low densities op opiate receptors, e.g., lamina X of the spinal cord, had high densities of enkephalin pentapeptide-LI.

Some of these apparent discrepancies have been shown by subsequent studies (e.g., Sar et al. 1978; Finley et al. 1981a) to be the result of technical defects. Some of the reported cases of high densities of enkephalin pentapeptide-LI occurring in regions with low densities of opiate receptors may result from staining of fibers *en passant*. However, other discrepancies still remain unresolved. The early immunohistochemical mapping studies were completed before the isolation and sequencing of prodynorphin-derived peptides (see 1.) and before the recognition that opiate receptors in the mammalian brain and spinal cord are heterogeneous (e.g., Chang et al. 1979; Chang and Cuatrecasas 1981). Opiate receptors in the CNS can be subdivided into μ-, δ-, and κ-receptors (Chang and Cuatrecasas 1981; Chang et al. 1981; Kosterlitz et al. 1981; Pfeiffer and Herz 1981; Wood 1982; Snyder 1984). Although there is a substantial variation in the regional distribution of the three subclasses of opiate receptors (e.g., Chang et al. 1979; Chang et al. 1981), some regions, e.g., the cerebral cortex (Goodman and Snyder 1982; Lewis et al. 1983; see 3.2. and 4.1.), contain all three subclasses of opiate receptors. The smaller proenkephalin-derived peptides bind preferentially to δ-receptors (Lord et al. 1977; Chang and Cuatrecasas 1981) while the peptides that are derived from prodynorphin all appear to bind preferentially to κ-receptors (James et al. 1982; Corbett et al. 1983). Some of the larger proenkephalin-derived peptides (e.g., peptide E and BAM 22P) bind with a similar high affinity to both μ- and κ-receptors (Quirion and Weiss 1983). β-Endorphin appears to bind with a similar high affinity to both μ- and δ-receptors (Lord et al. 1977).

The earliest studies on the autoradiographic localization of opiate receptors in the CNS (e.g., Pert et al. 1975; Atweh and Kuhar 1977) used in vivo injections of radioligands and tissue processing procedures that were similar to the methods traditionally used to localize steroid receptors in the brain (e.g., Pfaff 1968). Young and Kuhar (1979) introduced an in vitro method that permitted far better characterization of the binding properties of opiate receptors and with further modifications potentially higher sensitivity and spatial resolution (e.g., Herkenham and Pert 1982). This in vitro autoradiographic methodology should permit the distribution of proenkephalin-, prodynorphin- and PPOMC-containing neuronal processes to be correlated with the distribution of specific subclasses of opiate receptors at a high level of spatial resolution.

The distribution of perikarya and nerve terminals that store classical neurotransmitters such as acetylcholine, norepinephrine and GABA have been mapped with a high degree of specificity by immunohistochemistry using antisera directed against their biosynthetic enzymes, choline acetyltransferase (e.g., Houser et al. 1983), dopamine-β-hydroxylase (e.g., Hartman et al. 1972) and glutamic acid decarboxylase (e.g., Saito et al. 1974), respectively. Whether the enzymes responsible for the proteolytic processing of proenkephalin in the mammalian brain and spinal cord are restricted to enkephalin-containing neurons or even to very limited classes of neurons is unknown.

Fricker and Snyder (1982) purified an enzyme from bovine adrenal chromaffin granules that converts Met-ENK and Leu-ENK hexapeptides containing either arginine or lysine at their carboxyl terminus to Met- and Leu-ENK without any further degradation. This enzyme, enkephalin convertase, had a different subcellular distribution and a different sensitivity to inhibitors from carboxypeptidase B. Enkephalin convertase, a 50,000-dalton glycoprotein, was purified to apparent homogeneity from lysates of the adrenal gland, brain and pituitary gland (Fricker et al. 1982). A number of peripheral tissues had negligible enzyme activity. The gross regional distribution of enkephalin convertase activity in the brain varied over a 10-fold range and resembled the regional distribution of enkephalin pentapeptides (Fricker and Snyder 1982; Fricker et al. 1982). However, enkephalin convertase activity was 20-fold higher in the anterior than the posterior lobes of the pituitary, possibly reflecting a role in the processing of other peptide hormones. A membrane-bound form of enkephalin convertase having a higher molecular weight (52,500) but an identical pH optimum (pH 5.4–5.8) and substrate and inhibitor specificity has been purified to apparent homogeneity from bovine pituitary gland and adrenal chromaffin granule membranes (Supattapone et al. 1984). An enzyme(s) with a similar pH optimum and similar substrate and inhibitor specificity to enkephalin convertase has been purified from the secretory granules of the anterior, intermediate and neural lobes of the rat pituitary (Hook and Loh 1984). This enzyme also cleaves basic amino acid residues from the carboxyl terminus of putative PPOMC and provasopressin 'intermediates'. Immunohistochemical studies using polyclonal antisera against enkephalin convertase are currently in progress (S.H. Snyder, personal communication). It will be interesting to know whether antisera against enkephalin convertase discriminate between proenkephalin- and prodynorphin-containing neurons.

Lindberg et al. (1982) purified an enzyme 200-fold from bovine adrenal chromaffin granules that converted peptide F to free Met-ENK (see Fig. 1). The partially purified enzyme had a different pH optimum (7.5–8.0) and a different sensitivity to inhibitors from lysosomal cathepsins. The enzyme appeared to be serine protease with a molecular weight of 20–30,000 daltons. The protease did not convert β-lipotropin to lower molecular weight peptides (Lindberg et al. 1982). Troy and Musacchio (1982) and Evangelista et al. (1982) purified an enzyme(s) from bovine adrenal chromaffin granules that cleaved peptide E and BAM 12P, respectively, at the paired basic amino acid residues (see Fig. 1). The partially purified enzyme(s) had a pH optimum of 5–6 and appeared to be a thiol protease. The subcellular distribution of the enzyme activity was completely separate from the distribution of the lysosomal marker, acid phosphatase (Troy and Mussacchio 1982). Since proenkephalin is processed in the chromaffin granules (Fleminger et al. 1983) and the intragranular pH of secretory granules is acid (pH 5–6), the physiological significance of the enzyme activity described by Lindberg et al. (1982) is questionable. It would be valuable to determine whether serine protease inhibitors such as diisopropyl fluorophosphate inhibit the processing of proenkephalin in situ. Whether either the serine or the thiol protease occur in the mammalian CNS is unknown.

4.5. DISTRIBUTION OF ENKEPHALIN-CONTAINING NEURONS IN SUBMAMMALIAN VERTEBRATES

Opiate receptors are present in the brains of representatives of all major classes of submammalian vertebrates (Pert et al. 1974). However, evidence for the presence of a precursor protein that is structurally homologous to mammalian preproenkephalin in either the adrenal gland or the brain of submammalian vertebrates is, with one exception (Herbert et al. 1983), fragmentary. Although several preliminary studies detected enkephalin-like substances in the brain of submammalian vertebrates with either radioreceptor assays (e.g., Simantov et al. 1976) or RIA (e.g., Bayon et al. 1980a), these substances were not characterized with biochemical methods. Humbert et al. (1979) detected free Met-ENK in extracts of the retina of 11-day chicken embryos by using HPLC and RIA. Free Met-ENK, Leu-ENK and ENK-7 have been detected in extracts of the brain of 10-day post-hatch chickens (S. Udenfriend, personal communication) and in extracts of the spinal cord and the adrenal medulla of 18-day chicken embryos (Maderdrut et al. 1984) by using HPLC and RIA. Free Met-ENK, Leu-ENK and ENK-7 have also been detected in extracts of the brain of the toad, *Bufo marinus*, by HPLC, sequential proteolytic digestion and RIA (Kilpatrick et al. 1983a). Kilpatrick et al. (1983a) could not detect either free ENK-8 or high molecular weight ENK-8-LI in toad brain extracts using a specific RIA (*vide infra*).

Although a number of investigators have localized enkephalin-containing perikarya and/or nerve terminals in the brain and spinal cord of representatives of all major classes of submammalian vertebrates, all of these studies, with two exceptions (Reiner 1983; Maderdrut et al. 1984), used antisera with unknown degrees of cross-reactivity with pro-dynorphin-derived peptides (see 1.). The distribution of Leu-ENK-LI in the brain and spinal cord of the lizard (Naik et al. 1981), the crocodile (Brauth 1984) and the turtle (Eldred and Karten 1982; Reiner 1983) was similar to the distribution reported for mammals. However, unlike their distribution in mammals, enkephalin-containing peri-karya were rare in the dorsal ventricular ridge (homologue of the mammalian isocortex) and were numerous in the large-celled division of the ventrolateral area of the telen-cephalon (homologue of the mammalian globus pallidus) of the crocodile (Brauth 1984). Finally, some nuclei containing Leu-ENK-positive perikarya, e.g., the dorsal nucleus of the posterior commissure (homologue of the avian lateral spiriform nucleus) of several species of reptiles (Brauth and Rainer 1982), have no concensus mammalian homo-logues. Reiner (1983) also used antisera against BAM 22P and dynorphin. The distribu-tion of BAM-22P-LI in the turtle was similar to the distribution of Leu-ENK-LI and different from the distribution of dynorphin-LI. A substantial subpopulation of ama-crine cells in the retina of the turtle contain enkephalin pentapeptide-LI (Eldred and Karten 1982, 1983; cf. Altschuler et al. 1982). Although pre-treatment with colchicine is required to reveal Leu-ENK-LI in most perikarya in the mammalian brain (Hökfelt et al. 1977a; Finley et al. 1981a; cf. Bayon et al. 1980b), an extensive distribution of enkephalin-containing perikarya was seen in the brain of untreated reptiles (Naik et al. 1981; Brauth 1984). However, pre-treatment with colchicine dramatically increased the number of labeled perikarya in some areas of the crocodilian telencephalon (Brauth 1984). Dores (1982) detected β-endorphin-LI and α-melanocyte-stimulating hormone-LI in the *pars intermedia* of the lizard.

The distribution of enkephalin pentapeptide-LI in the brain of the chicken (De Lane-rolle et al. 1981) and the pigeon (Bayon et al. 1980a; Erichsen et al. 1982a; Reiner et al. 1982b) apparently differs substantially from the distribution reported for mammals. However, many areas (e.g., the anterior hypothalamus and the substantia gelatinosa of the caudal medulla) showed a distribution of enkephalin-containing perikarya and nerve terminals (Bayon et al. 1980a; De Lanerolle et al. 1981) that was similar to the distribu-tion reported for mammals. The mammalian homologues of some avian nuclei contain-ing enkephalin pentapeptide-positive perikarya, e.g., the lateral spiriform nucleus (Davis et al. 1980; Reiner et al. 1982a), are a subject of controversy. The distribution of perika-rya and nerve terminals containing enkephalin pentapeptide-LI in the pigeon brain was distinct from the distribution of perikarya and nerve terminals containing β-endorphin-LI (Bayon et al. 1980a). The distribution of β-endorphin-LI in the pigeon brain was sim-ilar to the distribution reported for mammals. A substantial subpopulation of amacrine cells in the retina of the pigeon and the chicken contain enkephalin pentapeptide-LI (Brecha et al. 1979; *vide supra*). The distribution of enkephalin pentapeptide-LI (see Fig. 27 and 3.7.; LaValley and Ho 1983), ENK-7-LI (Maderdrut et al. 1984) and BAM-22P-LI (I. Merchenthaler and J.L. Maderdrut, unpublished observations) in the spinal cord of the chicken showed both similarities to and differences from the distribution reported for mammals.

Herbert et al. (1983) provided partial information on the structure of the preproenkephalin gene from the toad, *Xenopus laevis*. The deduced amphibian proenkephalin precursor contains five copies of Met-ENK (and no copies of Leu-ENK), a single copy of ENK-7 at the carboxyl terminus, and a single copy of the octapeptide. (Met^5)-enkephalin-Arg^6-Gly^7-Tyr^8, in the same relative position as ENK-8 in the mammalian proenkephalin precursor; each internal opioid peptide sequence is flanked by pairs of basic amino acids (cf. Fig. 1)*.

Enkephalin pentapeptide-LI has been detected in the brain (Doerr-Schott et al. 1981; Kuljis and Karten 1982, 1983; Kuljis et al. 1984), spinal cord (Lorez and Kemali 1981) and the adrenal gland (Leboulenger et al. 1983) of the frog. The distribution of Met-ENK-LI in the brain of the frog was distinct from the distribution of α- and β-endorphin-LI (Doerr-Schott et al. 1981). The antisera against α- and β-endorphin labeled the same two populations of perikarya: one group of perikarya were located in the *pars ventralis* of the *tuber cinereum* and the second group of perikarya were located in the preoptic nucleus. Whether the α- and β-endorphin-containing perikarya in the preoptic nucleus are either vasotocin- or mesotocin-containing perikarya is unknown. A dynorphin-like opioid peptide has been isolated from the brain and the neurointermediate lobe of the toad pituitary (Cone 1982; Cone and Goldstein 1982b). A PPOMC-like prohormone has been identified in the neurointermediate lobe of the frog pituitary (Loh 1979; Martens et al. 1982).

The distribution of enkephalin pentapeptide-LI in the brain of the lamprey shows some similarities to the distribution reported for mammals (Gold and Finger 1981). Schulman et al. (1981) reported that Golgi cells and mossy fibers in the cerebellum of two species of teleosts contained Leu-ENK-LI. Separate anatomical systems of Met-ENK- and α-endorphin-containing neurons appear to also occur in the brain of teleosts (Follénius and Dubois 1979). Reaves and Hayward (1979a) described separate populations of vasotocin-, isotocin- and Met-ENK-containing perikarya in the preoptic nucleus of the goldfish. Whether the Met-ENK-containing perikarya described by Reaves and Hayward (1979a,b) are proenkephalin- or prodynorphin-containing perikarya is unknown (see 4.3.). Dores et al. (1984) were unable to stain the meta-adenohypophysis (homologue of the mammalian *pars intermedia*) of the lamprey using several antisera against either β-endorphin or β-lipotropin. However, antisera against either the amino terminus of adrenocorticotropin or enkephalin pentapeptides stained all of the cells in the meta-adenohypophysis.

Leung and Stefano (1984) and Stefano and Leung (1984) have provided suggestive evidence for the existence of a proenkephalin-like precursor in the pedal ganglion of a mollusc, *Mytilus edulis*.

Several homologous nuclear groups and several homologous pathways appear to contain enkephalin-immunoreactive perikarya and fibers, respectively, in the CNS of repre-

---

*The apparent discrepancy between the results reported by Kilpatrick et al. (1983a) and Herbert et al. (1983) could be due to either the different amphibian species investigated or the processing of prodynorphin in the amphibian brain (*vide infra*) to yield free Leu-ENK.

sentatives of all major classes of vertebrates. The current data (albeit fragmentary) are consistent with the hypothesis that opioid peptide synthesis is parcelled between three separate genes in all tetrapods. Whether the existence of three separate genes that code for the synthesis of opioid peptides is a characteristic of all vertebrates needs to be determined (cf. Comb et al. 1983).

5. CONCLUSIONS

The evidence (albeit indirect) for a preproenkephalin-like precursor in the brain and spinal cord of mammals that is structurally similar (or identical) to the preproenkephalin polyhormone in the adrenal medulla of the same species is compelling. However, the proteolytic processing of this precursor polyhormone in the mammalian CNS and adrenal medulla appears to differ substantially.

Although the distribution of perikarya and neuronal processes in the mammalian brain and spinal cord that contain proenkephalin-derived peptides was overestimated by earlier investigators who used antisera against enkephalin pentapeptides, the number of major errors that were made in the gross distribution of enkephalin-containing perikarya and neuronal processes is surprisingly low. The number of neuronal aggregates in the CNS that contain perikarya expressing the preproenkephalin gene appears to still be greater than the number of neuronal aggregates that contain perikarya expressing the gene that codes for the synthesis of any other peptide transmitter candidate.

Although most enkephalin-containing neurons appear to be interneurons (Golgi type II cells), many others are clearly projection neurons (Golgi type I cells) and some enkephalin-containing fibers traverse very long distances (e.g., from the hypothalamus to the lumbar spinal cord).

Proenkephalin-derived peptides appear to co-exist in the same perikarya with acetylcholine, indolamines, catecholamines, GABA, and/or various other peptide transmitter candidates. The functional significance of the co-localization of proenkephalin-derived peptides with other established and/or suspected neurotransmitters remains to be determined.

There is a high correlation between the density of opiate receptors in different regions of the mammalian brain and spinal cord and the density of enkephalin-containing neuronal processes in the same regions. There are, however, some regions where the correlation between these two measures is apparently low. Further clarification of this relationship will require the use of proenkephalin-specific antisera and high resolution autoradiography of opiate receptor subclasses. Whether any enzyme(s) responsible for the proteolytic processing of proenkephalin has a distribution in the mammalian brain and spinal cord that is restricted to proenkephalin-containing neurons remains to be determined.

Enkephalin-containing perikarya and nerve terminals appear to be present in some homologous nuclei and terminal fields, respectively, in representatives of all major classes of vertebrates. A proenkephalin-like precursor appears to be present in the CNS of representatives of all major classes of tetrapods.

Note added in proof

Since the manuscript for this chapter was submitted, there have been a number of scientific developments that are directly relevant to the central themes described therein.

322

Two laboratories have, independently, cloned and sequenced DNA complementary to rat brain preproenkephalin messenger RNA (Howells et al. 1984; Yoshikawa et al. 1984). Rosen et al. (1984) have sequenced the rat brain preproenkephalin gene. The deduced sequence of rat brain preproenkephalin is functionally identical to the sequence of bovine adrenal medullary preproenkephalin (see 1.).

Two laboratories have, independently, identified an amidated opioid octapeptide, (Met^5)-enkephalin-Arg^6-Arg^7-Val^8-NH$_2$ (metorphamide), as a product of preproenkephalin processing in mammalian tissues (Matsuo et al. 1983; Weber et al. 1983b).

We have confirmed the distribution of preproenkephalin described in this chapter using specific antisera directed against ENK-8 and the carboxyl termini of Met-ENK and metorphamide (Merchenthaler et al. 1985). We have also identified preproenkephalin-containing perikarya in the medial and lateral habenula (Merchenthaler et al. 1985).

6. ACKNOWLEDGMENTS

Many of our colleagues at other universities and research centers provided copies of manuscripts and page proofs that were of inestimable value in the preparation of an 'up-to-date' review chapter. We would like to extend our thanks to all of these colleagues (who are too numerous to list separately) for this courtesy. We would also like to thank our colleagues cited in the 'Materials and Methods' section for supplying the antisera that were used in the previously unreported experiments described in this chapter.

7. REFERENCES

Altschuler RA, Mosinger JL, Hoffman DW, Parakkal MH (1982): Immunocytochemical localization of enkephalin-like immunoreactivity in the retina of the guinea pig. *Proc. Natl Acad. Sci. USA, 79*, 2398–2400.
Altschuler RA, Parakkal MH, Fex J (1983): Localization of enkephalin-like immunoreactivity in acetylcholinesterase-positive cells in the guinea pig lateral superior olivary complex that project to the cochlea. *Neuroscience, 9*, 621–630.
Armstrong DM, Pickel VM, Joh TH, Reis DJ, Miller RJ (1981): Immunocytochemical localization of catecholamine synthesizing enzymes and neuropeptides in area postrema and medial nucleus tractus solitarius of rat brain. *J. Comp. Neurol., 196*, 505–517.
Aronin N, DiFiglia M, Liotta AS, Martin JB (1981): Ultrastructural localization and biochemical features of immunoreactive Leu-enkephalin in monkey dorsal horn. *J. Neurosci.*, 1, 561–577.
Aronin N, DiFiglia M, Graveland GA, Schwartz WJ, Wu JY (1984): Localization of immunoreactive enkephalins in GABA synthesizing neurons of the rat neostriatum. *Brain Res., 300*, 376–380.
Atweh SF, Kuhar MJ (1977): Autoradiographic localization of opiate receptors in rat brain. I. Spinal cord and lower medulla. *Brain Res., 124*, 53–67.
Baird A, Ling N, Böhlen P, Benoit R, Klepper R, Guillemin R (1982): Molecular forms of the putative enkephalin precursor BAM-22P in bovine adrenal, pituitary, and hypothalamus. *Proc. Natl Acad. Sci. USA, 79*, 2023–2025.
Basbaum AI, Fields HL (1978): Endogenous pain control mechanisms: review and hypothesis. *Ann. Neurol., 4*, 451–462.
Bayon A, Koda L, Battenberg E, Azad R, Bloom FE (1980a): Regional distribution of endorphin, Met^5-enkephalin and Leu^5-enkephalin in the pigeon brain. *Neurosci. Lett., 16*, 75–80.
Bayon A, Koda L, Battenberg E, Bloom FE (1980b): Redistribution of endorphin and enkephalin immunoreactivity in the rat brain and pituitary after *in vivo* treatment with colchicine or cytochalasin B. *Brain Res., 183*, 103–111.
Beauvillain JC, Tramu G, Croix D (1980): Electron microscopic localization of enkephalin in the median eminence and the adenohypophysis of the guinea pig. *Neuroscience, 5*, 1705–1716.
Beauvillain JC, Tramu G, Poulain P (1982): Enkephalin-immunoreactive neurons in the guinea pig hypothalamus. *Cell Tissue Res., 224*, 1–13.
Beauvillain JC, Poulain P, Tramu G (1983): Immunocytochemical localization of enkephalin in the lateral septum of the guinea-pig brain. A light- and electron-microscopic study. *Cell Tissue Res., 228*, 265–276.
Beauvillain JC, Tramu G, Garaud JC (1984): Coexistence of substances related to enkephalin and somatostatin in granules of the guinea-pig median eminence: demonstration by use of colloidal gold immunocytochemical methods. *Brain Res., 301*, 389–393.

Beitz AJ (1982): The nuclei of origin of brain stem enkephalin and substance P projections to the rodent nucleus raphe magnus. *Neuroscience, 7,* 2753–2768.

Bennett GJ, Ruda MA, Gobel S, Dubner R (1982): Enkephalin immunoreactive stalked cells and lamina IIb cells in the cat substantia gelatinosa. *Brain Res., 240,* 162–166.

Bloch B, Baird A, Ling N, Benoit R, Guillemin R (1983): Immunohistochemical evidence that brain enkephalins arise from a precursor similar to adrenal preproenkephalin. *Brain Res., 263,* 251–257.

Bloom FE, Battenberg E, Rossier J, Ling N, Guillemin R (1978): Neurons containing beta-endorphin in rat brain exist separately from those containing enkephalins: immunocytochemical studies. *Proc. Natl Acad. Sci. USA, 75,* 1591–1595.

Boarder MR, Lockfield AJ, Barchas JD (1982): Measurement of methionine-enkephalin [Arg^6,Phe^7] in rat brain by specific radioimmunoassay directed at methionine sulphoxide enkephalin [Arg^6,Phe^7]. *J. Neurochem., 38,* 299–304.

Bogan N, Brecha N, Gall C, Karten HJ (1982): Distribution of enkephalin-like immunoreactivity in the rat main olfactory bulb. *Neuroscience, 7,* 895–906.

Boone TB, Aldes LD (1984): The ultrastructure of two distinct neuron populations in the hypoglossal nucleus of the rat. *Exp. Brain Res., 54,* 321–326.

Botticelli LJ, Cox BM, Goldstein A (1981): Immunoreactive dynorphin in mammalian spinal cord and dorsal root ganglia. *Proc. Natl Acad. Sci. USA, 78,* 7783–7786.

Bouras C, Taban CH, Constantinidis J (1984): Mapping of enkephalins in human brain. An immunohistofluorescence study on brains from patients with senile and presenile dementia. *Neuroscience, 12,* 179–190.

Bouyer JJ, Miller RJ, Pickel VM (1984): Ultrastructural relation between cortical efferents and terminals containing enkephalin-like immunoreactivity in rat neostriatum. *Regul. Peptides, 8,* 105–115.

Bowker RM, Steinbusch HWM, Coulter JD (1981): Serotonergic and peptidergic projections to the spinal cord demonstrated by a combined retrograde HRP histochemical and immunocytochemical method. *Brain Res., 211,* 412–417.

Brann MR, Emson PC (1980): Microiontophoretic injection of fluorescent tracer with simultaneous immunofluorescence histochemistry for the demonstration of efferents from the caudate-putamen projecting to the globus pallidus. *Neurosci. Lett., 16,* 61–65.

Brauth SE (1984): Enkephalin-like immunoreactivity within the telencephalon of the reptile *Caiman crocodilus. Neuroscience, 11,* 345–358.

Brauth SE, Rainer E (1982): A pretectal-tectal enkephalin connection: immunohistochemical studies of homologous systems in reptiles. *Neurosci. Abstracts, 8,* 766.

Brecha NC, Karten HJ, Laverack C (1979): Enkephalin-containing amacrine cells in the avian retina: immunohistochemical localization. *Proc. Natl Acad. Sci. USA, 76,* 3010–3014.

Burns J (1978): Immunohistochemical methods and their application in the routine laboratory. In: Anthony PP, Wolf N (Eds), *Recent Advances in Histopathology, 10th Ed.,* pp. 337–350. Churchill-Livingstone, New York.

Chang KJ, Cuatrecasas P (1981): Heterogeneity and properties of opiate receptors. *Fed. Proc., 40,* 2729–2734.

Chang KJ, Cooper BR, Hazum E, Cuatrecasas P (1979): Multiple opiate receptors: different regional distribution in the brain and differential binding of opiates and opioid peptides. *Mol. Pharmacol., 16,* 91–104.

Chang KJ, Hazum E, Cuatrecasas P (1981): Novel opiate binding sites selective for benzomorphan drugs. *Proc. Natl Acad. Sci. USA, 78,* 4141–4145.

Charnay Y, Léger L, Dray F, Berod A, Jouvet M, Pujol JF, Dubois PM (1982): Evidence for the presence of enkephalin in catecholaminergic neurones of cat locus coeruleus. *Neurosci. Lett., 30,* 147–151.

Charnay Y, Paulin C, Dray F, Dubois PM (1984): Distribution of enkephalin in human fetus and infant spinal cord: an immunofluorescence study. *J. Comp. Neurol., 223,* 415–423.

Comb M, Seeburg PH, Adelman J, Eiden L, Herbert E (1982): Primary structure of the human met- and leu-enkephalin precursor and its mRNA. *Nature (London), 295,* 663–666.

Comb M, Rosen H, Seeburg P, Adelman J, Herbert E (1983): Primary structure of the human proenkephalin gene. *DNA, 2,* 213–229.

Cone RI (1982): Dynorphin immunoreactivity in the toad neurointermediate lobe. *Life Sci., 31,* 1801–1804.

Cone RI, Goldstein A (1982a): A specific radioimmunoassay for the opioid peptide dynorphin B in neural tissues. *Neuropeptides, 3,* 97–106.

Cone RI, Goldstein A (1982b): A dynorphin-like opioid in the central nervous system of an amphibian. *Proc. Natl Acad. Sci. USA, 79,* 3345–3349.

Corbett AD, Paterson SJ, McKnight AT, Magnan J, Kosterlitz HW (1983): Dynorphin$_{1-8}$ and dynorphin$_{1-9}$ are ligands for the κ-subtype of opiate receptor. *Nature (London), 299,* 79–81.

Correa FMA, Innis RB, Hester LD, Snyder SH (1981): Diffuse enkephalin innervation from caudate to globus pallidus. *Neurosci. Lett., 25,* 63–68.

Cuello AC (1983): Central distribution of opioid peptides. *Br. Med. Bull., 39,* 11–16.

Cuello AC, Paxinos G (1978): Evidence for a long Leu-enkephalin striopallidal pathway in rat brain. *Nature (London), 271*, 178–180.

Dalsgaard CJ, Hökfelt T, Johansson O, Elde R (1981): Somatostatin immunoreactive cell bodies in the dorsal horn and the parasympathetic intermediolateral nucleus of the rat spinal cord. *Neurosci. Lett., 27*, 335–339.

Dalsgaard CJ, Hökfelt T, Elfvin LG, Terenius L (1982): Enkephalin-containing sympathetic preganglionic neurons projecting to the inferior mesenteric ganglion: evidence from combined retrograde tracing and immunohistochemistry. *Neuroscience, 7*, 2039–2050.

Dalsgaard CJ, Vincent SR, Hökfelt T, Christensson I, Terenius L (1983): Separate origins for the dynorphin and enkephalin immunoreactive fibers in the inferior mesenteric ganglion of the guinea pig. *J. Comp. Neurol., 221*, 482–489.

Dandekar S, Sabol SL (1982): Cell-free translation and partial characterization of proenkephalin messenger RNA from bovine striatum. *Biochem. Biophys. Res. Commun., 105*, 67–74.

Davis BM, Brecha N, Karten HJ (1980): Enkephalin-like immunoreactivity in developing avian basal ganglia and nucleus spiriformis lateralis. *Neurosci. Abstracts, 6*, 744.

Davis BJ, Burd GD, Macrides E (1982): Localization of methionine-enkephalin, substance P, and somatostatin immunoreactivities in the main olfactory bulb of the hamster. *J. Comp. Neurol., 204*, 377–383.

De Lanerolle NC, LaMotte CC (1982): The human spinal cord: substance P and methionine-enkephalin immunoreactivity. *J. Neurosci., 2*, 1369–1386.

De Lanerolle NC, Elde RP, Sparber SB, Frick M (1981): Distribution of methionine-enkephalin immunoreactivity in the chick brain: an immunohistochemical study. *J. Comp. Neurol., 199*, 513–533.

Del Fiacco M, Cuello AC (1980): Substance P and enkephalin-containing neurones in the rat trigeminal system. *Neuroscience, 5*, 803–815.

Del Fiacco M, Paxinos G, Cuello AC (1982): Neostriatal enkephalin-immunoreactive neurons project to the globus pallidus. *Brain Res., 231*, 1–17.

DiFiglia M, Aronin N (1984): Immunoreactive Leu-enkephalin in the monkey hypothalamus including observations on its ultrastructural localization in the paraventricular nucleus. *J. Comp. Neurol., 225*, 313–326.

DiFiglia M, Aronin N, Martin JB (1982): Light and electron microscopic localization of immunoreactive Leu-enkephalin in the monkey basal ganglia. *J. Neurosci., 2*, 303–320.

Docherty K, Steiner DF (1982): Post-translational proteolysis in polypeptide hormone biosynthesis. *Annu. Rev. Physiol., 44*, 625–638.

Doerr-Schott J, Dubois MP, Lichte C (1981): Immunohistochemical localization of substances reactive to antisera against α- and β-endorphin and Met-enkephalin in the brain of *Rana temporaria L. Cell Tissue Res., 217*, 79–92.

Dores RM (1982): Evidence for a common precursor for α-MSH and β-endorphin in the intermediate lobe of the pituitary of the reptile, *Anolis carolinensis. Peptides, 3*, 925–935.

Dores RM, Finger TE, Gold MR (1984): Immunohistochemical localization of enkephalin- and ACTH-related substances in the pituitary of the lamprey. *Cell Tissue Res., 235*, 107–115.

Douglass J, Civelli O, Herbert E (1984): Polyprotein gene expression: generation of diversity of neuroendocrine peptides. *Annu. Rev. Biochem., 53*, 665–715.

Eccles JC, Ito M, Szentágothai J (1967): *The Cerebellum as a Neuronal Machine.* Springer-Verlag, Berlin.

Eipper BA, Mains RE (1981): Further analysis of post-translational processing of β-endorphin in rat intermediate pituitary. *J. Biol. Chem., 256*, 5689–5695.

Elde RT, Hökfelt T, Johansson O, Terenius L (1976): Immunohistochemical studies using antibodies to leucine-enkephalin: initial observations on the nervous system of the rat. *Neuroscience, 1*, 349–351.

Eldred WD, Karten HJ (1982): Synaptic contacts of enkephalinergic amacrine cells in the retina of the turtle (*Pseudemys scripta*). *Neurosci. Abstracts, 8*, 45.

Eldred W, Karten HJ (1983): Characterization and quantification of peptidergic amacrine cells in the turtle retina: enkephalin, neurotensin, and glucagon. *J. Comp. Neurol., 221*, 371–381.

Erichsen JT, Reiner A, Cabot J, Karten HJ (1981): Neurons of the nucleus of Edinger-Westphal are the source of enkephalinergic and substance P-containing terminals in the avian ciliary ganglion. *Neurosci. Abstracts, 7*, 777.

Erichsen JT, Karten HJ, Eldred WD, Brecha NC (1982a): Localization of substance P-like and enkephalin-like immunoreactivity within preganglionic terminals of the avian ciliary ganglion: light and electron microscopy. *J. Neurosci., 2*, 994–1003.

Erichsen JT, Reiner A, Karten HJ (1982b): Co-occurence of substance P-like and Leu-enkephalin-like immunoreactivities in neurons and fibres of avian nervous system. *Nature (London), 295*, 407–410.

Evangelista R, Ray P, Lewis RV (1982): A 'trypsin-like' enzyme in adrenal chromaffin granules: a proenkephalin processing enzyme. *Biochem. Biophys. Res. Commun., 106*, 895–902.

325

Fex J, Altschuler RA (1981): Enkephalin-like immunoreactivity of olivocochlear fibers in the cochlea of the guinea-pig and cat. *Proc. Natl Acad. Sci. USA, 78*, 1255–1259.

Finley JCW, Maderdrut JL, Petrusz P (1981a): The immunocytochemical localization of enkephalin in the central nervous system of the rat. *J. Comp. Neurol., 198*, 541–565.

Finley JCW, Lindström P, Petrusz P (1981b): Immunocytochemical localization of β-endorphin-containing neurons in the rat brain. *Neuroendocrinology, 33*, 28–42.

Fitzpatrick D, Johnson RP (1981): Enkephalin-like immunoreactivity in the mossy fiber pathway of the hippocampal formation of the tree shrew (*Tupaia glis*). *Neuroscience, 6*, 2485–2494.

Fleminger G, Ezra E, Kilpatrick DL, Udenfriend S (1983): Processing of enkephalin-containing peptides in isolated bovine adrenal chromaffin granules. *Proc. Natl Acad. Sci. USA, 80*, 6418–6421.

Follénius E, Dubois MP (1979): Localisation des sites immunoréactifs avec un antisérum contre la met-enképhaline et contre l'α-endorphine dans le cerveau de la Carpe. *C.R. Acad. Sci. (Paris), 288D*, 903–906.

Fricker LD, Snyder SH (1982): Enkephalin convertase: purification and characterization of a specific enkephalin-synthesizing carboxypeptidase localized to adrenal chromaffin granules. *Proc. Natl Acad. Sci. USA, 79*, 3886–3890.

Fricker LD, Supattapone S, Snyder SH (1982): Enkephalin convertase: a specific enkephalin synthesizing carboxypeptidase in adrenal chromaffin granules, brain, and pituitary gland. *Life Sci., 31*, 1841–1844.

Gall C, Moore RY (1984): Distribution of enkephalin, substance P, tyrosine hydroxylase, and 5-hydroxytryptamine immunoreactivity in the septal region of the rat. *J. Comp. Neurol., 225*, 212–227.

Gall C, Brecha N, Karten HJ, Chang KJ (1981): Localization of enkephalin-like immunoreactivity to identified axonal and neuronal populations of the rat hippocampus. *J. Comp. Neurol., 198*, 335–350.

Gall C, Brecha N, Chang KJ, Karten HJ (1984): Ontogeny of enkephalin-like immunoreactivity in the rat hippocampus. *Neuroscience, 11*, 359–380.

Gallyas F, Görcs T, Merchenthaler I (1982): High grade intensification of the end-product of the diaminobenzidine reaction for peroxidase histochemistry. *J. Histochem. Cytochem., 30*, 183–184.

Gee CE, Chen CL, Roberts JL (1983): Identification of proopiomelanocortin neurones in the rat hypothalamus by *in situ* cDNA-mRNA hybridization. *Nature (London), 306*, 374–376.

Gibson SJ, Polak JM, Bloom SR, Wall PD (1981): The distribution of nine peptides in rat spinal cord with special emphasis on the substantia gelatinosa and on the area around the central canal (lamina X). *J. Comp. Neurol., 201*, 65–79.

Glazer EJ, Basbaum AI (1980): Leucine enkephalin: localization in and axoplasmic transport by sacral parasympathetic preganglionic neurons. *Science, 208*, 1479–1480.

Glazer EJ, Basbaum AI (1981): Immunohistochemical localization of Leucine-enkephalin in the spinal cord of the rat: enkephalin-containing marginal neurons and pain modulation. *J. Comp. Neurol., 196*, 377–389.

Glazer EJ, Basbaum AI (1983): Opioid neurons and pain modulation: an ultrastructural analysis of enkephalin in cat superficial dorsal horn. *Neuroscience, 10*, 357–376.

Glazer EJ, Steinbusch H, Verhofstad A, Basbaum AI (1981): Serotonin neurons in nucleus raphe dorsalis and paragigantocellularis of the cat contain enkephalin. *J. Physiol. (Paris), 77*, 241–245.

Gold MR, Finger TE (1981): Localization of enkephalin-like immunoreactivity in the brain of the lamprey. *Neurosci. Abstracts, 7*, 85.

Goldstein A, Tachibana A, Lowney LI, Hunkapiller M, Hood L (1979): Dynorphin (1-13), an extraordinarily potent opioid peptide. *Proc. Natl Acad. Sci. USA, 76*, 6666–6670.

Goodman RR, Snyder SH (1982): Kappa-opiate receptors localized by autoradiography to deep layers of cerebral cortex: relation to sedative effects. *Proc. Natl Acad. Sci. USA, 79*, 5703–5707.

Gramsch C, Kleber G, Höllt V, Pasi A, Mehraein P, Herz A (1980): Proopiocortin fragments in human and rat brain: β-endorphin and γ-MSH are the predominant peptides. *Brain Res., 92*, 109–114.

Graybiel AM, Ragsdale CW, Yoneoka ES, Elde RP (1981): An immunohistochemical study of enkephalins and other neuropeptides in the striatum of the cat with evidence that the opiate peptides are arranged to form mosaic patterns in register with the striosomal compartments visible by acetylcholinesterase staining. *Neuroscience, 6*, 377–397.

Graybiel AM, Brecha N, Karten HJ (1984): Cluster-and-sheet pattern of enkephalin-like immunoreactivity in the superior colliculus of the cat. *Neuroscience, 12*, 191–214.

Greenberg MJ, Price DA (1983): Invertebrate neuropeptides: native and naturalized. *Annu. Rev. Physiol., 45*, 271–288.

Grzanna R, Molliver ME, Coyle JT (1978): Visualization of central noradrenergic neurons in thick sections by the unlabelled antibody method: a transmitter specific Golgi image. *Proc. Natl Acad. Sci. USA, 75*, 2502–2506.

Gubler U, Seeburg P, Hoffman BJ, Gage LP, Udenfriend S (1982): Molecular cloning establishes proenkephalin as precursor of enkephalin-containing peptides. *Nature (London), 295*, 206–208.

326

Haber S, Elde R (1981): Correlation between Met-enkephalin and substance P immunoreactivity in the primate globus pallidus. *Neuroscience, 7*, 1291–1297.

Haber S, Elde R (1982a): The distribution of enkephalin immunoreactive fibers and terminals in the monkey central nervous system: an immunohistochemical study. *Neuroscience, 7*, 1049–1095.

Haber S, Elde R (1982b): The distribution of enkephalin immunoreactive neuronal cell bodies in the monkey brain: preliminary observations. *Neurosci. Lett., 32*, 247–252.

Haber SN, Nauta WJH (1983): Ramifications of the globus pallidus in the rat as indicated by patterns of immunohistochemistry. *Neuroscience, 9*, 245–260.

Hancock MB (1982): Leu-enkephalin, substance P and somatostatin immunohistochemistry combined with the retrograde transport of horseradish peroxidase in sympathetic preganglionic neurons. *J. Autonom. Nerv. Syst., 6*, 263–272.

Hartman BK, Zide D, Udenfriend S (1972): The use of dopamine-β-hydroxylase as a marker for the noradrenergic pathways of the central nervous system in the rat. *Proc. Natl Acad. Sci. USA, 69*, 2722–2726.

Haynes LW, Zakarian S (1981): Microanatomy of enkephalin-containing neurons in developing rat spinal cord in vitro. *Neuroscience, 6*, 1899–1916.

Haynes LW, Smyth DG, Zakarian S (1982): Immunocytochemical localization of β-endorphin (lipotropin C-fragment) in the developing rat spinal cord and hypothalamus. *Brain Res., 232*, 115–128.

Herbert E, Oates E, Martens G, Comb M, Rosen H, Uhler M (1983): Generation of diversity and evolution of opioid peptides. *Cold Spring Harbor Symp. Quant. Biol., 48*, 375–384.

Herkenham M, Pert CB (1980): In vitro autoradiography of opiate receptors in rat brain suggest loci of 'opiatergic' pathways. *Proc. Natl Acad. Sci. USA, 77*, 5532–5536.

Herkenham M, Pert CB (1982): Light microscopic localization of brain opiate receptors: a general autoradiographic method which preserves tissue quality. *J. Neurosci., 2*, 1129–1149.

Hiller J, Pearson J, Simon E (1973): Distribution of stereospecific binding of the potent narcotic analgesic etorphine in human brain: predominance in the limbic system. *Res. Commun. Chem. Pathol. Pharmacol., 6*, 1052–1062.

Hoffman DW, Altschuler RA, Gutierrez J (1983): Multiple molecular forms of enkephalins in the guinea pig hippocampus. *J. Neurochem., 41*, 1641–1647.

Hökfelt T, Fuxe K, Goldstein M, Johansson O (1974): Immunohistochemical evidence for the existence of adrenaline neurons in the rat brain. *Brain Res., 66*, 235–251.

Hökfelt T, Elde R, Johansson O, Terenius L, Stein L (1977a): The distribution of enkephalin-immunoreactive cell bodies in the rat central nervous system. *Neurosci. Lett., 5*, 25–31.

Hökfelt T, Ljungdahl A, Terenius L, Elde R, Nilsson G (1977b): Immunohistochemical analysis of peptide pathways possibly related to pain and analgesia: enkephalin and substance P. *Proc. Natl Acad. Sci. USA, 74*, 3081–3085.

Hökfelt T, Ljungdahl A, Steinbusch H, Verhofstad A, Nilsson G, Brodin E, Pernow B, Goldstein M (1978): Immunohistochemical evidence of substance P-like immunoreactivity in some 5-hydroxytryptamine-containing neurons in the rat central nervous system. *Neuroscience, 3*, 517–538.

Hökfelt T, Terenius L, Kuypers HGM, Dann O (1979): Evidence for enkephalin immunoreactive neurons in the medulla oblongata projecting to the spinal cord. *Neurosci. Lett., 14*, 55–60.

Hökfelt T, Fahrenkrug J, Tatemoto K, Mutt V, Werner S, Hulting AL, Terenius L, Chang KJ (1983): The PHI (PHI-27)/corticotropin-releasing factor/enkephalin immunoreactive hypothalamic neuron: possible morphological basis for integrated control of prolactin, corticotropin, and growth hormone secretion. *Proc. Natl Acad. Sci. USA, 80*, 895–898.

Holets V, Elde R (1982): The differential distribution and relationship of serotonergic and peptidergic fibers to sympathoadrenal preganglionic neurons in the intermediolateral cell column of the rat: a combined retrograde axonal transport and immunofluorescence study. *Neuroscience, 7*, 1155–1174.

Höllt V, Haarmann I, Grimm C, Herz A, Tulunay FC, Loh HH (1982): Proenkephalin intermediates in bovine brain and adrenal medulla: characterization of immunoreactive peptides related to BAM-22P and peptide F. *Life Sci., 31*, 1883–1886.

Hook VYH, Loh YP (1984): Carboxypeptidase B-like converting enzyme activity in secretory granules of rat pituitary. *Proc. Natl Acad. Sci. USA, 81*, 2776–2780.

Houser CR, Crawford GD, Barber RP, Salvaterra PM, Vaughn JE (1983): Organization and morphological characteristics of cholinergic neurons: an immunocytochemical study with a monoclonal antibody to choline acetyltransferase. *Brain Res., 266*, 97–119.

Howells RD, Kilpatrick DL, Bhatt R, Monahan JJ, Poonian M, Udenfriend S (1984): Molecular cloning and sequence determination of rat preproenkephalin cDNA: sensitive probe for studying transcriptional changes in rat tissues. *Proc. Natl Acad. Sci. USA, 81*, 7651–7655.

Hughes J, Smith TW, Kosterlitz HW, Fothergill LA, Morgan BA, Morris HR (1975): Identification of two related pentapeptides from brain with potent opiate agonist activity. *Nature (London), 258*, 577–579.

Humber J, Pradelles P, Gros C, Dray F (1979): Enkephalin-like products in embryonic chicken retina. *Neurosci. Lett., 12*, 259–263.

Hunt SP, Lovick TA (1982): The distribution of serotonin, Met-enkephalin and β-lipotropin-like immunore-activity in neuronal perikarya of the cat brainstem. *Neurosci. Lett., 30*, 139–145.

Hunt SP, Emson PC, Gilbert R, Goldstein M, Kimmel JR (1981a): Presence of avian pancreatic polypeptide-like immunoreactivity in catecholamine and methionine-enkephalin-containing neurons within the central nervous system. *Neurosci. Lett., 21*, 125–130.

Hunt SP, Kelly JS, Emson PC, Kimmel JR, Miller RJ, Wu JY (1981b): An immunohistochemical study of neuronal populations containing neuropeptides or γ-aminobutyrate within the superficial layers of the rat dorsal horn. *Neuroscience, 6*, 1883–1898.

Ikeda Y, Nakao K, Yoshimasa T, Yanaihara N, Numa S, Imura H (1982): Existence of met-enkephalin-Arg^6-Gly^7-Leu^8 with met-enkephalin, leu-enkephalin and met-enkephalin-Arg^6-Phe^7 in the brain of guinea pig, rat and golden hamster. *Biochem. Biophys. Res. Commun., 107*, 656–662.

Innocenti GM (1981): Growth and reshaping of axons in the establishment of visual callosal connections. *Science, 212*, 824–827.

James IF, Chavkin C, Goldstein A (1982): Preparation of brain membranes containing a single type of opioid receptor highly selective for dynorphin. *Proc. Natl Acad. Sci. USA, 79*, 7570–7574.

Jancsó G, Hökfelt T, Lundberg JM, Király E, Halász N, Nilsson G, Terenius L, Rehfeld J, Steinbush H, Verhofstad A, Elde R, Said S, Brown M (1981): Immunohistochemical studies on the effect of capsaicin on spinal and medullary peptide and monoamine neurons using antisera to substance P, gastrin/CCK, somatostatin, VIP, enkephalin, neurotensin and 5-hydroxytryptamine. *J. Neurocytol., 10*, 963–980.

Johansson O, Hökfelt T, Elde RP, Schultzberg M, Terenius L (1978): Immunohistochemical distribution of enkephalin neurons. *Adv. Biochem. Psychopharmacol., 18*, 51–70.

Johansson O, Hökfelt T, Pernow B, Jeffcoate SL, White N, Steinbusch HWM, Verhofstad AAJ, Emson PC, Spindel E (1981): Immunohistochemical support for three putative transmitters in one neuron: coexistence of 5-hydroxytryptamine, substance P- and thyrotropin releasing hormone-like immunoreactivity in medullary neurons projecting to the spinal cord. *Neuroscience, 6*, 1857–1881.

Joseph SA, Sternberger LA (1979): The unlabelled antibody method. Contrasting color staining of β-lipotropin and ACTH-associated hypothalamic peptides without antibody removal. *J. Histochem. Cytochem., 27*, 1430–1437.

Kakidani HY, Furutani Y, Takahashi H, Noda M, Motimoto Y, Hirose T, Asai M, Inayama S, Nakanishi S, Numa S (1982): Cloning and sequence analysis of cDNA for porcine β-neo-endorphin/dynorphin precursor. *Nature (London), 298*, 245–249.

Kalia M, Fuxe K, Hökfelt T, Johansson O, Lang R, Ganten D, Cuello C, Terenius L (1984): Distribution of neuropeptide immunoreactive nerve terminals within the subnuclei of the nucleus of the tractus solitarius of the rat. *J. Comp. Neurol., 222*, 409–444.

Kangawa K, Matsuo H, Igarashi M (1979): α-Neo-endorphin: a 'big' Leu-enkephalin with potent opiate activity from porcine hypothalami. *Biochem. Biophys. Res. Commun., 95*, 1475–1481.

Kapadia SE, De Lanerolle NC (1984): Populations of substance P, Met-enkephalin and serotonin immunoreactive neurons in the interpeduncular nucleus of cat: cytoarchitectonics. *Brain Res., 302*, 33–43.

Kawatani M, Lowe IP, Booth AM, Backes MG, Erdman SL, De Groat WC (1983): The presence of Leucine-enkephalin in the sacral preganglionic pathway to the urinary bladder of the cat. *Neurosci. Lett., 39*, 143–148.

Khachaturian H, Lewis ME, Höllt V, Watson SJ (1983a): Telencephalic enkephalinergic systems in the rat. *J. Neurosci., 3*, 844–855.

Khachaturian H, Lewis ME, Watson SJ (1983b): Enkephalin systems in diencephalon and brainstem of the rat. *J. Comp. Neurol., 220*, 310–320.

Kilpatrick DL, Jones BN, Kojima K, Udenfriend S (1981): Identification of the octapeptide [Met]enkephalin-Arg^6-Gly^7-Leu^8 in extracts of bovine adrenal medulla. *Biochem. Biophys. Res. Commun., 103*, 698–705.

Kilpatrick DL, Howells RD, Lahm HW, Udenfriend S (1983a): Evidence for a proenkephalin-like precursor in amphibian brain. *Proc. Natl Acad Sci. USA, 80*, 5772–5775.

Kilpatrick DL, Eisen M, Ezra E, Udenfriend S (1983b): Processing of dynorphin at single and paired basic residues in porcine neurointermediate lobe. *Life Sci., 33, Suppl. 1*, 93–96.

Kiss JZ, Williams TH (1983): ACTH-immunoreactive boutons form synaptic contacts in the hypothalamic arcuate nucleus of rat: evidence for local opiocortin connections. *Brain Res., 263*, 142–146.

Kojima K, Kilpatrick DL, Stern AS, Jones BN, Udenfriend S (1982): Proenkephalin: a general pathway for enkephalin biosynthesis in animal tissues. *Arch. Biochem. Biophys., 215*, 638–643.

Kosterlitz HW, Paterson SJ, Robson LE (1981): Characterization of the kappa subtype of the opiate receptor in the guinea-pig brain. *Br. J. Pharmacol., 73*, 939–949.

Kuhar MJ, Pert CB, Snyder SH (1973): Regional distribution of opiate receptor binding in monkey and human brain. *Nature (London)*, *245*, 447–450.

Kuljis RO, Karten HJ (1982): Laminar organization of peptide-like immunoreactivity in the anuran optic tectum. *J. Comp. Neurol.*, *212*, 188–201.

Kuljis RO, Karten HJ (1983): Modification in the laminar organization of peptide-like immunoreactivity in the anuran optic tectum following retinal deafferentation. *J. Comp. Neurol.*, *217*, 239–251.

Kuljis RO, Krause JE, Karten HJ (1984): Peptide-like immunoreactivity in anuran optic nerve fibers. *J. Comp. Neurol.*, *226*, 222–237.

LaMotte CC, De Lanerolle NC (1981): Human spinal neurons: innervation by both substance P and enkephalin. *Neuroscience*, *6*, 713–723.

Landmesser L, Pilar G (1970): Selective reinnervation of two cell populations in the adult pigeon ciliary ganglion. *J. Physiol. (London)*, *211*, 203–216.

LaValley AL, Ho RH (1983): Substance P, somatostatin, and methionine enkephalin immunoreactive elements in the spinal cord of the domestic fowl, *Gallus domesticus*. *J. Comp. Neurol.*, *213*, 406–413.

Leboulenger F, Leroux P, Delarue C, Tonon MC, Charnay Y, Dubois PM, Coy DH, Vaudry H (1983): Colocalization of vasoactive intestinal peptide (VIP) and enkephalins in chromaffin cells of the adrenal gland of amphibia. Stimulation of cortico-steroid production by VIP. *Life Sci.*, *32*, 375–383.

Léger L, Charnay Y, Chayvialle, Bérod A, Dray F, Pujol JF, Jouvet M, Dubois PM (1983): Localization of substance P- and enkephalin-like immunoreactivity in relation to catecholamine-containing cell bodies in the cat dorsolateral pontine tegmentum: an immunofluorescence study. *Neuroscience*, *8*, 525–546.

Legon S, Glover DM, Hughes J, Lowry PJ, Rigby PWJ, Watson CJ (1982): The structure and expression of the preproenkephalin gene. *Nucleic Acid Res.*, *10*, 7905–7918.

Leung MK, Stefano GB (1984): Isolation and identification of enkephalins in pedal ganglia of *Mytilus edulis* (Mollusca). *Proc. Natl Acad. Sci. USA*, *81*, 955–958.

Lewis ME, Pert A, Pert CB, Herkenham M (1983): Opiate receptor localization in rat cerebral cortex. *J. Comp. Neurol.*, *216*, 339–358.

Lindberg I, Yang HYT, Costa E (1982): Characterization of a partially purified trypsin-like enkephalin-generating enzyme in bovine adrenal medulla. *Life Sci.*, *31*, 1713–1716.

Lindberg I, Yang HYT (1984): Distribution of Met^5-enkephalin-Arg^6-Gly^7-Leu^8-immunoreactive peptides in rat brain: presence of multiple molecular forms. *Brain Res.*, *299*, 73–78.

Liston D, Rossier J (1984): Distribution and characterization of synenkephalin immunoreactivity in the bovine brain and pituitary. *Regul. Peptides*, *8*, 79–87.

Liston DR, Vanderhaeghen JJ, Rossier J (1983): Presence in brain of synenkephalin, a proenkephalin-immunoreactive protein which does not contain enkephalin. *Nature (London)*, *302*, 62–65.

Livett BG, Day R, Elde RP, Howe PRC (1982): Co-storage of enkephalins and adrenaline in the bovine adrenal medulla. *Neuroscience*, *7*, 1323–1332.

Loh YP (1979): Immunological evidence for two common precursors to corticotropins, endorphins, and melanotropin in the neurointermediate lobe of the toad pituitary. *Proc. Natl Acad. Sci. USA*, *76*, 796–800.

Loh YP, Brownstein MJ, Gainer H (1984): Proteolysis in neuropeptide processing and other neural functions. *Annu. Rev. Neurosci.*, *7*, 189–222.

Lord JAH, Waterfield AA, Hughes J, Kosterlitz HW (1977): Endogenous opioid peptides: multiple agonists and receptors. *Nature (London)*, *267*, 495–500.

Lorez HP, Kemali M (1981): Substance P-, Met-enkephalin and somatostatin-like immunoreactivity distribution in frog spinal cord. *Neurosci. Lett.*, *26*, 119–124.

Maderdrut JL, Yaksh TL, Petrusz P, Go VLW (1982): Origin and distribution of cholecystokinin-containing nerve terminals in the lumbar dorsal horn and nucleus caudalis of the cat. *Brain Res.*, *243*, 363–368.

Maderdrut JL, Sundberg DK, Merchenthaler I, Okado N, Oppenheim RW (1984): Development of proenkephalin-like immunoreactivity in the lumbar spinal cord and the adrenal medulla of the chick embryo. *Eur. Soc. Neurochem.*, *5* (Abstract).

Majane EA, Iadarola MJ, Yang HYT (1983): Distribution of Met^5-enkephalin-Arg^6,Phe^7 in rat spinal cord. *Brain Res.*, *264*, 336–339.

Makara GB, Palkovits M, Antoni FA, Kiss JZ (1983): Topography of the somatostatin-immunoreactive fibers to the stalk-median eminence of the rat. *Neuroendocrinology*, *37*, 1–8.

Maley B, Mullett T, Elde R (1983): The nucleus tractus solitarii of the cat: a comparison of Golgi impregnated neurons with methionine-enkephalin- and substance P-immunoreactive neurons. *J. Comp. Neurol.*, *217*, 405–417.

Mantyh PW, Hunt SP (1984): Neuropeptides are present in projection neurones at all levels in visceral and taste pathways: from periphery to sensory cortex. *Brain Res.*, *299*, 297–311.

Martens GJM, Jenks BG, Van Overbeeke AP (1982): Biosynthesis of pairs of peptides related to melanotropin, corticotropin and endorphin in the pars intermedia of the amphibian pituitary gland. *Eur. J. Biochem.*, *122*, 1–10.

Martin R, Voigt KH (1981): Enkephalins co-exist with oxytocin and vasopressin in nerve terminals of rat neurohypophysis. *Nature (London), 289*, 502–504.

Martin R, Geis R, Holl R, Schafer M, Voigt KH (1983): Co-existence of unrelated peptides in oxytocin and vasopressin terminals of rat neurohypophyses: immunoreactive methionine[5]-enkephalin-, leucine[5]-enkephalin- and cholecystokinin-like substances. *Neuroscience, 8*, 213–227.

Matsuo H, Miyata A, Mizuno K (1983): Novel C-terminally amidated opioid peptide in human phaeochromocytoma tumour. *Nature (London), 305*, 721–723.

McGinty JF (1983): Immunocytochemical distribution of opioid peptidergic neurons in rat neocortex. *Neurosci. Abstracts, 9 (Part 1)*, 439.

McGinty JF, Bloom FE (1983): Double immunostaining reveals distinctions among opioid peptidergic neurons in the medial basal hypothalamus. *Brain Res., 278*, 145–153.

McGinty JF, Henriksen SJ, Goldstein A, Terenius L, Bloom FE (1983): Dynorphin is contained within hippocampal mossy fibers: immunocytochemical alterations after kainic acid administration and colchicine-induced neurotoxicity. *Proc. Natl Acad. Sci. USA, 80*, 589–593.

McGinty JF, Van der Kooy D, Bloom FE (1984): The distribution and morphology of opioid peptide immunoreactive neurons in the cerebral cortex of rats. *J. Neurosci., 4*, 1104–1117.

McLean S, Skirboll LR, Pert CB (1983): Opiatergic projection from the bed nucleus to the habenula: demonstration by a novel radioimmunohistochemical method. *Brain Res., 278*, 255–257.

Merchenthaler I, Görcs T, Petrusz P (1982a): Silver intensification of the diaminobenzidine reaction product for peroxidase immunocytochemistry. *J. Histochem. Cytochem., 30*, 607.

Merchenthaler I, Vigh S, Petrusz P, Schally AV (1982b): Immunocytochemical localization of corticotropin releasing factor (CRF) in the rat brain. *Am. J. Anat., 165*, 385–396.

Merchenthaler I, Maderdrut JL, Altschuler RA, Petrusz P (1985): Immunocytochemical localization of proenkephalin-derived peptides in the central nervous system of the rat. *Neuroscience,* in press.

Micevych P, Elde R (1980): Relationship between enkephalinergic neurons and the vasopressin-oxytocin neuroendocrine systems of the cat: an immunohistochemical study. *J. Comp. Neurol., 190*, 135–146.

Millan MJ, Millan MH, Herz A (1983): Contribution of the supra-optic nucleus to brain and pituitary pools of immunoreactive vasopressin and particulair opioid peptides, and the interrelationships between these, in the rat. *Neuroendocrinology, 36*, 310–319.

Miller RJ, Chang KJ, Cooper B, Cuatrecasas P (1978): Radioimmunoassay and characterization of enkephalin in rat tissues. *J. Biol. Chem., 253*, 531–538.

Mizuno K, Minamino N, Kangawa K, Matsuo H (1980a): A new endogenous opioid peptide from bovine adrenal medulla: isolation and amino acid sequence of a dodecapeptide (BAM 12P). *Biochem. Biophys. Res. Commun., 95*, 1482–1488.

Mizuno K, Minamino N, Kangawa K, Matsuo H (1980b): A new family of endogenous big Met-enkephalins from bovine adrenal medulla: purification and structure of docosa (BAM22P) and eicosapeptide (BAM20P) with very potent opiate activity. *Biochem. Biophys. Res. Commun., 97*, 1283–1290.

Moss MS, Basbaum AI (1983): The fine structure of the caudal periaqueductal gray of the cat: morphology and synaptic organization of normal and immunoreactive enkephalin-labelled profiles. *Brain Res., 289*, 27–43.

Moss MS, Glazer EJ, Basbaum AI (1981): Enkephalin-immunoreactive perikarya in the cat raphe dorsalis. *Neurosci. Lett., 21*, 33–37.

Moss MS, Glazer EJ, Basbaum AI (1983): The peptidergic organization of the cat periaqueductal gray. I. The distribution of immunoreactive enkephalin-containing neurons and terminals. *J. Neurosci., 3*, 603–616.

Mulcahy J, Lee HS, Basbaum AI (1983): Coexistence of immunoreactive enkephalin (I-Enk) and dynorphin (I-Dyn) in the nucleus of the solitary tract of the rat. *Neurosci. Abstracts, 9 (Part 1)*, 461.

Naik DR, Sar M, Stumpf WE (1981): Immunohistochemical localization of enkephalin in the central nervous system and pituitary of the lizard, *Anolis carolinensis. J. Comp. Neurol., 198*, 583–601.

Nakanishi S, Inoue A, Kita T, Nakamura M, Chang ACY, Cohen SN, Numa S (1979): Nucleotide sequence of cloned cDNA for bovine corticotropin-β-lipotropin precursor. *Nature (London), 278*, 423–427.

Noda M, Furutani Y, Takahashi H, Toyosato M, Hirose T, Inayama S, Shigetada S, Numa S (1982): Cloning and sequence analysis of cDNA for bovine adrenal preproenkephalin. *Nature (London), 295*, 202–206.

Oertel WH, Schmechel DE, Mugnaini E, Tappaz ML, Kopin IJ (1981): Immunocytochemical localization of glutamate decarboxylase in rat cerebellum with a new antiserum. *Neuroscience, 6*, 2715–2735.

Oppenheim RW, Maderdrut JL, Wells DJ (1982): Cell death of motoneurons in the chick embryo spinal cord. VI. Reduction of naturally-occurring cell death in the thoracolumbar column of Terni by nerve growth factor. *J. Comp. Neurol., 210*, 174–189.

Ordronneau P, Petrusz P (1980): Immunocytochemical demonstration of anterior pituitary hormones in the pars tuberalis of long-term hypophysectomized rats. *Am. J. Anat., 158*, 491–506.

330

Ordronneau P, Lindström PBM, Petrusz P (1981): Four unlabelled antibody bridge techniques: a comparison. *J. Histochem. Cytochem., 29*, 1397–1404.

Palkovits M, Epelbaum J, Gros C (1981): Met-enkephalin concentrations in individual brain nuclei of ansa lenticularis and stria terminalis transected rats. *Brain Res., 216*, 203–209.

Palmer MR, Miller RJ, Olson L, Seiger A (1982): Prenatal ontogeny of neurons with enkephalin-like immunoreactivity in the rat central nervous system: an immunohistochemical mapping investigation. *Med. Biol., 60*, 61–88.

Panula P, Lindberg I, Yang HYT, Costa E (1983): Enkephalins in the pituitary gland: immunohistochemical and biochemical characterization. *Neurosci. Abstracts, 9 (Part 1)*, 438.

Pert CB, Snyder SH (1973): Opiate receptors: demonstration in nervous tissues. *Science, 179*, 1011–1014.

Pert CB, Aposhian D, Snyder SH (1974): Phylogenetic distribution of opiate receptor binding. *Brain Res., 75*, 356–361.

Pert CB, Kuhar MJ, Snyder SH (1975): Autoradiographic localization of the opiate receptor in rat brain. *Life Sci., 16*, 1849–1854.

Petrusz P, Sar M, Ordronneau P, DiMeo P (1976): Specificity in immunocytochemical staining. *J. Histochem. Cytochem., 24*, 1110–1115.

Petrusz P, Ordronneau P, Finley JCW (1980): Criteria of reliability for light microscopic immunocytochemical staining. *Histochem. J., 12*, 333–348.

Pfaff DW (1968): Autoradiographic localization of radioactivity in rat brain after injection of tritiated sex hormones. *Science, 161*, 1355–1356.

Pfeiffer A, Herz A (1981): Demonstration and distribution of an opiate binding site with high affinity for ethylketocyclazocine and SKF 10,047. *Biochem. Biophys. Res. Commun., 101*, 38–44.

Pickel VM, Joh TH, Reis DJ, Leeman SF, Miller RJ (1979): Electron microscopic localization of substance P and enkephalin in axon terminals related to dendrites of catecholaminergic neurons. *Brain Res., 160*, 387–400.

Pickel VM, Sumal KK, Beady SC, Miller RJ, Reis DJ (1980a): Immunocytochemical localization of enkephalin in the neostriatum of rat brain: a light and electron microscopic study. *J. Comp. Neurol., 189*, 721–740.

Pickel VM, Sumal KK, Reis DJ, Miller RJ, Hervonen A (1980b): Immunocytochemical localization of enkephalin and substance P in the dorsal tegmental nuclei in human fetal brain. *J. Comp. Neurol., 193*, 805–814.

Pickel VM, Miller R, Chan J, Sumal KK (1983): Substance P and enkephalin in transected axons of medulla and spinal cord. *Regul. Peptides, 6*, 121–135.

Pittius CW, Seizinger BR, Mehraein P, Pasi A, Herz A (1983): Proenkephalin-A-derived peptides are present in human brain. *Life Sci., 33, Suppl. 1*, 41–44.

Poulain P, Martin-Bouyer L, Beauvillain JC, Tramu G (1984): Study of the efferent connections of the enkephalinergic magnocellular dorsal nucleus in the guinea-pig hypothalamus using lesions, retrograde tracing and immunohistochemistry: evidence for a projection to the lateral septum. *Neuroscience, 11*, 331–343.

Przewlocki R, Gramsch C, Pasi A, Herz A (1983): Characterization and localization of immunoreactive dynorphin, α-endorphin, Met-enkephalin and substance P in human spinal cord. *Brain Res., 280*, 95–103.

Quirion R, Weiss AS (1983): Peptide E and other proenkephalin-derived peptides are potent kappa opiate receptor agonists. *Peptides, 4*, 445–449.

Reaves TA, Hayward JN (1979a): Immunocytochemical identification of enkephalinergic neurons in the hypothalamic magnocellular preoptic nucleus of the goldfish, *Carassius auratus. Cell Tissue Res., 200*, 147–151.

Reaves TA, Hayward JN (1979b): Intracellular dye-marked enkephalin neurons in the magnocellular preoptic nucleus of the goldfish hypothalamus. *Proc. Natl Acad. Sci. USA, 76*, 6009–6011.

Reiner A (1983): Comparative studies of opioid peptides: enkephalin distribution in turtle central nervous system. *Neurosci. Abstracts, 9 (Part 1)*, 439.

Reiner A, Brecha NC, Karten HJ (1982a): Basal ganglia pathways to the tectum: the afferent and efferent connections of the lateral spiriform nucleus of the pigeon. *J. Comp. Neurol., 208*, 16–36.

Reiner A, Karten HJ, Brecha NC (1982b): Enkephalin-mediated basal ganglia influences over the optic tectum: immunohistochemistry of the tectum and the lateral spiriform nucleus in pigeon. *J. Comp. Neurol., 208*, 37–53.

Roberts GW, Woodhams PL, Polak JM, Crow TJ (1982): Distribution of neuropeptides in the limbic system of the rat: the amygdaloid complex. *Neuroscience, 7*, 99–131.

Roberts GW, Allen Y, Crow TJ, Polak JM (1983): Immunocytochemical localization of neuropeptides in the fornix of the rat, monkey and man. *Brain Res., 263*, 151–155.

Roberts GW, Woodhams PL, Polak JM, Crow TJ (1984): Distribution of neuropeptides in the limbic system of the rat: the hippocampus. *Neuroscience, 11*, 35–77.

Roisin MP, Artola A, Henry JP, Rossier J (1983): Enkephalins are associated with adrenergic granules in bovine adrenal medulla. *Neuroscience, 10*, 83–88.

Romagnano MA, Chafel TL, Pilcher WH, Joseph SA (1982): The distribution of enkephalin in the mediobasal hypothalamus of the mouse brain: effects of neonatal administration of MSG. *Brain Res., 236*, 497–504.

Romagnano MA, Hamill RW (1983): The immunocytochemical distribution of enkephalin in the thoracolumbar spinal cord of the rat: coincidence with sympathetic preganglionic nuclear regions. *Neurosci. Abstracts, 9 (Part 1)*, 440.

Rosen H, Douglass J, Herbert E (1984): Isolation and characterization of the rat proenkephalin gene. *J. Biol. Chem., 259*, 14309–14313.

Rossier J, Battenberg E, Pittman Q, Bayon A, Koda L, Miller R, Guillemin R, Bloom FE (1979): Hypothalamic enkephalin neurons may regulate the neurohypophysis. *Nature (London), 277*, 653–654.

Rossier J, Audigier Y, Ling N, Cros J, Udenfriend S (1980a): Met-enkephalin-Arg[6]-Phe[7], present in high amounts in brain of rat, cattle and man, is an opioid agonist. *Nature (London), 288*, 88–90.

Rossier J, Pittman Q, Bloom F, Guillemin R (1980b): Distribution of opioid peptides in the pituitary: a new hypothalamic-pars nervosa enkephalinergic pathway. *Fed. Proc., 39*, 2555–2560.

Rossier J, Liston D, Patey G, Chaminade M, Foutz AS, Cupo A, Giraud P, Roisin MP, Henry JP, Verbanck P, Vanderhaeghen JJ (1983): The enkephalinergic neuron: implications of a polyenkephalin precursor. *Cold Spring Harbor Symp. Quant. Biol., 48*, 393–404.

Ruda M (1982): Opiates and pain pathways: demonstration of enkephalin synapses on dorsal horn projection neurons. *Science, 215*, 1523–1525.

Ruda MA, Coffield J, Bennett GJ, Dubner R (1983): Role of serotonin (5-HT) and enkephalin (ENK) in trigeminal and spinal pain pathways. *J. Dent. Res., 62*, 691.

Sabol SL, Yoshikawa K, Hong JS (1983): Regulation of methionine-enkephalin precursor messenger RNA in rat striatum by haloperidol and lithium. *Biochem. Biophys. Res. Commun., 113*, 391–399.

Saito K, Barber R, Wu JY, Matsuda T, Roberts E, Vaughn JE (1974): Immunohistochemical localization of glutamic acid decarboxylase in rat cerebellum. *Proc. Natl Acad. Sci. USA, 71*, 269–273.

Sakanaka M, Senba E, Shiosaka S, Takatsuki K, Inagaki S, Takagi H, Hara Y, Tohyama M (1982): Evidence for the existence of an enkephalin-containing pathway from the area just ventrolateral to the anterior hypothalamic nucleus to the lateral septal area of the rat. *Brain Res., 239*, 240–244.

Sar M, Stumpf WE, Miller RJ, Chang KJ, Cuatrecasas P (1978): Immunohistochemical localization of enkephalin in rat brain and spinal cord. *J. Comp. Neurol., 182*, 17–38.

Sawchenko PE, Swanson LW (1982): Immunohistochemical identification of neurons in the paraventricular nucleus of the hypothalamus that project to the medulla or to the spinal cord in the rat. *J. Comp. Neurol., 205*, 260–272.

Schulman JA, Finger TE, Brecha NC, Karten HJ (1981): Enkephalin immunoreactivity in Golgi cells and mossy fibers of mammalian, avian, amphibian and teleost cerebellum. *Neuroscience, 6*, 2407–2416.

Seizinger BR, Grimm C, Höllt V, Herz A (1984): Evidence for a selective processing of proenkephalin B into different opioid peptide forms in particular regions of rat brain and pituitary. *J. Neurochem., 42*, 447–457.

Senba E, Tohyama M (1983): Reticulo-facial enkephalinergic pathway in the rat: an experimental immunohistochemical study. *Neuroscience, 10*, 831–839.

Seybold V, Elde RP (1980): Immunohistochemical studies of peptidergic neurons in the dorsal horn of the spinal cord. *J. Histochem. Cytochem., 28*, 267–370.

Simantov R, Goodman R, Aposhian D, Snyder SH (1976): Phylogenetic distribution of a morphine-like peptide 'enkephalin'. *Brain Res., 111*, 204–211.

Simantov R, Kuhar MJ, Uhl GR, Snyder SH (1977): Opioid peptide enkephalin: immunohistochemical mapping in rat central nervous system. *Proc. Natl Acad. Sci. USA, 74*, 2167–2171.

Simon EJ, Hiller JM, Edelman I (1973): Stereospecific binding of the potent narcotic analgesic [³H]-etorphine to rat brain homogenates. *Proc. Natl Acad. Sci. USA, 70*, 1947–1949.

Snyder SH (1984): Drug and neurotransmitter receptors in the brain. *Science, 224*, 22–31.

Sofroniew MV, Glassman W (1981): Golgi-like immunoperoxidase staining of hypothalamic magnocellular neurons that contain vasopressin, oxytocin or neurphysin in the rat. *Neuroscience, 6*, 619–643.

Somogyi P, Priestley JV, Cuello AC, Smith AD, Takagi H (1982): Synaptic connections of enkephalin-immunoreactive nerve terminals in the neostriatum: a correlated light and electron microscopic study. *J. Neurocytol., 11*, 779–807.

Stefano GB, Leung MK (1984): Presence of Met-enkephalin-Arg[6]-Phe[7] in molluscan neural tissues. *Brain Res., 298*, 362–365.

Stengaard-Pedersen K, Larsson LI (1981): Comparative immunocytochemical localization of putative opioid ligands in the central nervous system. *Histochemistry, 73*, 89–114.

Stengaard-Pedersen K, Larsson LI (1983): Met- and Leu-enkephalinergic innervation of the lateral septal nucleus. *Brain Res., 264,* 152–156.

Stern AS, Lewis RV, Kimura LS, Rossier J, Gerber LD, Brink L, Stein S, Udenfriend S (1979): Isolation of the opioid heptapeptide Met-enkephalin (Arg^6,Phe^7) from bovine adrenal medullary granules and striatum. *Proc. Natl Acad. Sci. USA, 76,* 6680–6683.

Sternberger LA (1979): *Immunocytochemistry. 2nd Ed.* John Wiley, New York.

Sumal KK, Pickel VM, Miller RJ, Reis DJ (1982): Enkephalin-containing neurons in substantia gelatinosa of spinal trigeminal complex: ultrastructure and synaptic interactions with primary sensory afferents. *Brain Res., 248,* 223–236.

Supattapone S, Fricker LD, Snyder SH (1984): Purification and characterization of a membrane-bound enkephalin-forming carboxypeptidase, 'enkephalin convertase'. *J. Neurochem., 42,* 1017–1023.

Swanson LW, Kuypers HGJM (1980): The paraventricular nucleus of the hypothalamus: cytoarchitectonic subdivisions and the organization of projections to the pituitary, dorsal vagal complex and spinal cord as demonstrated by retrograde fluorescence double-labelling methods. *J. Comp. Neurol., 194,* 555–570.

Tang F, Costa E, Schwartz JP (1983): Increase of proenkephalin mRNA and enkephalin content of rat striatum after daily injection of haloperidol for 2 to 3 weeks. *Proc. Natl Acad. Sci. USA, 80,* 3841–3844.

Tatemoto K, Mutt V (1981): Isolation and characterization of the intestinal peptide porcine PHI (PHI-27), a new member of the glucagon-secretin family. *Proc. Natl Acad. Sci. USA, 78,* 6603–6607.

Terenius L (1973): Stereospecific interaction between narcotic analgesics and a synaptic plasma membrane fraction of rat cerebral cortex. *Acta Pharmacol. Toxicol., 32,* 317–320.

Tielen AM, Van Leeuwen FW, Lopes da Silva FH (1982): The localization of leucine-enkephalin immunoreactivity within the guinea pig hippocampus. *Exp. Brain Res., 48,* 288–295.

Tramu G, Leonardelli J (1979): Immunohistochemical localization of enkephalins in median eminence and adenohypophysis of the guinea pig. *Brain Res., 168,* 457–471.

Tramu G, Pillez A, Leonardelli J (1978): An efficient method of antibody elution for the successive or simultaneous localization of two antigens by immunocytochemistry. *J. Histochem. Cytochem., 26,* 322–324.

Tramu G, Beauvillain JC, Croix D, Leonardelli J (1981): Comparative immunocytochemical localization of enkephalin and somatostatin in the median eminence, hypothalamus and adjacent areas of the guinea pig brain. *Brain Res., 215,* 235–255.

Troy CM, Musacchio JM (1982): Processing of enkephalin precursors by chromaffin granule enzymes. *Life Sci., 31,* 1717–1720.

Udenfriend S, Kilpatrick DL (1983): Biochemistry of the enkephalins and enkephalin-containing peptides. *Arch. Biochem. Biophys., 221,* 309–323.

Uhl GR, Kuhar MJ, Snyder SH (1978): Enkephalin-containing pathway: amygdaloid efferents in the stria terminalis. *Brain Res., 149,* 223–228.

Uhl GR, Goodman RR, Kuhar MJ, Childers SR, Snyder SH (1979): Immunocytochemical mapping of enkephalin containing cell bodies, fibers and nerve terminals in the brain stem of the rat. *Brain Res., 116,* 75–94.

Vanderhaeghen JJ, Lotstra F, Liston DR, Rossier J (1983): Proenkephalin, [Met]-enkephalin, and oxytocin immunoreactivities are colocalized in bovine hypothalamic magnocellular neurons. *Proc. Natl Acad. Sci. USA, 80,* 5139–5143.

Vandesande R, Dierickx K (1975): Identification of the vasopressin producing and of the oxytocin producing neurons in the hypothalamic magnocellular neurosecretory system of the rat. *Cell Tissue Res., 164,* 153–162.

Van Leeuwen FW, Pool CW, Sluiter AA (1983): Enkephalin immunoreactivity in synaptoid elements on glial cells in the rat neural lobe. *Neuroscience, 8,* 229–241.

Veening JG, Swanson LW, Sawchenko PE (1984): The organization of projections from the central nucleus of the amygdala to brainstem sites involved in central autonomic regulation: a combined retrograde transport-immunohistochemical study. *Brain Res., 303,* 337–357.

Vigh S, Merchenthaler I, Torres-Aleman I, Sueiras-Diaz J, Coy DH, Carter WH, Petrusz P, Schally AV (1982): Corticotropin releasing factor (CRF): immunocytochemical localization and radioimmunoassay (RIA). *Life Sci., 31,* 2441–2448.

Vincent SR, Hökfelt T, Christensson I, Terenius L (1982): Dynorphin-immunoreactive neurons in the central nervous system of the rat. *Neurosci. Lett., 33,* 185–190.

Watson SJ, Akil H, Sullivan S, Barchas JD (1977): Immunocytochemical localization of methionine-enkephalin: preliminary observations. *Life Sci., 25,* 733–738.

Watson SJ, Akil H, Fischli W, Goldstein A, Zimmerman E, Nilaver G, Van Wimersma Greidanus TB (1982): Dynorphin and vasopressin: common localization in magnocellular neurons. *Science, 216,* 85–87.

Watson SJ, Khachaturian H, Taylor L, Fischli W, Goldstein A, Akil H (1983): Pro-dynorphin peptides are found in the same neurons throughout rat brain: immunocytochemical study. *Proc. Natl Acad. Sci. USA, 80,* 891–894.

Wamsley JK, Young WS, Kuhar MJ (1980): Immunohistochemical localization of enkephalin in rat forebrain. *Brain Res., 190*, 153–174.

Weber E, Barchas JD (1983): Immunohistochemical distribution of dynorphin B in rat brain: relation to dynorphin A and α-neo-endorphin systems. *Proc. Natl Acad. Sci. USA, 80*, 1125–1129.

Weber E, Voigt KH, Martin R (1978): Pituitary somatotrophs contain (Met)-enkephalin-like immunoreactivity. *Proc. Natl Acad. Sci. USA, 75*, 6134–6138.

Weber E, Evans CJ, Samuelsson SJ, Barchas JD (1981a): Novel peptide neuronal system in rat brain and pituitary. *Science, 214*, 1248–1251.

Weber E, Roth KA, Barchas JD (1981b): Colocalization of α-neo-endorphin and dynorphin immunoreactivity in hypothalamic neurons. *Biochem. Biophys. Res. Commun., 103*, 951–958.

Weber E, Evans CJ, Chang JK, Barchas JD (1982): Brain distribution of α-neo-endorphin and β-neo-endorphin: evidence for regional processing difference. *Biochem. Biophys. Res. Commun., 108*, 81–88.

Weber E, Evans CJ, Barchas JD (1983a): Multiple endogenous ligands for opioid receptors. *Trends Neurosci., 6*, 333–336.

Weber E, Esch FS, Böhlen P, Paterson S, Corbett A, McKnight AT, Kosterlitz HW, Barchas JD, Evans CJ (1983b): Metorphamide: isolation, structure and biologic activity of an amidated opioid octapeptide from bovine brain. *Proc. Natl Acad. Sci. USA, 80*, 7362–7366

Whitnall MH, Gainer H, Cox BM, Molineaux CJ (1983): Dynorphin-A-(1–8) is contained within vasopressin neurosecretory vesicles in rat pituitary. *Science, 222*, 1137–1138.

Willard FH, Ho RH, Martin GF (1984): The neuronal types and the distribution of 5-hydroxytryptamine and enkephalin-like immunoreactive fibers in the dorsal cochlear nucleus of the North American opossum. *Brain. Res. Bull., 12*, 253–266.

Williams RG, Dockray GJ (1982): Differential distribution in rat basal ganglia of Met-enkephalin- and Met-enkephalin Arg[6]Phe[7]-like peptides revealed by immunohistochemistry. *Brain Res., 240*, 167–170.

Williams RG, Dockray GJ (1983a): Distribution of enkephalin-related peptides in rat brain: immunohistochemical studies using antisera to Met-enkephalin and Met–enkephalin Arg[6]Phe[7]. *Neuroscience, 9*, 563–586.

Williams RG, Dockray GJ (1983b): Immunohistochemical studies of FMRF-amide-like immunoreactivity in rat brain. *Brain Res., 276*, 213–229.

Wilson SP, Chang KJ, Viveros OH (1982): Proportional secretion of opioid peptides and catecholamines from adrenal chromaffin cells in culture. *J. Neurosci., 2*, 1150–1156.

Wood PL (1982): Multiple opiate receptors: support for unique mu, delta and kappa sites. *Neuropharmacology, 21*, 487–497.

Woodhams RL, Roberts GW, Polak JM, Crow TJ (1983): Distribution of neuropeptides in the limbic system of the rat: the bed nucleus of the stria terminalis, septum and preoptic area. *Neuroscience, 8*, 677–703.

Wray S, Hoffman GE (1983): Organization and interrelationships of neuropeptides in the central amygdaloid nucleus of the rat. *Peptides, 4*, 525–541.

Wray S, Schwaber J, Hoffman G (1981): Neuropeptide localization in the rat central amygdaloid nucleus. *Anat. Rec., 199*, 282A.

Yang HYT, Panula P, Tang J, Costa E (1983): Characterization and location of Met[5]-enkephalin-Arg[6]-Phe[7] stored in various rat brain regions. *J. Neurochem., 40*, 969–976.

Yoshikawa K, Williams C, Sabol SL (1984): Rat brain preproenkephalin messenger RNA: cDNA cloning, primary structure, and distribution in the central nervous system. *J. Biol. Chem., 259*, 14301–14308.

Yoshikawa K, Hong JS, Sabol SL (1985): Electroconvulsive shock increases preproenkephalin messenger RNA abundance in rat hypothalamus. *Proc. Natl Acad. Sci. USA, 82*, 589–593.

Young WS, Kuhar MJ (1979): A new method for receptor autoradiography: [³H]-opioid receptors in rat brain. *Brain Res., 179*, 255–270.

Zamir N, Palkovits M, Brownstein M (1983a): Comparison of the distribution of prodynorphin and proenkephalin derived peptides in the rat central nervous system. *Neurosci. Abstracts, 9 (Part 1)*, 440.

Zamir N, Palkovits M, Brownstein MJ (1983b): Distribution of immunoreactive dynorphin in the central nervous system of the rat. *Brain Res., 280*, 81–93.

Zamir N, Palkovits M, Weber E, Mezey E, Brownstein MJ (1984): A dynorphinergic pathway of Leu-enkephalin production in rat substantia nigra. *Nature (London), 307*, 643–645.

CHAPTER VII

VIP-containing neurons*

GARY M. ABRAMS, GAJANAN NILAVER AND EARL A. ZIMMERMAN

1. INTRODUCTION

Vasoactive intestinal polypeptide (VIP) is a 28 amino acid peptide, originally isolated from porcine duodenum (Said and Mutt 1970a). It was initially noted to have potent vasodilatory activity on peripheral and splanchnic circulations (Said and Mutt 1970b), thus accounting for its name. The amino acid sequence was established (Mutt and Said 1974) and VIP was subsequently synthesized (Bodanszky et al. 1974). Porcine VIP is a basic, linear polypeptide which shares structural homologies with secretin, glucagon, gastric inhibitory peptide (Mutt and Said 1974), and PHI(1–27) (Tatemoto and Mutt 1980). Avian VIP (Nilsson 1977), bovine VIP (Carlquist et al. 1979), and human VIP (Carlquist et al. 1982) have also been characterized. A number of molecular variants of VIP have been isolated from intestines of several species, however, the octacosapeptide is the predominant form found in the central nervous system (Dimaline and Dockray 1979; Maletti et al. 1980).

VIP was originally localized in gastrointestinal nerves and the central nervous system of several mammalian species using radioimmunoassay (RIA) and immunohistochemical techniques (Bryant et al. 1976; Larsson et al. 1976a; Fuxe et al. 1977). Immunoreactive VIP is now known to be widely distributed throughout the central nervous system (Said and Rosenberg 1976; Bryant et al. 1976; Fahrenkrug and Schaffalitzky de Muckadell 1978). It is also present in the nervous system of invertebrates (Sundler et al. 1977), and is widespread in vertebrate peripheral nervous system (Larsson et al. 1976a; Bryant et al. 1976; Fuxe et al. 1977). Several comprehensive immunohistochemical mapping studies of VIP in rat central nervous system have been reported and will be reviewed (Lorén et al. 1979; Roberts et al. 1980a; Sims et al. 1980).

The evidence that VIP may function as a neurotransmitter or neuromodulator in the central nervous system has become increasingly compelling. Giachetti et al. (1977) showed that intraneuronal VIP was predominantly localized in purified synaptosomal fractions and could be released by potassium depolarization in a calcium-dependent manner. Emson et al. (1977) also demonstrated VIP in an enriched synaptosomal preparation from hypothalamus and showed potassium-induced calcium-dependent release of the peptide from superfused hypothalamic slices. VIP can also be released from similar preparations by a variety of depolarizing agents, and this neuropharmacological profile

*Work in our laboratories is supported by USPHS grants HD 13147 and NS18324, and a Parkinson's Disease Foundation Grant to Columbia University. G.M.A. is a recipient of a Teacher Investigator Development Award K07-00478.

Handbook of Chemical Neuroanatomy. Vol. 4: GABA and Neuropeptides in the CNS, Part I.
A. Björklund and T. Hökfelt, editors.
© Elsevier Science Publishers B.V., 1985.

is consistent with a neurotransmitter type of release (Besson et al. 1982).

VIP binds specifically and reversibly to receptors in guinea pig and rat brain membranes (Robberecht et al. 1978; Taylor and Pert 1979). The regional distribution of VIP receptors in brain is heterogeneous, with high concentrations in striatum, hippocampus, and cortex, and very low levels in cerebellum and lower brainstem (Taylor and Pert 1979). Some VIP receptors are linked with the adenylate cyclase-cAMP system. VIP activates an adenylate cyclase from synaptosomal fraction of guinea pig brain (Deschodt-Lanckman et al. 1977). Rat brain slices from cortex, hypothalamus, and striatum will accumulate cAMP when incubated with VIP (Quik et al. 1978). Homogenates of rat cortex, hypothalamus, hippocampus, and cerebellum show increased adenylate cyclase activity when stimulated with VIP, while no stimulation occurs in caudate nucleus or brain stem (Borghi et al. 1979). Adenylate cyclase is reportedly most sensitive to VIP stimulation in the olfactory bulb and hippocampus, and least sensitive in cerebellum and spinal cord. In the hypothalamus, VIP-sensitive adenylate cyclase seems partially localized on noradrenergic neurons (Kerwin et al. 1980). Paradoxically, VIP receptors seem to be most highly concentrated in the striatum, an area neither rich in VIP content by RIA or in VIP-linked adenylate cyclase activity. A recent study has shown that microinjections of VIP into the caudate nucleus can increase glucose utilization in selected brain regions (McCulloch et al. 1983).

Phillis initially demonstrated an excitatory action for VIP when iontophoretically applied to cortical neurons (Phillis et al. 1978). Dodd et al. (1979) reported excitation of hippocampal CA1 neurons by VIP. VIP shows excitatory and inhibitory effects when applied to selected neurons in the preoptic, midbrain central gray, or septal regions. The latency and duration of the VIP-induced response is generally characterized by a rapid onset which occasionally may persist beyond the duration of the ejection (Haskins et al. 1982). VIP will induce long duration excitation of nociceptive and non-nociceptive neurons in the trigeminal nucleus caudalis (Salt and Hill 1981). In the spinal cord, iontophoresis or pressure ejection of VIP causes excitation of 75% of all neurons in laminae I–VII of cat and rat spinal cord preparations. VIP depolarizes dorsal horn neurons in the rat and increases their firing rate (Jeftinija et al. 1982). Most neurons seem to be excited by VIP, although inhibitory responses have been observed at selected sites (Haskins et al. 1982).

The mechanism for inactivation of VIP is unknown. Quik and Fahrenkrug reported 50% degradation of VIP in 4–15 minutes when incubated with various slices of rat brain (Fahrenkrug 1979). A highly specific enzyme for degrading VIP has been found in brain extracts (Keltz et al. 1980). However, the mechanism for the physiological inactivation of VIP at the synaptic level is a matter of speculation. VIP is similar to other putative peptide neurotransmitters in that there is no presynaptic re-uptake system. At present it is evident that VIP fulfills many of the agreed specifications for a potential neurotransmitter or neuromodulator in the central nervous system (Gainer 1977).

The broad biological activity of VIP in the central nervous system is an area of active investigation. VIP-containing neurons have a close association with the vasculature based on morphological studies (Larsson 1976b), and it has been suggested that VIP plays a local vasoregulatory role in the brain (Heistad et al. 1980; McCulloch and Edvinsson 1980; Wilson et al. 1981). VIP induces dose-dependent relaxation of isolated middle cerebral arteries in vitro (Larsson et al. 1976b) and is a potent dilator of pial arterioles when topically applied in vivo (Wei et al. 1980). The latter effect is abolished by cyclo-oxygenase inhibitors, and thus appears to be mediated by the prostaglandin system (Wei et al. 1980).

A direct neuroendocrine role has been postulated for VIP neurons which project to the hypothalamus and portal hypophyseal system. Intraventricular VIP induces release of prolactin, growth hormone and luteinizing hormone from the pituitary of ovariectomized rats (Kato et al. 1978; Vijayan et al. 1979). Consistent with these observations, VIP inhibits the release of somatostatin from hypothalamus in vitro (Epelbaum et al. 1979; Shimatsu et al. 1982), and stimulates release of LH-RH from median eminence synaptosomes (Samson et al. 1981). VIP is present in the median eminence (Samson et al. 1979) and also in portal capillary blood (Said and Porter 1979; Shimatsu et al. 1981). Pituitary adenylate cyclase activity is stimulated by VIP (Borghi et al. 1979) and VIP will directly release prolactin from the pituitary gland (Ruberg et al. 1978). Corticosteroids and estrogen have been reported to modulate VIP content in discrete brain regions, suggesting a regulatory system for VIP neurons which is influenced by peripheral endocrine secretion (Rotsztejn et al. 1980; Maletti et al. 1982). Nevertheless, a distinct role for VIP in modulation of hypothalamic pituitary function has not been fully established.

Finally, VIP may play a role in local regulation of energy metabolism in the brain. VIP stimulates enzymatic breakdown of glycogen in mouse cerebral cortex slices (Magistretti et al. 1981). Recent studies have demonstrated that microinjections of VIP into the striatum, an area rich in VIP receptors (Taylor and Pert 1979) can increase glucose utilization in selected brain regions (McCulloch et al. 1983). This concept of VIP as a potential modulator of local brain energy metabolism is also supported by observations in baboon, where direct intracarotid infusions of VIP increase cerebral blood flow and activate the EEG, if the blood–brain barrier is compromised.

In summary, diverse roles have been proposed for VIP in the central nervous system. The scant experimental evidence available at present suggests that this neuropeptide may be a regulator of neuroendocrine function, as well as a local modulator of cerebral blood flow and metabolic activity. The true physiological functions of intraneuronal VIP, however, are still unclear and await further investigation.

2. ANATOMY

2.1. GENERAL OVERVIEW

The localization of VIP in the mammalian central nervous system has been accomplished using both RIA and immunohistochemical techniques. Initial reports found the bulk of immunoreactive VIP to be localized in the forebrain, predominantly in the cortex (Said and Rosenberg 1976; Bryant et al. 1976; Fahrenkrug and Schaffalitzky de Muckadell 1978). Immunohistochemical studies showed VIP in cortical (Fuxe et al. 1977) and hypothalamic neurons (Larsson et al. 1976a). More detailed examinations of VIP anatomy in rat brain have subsequently been reported (Lorén et al. 1979; Roberts et al. 1980a; Sims et al. 1980). VIP-rich regions such as the suprachiasmatic nucleus and amygdala have been closely scrutinized using light and electron microscopic techniques (Pelletier et al. 1981; Card et al. 1981; Gray et al. 1982).

Several analyses of specific VIP neuronal pathways have been done using selective stereotaxic lesions (Roberts et al. 1980b; Marley et al. 1981; Palkovits et al. 1981, 1982). A developmental study of VIP neurons has been reported (McGregor et al. 1982) and several groups have detected VIP immunoreactivity in dissociated cell cultures of hypothalamus, midbrain, and spinal cord (Jirikowsky et al. 1982; E. Matthew, personal communication). VIP is present in spinal cord as well as brain, but considerably less is known about its specific anatomical organization (Gibson et al. 1981).

2.2. RADIOIMMUNOASSAY

A summary of the regional distribution of VIP in rat central nervous system is presented in Table 1. The highest concentration of VIP is found in the cerebral cortex (Fahrenkrug and Schaffalitzky de Muckadell 1978). All cortical regions are rich in VIP and this appears to be true in all species that have been examined (Fahrenkrug 1979). On a weight basis, the hippocampus contains substantially less VIP than neocortex in rodents; this, however, does not appear to be true in porcine or human brain (Fahrenkrug 1979). The amygdaloid complex is the area with the highest concentrations of VIP and the central amygdaloid nucleus contains the bulk of immunoreactivity. The bed nucleus of the stria terminalis also has large amounts of the octacosapeptide. Ipsilateral transection of the stria terminalis will markedly reduce VIP in this region (Roberts et al. 1980b; Palkovits et al. 1981) suggesting that this established amygdalofugal pathway is at least partially VIPergic.

The striatum and thalamus, although rich in VIP receptors (Taylor and Pert 1979), do not contain large quantities of VIP. The hypothalamus has a heterogeneous distribution of VIP with the highest concentrations being found in the suprachiasmatic and supraoptic nuclei, as well as the anterior and preoptic areas. Unilateral lesions of the stria terminalis reduce the amount of VIP in both ipsilateral and contralateral suprachiasmatic nuclei. This has been proposed as indicating amygdaloid regulation of VIP synthesis in the suprachiasmatic nucleus (Palkovits et al. 1981). Curiously, the supraoptic nucleus is not an area which is rich in VIP by cytochemical techniques, and the high concentrations of VIP found in this region by RIA may represent limitations of dissection techniques. The median eminence or hypophysiotropic region of the hypothalamus contains modest amounts of VIP (Palkovits et al. 1981), with high levels being detected in portal blood (Said and Porter 1979; Shimatsu et al. 1981).

The distribution of VIP in the brainstem has been studied in detail (Table 2). The dorsal brainstem contains the most VIP, particularly the midbrain gray. The periaqueductal mesencephalon and parabrachial nucleus contain approximately 10–20% as much VIP as the cortex, when measured by RIA employing identical extraction procedures (Eiden et al. 1982). Many other selected brainstem regions have detectable amounts of VIP, although the cerebellum is nearly devoid of this peptide (Eiden et al. 1982). The spinal cord contains modest amounts of VIP. Lorén et al. (1979) have shown that rat cortical VIP is chromatographically identical to porcine duodenal VIP. At present, there have been no reports suggesting that central nervous system VIP immunoreactivity may be due to substances other than the native 28 amino acid peptide.

2.3. IMMUNOCYTOCHEMISTRY

Immunocytochemical mapping of VIP in the central nervous system has been carried out in both rat and mouse. The following anatomical data is primarily based on extensive studies from our laboratory (Sims et al. 1980), and 2 additional comprehensive reports (Lorén et al. 1979; Roberts et al. 1980a). It should be noted that the mapping studies have included the use of axon transport inhibitors (such as colchicine) for demonstration of peptidergic cell bodies at selected sites, and light microscopic observations have been made on both thick (cryostat or Vibratome cut) and paraffin-embedded

TABLE 1. *Regional distribution of vasoactive intestinal polypeptide in rat brain*

Region	VIP (pmol/g weight)		
	Lorén et al. (1979)	Roberts et al. (1980a)	Besson et al. (1979)
Forebrain			
Frontal cortex	111.70 ± 16.58 (5)	37.6 ± 3.7	50.7 ± 6.0 (5)
Parietal cortex	69.43 ± 3.72 (4)	40.1 ± 5.4	79.5 ± 4.5 (5)
Occipital cortex	99.47 ± 7.3 (4)	42.0 ± 4.0	90.0 ± 4.8 (5)
Anterior cingulate cortex	153.85 ± 28.64 (3)		
Posterior cingulate cortex	85.41 ± 9.90 (5)		
Temporal cortex	103.32 ± 18.76 (5)		
Entorhinal cortex	136.61 ± 8.95 (4)		
Pyriform cortex	66.14 ± 23.79 (5)	42.0 ± 4.0	
Insular cortex	143.30 ± 16.25 (4)		
Hippocampus	26.69 ± 6.54 (7)	17.0 ± 3.0	20.7 ± 0.3 (6)
Dentate gyrus	24.24 ± 5.78 (6)		
Subiculum	29.13 ± 9.47 (3)		
Olfactory tubercle	6.80 ± 1.15 (8)		
Olfactory bulb	6.69 ± 0.9 (4)		17.4 ± 2.4 (4)
Lateral olfactory nucleus	20.73 ± 1.54 (4)		
Septum	20.88 ± 6.6 (7)	26.5 ± 5.0	
Bed nucleus	97.04 ± 5.32 (8)		
Nucleus accumbens	11.92 ± 3.58 (6)		
Globus pallidus	10.49 ± 1.78 (8)		
Caudate-putamen	5.51 ± 1.07	8.2 ± 1.1	17.4 ± 2.7 (6)
Amygdala		52.0 ± 7.0	
Central nucleus	104.14 ± 18.66 (4)		
Corticomedial nucleus	29.54 ± 9.53 (8)		
Anterior nucleus	19.14 ± 7.42 (4)		
Basolateral nucleus	33.10 ± 5.79 (4)		
Hypothalamus		10.9 ± 1.0	
Anterior area	15.85 ± 2.37 (8)		
Lateral area	5.10 ± 2.01 (8)		
Magnocellular preoptic	13.68 ± 4.91 (3)		
Lateral preoptic	27.48 ± 18.50 (3)		
Suprachiasmatic nucleus	34.03 ± 20.91 (4)		
Supraoptic nucleus	32.77 ± 15.47 (4)		
Dorsomedial nucleus	6.65 ± 4.12 (4)		
Ventromedial nucleus	5.86 ± 1.13 (3)		
Periventricular nucleus	8.22 ± 3.13 (4)		
Arcuate nucleus	4.70 ± 1.13 (4)		
Mammillary body	2.58 ± 0.96 (4)		
Thalamus		10.0 ± 1.7	10.2 ± 0.9
Dorsal thalamus	8.58 ± 1.11 (7)		
Ventral thalamus	10.73 ± 1.64 (7)		
Habenular nucleus	6.29 ± 1.30 (8)		
Pons		3.9 ± 0.5	
Cerebellum	0.84 ± 0.22 (5)	0.9 ± 0.2	n.d.
Spinal cord	6.21 ± 1.55 (5)		

n.d.: not detectable.

sections. Although a variety of fixatives and antisera have been employed, the immuno-cytochemical studies in general have yielded comparable results. Since the mapping of VIP in all these studies is based on immunoreactivity alone, the localization properly

TABLE 2. *Distribution of vasoactive intestinal polypeptide in rat brainstem nuclei*

Region	VIP (pmol/g weight)
Midbrain	
Central gray (rostral)	33.38 ± 3.45 (6)
Central gray (middle)	52.09 ± 5.98 (6)
Ventral tegmental area	14.40 ± 0.97 (6)
Red nucleus	6.82 ± 1.52 (6)
Pons	
Dorsal raphae nucleus	41.19 ± 3.31 (6)
Parabrachial nucleus	33.38 ± 3.31 (5)
Locus ceruleus	26.25 ± 2.02 (5)
Dorsal tegmental nucleus	20.66 ± 1.80 (6)
Motor nucleus of V	13.08 ± 1.25 (6)
Motor nucleus of VII	15.07 ± 2.54 (6)
Pontine reticular nucleus	8.93 ± 1.34 (6)
Cuneiform nucleus	8.27 ± 0.44 (6)
Sensory nucleus of V	5.53 ± 1.37 (6)
Medulla	
Nucleus of the solitary tract	26.07 ± 4.69 (6)
Area postrema	25.89 ± 2.48 (5)
Gracile nucleus	26.46 ± 3.13 (5)
Nucleus raphae magnus	15.79 ± 2.70 (6)
Lateral reticular nucleus	15.31 ± 1.25 (6)
Gigantocellular reticular nucleus	9.44 ± 2.12 (6)
Superior olive	4.00 ± 0.52 (6)
Inferior olive	8.09 ± 1.59 (6)
Nucleus of spinal tract of V	3.67 ± 0.33 (6)
Lateral vestibular nucleus	7.55 ± 1.92 (6)
Motor nucleus of XII	25.41 ± 2.84 (6)

(From Eiden et al. (1982), by courtesy of the Editors of *Brain Research*.)

refers only to 'VIP-like' (or VIP-related) immunoreactivity, although well characterized specific antisera to VIP have been employed. Distribution of VIP neurons in various brain regions is schematically represented in the Atlas.

Atlas. Coronal plane sections of rat brain schematic mapping of VIP neurons (*), fibers ($\cdots$), and tracts (====). *For abbreviations*, see the General Abbreviations List, p. 609.

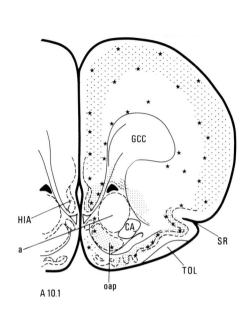

A 10.1

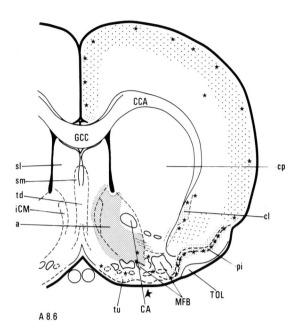

A 8.6

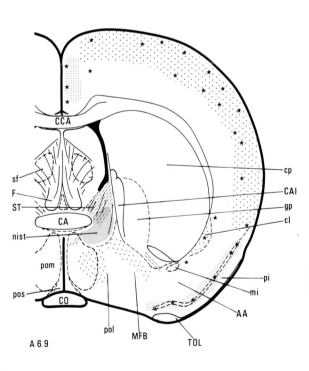

A 6.9

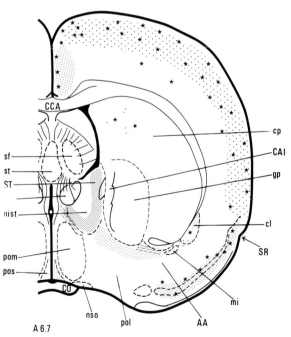

A 6.7

341

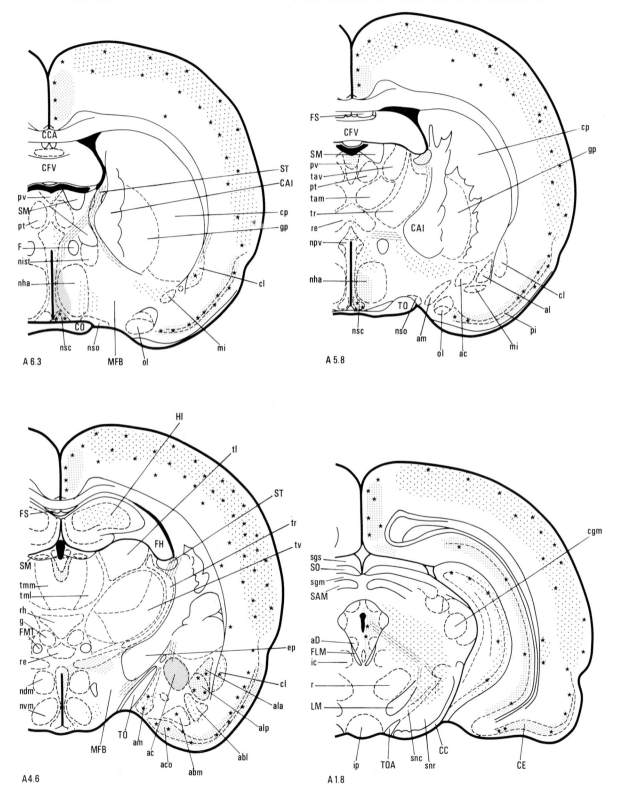

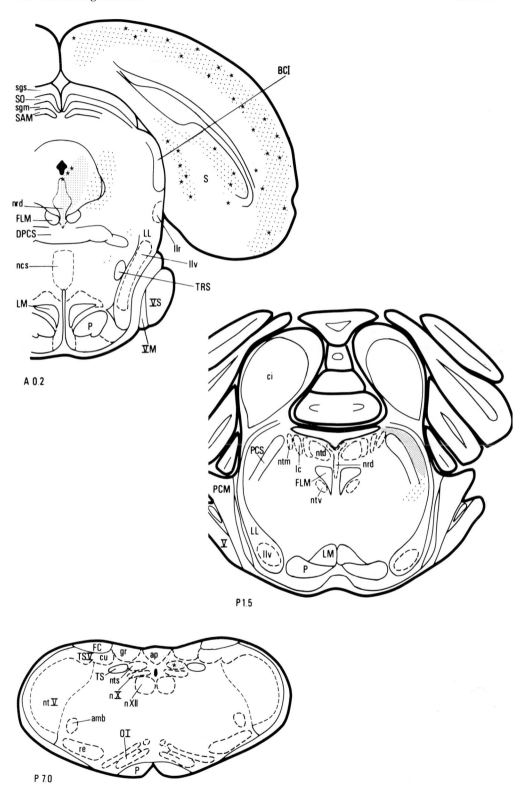

A 0.2

P 1.5

P 7.0

3. LOCALIZATION OF CELL BODIES

3.1. CEREBRAL CORTEX (*Fig. 1*)

The cerebral cortex has the greatest number of VIP immunoreactive neurons. Neocortical VIP perikarya are seen in lamina II–IV with the largest concentration being found in layers II and III. The typical immunoreactive neurons in these layers are fusiform and bipolar with long radially oriented processes. Many are perpendicular to the cortical surface and the processes from these cells frequently run through the upper cortical layers to the pial margin. A second cell type described by Lorén et al. (1979) is a stellate-shaped neuron with multiple processes, also localized in layers II and III.

The older 'limbic' cortex has a moderate, uneven distribution of VIP neurons. The pyriform cortex has a dense concentration of immunoreactive neurons oriented similarly to the ones in the neocortex. The cingulate cortex has a moderate number of VIP neurons predominantly located in lamina II. A cingulate bundle, lying dorsal to the corpus callosum, appears to connect the prefrontal with more caudal areas of the cortex when brains are examined in sagittal sections. The entorhinal cortex contains a homogeneous group of cells with fibers that appear to course towards the hippocampus. The anterior olfactory nucleus is rich in VIP cells with fibers projecting to the olfactory bulb. Sims et al. (1980) reported the presence of VIP cell bodies in the olfactory tubercle. The claustrum is densely filled with VIP neurons and many of these are multi-processed with morphology similar to the stellate cells of the neocortex.

Lorén et al. (1979) have speculated that the dominant VIP neuron seen in the cortex corresponds to the non-spiny bipolar neuron described in Golgi studies (Feldman and Peters 1978). These neurons would be classified as interneurons and give rise to intracortical projections. Lorén et al. (1979) have also described a long cortical projection via the corpus callosum. Lesion studies isolating the cortex, however, suggest that the VIP neuronal population in this region are exclusively interneurons and have local ipsilateral terminations.

3.2. HIPPOCAMPUS (*Fig. 1*)

The dorsal hippocampus is packed with medium-sized VIP neurons which are neither characteristically fusiform nor bipolar. The typical neurons seen in the remainder of the hippocampus are morphologically similar to those that are found in other cortical regions. The dentate gyrus contains smaller VIP cells than the hippocampus proper, some of which seem to correspond to basket cells (Lorén et al. 1979). The subiculum is densely packed with VIP perikarya and appears to be a transition zone from the neocortex.

On a cytoarchitectonic level, the CA1 region contains the largest number of VIP neurons with many of the multipolar variety. Lorén et al. (1979) have noted that the VIP neurons in stratum oriens and stratum pyramidale resemble the short-axoned polygonal cells described by Lorente de No (1934) and Ramón y Cajal (1955). Some are thought to be basket cells with terminals in the pyramidal layer and others may be polygonal cells with terminations in the dendritic region. Lorente de No (1934), using Golgi methods, described locally projecting cells in the stratum lacunosum moleculare of CA1 which also appear to be reactive for VIP. The CA3 region seems to have lesser numbers of VIP-positive neurons than CA1. In the dentate region, VIP reactivity is seen in three types of neurons: short axon neurons in the molecular layer, the basket cells, and horizontal cells in the subgranular and polymorph layers (Lorén et al. 1979). Extrahippocampal projections from these neurons have not been described.

344

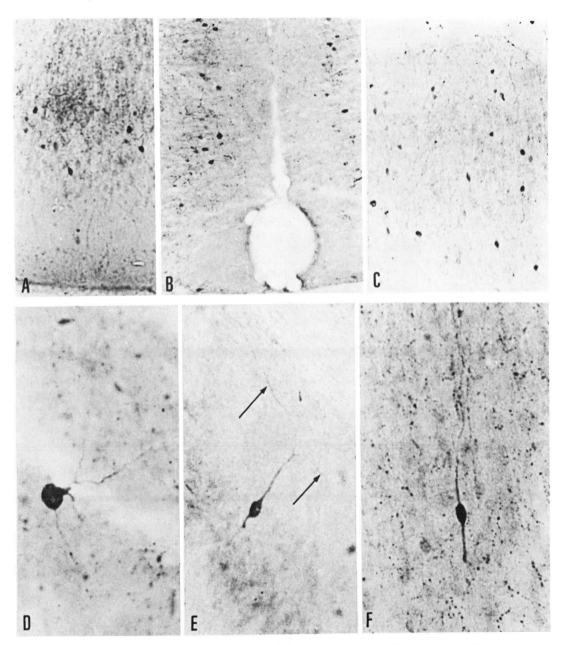

Fig. 1 A–F. Neurons containing VIP in different regions of the rodent cortex stained by immunoperoxidase technique. *A.* Typical distribution of VIP cell bodies in pyriform cortex. *B.* Cingulate cortex. *C.* Neocortex. *D.* Multiprocessed cells densely fill claustrum, while bipolar cells are most commonly seen in hippocampus (E) and neocortex (F). Arrows denote branching of proximal axon in hippocampus. Dense terminals are seen in laminae II–IV of neocortex. (Reproduced from Sims et al. (1980), by courtesy of the Editors of *Brain Research*.)

3.3. AMYGDALA

VIP neurons are seen in most regions of the amygdaloid complex. The lateral and corti-cal amygdaloid nuclei have the greatest number of cell bodies with moderate numbers seen in the medial, basolateral, and basomedial amygdaloid nuclei. The central amygda-loid nucleus is positive for VIP cell bodies, although they are often obscured by the heavy VIP innervation of this region.

3.4. OTHER TELENCEPHALIC AREAS

In colchicine-treated rats VIP cell bodies have been described in the bed nucleus of the stria terminalis and the lateral septum.

3.5. HYPOTHALAMUS (*Fig. 2*)

The suprachiasmatic nucleus has a very dense concentration of VIP containing peri-karya. Card et al. (1981) found the VIP neurons to be concentrated in the ventral half of the nucleus, immediately adjacent to the optic chiasm. Sims et al. (1980) reported a number of these neurons to be embedded within the chiasm. Ultrastructurally, these VIP neurons have a spherical or slightly elongated soma and an invaginated nucleus that occupies most of the cell body. Within the soma, the VIP immunoreactivity appears to be located on the outer surface of all cellular organelles and in vesicles located at termi-nal boutons (Card et al. 1981). We have recently observed VIP cell bodies in the lateral magnocellular portion of the paraventricular nucleus which seem to send projections to the median eminence (Nilaver and Abrams, unpublished data). Scattered cells have also been observed in the preoptic area of the hypothalamus.

3.6. MESENCEPHALON (*Fig. 3*)

Numerous small VIP neurons are found immediately adjacent to the aqueduct and fourth ventricle on the ventral and lateral aspects of the midbrain central gray. In sagit-tal sections the cells appear to cluster in a poorly defined rostral grouping, and more caudally, near the dorsal raphae nucleus. The superior colliculus also contains a few VIP cell bodies.

3.7. OTHER NON-TELENCEPHALIC AREAS (*Fig. 3*)

A few VIP cell bodies have been reported in the caudal thalamus. These neurons proba-bly represent a rostral extension of the dense cluster of cells in the mesencephalon. In recent studies conducted in our laboratory we have found VIP cell bodies in moderate

Fig. 2. VIP neurons in suprachiasmatic nucleus of hypothalamus (sc). *A* and *B*. Neuronal perikarya seen in ventromedial portion of the nucleus at low and high magnification. Arrow denotes dorsal fiber projection. *C*. Caudal section through suprachiasmatic nucleus showing dense cluster of cells. Arrow again denotes dorsal entry or exit of axon projection. *D*. Thick (50 μm) section shows dense terminal innervation pattern. *E*. VIP-containing cells can be seen extending into the optic chiasm (CO). (Reproduced from Sims et al. (1980), by courtesy of the Editors of *Brain Research*.)

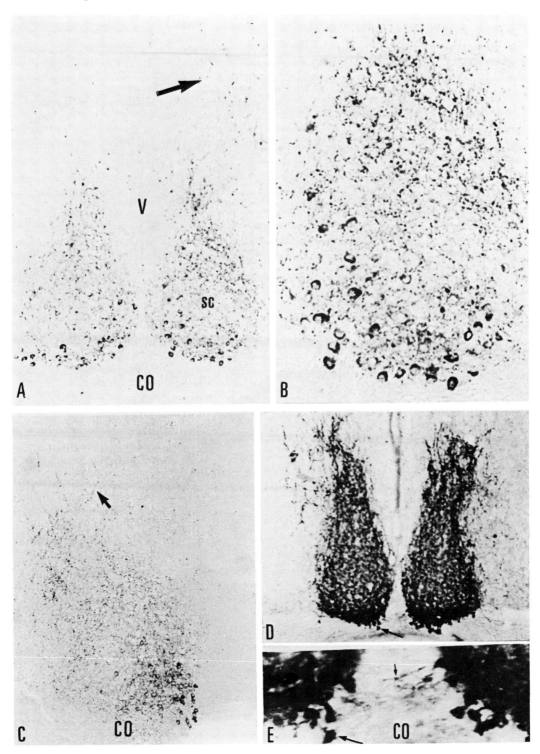

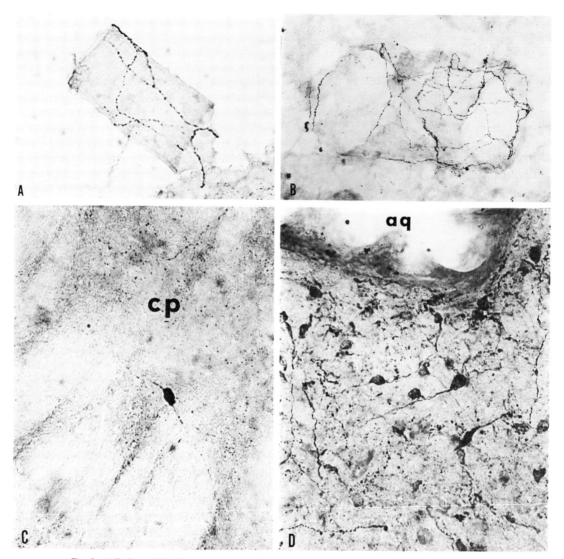

Fig. 3. A. Delicate VIP fibers envelop pial blood vessels of posterior, and *B* anterior circulation. *C.* Bipolar VIP perikaryon and moderate numbers of fibers are seen in caudate-putamen (cp). *D.* Numerous VIP cell bodies are visualized in mesencephalic gray, adjacent to the aqueduct (aq).

numbers in the caudate-putamen of the rat (Nilaver and Abrams, unpublished data). Palkovits et al. (1982) have observed VIP neurons within the nucleus of the solitary tract. In the guinea pig, VIP-containing perikarya have been reported in the nucleus of the solitary tract, reticular formation of the medulla, and the nucleus of the vagal nerve. Some of the VIP neurons in the latter area were reported to have the typical morphology of motor neurons (Triepel 1982).

4. FIBERS

4.1. CORTEX

The striking feature of VIP-containing neurons in the cortex is the radial orientation of their axons in relation to the cortical surface. It is often difficult to distinguish between axons and dendritic arborizations, but it appears that most VIP neurons in the cortex are locally projecting and could be described as interneurons. Fiber density is heavy and relatively evenly distributed throughout the neocortical layers, with laminae II–IV showing the greatest abundance. The 'limbic cortex' including the pyriform, cingulate, and entorhinal areas contains many fibers. The anterior olfactory nucleus appears to send a rich projection of VIP fibers to the olfactory bulbs. Ultrastructural studies have shown that VIP terminals tend to form asymmetrical axo-dendritic contacts in the cortex (Pelletier et al. 1981).

4.2. HIPPOCAMPUS

VIP fibers are numerous in the dorsal hippocampus. They are also abundant in the molecular, granular, and hilar layers of the dentate gyrus; the stratum oriens, stratum radiatum, stratum moleculare, and especially stratum pyramidale of both regio superior and inferior, and the subicular region (Roberts et al. 1980b; Sloviter et al. personal communication).

4.3. AMYGDALA (*Fig. 3*)

The most prominent feature of the amygdaloid complex is the density of VIP terminals found in the central amygdaloid nucleus. An amygdalofugal projection arising from the lateral basal and cortical nuclei of the amygdala runs in the stria terminalis and terminates in the bed nucleus and the preoptic area of the hypothalamus (Roberts et al. 1980b). Transection of the stria terminalis results in reduced VIP immunoreactivity in the ipsilateral bed nucleus of the stria terminalis, preoptic area, anterior hypothalamus and both suprachiasmatic nuclei (Roberts et al. 1980b; Palkovits et al. 1981). The caudal, medial nucleus accumbens, lateral septum, and the pericallosal area of the anterior commissure also receive dense VIP innervation, presumably via the stria terminalis projection. Evidence for an amygdalopetal VIP pathway is suggested by the reduction of VIP in the lateral amygdaloid nucleus following unilateral stria terminalis lesions (Palkovits et al. 1981).

The synaptology of VIP neurons in the central nucleus of the amygdala has been studied at the ultrastructural level. VIP terminals containing many round and oval vesicles have been shown to form symmetrical axo-somatic and asymmetrical axo-dendritic contacts. The post-synaptic cell type for these terminals has more recently been shown to be also VIPergic (Gray et al. personal communication). It has further been shown that such VIPergic terminals do not interact with neurotensin- or somatostatin-containing cellular elements, which are also concentrated in this area (Gray et al. 1982).

4.4. HYPOTHALAMUS

The suprachiasmatic nucleus is the most densely innervated area of the hypothalamus. Many other hypothalamic areas contain VIP nerve fibers including the anterior hypothalamus, the paraventricular nucleus, the dorsomedial and ventromedial nuclei, the periventricular nucleus and the premammillary nuclei. Complete deafferentation of the hypothalamus results in a 40% decrease in VIP content (Besson et al. 1979). The pathway in the stria terminalis is an important source of hypothalamic innervation. Section of the median forebrain bundle also results in reduced ipsilateral hypothalamic VIP suggesting significant contributions from this pathway as well (Marley et al. 1981). The median eminence, particularly the zona externa, has a moderate concentration of VIP fibers (Nilaver and Abrams, unpublished data). Median eminence VIP is unaffected by stria terminalis transection (Palkovits et al. 1981) consistent with a local projection from within the hypothalamus. VIP cells recently found in the paraventricular nucleus may be the source of zona externa projections (Nilaver and Abrams, unpublished data); other fibers projecting to this neurosecretory region containing vasopressin- (Silverman and Zimmerman 1983) and corticotropin-releasing factor (Swanson et al. 1983) are known to originate in the paraventricular region.

4.5. STRIATUM

The corpus striatum has scattered VIP fibers with no recognizable organization. Lorén et al. (1979) have noted a fairly dense network of varicose fibers ventral to the posterior limb of the anterior commissure. Roberts et al. (1980a) reported the heaviest concentration of striatal VIP fibers in the dorso-caudal regions of the caudate nucleus. The globus pallidus has a few scattered immunoreactive axons.

4.6. THALAMUS

The medial thalamus contains a few VIP fibers. In contrast, the lateral geniculate body has a moderately dense band of fibers running along its lateral border. These fibers appear to be continuous with a band of axons extending into the pretectal areas and superior colliculus of the mesencephalon.

4.7. MESENCEPHALON

Moderately dense numbers of VIP fibers are seen in the mesencephalic region. At the level of the interpeduncular nucleus, the fibers cross laterally to both the lateral lemniscal system and the substantia nigra. The dorsal raphae nucleus receives fibers apparently originating from the dense cluster of VIP cells in the periaqueductal region. In sagittal sections, some VIP fibers emanate from the mesencephalon and appear to cross rostrally through the thalamic central gray. A mesencephalic VIP projection via the median forebrain bundle has been proposed, with axons innervating the nucleus accumbens, the hypothalamus, amygdala, and the bed nucleus of the stria terminalis (Marley et al. 1981).

4.8. OTHER NON-TELENCEPHALIC AREAS

The parabrachial nucleus contains a moderately dense concentration of VIP fibers. Scattered fibers are also seen in the area postrema, cuneate nucleus, and nucleus solitarius. Fibers have also been observed within the olivary complex. The cerebellum is devoid of VIP innervation. The VIP innervation of the spinal cord appears to be relatively sparse. VIP fibers have been observed within the dorsal and ventral horns of the cord, with the heaviest concentrations present in the gray matter surrounding the central canal

(Rexed lamina X) (Gibson et al. 1981; Hoffman et al. unpublished data). The source of these fibers is still uncertain, although unilateral lumbar dorsal rhizotomy in the cat has been shown to result in marked depletion of immunoassayable VIP in the ipsilateral dorsal horn (Yaksh et al. 1982). In these studies no change was found in the VIP content of the ventral horn. This finding would be consistent with previous reports of VIP immunoreactivity in small cells of sensory ganglia (Lundberg et al. 1978).

5. NON-NEURAL INNERVATION

A uniform feature of VIP innervation in all organ systems is its association with the vasculature (Fig. 3). VIP fibers are seen in the adventitia or adventitia-media border of most pial vessels, with the heaviest concentration found more proximally in the major intracranial arteries. VIP fibers have also been encountered adjacent to small intracerebral vascular branches (Larsson et al. 1976b; Edvinsson et al. 1980). The source of such VIP innervation is unclear, but fibers containing VIP have been observed crossing directly from brain parenchyma to pial vessels (Lorén et al. 1979; Nilaver and Abrams, unpublished data). In addition, VIP cell bodies within the cortex occasionally appear to project directly to intracerebral vasculature (Nilaver and Abrams, unpublished data).

VIP has been reported in nerves in the choroid plexus (Lindvall et al. 1978). Nerves in the pineal gland of rabbit, cat, and pig have been reported to contain VIP. While most of these fibers are associated with small blood vessels, some fibers are seen crossing directly into the pineal parenchyma with no obvious site of termination (Uddman et al. 1980).

6. CONCLUSIONS

VIP is one of many peptides found in both gut and brain. In the brain, the physiological function of VIP is still unknown, although present evidence suggests possible modulatory roles in neural communication, cortical energy metabolism, cerebral blood flow, and modulation of hypothalamic-pituitary function. VIP pathways in the spinal cord may be involved in the processing of autonomic or peripheral sensory information (DeGroat et al. 1983). Clearly, our understanding of the functional anatomy of VIP neurons is limited. It is expected that the proposed roles for VIP in central nervous system activity will be further clarified, and that additional pathways and functions will be discovered in future studies.

7. ACKNOWLEDGMENTS

We thank Dr S. Rosario and Ms Anne Sollas for their technical assistance.

8. REFERENCES

Besson J, Rotsztejn W, Laburthe M, Epelbaum J, Beaudet A, Kordon C, Rosselin G (1979): Vasoactive intestinal peptide (VIP): brain distribution, subcellular localization and effect of deafferentation of the hypothalamus in male rats. *Brain Res., 165*, 79–85.

Besson J, Rotsztejn W, Poussin B, Lhiaubet AM, Rosselin G (1982): Release of vasoactive intestinal peptide from rat brain slices by various depolarizing agents. *Neurosci. Lett., 28,* 281–285.

Bodanszky M, Klausner YS, Yang Lin C, Mutt V, Said SI (1974): Synthesis of vasoactive intestinal peptide (VIP). *J. Am. Chem. Soc., 96,* 4973–4978.

Borghi C, Nicosia S, Giachetti A, Said SI (1979): Vasoactive intestinal polypeptide (VIP) stimulates adenylate cyclase in selected areas of rat brain. *Life Sci., 24,* 65–70.

Bryant MG, Polak JM, Modlin I, Bloom SR, Albuquerque RH, Pearse AGE (1976): Possible dual role for vasoactive intestinal peptide as gastrointestinal hormone and neurotransmitter substance. *Lancet, 1,* 991–993.

Card JP, Brecha N, Karten H, Moore RY (1981): Immunocytochemical localization of vasoactive intestinal polypeptide-containing cells and processes in the suprachiasmatic nucleus of the rat. Light and electron microscopic analysis. *J. Neurosci., 1,* 1289–1303.

Carlquist M, Mutt V, Jornvall H (1979): Isolation and characterization of bovine vasoactive intestinal peptide (VIP). *FEBS Lett., 108,* 457–460.

Carlquist M, McDonald TS, Go VLW, Bataille D, Johansson C, Mutt V (1982): Isolation and aminoacid composition of human vasoactive intestinal polypeptide. *Horm. Metab. Res., 14,* 28–29.

DeGroat W, Kawatani M, Hisamistu T, Lowe I, Morgan C, Roppolo J, Booth AM, Nadelhaft I, Kuo D, Thor K (1983): The role of neuropeptides in the sacral autonomic reflex pathways of the cat. *J. Autonom. Nerv. Syst., 7,* 339–350.

Deschodt-Lanckman M, Robberecht P, Christophe J (1977): Characterization of VIP-sensitive adenylate cyclase in guinea pig brain. *FEBS Lett., 83,* 76–80.

Dimaline R, Dockray GS (1979): Molecular variants of vasoactive intestinal polypeptide in dog, rat, and hog. *Life Sci., 25,* 1893–1900.

Dodd J, Kelly JS, Said SI (1979): Excitation of CA1 neurons of the rat hippocampus by the octacosapeptide, vasoactive intestinal polypeptide (VIP). *Br. J. Pharmacol., 66,* 125P.

Edvinsson L, Fahrenkrug J, Hanko J, Owman C, Sundler F, Uddman R (1980): VIP (vasoactive intestinal polypeptide)-containing nerves of intracranial arteries in mammals. *Cell Tissue Res., 208,* 135–142.

Eiden L, Nilaver G, Palkovits M (1982): Distribution of vasoactive intestinal polypeptide (VIP) in the rat brainstem nuclei. *Brain Res., 231,* 472–477.

Emson PC, Fahrenkrug J, Schaffalitzky de Muckadell OB, Jessell TM, Iversen LI (1977): Vasoactive intestinal polypeptide (VIP): vesicular localization and potassium evoked release from rat hypothalamus. *Brain Res., 143,* 174–178.

Epelbaum J, Tapia-Arancibia L, Besson J, Rotsztejn W, Kordon C (1979): Vasoactive intestinal peptide inhibits release of somatostatin from hypothalamus in vitro. *Eur. J. Pharmacol., 58,* 493–495.

Fahrenkrug J (1979): Vasoactive intestinal polypeptide. Measurement, distribution, and putative neurotransmitter function. *Digestion, 19,* 149–169.

Fahrenkrug J, Schaffalitzky de Muckadell OB (1978): Distribution of vasoactive intestinal polypeptide (VIP) in the porcine central nervous system. *J. Neurochem., 31,* 1445–1451.

Feldman ML, Peters A (1978): The forms of nonpyramidal neurons in the visual cortex. *J. Comp. Neurol., 179,* 761–794.

Fuxe K, Hökfelt T, Said SI, Mutt V (1977): Vasoactive intestinal polypeptide and the nervous system: immunohistochemical evidence for localization in central and peripheral neurons, particularly intracortical neurons of the cerebral cortex. *Neurosci. Lett., 5,* 241–246.

Gainer H (1977): *Peptides in Neurobiology.* Plenum Press, New York.

Giachetti A, Said SI, Reynolds RC, Koniges FC (1977): Vasoactive intestinal polypeptide in brain. Localization in and release from isolated nerve terminals. *Proc. Natl Acad. Sci. USA, 74,* 3424–3428.

Gibson SI, Polak JM, Bloom SR, Wall PD (1981): The distribution of nine peptides in the rat spinal cord with special emphasis on the substantia gelatinosa and on the area around the central canal (lamina X). *J. Comp. Neurol., 201,* 65–79.

Gray TS, Cassell MD, Williams TH (1982): Synaptology of three peptidergic neuron types in the central nucleus of the rat amygdala. *Peptides, 3,* 273–281.

Haskins JT, Samson WK, Moss RL (1982): Evidence for vasoactive intestinal polypeptide (VIP) altering the firing rate of preoptic, septal and midbrain central gray neurons. *Regul. Peptides, 3,* 113–123.

Heistad DD, Marcus ML, Said SI, Gross PM (1980): Effect of acetylcholine and vasoactive intestinal peptide on cerebral blood flow. *Am. J. Physiol., 239,* H73–H80.

Jeftinija S, Murase K, Nedeljkov V, Randic M (1982): Vasoactive intestinal polypeptide excites mammalian dorsal horn neurons in vivo and in vitro. *Brain Res., 243,* 158–164.

Jirikowski G, Reisert I, Pilgrim C (1982): Nerve cells immunoreactive for vasoactive intestinal polypeptide in dissociated cultures of the rat hypothalamus and midbrain. *Neurosci. Lett., 31,* 75–79.

352

Kato Y, Iwasaki Y, Iwasaki J, Abe H, Yanaihara N, Imura H (1978): Prolactin release by vasoactive intestinal peptide in rats. *Endocrinology, 103*, 554–558.

Keltz TN, Straus E, Yalow RS (1980): Degradation of vasoactive intestinal polypeptide by tissue homogenates. *Biochem. Biophys. Res. Commun., 92*, 669–674.

Kerwin RW, Pay S, Bhoola K, Pycock C (1980): Vasoactive intestinal polypeptide (VIP) sensitive adenylate cyclase in rat brain: regional distribution and localization on hypothalamic neurons. *J. Pharm. Pharmacol., 32*, 561–566.

Larsson L-I, Fahrenkrug J, Schaffalitzky de Muckadell OB, Sundler F, Håkanson R, Rehfeld JF (1976a): Localization of vasoactive intestinal polypeptide to central and peripheral neurons. *Proc. Natl Acad. Sci. USA, 73*, 3197–3200.

Larsson L-I, Fahrenkrug J, Håkanson R, Hanko J, Schaffalitzky de Muckadell OB, Sundler F (1976b): Immunohistochemical localization of a vasodilatory peptide (VIP) in cerebrovascular nerves. *Brain Res., 113*, 400–404.

Lindvall M, Alumets J, Edvinsson L, Fahrenkrug J, Håkanson R, Hanko J, Schaffalitzky de Muckadell OB, Sundler F (1978): Peptidergic (VIP) nerves in the mammalian choroid plexus. *Neurosci. Lett., 9*, 77–82.

Lorén I, Emson PC, Fahrenkrug J, Bjorklünd A, Alumets J, Håkanson R, Sundler F (1979): Distribution of vasoactive intestinal polypeptide in the rat and mouse brain. *Neuroscience, 4*, 1953–1976.

Lorente de No R (1934): Studies on the structure of the cerebral cortex. Continuation of the study of the ammonic system. *J. Physiol. Neurol., 46*, 113–177.

Lundberg J, Hökfelt T, Nilsson G, Terenius L, Rehfeld J, Elde R, Said S (1978): Peptide neurons in the vagus, splanchnic, and sciatic nerves. *Acta Physiol. Scand., 104*, 499–501.

Magistretti PJ, Morrison JH, Shoemaker WJ, Sapin V, Bloom FE (1981): Vasoactive intestinal polypeptide induces glycogenolysis in mouse cortical slices: a possible regulatory mechanism for the local control of energy metabolism. *Proc. Natl Acad. Sci. USA, 78*, 6535–6539.

Maletti M, Besson J, Bataille D, Laburthe M, Rosselin G (1980): Ontogeny and immunoreactive forms of vasoactive intestinal peptide in rat brain. *Acta Endocrinol. (Copenhagen), 93*, 479–487.

Maletti M, Rostene WH, Carr L, Scherrer H, Rotten D, Kordon C, Rosselin G (1982): Interaction between estradiol and prolactin on vasoactive intestinal polypeptide concentrations in the hypothalamus and in the anterior pituitary of the female rat. *Neuroendocrinology, 32*, 307–313.

Marley PD, Emson PC, Hunt SP, Fahrenkrug J (1981): A long ascending projection in the rat brain containing vasoactive intestinal polypeptide. *Neurosci. Lett., 27*, 261–266.

McCulloch J, Edvinsson L (1980): Cerebral circulatory and metabolic effects of vasoactive intestinal polypeptide. *Am. J. Physiol., 238*, H449–H456.

McCulloch J, Kelly PAT, Uddman R, Edvinsson L (1983): Functional role of vasoactive intestinal polypeptide in the caudate nucleus: a 2-deoxy (^{14}C) glucose investigation. *Proc. Natl Acad. Sci. USA, 80*, 1472–1476.

McGregor GP, Woodhams PL, O'Shaughnessy DJ, Ghatei MA, Polak JM, Bloom SR (1982): Developmental changes in bombesin, somatostatin, and vasoactive intestinal polypeptide in the rat brain. *Neurosci. Lett., 28*, 21–27.

Mutt V, Said SI (1974): Structure of the porcine vasoactive intestinal octacosapeptide. *Eur. J. Biochem., 42*, 581–584.

Nilsson A (1977): Structure of the vasoactive intestinal octacosapeptide from chicken intestine. The aminoacid sequence. *FEBS Lett., 60*, 322–326.

Palkovits M, Besson J, Rotsztejn W (1981): Distribution of vasoactive intestinal polypeptide in intact, stria terminalis transected, and cerebral cortex isolated rats. *Brain Res., 213*, 455–459.

Palkovits M, Leranth C, Eiden LE, Rotsztejn W, Williams TH (1982): Intrinsic vasoactive intestinal polypeptide (VIP)-containing neurons in the baroreceptor nucleus of the solitary tract in the rat. *Brain Res., 244*, 351–355.

Pelletier G, LeClerc R, Povianni R, Polak JM (1981): Electron immunocytochemistry of vasoactive intestinal polypeptide in the rat brain. *Brain Res., 210*, 356–360.

Phillis J, Kirkpatrick JR, Said SI (1978): Vasoactive intestinal polypeptide excitation of central neurons. *Can. J. Physiol. Pharmacol., 56*, 337–340.

Quik M, Iversen LI, Bloom SR (1978): Effect of vasoactive intestinal peptide (VIP) and other peptides on cAMP accumulation in rat brain. *Biochem. Pharmacol., 27*, 2209–2213.

Ramón y Cajal S (1955): *Histologie du Système Nerveux de l'Homme et des Vertébrés. Vol. 2*. Consejo Superior de Investigaciones Cientificas, Inst. Ramón y Cajal, Madrid.

Robberecht P, DeNeef P, Lammens M, Deschodt-Lanckman M, Christophe JP (1978): Specific binding of vasoactive intestinal peptide to brain membranes from guinea pig. *Eur. J. Biochem., 90*, 147–154.

Roberts GW, Woodhams PL, Bryant MG, Crow T, Bloom SR, Polak JM (1980a): VIP in the rat brain: evidence for a major pathway linking the amygdala and hypothalamus via the stria terminalis. *Histochemistry, 65*, 103–119.

Roberts GW, Woodhams PL, Crow TJ, Polak JM (1980b): Loss of immunoreactive VIP in the bed nucleus following lesions of the stria terminalis. *Brain Res., 195*, 471–475.

Rotsztejn WH, Besson J, Briaud B, Gagnant L, Rosselin G, Kordon C (1980): Effect of steroids on vasoactive intestinal peptide in discrete brain regions and peripheral tissue. *Neuroendocrinology, 31*, 287–291.

Ruberg M, Rotsztejn WH, Arancibia S, Besson J, Enjalbert A (1978): Stimulation of prolactin release by vasoactive intestinal polypeptide (VIP). *Eur. J. Pharmacol., 51*, 319–320.

Said SI, Mutt A (1970a): Polypeptide with broad biological activity: isolation from small intestine. *Science, 169*, 1217–1218.

Said SI, Mutt A (1970b): Potent peripheral and splanchnic vasodilator peptide from normal gut. *Nature (London), 225*, 863–864.

Said SI, Porter JC (1979): Vasoactive intestinal polypeptide: release into hypophysial portal blood. *Life Sci., 24*, 227–230.

Said SI, Rosenberg R (1976): Vasoactive intestinal polypeptide: abundant immunoreactivity in neural cell lines and normal nervous tissue. *Science, 192*, 907–908.

Salt TE, Hill RG (1981): Vasoactive intestinal polypeptide (VIP) applied by microiontophoresis excites single neurons in the trigeminal nucleus caudalis of the rat. *Neuropeptides, 1*, 403–408.

Samson WK, Said SI, McCann SM (1979): Radioimmunologic localization of vasoactive intestinal polypeptide in hypothalamic and extrahypothalamic sites in the rat brain. *Neurosci. Lett., 12*, 265–269.

Samson WK, Burton KP, Reeves JP, McCann SM (1981): Vasoactive intestinal peptide stimulates luteinizing hormone-releasing hormone from median eminence synaptosomes. *Regul. Peptides, 2*, 253–264.

Shimatsu A, Kato Y, Matushita N, Katakami H, Yanaihara N, Imura H (1981): Immunoreactive vasoactive intestinal polypeptide in rat hypophysial portal blood. *Endocrinology, 108*, 395–398.

Shimatsu A, Kato Y, Matushita N, Katakami H, Yanaihara H, Imura H (1982): Effects of glucagon, neurotensin, and vasoactive intestinal polypeptide on somatostatin release from perfused rat hypothalamus. *Endocrinology, 110*, 2113–2117.

Silverman A-J, Zimmerman EA (1983): Magnocellular neurosecretory system. *Annu. Rev. Neurosci., 6*, 357–380.

Sims KB, Hoffman DL, Said SI, Zimmerman EA (1980): Vasoactive intestinal peptide (VIP) in mouse and rat brain: an immunocytochemical study. *Brain Res., 186*, 165–183.

Sundler F, Håkanson R, Alumets J, Walles B (1977): Neuronal localization of pancreatic polypeptide and vasoactive intestinal peptide immunoreactivity in the earthworm *(Lumbricus terrestris)*. *Brain Res. Bull., 2*, 61–65.

Swanson LW, Sawchenko PE, Rivier J, Vale WW (1983): The organization of ovine corticotropin releasing factor (CRF) immunoreactive cells and fibers in the rat brain: an immunohistochemical study. *Neuroendocrinology, 36*, 165–186.

Tatemoto K, Mutt V (1980): Isolation of two novel candidate hormones using a chemical method for finding naturally occurring polypeptides. *Nature (London), 285*, 417–418.

Taylor DP, Pert CB (1979): Vasoactive intestinal polypeptide. Specific binding to rat brain membranes. *Proc. Natl Acad. Sci. USA, 76*, 660–664.

Triepel J (1982): Vasoactive intestinal polypeptide in the medulla oblongata of the guinea pig. *Neurosci. Lett., 29*, 73–78.

Uddman R, Alumets H, Håkanson R, Lorén I, Sundler F (1980): Vasoactive intestinal polypeptide (VIP) in nerves of the pineal gland. *Experientia, 36*, 1119–1120.

Vijayan E, Samson WK, Said SI, McCann SM (1979): Vasoactive intestinal polypeptide: evidence for a hypothalamic site of action to release growth hormone, luteinizing hormone and prolactin in conscious ovariectomized rats. *Endocrinology, 104*, 53–57.

Wei EP, Kontos HA, Said SI (1980): Mechanism of action of vasoactive intestinal polypeptide on cerebral arterioles. *Am. J. Physiol., 235*, H765–H768.

Wilson D, O'Neill JT, Said SI, Traystman RJ (1981): Vasoactive intestinal polypeptide and the canine cerebral circulation. *Circ. Res., 48*, 138–148.

Yaksh T, Abay EO, Go VL (1982): Studies on the localization and release of cholecystokinin and vasoactive intestinal polypeptide in the rat and cat spinal cord. *Brain Res., 242*, 279–290.

CHAPTER VIII

Neurotensin-containing neurons

PIERS C. EMSON, MICHEL GOEDERT AND PATRICK W. MANTYH

1. INTRODUCTION

Neurotensin (NT) is a 13 amino acid peptide originally isolated and sequenced by Carraway and Leeman from bovine hypothalamic extracts (Carraway and Leeman 1973, 1975a,b) and subsequently from bovine and human small intestine (Table 1) (Carraway et al. 1978; Hammer et al. 1980). The availability of the synthetic peptide (Carraway and Leeman 1975b) soon led to the production of NT antibodies (Carraway and Leeman 1974, 1975a,b; Carraway 1982); and NT-like immunoreactivity (NT-LI) has been shown to be widely distributed in the central and peripheral nervous system of a number of mammalian species by using both radioimmunoassays (RIA) and immunohistochemical techniques (see review by Nemeroff and Prange 1982).

Initial biochemical investigations using NT-directed RIA demonstrated that NT-LI is concentrated in synaptosomes (Uhl and Snyder 1976) and further work has established that synaptic membrane fractions are enriched in specific binding sites for ^{125}I- or ^{3}H-NT being consistent with the presence of NT receptors in the mammalian central nervous system (CNS) (Uhl and Snyder 1977; Lazarus et al. 1977; Kitabgi et al. 1977, 1980; Young and Kuhar 1981; Checler et al. 1982; Quirion et al. 1982; Goedert et al. 1984d). The demonstration of an evoked release of NT (Iversen et al. 1978; Maeda and Frohman 1981), and its ability to influence neuronal excitability (Zieglgänsberger et al. 1978; Miletic and Randic 1979; Andrade and Aghajanian 1981; Henry 1982; Stanzione and Zieglgänsberger 1983) are consistent with the peptide being a neurotransmitter or neuromodulator. When injected into the CNS, NT has been reported (Nemeroff et al. 1980) to produce antinociception and hypothermia, to influence dopaminergic transmission and to modify anterior pituitary function (Clineschmidt and McGuffin 1977; Loosen et al. 1978; Nemeroff et al. 1979, 1980; Rioux et al. 1981, Kalivas et al. 1981, 1982a,b, 1983; Enjalbert et al. 1982; Beitz 1982; Haubrich et al. 1982; De Quidt and Emson 1983; Okuma et al. 1983). However, although behavioral and pharmacological effects of NT can be readily demonstrated, we currently lack the specific receptor antagonists which would enable us to establish unambiguously a physiological role for NT.

Three neuropeptides structurally related to mammalian NT have been isolated and sequenced from non-mammalian sources (Table 1) (Araki et al. 1973; Carraway and Bhatnagar 1980; Carraway and Ferris 1983). It is unknown whether chicken intestinal NT(1–13) is present in mammalian tissues or whether it simply represents the avian counterpart of mammalian NT. The chicken intestinal peptide [Lys^{8}Asn^{9}]NT(8–13) is found in central and peripheral tissues of the chicken (Carraway et al. 1983), however, there exists no conclusive evidence demonstrating its presence in mammalian tissues.

Handbook of Chemical Neuroanatomy. Vol. 4: GABA and Neuropeptides in the CNS, Part I.
A. Björklund and T. Hökfelt, editors.
© Elsevier Science Publishers B.V., 1985.

TABLE 1. *Amino acid sequences of peptides of the neurotensin family*

	1	2	3	4	5	6	7	8	9	10	11	12	13
NT(1–13) (bovine hypothalamus, bovine and human small intestine)	pGlu -	Leu -	Tyr -	Glu -	Asn -	Lys -	Pro -	Arg -	Arg -	Pro -	Tyr -	Ile -	Leu - OH
NT(1–13) (chicken intestine)	pGlu -	Leu -	His -	Val -	Asn -	Lys -	Ala -	Arg -	Arg -	Pro -	Tyr -	Ile -	Leu - OH
[Lys8Asn9]NT(8–13) (chicken intestine)							H -	Lys -	Asn -	Pro -	Tyr -	Ile -	Leu - OH
Xenopsin (*Xenopus laevis* skin)						pGlu -	Gly -	Lys -	Arg -	Pro -	Trp -	Ile -	Leu - OH

TABLE 2. *Regional distribution of immunoreactive NT in the mammalian CNS*

	Rat[1]	Rat[2]	Calf[3]	Cat[4]	Monkey[5]	Man[6]	Man[7,8,9]
Cerebral cortex	12.0	4.0	2.0	4.0	6.0	0.8	0.6
Olfactory bulb	3.6	3.5	–	–	12.7	4.4	–
Nucleus accumbens	83.5	29.2	–	91	–	–	2.6
Septum	41.4	73.0	–	–	5.2	–	–
Caudate nucleus	1.8	10.2	11.1	23.0	8.0	2.5	5.4
Lateral preoptic nucleus	155	124	–	–	44.5	–	–
Medial preoptic nucleus	136	143	–	–	51.5	–	–
Globus pallidus	–	12.6	9.3	–	–	9.8	12.1 (lateral segment)
Bed nucleus of the stria terminalis	–	171.8	–	–	–	–	–
Amygdala (whole)	39.6	–	1.9	–	–	5.5	21.7
Medial amygdaloid nucleus	–	40	–	–	18.8	–	–
Central amygdaloid nucleus	–	106	–	–	19.2	–	–
Anterior hypothalamic nucleus	–	113	17.3	–	–	–	–
Arcuate nucleus	59	–	–	–	70.8	–	–
Median eminence	202	128	–	–	85.5	–	–
Mammillary bodies	–	128	11.1	–	26.0	–	–
Ventral tegmental area	51	35	–	–	48.7	23.4	–
Substantia nigra	17	13	–	36	–	–	19.3
Spinal cord (whole)	8.5	–	1.1	4	–	–	–
Spinal cord (dorsal)	–	23	–	4	–	–	–
Spinal cord (ventral)	–	2.0	–	3	–	–	–
Cerebellum	<1.2	<0.9	<0.32	<0.3	4.5	0.8	0.6

Modified from [1]Kobayashi et al. (1977), [2]Emson et al. (1982), [3]Uhl and Snyder (1976), [4]Goedert and Emson (1983), [5]Kataoko et al. (1979), [6]Cooper et al. (1981), [7]Manberg et al. (1982), [8]Langevin and Emson (1982), [9]Emson et al. (1985). All units pmol/gram wet weight.

NT-LI and xenopsin-LI are both present in central and peripheral tissues of *Xenopus laevis*, indicating that xenopsin does not represent the amphibian counterpart of NT (Carraway et al. 1982a; Goedert et al. 1984e). However, xenopsin-LI is not present in mammalian tissues (Goedert et al. 1984e).

2. STRUCTURE–ACTIVITY RELATIONSHIPS AND MECHANISM OF ACTION OF NEUROTENSIN

The availability of synthetic NT and of partial NT sequences has allowed the characterization of the structure–activity profile in both biological assays and receptor binding studies (Kitabgi 1982). The results clearly indicate that the carboxy-terminal end of NT is responsible for the biological effects of the molecule, whereas amino-terminal fragments, such as NT(1–11) and NT(1–12) are completely inactive. Of the carboxy-terminal fragments NT(8–13) is equipotent with the whole molecule, whereas removal of the Arg residue in position 8 leads to a more than 90% loss in potency and removal of the Arg residue in position 9 results in a complete loss of biological activity and receptor binding capacity. It therefore appears that 2 basic amino acids in positions 8 and 9 are required for biological activity. This is further supported by the finding that the chicken intestinal peptide [Lys^{8}Asn^9]NT(8–13) possesses less than 2% of the potency of NT(8–13) in competing with ^{3}H-NT for its specific binding site in rat brain membranes (Goedert et al. 1984d).

The specific binding of ^{3}H-NT to rat brain membranes is unaffected by either divalent cations or guanyl nucleotides, thereby providing indirect evidence that NT receptor activation is not coupled to stimulation of adenylate cyclase (Goedert et al. 1984d). This is further supported by experiments indicating that NT does not influence basal or stimulated cAMP levels in brain or intestinal slices (Kitagbi and Freychet 1979a; our unpublished observations). Conversely, several lines of evidence indicate that NT receptor activation leads to calcium mobilization (Kachur et al. 1982; Goldman et al. 1983) and the intestinal smooth muscle relaxation effected by NT is prevented by the bee venom apamin which blocks calcium-dependent potassium channels (Kitabgi and Vincent 1981; Huidobro-Toro and Yoshimura 1983). As there exists extensive circumstantial evidence in favor of a link between calcium mobilization and the hydrolysis of inositol phospholipids (Michell 1983) we investigated the effects of NT on inositol phospholipid hydrolysis. It appears that NT stimulates inositol phospholipid hydrolysis in rat brain slices and that there exists a good correlation between the magnitude of the response and the number of specific NT binding sites in various brain regions (unpublished observations).

3. NEUROTENSIN IN THE CENTRAL NERVOUS SYSTEM

Before morphological studies of the cellular sites containing NT-LI were undertaken several early studies using RIA techniques had shown that NT-LI is regionally distributed in the mammalian CNS (Carraway and Leeman 1974, 1976; Kobayashi et al. 1977). These and subsequent studies (summarized in Table 2) have shown that in most mammals NT-LI is particularly concentrated in the hypothalamus, brainstem, amygdala and spinal cord. Characterization of mammalian NT-LI using gel chromatography or high performance liquid chromatography (HPLC) on reverse phase has revealed the presence

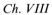

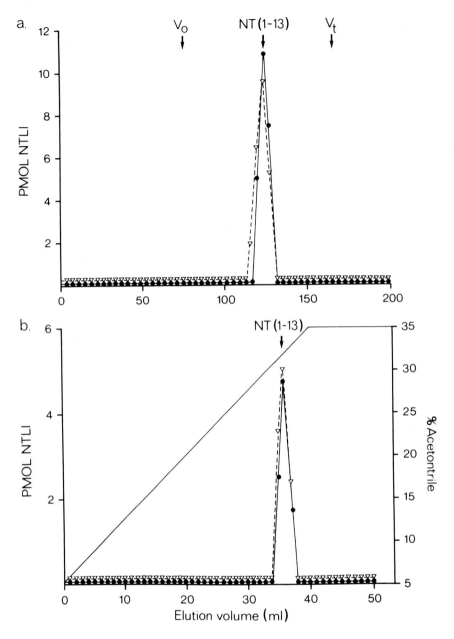

Fig. 1. a. Fractionation of neurotensin-like immunoreactivity (NT-LI) in acetic acid extracts from cat striatum on a Sephadex G-25 column. Fractions were assayed using RIAs specific for the amino- and carboxy-terminus of NT. V_o, void volume, NT(1–13), elution position of bovine synthetic neurotensin standard. V_t, total volume. *b.* Fractionation of NT-LI in acetic acid extracts from rat brain on a C_{18} reverse phase column using an acetonitrile gradient. NT(1–13) elution position of synthetic neurotensin. ●—● carboxy-terminal cross-reactivity. ▽—▽ amino-terminal cross-reactivity.

of only major immunoreactive form of NT which cross-reacts with antisera raised against synthetic NT (Fig. 1a,b), consistent with the presence of a peptide identical to, or very closely related to the mammalian NT sequence used as the standard. The possible presence of additional forms of NT or NT fragments that may be visualized immunohistochemically must be considered in any description of the cellular localization of NT. Abbreviations such as 'NT-LI' will be used in this chapter to indicate that the exact nature of the NT immunoreactivity visualized has not been determined.

Following the development of NT-directed RIA the antibodies used were also successfully employed for the immunohistochemical localization of NT-LI in the CNS (Uhl et al. 1977a,b, 1979). Subsequent studies confirmed these initial observations and extended their resolution to the electron microscopic level (Ninkovic et al. 1981) (see also Fig. 19). As with other histochemical methods, such as the fluorescent method for visualizing catecholamines which gradually developed and improved, it is likely that the currently used antibodies do not reveal all NT-containing systems in the CNS (even with colchicine pretreatment to enhance cell body content). This is well illustrated in the development of the rat CNS, where a number of NT-positive neurons can be visualized which are not readily demonstrable in the adult rat CNS (Minagawa et al. 1983; Hara et al. 1982). Whether all these neurons continue to produce and release small amounts of NT can not yet be determined and complete visualization of NT systems in the brain will have to wait for improvements in the sensitivity of the existing histochemical methods.

The distribution of NT-containing neurons in the rat brain is summarized schematically in The Atlas. The black dots are intended to illustrate the approximate locations and relative abundance of NT-containing neurons. The distributions are compiled from our own material and the studies of Uhl et al. (1977a,b), Kahn et al. (1981, 1982), Ninkovic et al. (1981), Jennes et al. (1982), Hara et al. (1982), Minagawa et al. (1983) and Hökfelt et al. (1984). Two reported cell groups which are not readily visualized have been omitted from the general scheme, these are the subicular neurons described by Roberts et al. (1981, 1982) and Hara et al. (1982), and the cingulate cortex neurons visualized by Hara et al. (1982). Because the majority of NT neurons is also found in regions with a reasonable density of NT fibers (presumably because many NT neurons are interneurons), only 3 terminal densities are included, so that the localization of cell bodies is not obscured by dense terminal shading. The 3 terminal densities correspond approximately to the following NT contents: $(3+) > 100$ pmol/g wet weight, $(2+) > 50$ pmol/g wet weight and $(1+)$ 10–15 pmol/g wet weight (see Table 2). The figures illustrating the distribution of specific ^{3}H-NT binding sites in the rat CNS are taken from our own studies (Fig. 2). They are in good agreement with the earlier studies of Young and Kuhar (1981), and Quirion et al. (1982). Previous structure–activity studies and those in our laboratory are consistent with the binding site being a physiological NT receptor (Kitabgi et al. 1977, 1980; Checler et al. 1982; Mazella et al. 1983; Goedert et al. 1984d). As with some classical neurotransmitters and neuropeptides, there exists no strict correlation between the number of specific NT binding sites and the amount of NT-LI in various regions of the mammalian brain (Table 3) (Goedert et al. 1984d).

3.1. RETINA

NT-LI has been detected in retinae from both mammalian and non-mammalian species and, at least in the pigeon, NT-LI is present in amacrine cells, as demonstrated by immunohistochemistry (Brecha et al. 1981). Specific NT binding sites have been found to be

TABLE 3. *Distribution of ³H-NT binding sites and NT-LI in the rat brain*

Brain region	³H-NT binding sites (fmol/mg protein)	K_D (nM)	NT-LI (pmol/g tissue)
Hypothalamus	565 ± 62 (5)	2.43 ± 0.10 (5)	76.15 ± 8.30 (5)
Frontal cortex	524 ± 56 (4)	3.09 ± 0.39 (4)	1.48 ± 0.25 (5)
Midbrain	448 ± 25 (3)	3.72 ± 0.63 (3)	45.84 ± 6.44 (5)
Striatum	418 ± 43 (4)	2.64 ± 0.40 (4)	19.02 ± 1.94 (5)
Thalamus	392 ± 35 (3)	3.08 ± 0.63 (3)	24.94 ± 2.70 (5)
Hippocampus	374 ± 22 (3)	2.37 ± 0.20 (3)	8.16 ± 0.92 (5)
Olfactory bulb	366 ± 18 (3)	3.64 ± 0.21 (3)	3.56 ± 0.28 (5)
Cerebellum	212 ± 18 (6)	3.71 ± 0.39 (6)	0.85 ± 0.18 (5)
Pons-medulla	202 ± 14 (4)	2.39 ± 0.25 (4)	22.75 ± 1.06 (5)

The brain dissections were performed as described in Goedert et al. (1984d). In individual experiments whole brain membranes were always run in parallel with membranes from the brain region under investigation. Specific ³H-NT binding and NT-LI were determined as described in Goedert et al. (1984d) and Emson et al. (1982). The maximum number of binding sites and the dissociation constants were calculated from the saturation curves. Each value represents the mean ± SEM (the number of experiments is indicated in parentheses).

localized in the inner plexiform layer of avian and mammalian retinae by receptor autoradiography (Fig. 3). The function of neurotensin in the retina is unknown at present.

3.2. OLFACTORY SYSTEM

The presence of NT-containing neurons has not been reported in the olfactory bulb in the adult rat; however, in a study on the ontogeny of NT-containing neurons (Hara et al. 1982), it was found that NT-LI-positive neurons can be observed in the olfactory bulb from gestational day 16 to post-natal day 21. It is not known whether these NT-containing neurons are the source of the NT-containing processes which are visible in the external plexiform layer. This localization of NT-containing nerve fibers is also consistent with the presence of a high density of specific ³H-NT binding sites in the external plexiform layer of the olfactory bulb and this density is among the highest in the rat CNS (Young and Kuhar 1981; Quirion et al. 1982). A lower density of NT receptors is localized over the internal part of the granule cell layer (Young and Kuhar 1981; Quirion et al. 1982).

Apart from intrinsic NT-containing cell bodies, NT-containing axons may also originate from regions such as the amygdala and the piriform cortex which are known to innervate the olfactory bulb and which contain NT-positive cell bodies. This possibility has recently been confirmed by the demonstration of NT-containing projections from the endopiriform nucleus and the prepiriform cortex to the anterior olfactory nucleus and the nucleus of the diagonal band (Inagaki et al. 1983b), the distribution of NT-LI-containing fibers in the olfactory nucleus being fairly even with the highest density of

Atlas

Schematic representation of NT-containing nerve terminals and cell bodies in the rat CNS as depicted in 18 frontal planes. The terminal densities are presented according to the scale beside level A 9.8, as dense (3+), medium dense (2+) and low density (1+). This staining density corresponding approximately to: (3+) > 100 pmol/g wet weight, (2+) 50–100 pmol/g wet weight, and (1+) 10–50 pmol/g wet weight. See Table 2 for exact figures.

For abbreviations, see the General Abbreviations List, p. 609.

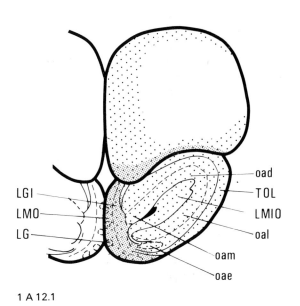

1 A 12.1

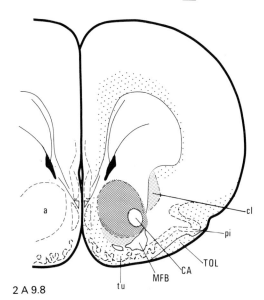

2 A 9.8

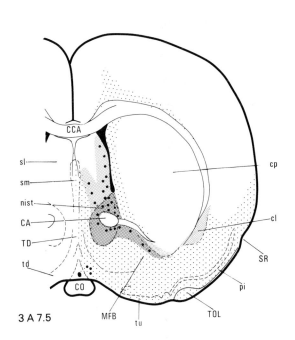

3 A 7.5

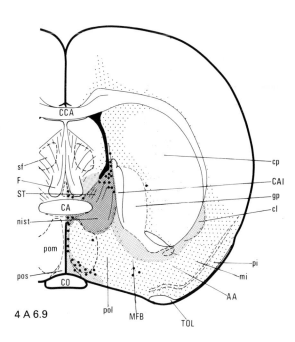

4 A 6.9

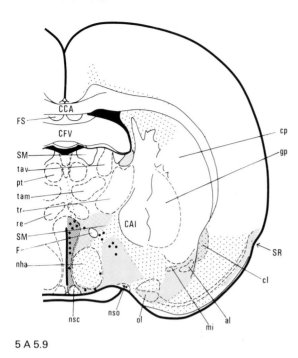

5 A 5.9

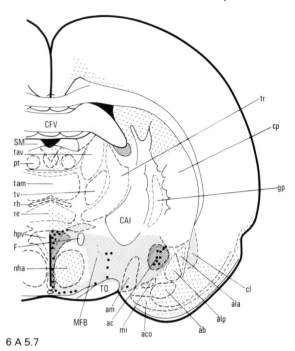

6 A 5.7

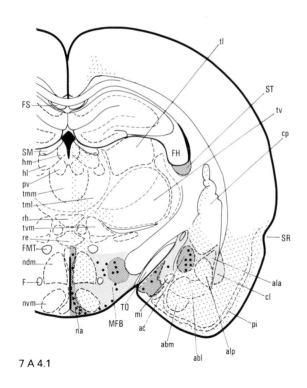

7 A 4.1

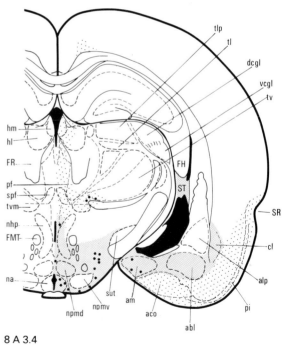

8 A 3.4

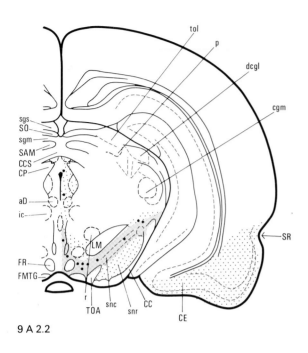

9 A 2.2

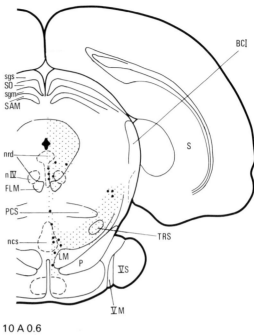

10 A 0.6

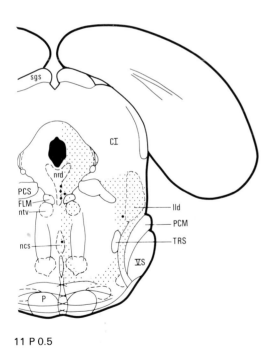

11 P 0.5

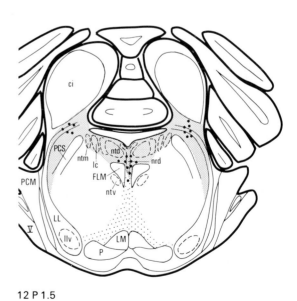

12 P 1.5

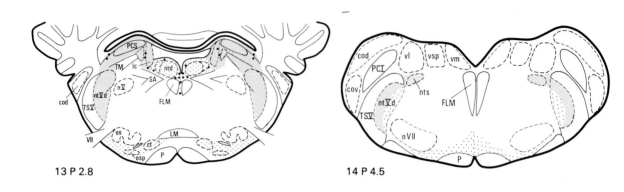

13 P 2.8

14 P 4.5

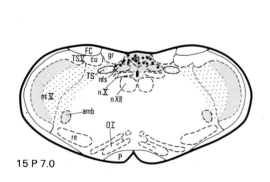

15 P 7.0

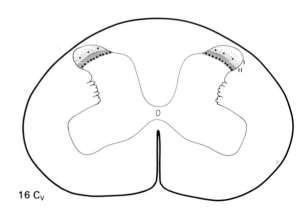

16 C_V

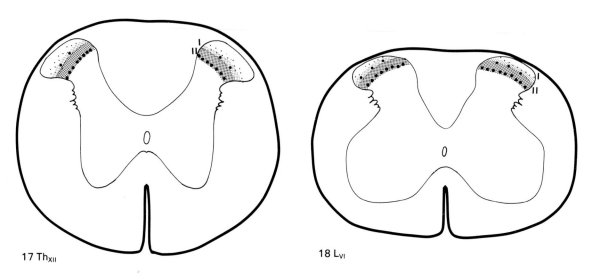

17 Th$_{XII}$ 18 L$_{VI}$

fibers apparent in the pars medialis. Cells could be labeled in the endopiriform and pre-piriform cortices following horseradish peroxidase injection into the anterior olfactory nucleus or the diagonal band, consistent with an origin of the NT projection from the NT-containing cells in this region. This group of NT-containing cells has also been reported to give rise to a NT-containing projection to the mediodorsal thalamic nucleus (Inagaki et al. 1983a). An olfactory cortex projection to the mediodorsal thalamic nucleus has been established by Heimer (1972); however, this is the first report of a peptidergic projection to this nucleus. The mediodorsal thalamus itself projects to the frontal as well as the cingulate and piriform cortices, so that it could form part of a feed-back loop passing information back to the olfactory bulb and the anterior olfactory nucleus.

3.3. SEPTUM, NUCLEUS ACCUMBENS AND BASAL FOREBRAIN

Both the medial and lateral septal nuclei contain NT-positive cell bodies (Atlas, level 3); some of these cells are fusiform with one or two major processes, whilst others are multipolar. The larger group of neurons is located in the lateral septum and it extends caudally to join neurons in the bed nucleus of the stria terminalis. The bed nucleus of the stria terminalis contains a large number of NT-positive neurons (Fig. 4a), especially in its dorsal and lateral parts running upwards towards the stria terminalis itself (Atlas, levels 3 and 4). Some of the NT-immunoreactive cells in this nucleus extend forwards and laterally, into the caudate-putamen, where they contribute fibers to a band of NT-positive fibers concentrated on the edge of the globus pallidus. The NT-positive neurons in the bed nucleus of the stria terminalis send axons into the stria terminalis which presumably project to the central nucleus of the amygdala and in turn they receive a reciprocal input from NT-containing neurons in the central nucleus (Roberts et al. 1982).

Below the anterior commissure there are fewer NT-positive cells and they form a band of neurons and fibers concentrated in the ventral pallidum and the medial forebrain bundle (MFB). This system of fibers is most obvious in the adult cat (Fig. 8) and the neonatal rat (Hara et al. 1982). Medially, the septal NT cells merge to join the medial

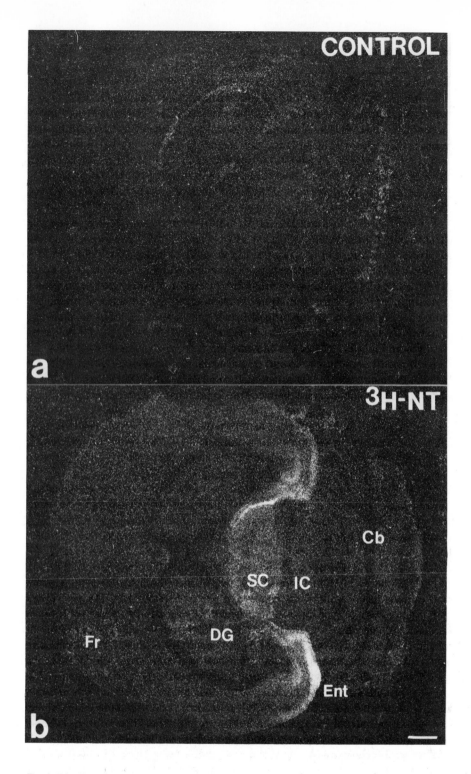

Fig. 2. Distribution of ³H-NT binding sites in the rat brain at different horizontal levels. *a.* Control section at level *b* incubated in the presence of 1 μM NT to determine nonspecific binding. *b–f.* Horizontal-longitudinal sections at different levels in the rat brain.

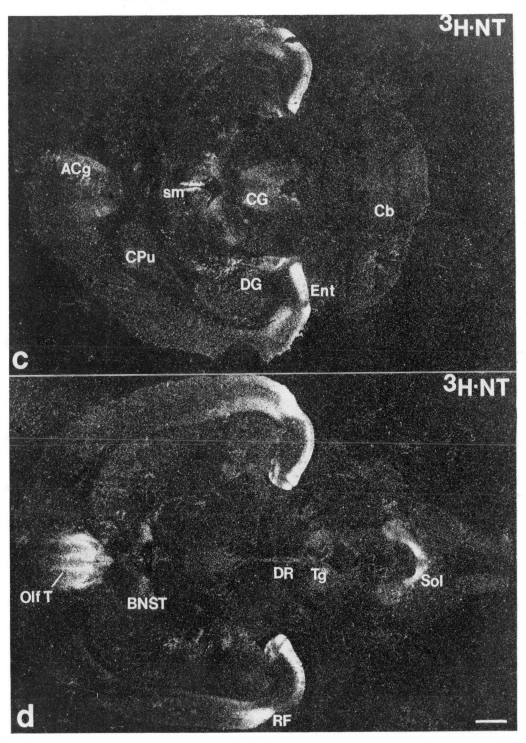

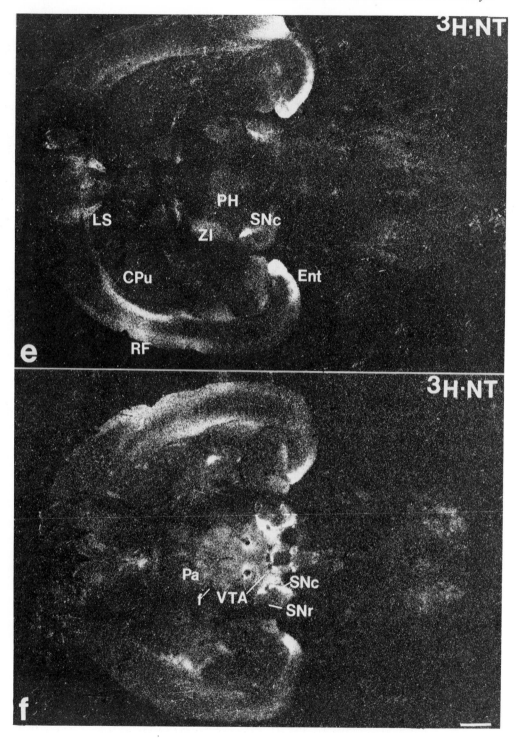

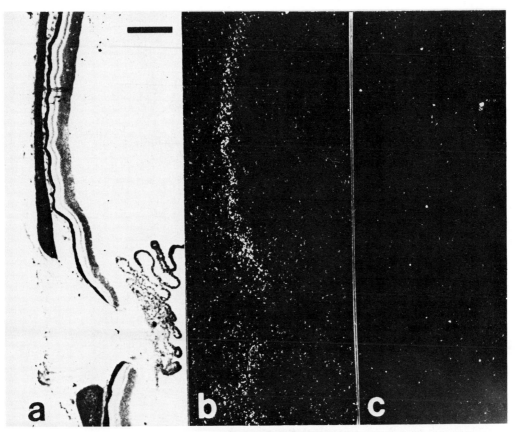

Fig. 3. Autoradiographic localization of specific ³H-NT binding sites in the retina of 2-day-old chicken: *a.* shows a Nissl stain of the section, *b.* incubated in the presence of ³H-NT, whereas *c.* represents an absorption control. Note the labeling of the inner plexiform layer in *b.*

preoptic nucleus and the periventricular hypothalamic nucleus (Atlas, level 4). In the nucleus accumbens and olfactory tubercle there are substantial numbers of coarse NT fibers and in the olfactory tubercle some of these NT fibers outline the islands of Calleja. It is tempting to speculate that some of these fibers originate in the NT cells in the midline ventral tegmental area (A10), where NT co-exists with dopamine (Hökfelt et al. 1984). Consistent with such an ascending projection is the observation that NT-LI does accumulate below a knife-cut lesion placed through the MFB (Fig. 4B); however, we have been unable to detect any significant depletions of NT-LI from septum, nucleus accumbens, olfactory tubercle or caudate-putamen following injections of the neurotoxin 6-hydroxydopamine into the ventral tegmental area and substantia nigra (our unpublished observations).

The concentration of specific NT binding sites in the septum, bed nucleus of the stria terminalis and olfactory tubercle (Fig. 2, levels c–f) is in good agreement with the presence of NT-containing fibers and cells in these areas. One anomaly is, however, the low density of binding sites in the rat nucleus accumbens, although this area contains a high NT-LI content (Atlas, level 2 and Table 2). The nucleus of the diagonal band (Fig. 2f) is moderately labeled in both vertical and horizontal limbs (Young and Kuhar 1981; Quirion et al. 1982).

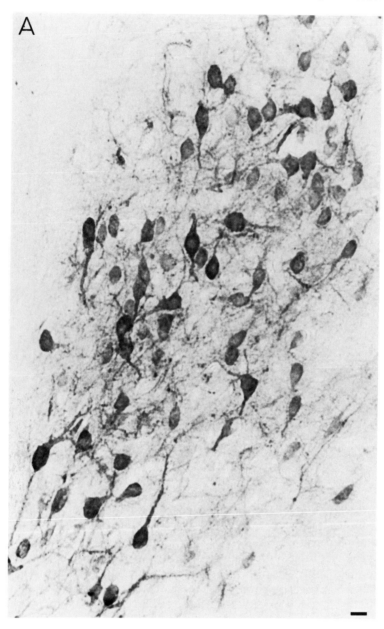

Fig. 4. A. NT-containing neurons in the bed nucleus of the stria terminalis of the rat. Bar 10 μm. *B.* Accumulation of NT-LI below a knife-cut severing the medial forebrain bundle (MFB). L, lesion. Bar = 50 μm. *C.* NT-containing neurons in the central nucleus of the amygdala of the rat. CEN, central nucleus; st, stria terminalis. Bar = 10 μm.

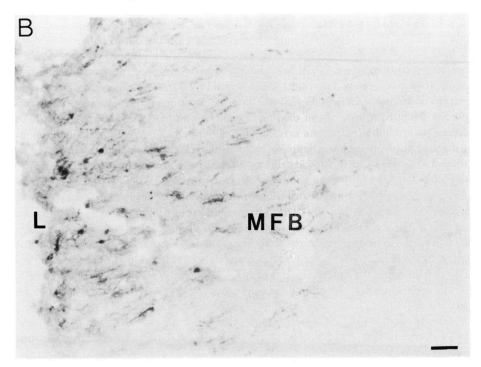

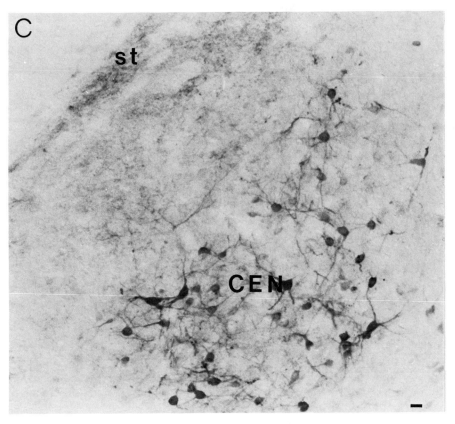

3.4. AMYGDALA, CINGULATE GYRUS, CEREBRAL CORTEX AND HIPPOCAMPUS

The amygdala contains a number of NT-immunoreactive neurons and these are particularly located in the central and medial nuclei (Atlas, levels 6–8, Fig. 4C). These cells which form a continuous rostrocaudal group are similar in morphological appearance to those in the bed nucleus of the stria terminalis (Fig. 4A). The NT cells are located in the more medial portions of the central and medial nucleus. At the more dorsal extension the cells merge into the ventral portion of the caudate nucleus and in a horizontal section it can be observed that NT-positive fibers form a continuous strip run around the edge of the pallidum to the bed nucleus of the stria terminalis. The stria terminalis contains a number of NT-positive nerve fibers which have been shown by lesion experiments severing the stria terminalis to project from the central nucleus to or through the bed nucleus of the stria terminalis (Uhl et al. 1979; Roberts et al. 1982). Additional lesion studies indicate that destruction of the amygdaloid complex, with the exclusion of the central nucleus and the stria terminalis, depletes the medial dorsal thalamic nucleus, the olfactory bulb and the diagonal band of NT-LI, suggesting that NT-containing cells outside the central nucleus provide the axons innervating these regions (Inagaki et al. 1983a,b; see also Fig. 17).

In a detailed study of the ontogeny of NT cells in the rat Hara et al. (1982) showed that NT cells could first be visualized at gestational day 16, and reached a maximum in the amygdaloid complex at post-natal day 7 (Fig. 5). At this time, NT-positive cells are found in the anterior and cortical nuclei, regions in which NT cells are not readily demonstrable in the adult rat. At gestational day 19 two NT-positive nerve fiber tracts, in addition to the stria terminalis, can be demonstrated, the first being in the lateral olfactory tract (Fig. 5C, TOL) and the second lying medial to the anterior amygdaloid nucleus and running towards the hypothalamus (Hara et al. 1982) (Fig. 5C, VAF).

Ontogenetic studies have also revealed the presence of NT-containing neurons in the subiculum (Fig. 6A) and cingulate gyrus (Fig. 6B) (Hara et al. 1982). These pyramidal shaped neurons are most readily demonstrated at gestational day 7 (Hara et al. 1982) and those in the dorsal subiculum provide a substantial NT projection via the fimbria and fornix (Fig. 7) to the hypothalamus and mammillary bodies (see also Fig. 15). This subiculum/fornix projection to the mammillary bodies can also be demonstrated in the adult rat by lesions severing the fornix which leads to accumulation of NT-LI above the lesion and bilateral depletion of NT-LI from the mammillary bodies (Cuello et al. 1983). Roberts et al. (1981) have reported that these subiculum NT-containing neurons project to the cingulate cortex; however, given the earlier presence of NT-containing cells in the anterior and posterior cingulate cortex contributing NT fibers to the cingulum, this conclusion must be considered suspect.

The neocortex and the hippocampus have not yet been shown to contain any NT-positive cells, although both regions contain NT receptors. The receptors in the neocortex have been reported to be concentrated in laminae I and IV (Young and Kuhar 1981; Quirion et al. 1982). In the cingulate, retrosplenial and frontal cortices there is a particular concentration of NT receptors in the superficial cortical layers (see Fig. 2b–f). It is of interest to note that in part this distribution coincides with the distribution of dopaminergic mesocortical fibers which are concentrated in frontal and cingulate cortices, as well as around the rhinal sulcus (for recent review, see Björklund and Lindvall, *Vol. 2,* Ch. III, This Series). However, the distribution of NT receptors in the cingulate cortex includes both anterior and posterior cingulate cortices and these receptors run

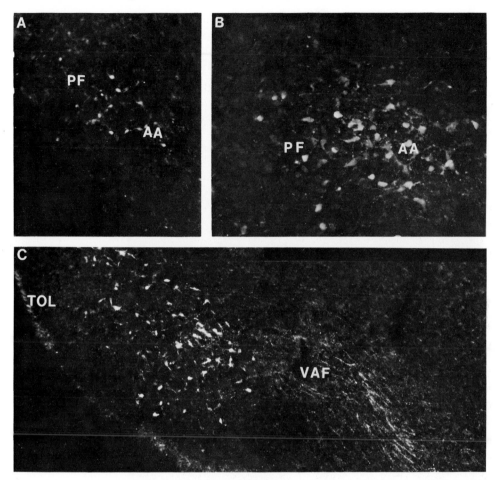

Fig. 5. Fluorescent photomicrographs to demonstrate the localization of NT-positive structures in the anterior amygdala (AA) and piriform cortex (PF) at *A*, gestational day 16, *B*, gestational day 17 and *C*, gestational day 19. Note the presence of NT-positive fibers in the lateral olfactory tract (TOL) and in the ventral amygdala (VAF). Scale: A × 100, B × 160 and C × 100. (Reproduced from Hara et al. (1982), by courtesy of the Editors of the *Journal of Comparative Neurology*.)

back into the retrosplenial cortex, dorsal subiculum, around the medial edge of the dentate gyrus, through the presubiculum into the entorhinal cortex. This is a much more widespread distribution than the mesocortical dopamine system and in the subiculum and ventral parts of the dentate gyrus includes regions not significantly innervated by the mesocortical dopamine system.

In the amygdala, moderate levels of receptor binding are found in the medial, basomedial and cortical nuclei (Fig. 2d,e) but it is interesting to note that the central nucleus, which is one of the areas with the highest concentration of NT cells and fibers, is not particularly rich in receptors.

3.5. CAUDATE-PUTAMEN, SUBSTANTIA NIGRA AND VENTRAL MESENCEPHALON

The caudate-putamen of the rat is only sparsely innervated by NT-containing fibers and

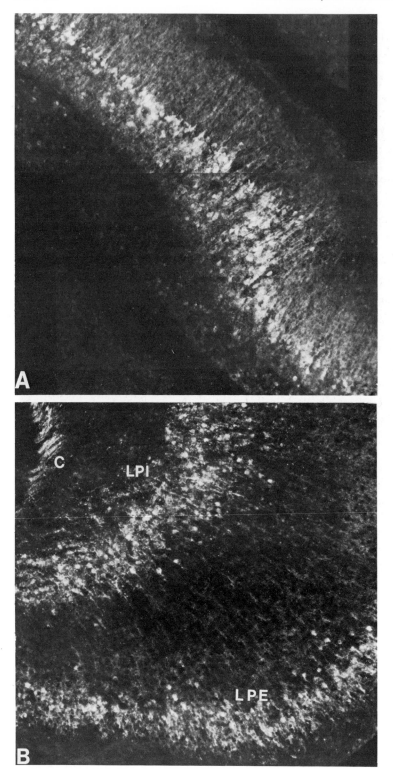

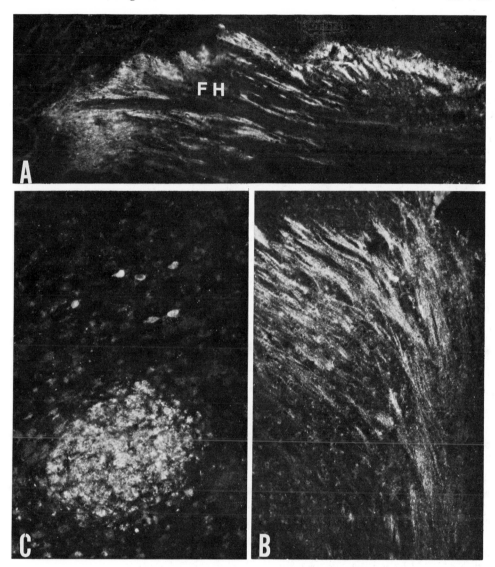

Fig. 7. Photomicrographs showing numerous NT-positive fibers located in various parts of the fornix in 7-day-old rats pretreated with colchicine. Frontal sections A. NT-positive nerve fibers in fimbria hippocampi (FH) and in the fornix at the level of the hypothalamus (B) and in the fornix of the septum (C). A × 90, B × 108, C × 170. (Reproduced from Hara et al. (1982), by courtesy of the Editors of the *Journal of Comparative Neurology*.)

contains only a few NT neurons (these being concentrated in the ventral and medial portions and representing extensions of the amygdaloid and bed nucleus cell groups) (Atlas, level 3–5). However, the rat caudate-putamen does show some evidence of a patchy distribution of NT fibers (Jennes et al. 1982) which may relate to the histochemi-

---

Fig. 6. NT-positive neurons in *A*, the subiculum and *B*, the cingulate gyrus of the rat at postnatal day 1 (A), or postnatal day 7 (B). LPI, lamina principalis interna; LPE, lamina principalis externa; C, cingulum bundle. A and B: × 120. (Reproduced from Hara et al. (1982), by courtesy of the Editors of the *Journal of Comparative Neurology*.)

cally distinct organization of afferent and efferent connections characteristic of the striatum (Graybiel et al. 1979, 1981). This patterning of NT-containing fibers is, however, better seen in the cat brain and we have recently studied the cat striatum using both immunocytochemistry to localize NT-containing fibers (Goedert et al. 1983a) and receptor autoradiography to localize ^{3}H-NT binding sites (Goedert et al. 1984b).

The cat striatum is relatively enriched in NT-containing fibers (Fig. 8) which are in register with the enkephalin-rich, cholinesterase-poor regions which have been termed 'striosomes' (Graybiel and Ragsdale 1978; Graybiel et al. 1979,1981; Graybiel 1982; Goedert et al. 1983a). These patches also coincide with patches of opiate receptors (Herkenham and Pert 1981) (Fig. 9) but interestingly these patches are not enriched in NT receptors which instead are concentrated in the AChE-rich, NT-poor tissue surrounding the striosomes (Goedert et al. 1984b).

Autoradiographic studies in both cat and rat show a concentration of NT receptors over the substantia nigra and the ventral tegmental area dopamine neurons (Fig. 2e,f, Fig. 10). That some, at least, of these dopamine cells do indeed carry NT receptors can be shown by use of the neurotoxin 6-hydroxydopamine (6-OHDA), intranigral injection of which results in degeneration of the dopamine cells and depletion of nigral NT binding sites (Palacios and Kuhar 1981). As would be expected from the location of these receptors over both A9 and A10 dopamine neurons a depletion of NT receptor binding sites can be detected in the rat striatum following 6-OHDA lesions (Table 4) (Goedert et al. 1984c). However, the majority of ^{3}H-NT binding sites in the caudate-putamen is localized on intrinsic cells, as kainic acid lesions destroy between 50–60% of ^{3}H-NT binding sites (Goedert et al. 1984c). The relationship between the striatal NT-containing axons and the NT-receptor binding sites is not known, but it is worth noting that chronic neuroleptic treatment which leads to dopamine receptor blockade results in a dramatic increase of the NT content (3–4-fold increase) in the rat striatum and nucleus accumbens (our unpublished observations). Striatal tissue from brains of patients dying with a diagnosis of schizophrenia (and exposed to long-term neuroleptic therapy) has also been reported to contain increased numbers of ^{3}H-NT binding sites (Quirion et al. 1982). All these data suggest that the basal ganglia NT system may be involved in the modulation of dopaminergic activity and that the increase in NT-LI content following neuroleptic treatment is related to chronic dopamine-receptor blockade (for further discussion, see review by Nemeroff and Prange 1982).

Immunohistochemical studies (Hökfelt et al. 1984) have recently established that a population of ventral tegmental and pars lateralis dopamine neurons also contain NT-LI (Atlas, level 9–10). These cells include the majority of the NT-positive cells in the ventral mesencephalic area (Fig. 11C,D), including the ventral tegmental area, pars compacta and pars lateralis of the substantia nigra and extending up from the ventral tegmental area to NT-positive cells in the midline. At more caudal levels these double-stained neurons include cells in the dorsal raphe and the vagal solitary nucleus (Fig. 11A,B) (see later). The projections of these cells, the majority of which is localized in the ventral tegmental area are not known, but it seems likely that they contribute to

---

Fig. 8. Photomicrographs *A* and *B* show the distribution of NT-LI (NT) in the striatum of the cat. Note that in the caudate nucleus (Cd) there is a patchy distribution, whereas the globus pallidus (GP) has a homogeneous distribution broken up by myelinated fiber bundles. Bars = 450 μm. Photomicrographs *C* and *D* show enkephalin (ENK) and NT-LI (NT) in adjacent sections of the caudate nucleus. The arrrows indicate patches of immunoreactivity which appear to overlap in the 2 adjacent 30-μm brain sections. Bars = 250 μm. Cd, caudate nucleus; CI, internal capsule; ENK, enkephalin; GP, globus pallidus; NT, neurotensin; Put, putamen.

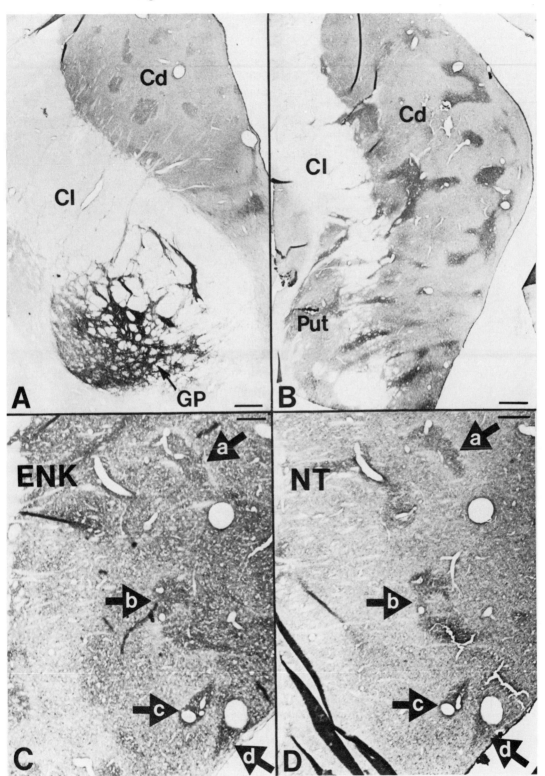

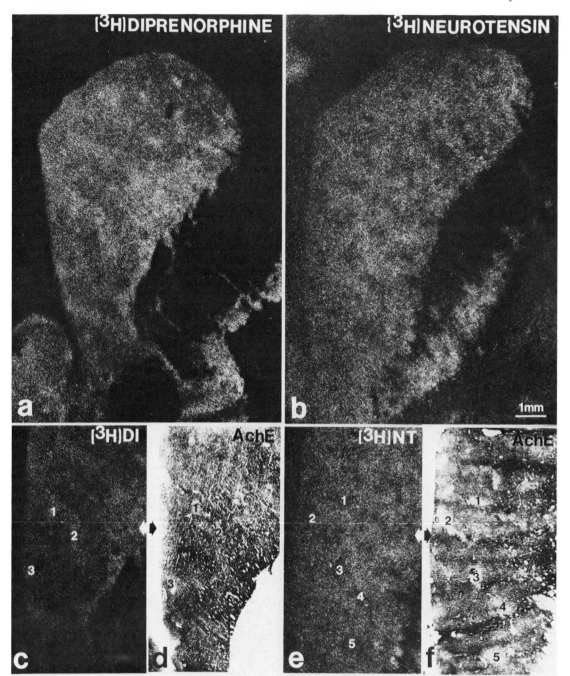

Fig. 9. Autoradiography of ³H-NT and ³H-diprenorphine in the cat caudate nucleus. *a,b.* The caudate nucleus labeled with ³H-diprenorphine and ³H-NT respectively. *c,d.* Section labeled with ³H-diprenorphine and stained for acetylcholinesterase. *e,f.* Section labeled with ³H-NT and stained for acetylcholinesterase. The numbers in *c–f* refer to the acetylcholinesterase-poor striosomes. Note the correspondence between striosomes and dense ³H-diprenorphine labeling and the inverse relationship between striosomes and ³H-NT binding sites.

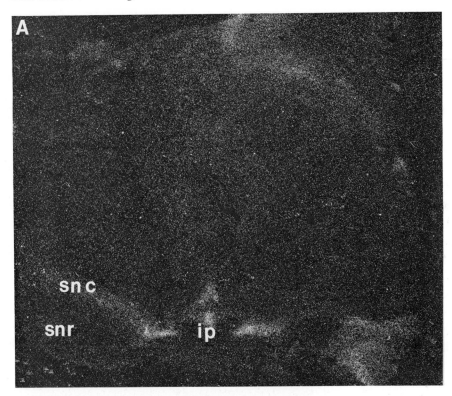

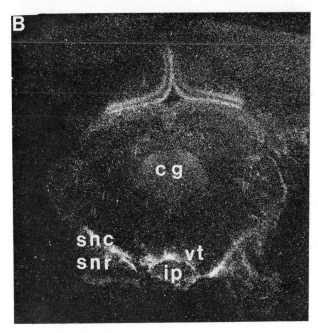

Fig. 10. Localization of ³H-NT binding sites in (A) the cat substantia nigra and (B) the rat substantia nigra. snc, substantia nigra, pars compacta; snr, substantia nigra, pars reticulata; vt, ventral tegmental area; ip, interpeduncular nucleus; cg, central gray.

P.C. Emson, M. Goedert and P.W. Mantyh

TABLE 4. *Effects of kainic acid, 6-hydroxydopamine and cortical ablation on specific ³H-NT binding in the rat striatum*

	³H-NT binding (fmol/mg protein)	Tyrosine hydroxylase activity (nmol DOPA/hr/mg protein)	Choline acetyltransferase activity (nmol acetylcholine/hr/mg protein)
Controls	177 ± 10 (6)	n.d.	175 ± 12 (6)
Kainic acid	76 ± 6* (6)	n.d.	37 ± 5* (6)
Controls	165 ± 12 (6)	3 ± 0.2 (6)	n.d.
6-Hydroxydopamine	108 ± 11** (6)	0.4 ± 0.008* (6)	n.d.
Controls	169 ± 10 (4)	n.d.	n.d.
Cortex ablation	138 ± 4** (4)	n.d.	n.d.

Each value represents the mean ± SEM of the number of determinations indicated in parentheses. The concentration of ³H-NT used was 2 nM.
*p < 0.001; **p < 0.05 (Student's *t* test). n.d., not determined.

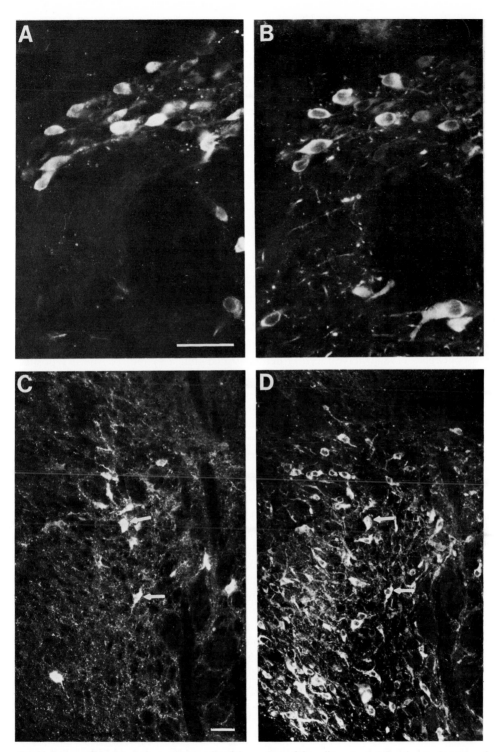

Fig. 11. Immunofluorescent photomicrographs of the nucleus of the solitary tract *A,B* and ventral mesencephalon *C,D*, after incubation with antiserum to NT (A,C) and after elution and restaining with antiserum to tyrosine hydroxylase (TOH) (B,D). Note the large number of cells in *A* and *C* which contain both NT, and TOH immunoreactivity. These cells are adrenergic neurons. Note also the presence of a few neurons staining for both neurotensin and TOH in the ventral mesencephalon (arrowed cells in *C* and *D*). Bar A–D 50 μm. (Reproduced from Hökfelt et al. (1984), by courtesy of the Editors of the *Journal of Comparative Neurology*.)

mesocortical and mesolimbic projections (for review, see Björklund and Lindvall, *Vol. 2*, Ch. III, This Series). Biochemical studies do not indicate any significant depletions of rat basal ganglia NT-LI following 6-OHDA lesions (our unpublished observations); thus, it may be that the co-existence of dopamine and NT-LI is confined to rather discrete regions of the telencephalon, as has previously been shown for dopamine and cholecystokinin-LI (Hökfelt et al. 1980a,b; Marley et al. 1982).

3.6. HYPOTHALAMUS AND THALAMUS

The rat hypothalamus contains by far the largest number of NT-containing cell bodies in the mammalian CNS (Atlas, levels 3–8). The neurons are particularly localized around the ventricles extending from the rostral preoptic periventricular nucleus through to the more caudal arcuate and paraventricular nuclei (Kahn et al. 1981, 1982; Jenner et al. 1982) (Fig. 12). Apart from these more medially concentrated NT neurons, the lateral preoptic nucleus and the lateral hypothalamus contain a number of NT-positive neurons. The neurons in the lateral hypothalamus run medially to join up with a group of NT-positive cells lying between the dorsomedial and ventromedial cell groups; the ventromedial nucleus is essentially devoid of positive cells. It has originally been reported that the ventromedial nucleus is also free of NT-positive fibers; however, Inagaki and colleagues (1983c) have recently demonstrated that a system of fine NT-positive nerve fibers apparently originating from the medial amygdala exists in this nucleus (Fig. 13).

At the very rostral end of the hypothalamus, Jennes et al. (1982) noted that the NT-positive neurons in the nuclei surrounding the ventricles are continuous with cells in the diagonal band. These nuclei include the preoptic nucleus, the periventricular and median preoptic nuclei, as well as a group of cells in the rostral preoptic suprachiasmatic nucleus (Kahn et al. 1981,1982; Jennes et al. 1982). The more laterally placed cells in this region merge with cells in the lateral preoptic region and horizontal limb of the diagonal band (Jennes et al. 1982). The most striking concentration of NT-positive cells is found in the paraventricular nucleus (Fig. 12), especially in its parvocellular part, and this system is continuous rostrally and caudally with cells in the periventricular nucleus and the arcuate nucleus (Atlas, level 6–7). Most of the NT-positive cells in the arcuate nucleus have also been shown to contain dopamine (Ibata et al. 1983; Hökfelt et al. 1984) (Fig. 14). The presence of NT and dopamine in these cells indicates that they correspond to the A12 dopamine neurons known to project to the median eminence and the intermediate and posterior lobes of the pituitary gland (for details, see Björklund and Lindvall, *Vol. 2*, Ch. III, This Series). In this respect, it is interesting to notice that neonatal administration of monosodium glutamate produces a 70% decrease in NT-LI in the neurointermediate lobe of the pituitary gland, indicating the existence of a NT projection from the arcuate nucleus to the neurointermediate pituitary (our unpublished results). The arcuate nucleus cells are multipolar with 4 or 5 main dendritic processes. The NT-positive cells in the paraventricular nucleus are located primarily in the medial parvocellular portion of the nucleus, although some NT cells are found in the magnocellular region (Kahn et al. 1981,1982; Jennes et al. 1982) (Fig. 12). These cells do not contain dopamine; however, it is likely that they may contain other neuropeptides, such as enkephalin and corticotropin-releasing factor (Gilbert and Emson 1981). It is not yet known if NT is found in any neurophysin-positive cells in the parvocellular portion of the paraventricular nucleus, but if this is the case the peptide would be expected to co-exist with oxytocin rather than with vasopressin, as this is the major neurohypophyseal

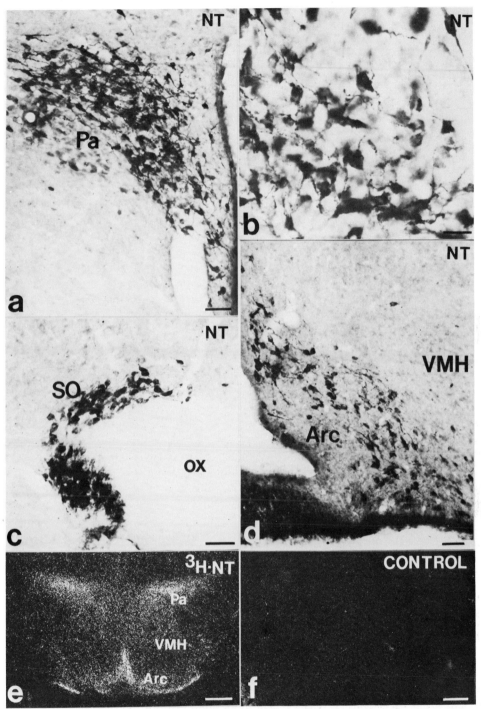

Fig. 12. Photomicrographs of NT neurons and binding sites for ³H-NT in the rat hypothalamus. *a.* Paraventricular nucleus, note that the majority of NT-positive neurons are in the parvocellular portion (Pa). *b.* Higher magnification of the paraventricular nucleus demonstrating neurons and fibers. *c.* Supraoptic nucleus (SO), note the reactive neurons in this nucleus (OX, optic chiasm). *d.* Arcuate nucleus (Arc) and median eminence, (VMH, ventromedial hypothalamus). *e.* Localization of specific ³H-NT binding sites in the hypothalamus. Note the presence of binding sites in the hypothalamus. Note the presence of binding sites in the paraventricular and arcuate regions. *f.* Control nonspecific binding in the presence of 1 μM NT.

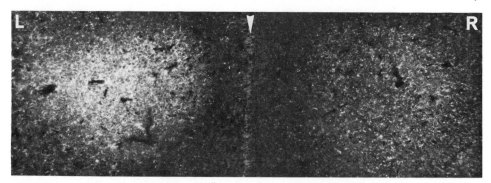

Fig. 13. Photomontage showing a reduction in NT-positive nerve fibers in the ventromedial hypothalamus after destruction of the amygdala. R, lesion side; L, control side. Note the marked decrease in NT fibers on the lesioned side (R). × 80. (Reproduced from Inagaki et al. (1984), by courtesy of the Editors of *Brain Research*.)

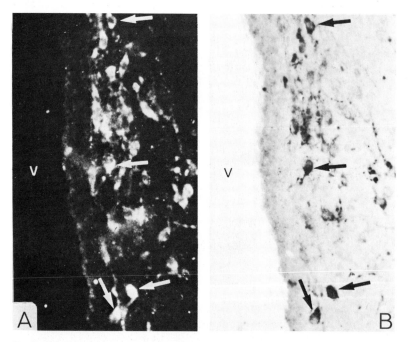

Fig. 14. Fluorescence histochemistry for dopamine and immunohistochemistry for NT when performed on the same section. *A.* Dopamine fluorescent neurons in the periventricular nucleus. *B.* NT-immunoreactive neurons in the same nucleus by peroxidase-antiperoxidase immunohistochemistry. Neuronal perikarya containing both NT and dopamine are indicated by arrows. V, third ventricle. × 180. (Reproduced from Ibata et al. (1983), by courtesy of the Editors of *Brain Research*.)

peptide in this region (see Chapter III by Sofroniew). Apart from the paraventricular nucleus it has been reported that the supraoptic nucleus is devoid of NT-positive cells (Jennes et al. 1982; Kahn et al. 1981,1982). However, we have been able to show the presence of NT-positive cells in this nucleus (see Fig. 12).

The hypothalamus contains several systems of NT-positive nerve fibers, including those in the ascending MFB (Fig. 4B) to which NT cells in the hypothalamus may contribute axons. A major NT projection descends in the fornix to innervate the mammillary body (Hara et al. 1982; Cuello et al. 1983), especially the posterior mammillary nucleus (Fig. 15). As was described earlier, these fibers apparently originate in the subiculum and they project bilaterally to the posterior mammillary nucleus (Hara et al. 1982; Cuello et al. 1983). The other major projection system is that from the paraventricular and arcuate nuclei to the median eminence and the neurointermediate lobe of the pituitary gland. It is not known what role the NT projection to the neurointermediate lobe may have, or indeed if the NT-LI released at the level of the median eminence is hypophysiotrophic. It is known, however, that the intraventricular injection of NT decreases prolactin release, whilst enhancing thyroid-stimulating hormone release; in contrast, NT releases both prolactin and thyroid-stimulating hormone from hemi-pituitaries 'in vitro' (Rivier et al. 1977; Maeda and Frohman 1978; Vijayan and McCann 1979; McCann et al. 1982). In view of the co-existence of NT with dopamine and the ability of NT to enhance dopamine release from some dopaminergic neurons it is possible that the effects of NT on prolactin secretion following intraventricular application are mediated via dopamine release. In agreement with this suggestion is the finding that

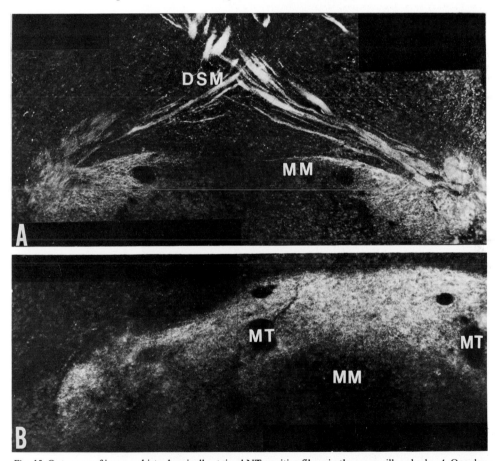

Fig. 15. Ontogeny of immunohistochemically stained NT-positive fibers in the mammillary body. *A.* One-day-old rat. *B.* Seven-day-old rat, colchicine-treated. Numerous NT-positive fibers are found in the nucleus mamillaris medialis (MM). Note that the fibers spread medially and caudally to include most of the MM by postnatal day 7. Descending NT fibers can be observed in the supramammillary decussation (DSM). MT, mammillo-thalamic tract. A, × 74; B, × 82. (Reproduced from Hara et al. (1982), by courtesy of the Editors of the *Journal of Comparative Neurology*.)

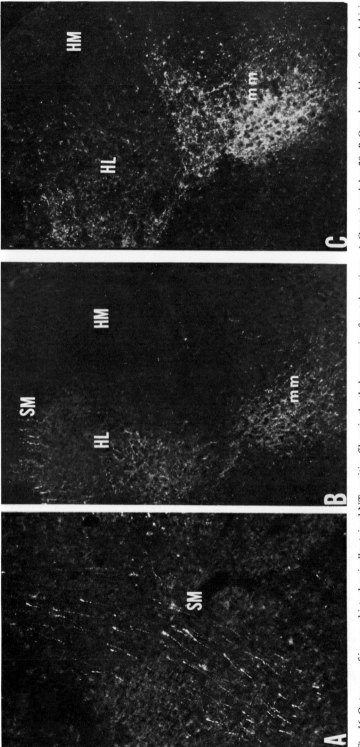

Fig. 16. Ontogeny of immunohistochemically stained NT-positive fibers in the thalamus using frontal sections. *A.* Gestational day 20. *B.* One-day-old rat after colchicine treatment. *C.* Seven-day-old rat. During the fetal period, numerous NT-positive fibers are seen in the stria medullaris (SM) (A). On the other hand, in the lateral habenular (HL) and nucleus medialis thalami pars medialis (mm), the density of NT-positive fibers increases progressively after gestational day 19. HM, medial habenular nucleus. A, × 170; B, × 170; C, × 107. (Reproduced from Hara et al. (1982), by courtesy of the Editors of the *Journal of Comparative Neurology.*)

NT receptors are localized over the arcuate and paraventricular nuclei and also in the intermediate lobe of the pituitary gland (Figs 12 and 22).

Outside the hypothalamus the thalamus is relatively devoid of cells except for a few medially located cells in the ventral posteromedial thalamic nucleus above the medial lemniscus (Jennes et al. 1982; Mantyh and Hunt 1984). NT-positive fibers are found in the medial and lateral habenular nuclei (Fig. 16B,C). The origin of these fibers may lie in the diagonal band or septum, as there are fibers in the stria medullaris running to the habenula (Fig. 16A). The habenula, zona incerta and stria medullaris are characterized by a high density of ^{3}H-NT binding sites (Young and Kuhar 1981; Quirion et al. 1982) (Fig. 2c,f). As mentioned earlier, there is also a NT projection to the mediodorsal thalamic nucleus which originates from the endopiriform nucleus and piriform cortex (Inagaki et al. 1983a,b). Destruction of the endopiriform nucleus and the piriform cortex results in a substantial loss in NT-positive fibers in the mediodorsal nucleus (Fig. 17).

3.7. BRAINSTEM AND SPINAL CORD

The central gray at the level of the substantia nigra (Atlas, levels 8–11) contains a number of scattered NT neurons which at more caudal levels become concentrated into a group lying immediately below the fourth ventricle and including the dorsal raphe nucleus (Jennes et al. 1982; Hökfelt et al. 1984). This system of central gray NT neurons continues down to the level of the facial nerve. The caudal extension of the dorsal raphe NT cells is so conspicuous that Jennes et al. (1982) have suggested that this group of cells forms a distinct nucleus which they termed the nucleus recessus sulci mediani ponti.

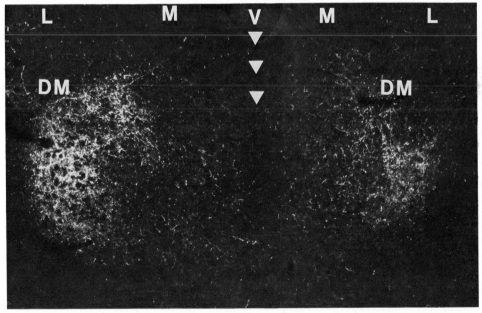

Fig. 17. Photomontage showing the changes of NT-positive fibers in the mediodorsal thalamic nucleus after destruction of the endopiriform nucleus and the adjacent piriform cortex. Note the substantial loss of NT-positive fibers from the central segment of the nucleus. Arrowheads indicate the midline. Left is control side, and right the lesioned side. L, lateral habenular nucleus; M, medial habenular nucleus; V, ventricle. Frontal section, × 96. (Reproduced from Inagaki et al. (1983a), by courtesy of the Editors of *Brain Research*.)

In the midline, below the dorsal raphe nuclei, the medial raphe nucleus contains scattered NT cells. The distribution of these cells places them among the serotonin (5-HT)-containing cell groups of the raphe and periaqueductal gray. However, it is not known if any of the 5-HT cells also contain NT, although this seems a possibility. In the brainstem, NT has been shown to co-exist with dopamine (Hökfelt et al. 1984). The midline NT- and dopamine-containing neurons lie above the interpeduncular nucleus and extend up to the aqueduct; they represent the caudal extensions of the catecholamine-containing regions A9 and A10, whilst the more lateral cells in the retrorubral nucleus represent A8.

In the more caudal parts of the pontine central gray the cells of the dorsal raphe group are continuous laterally with NT cell bodies located around the edge of the fourth ventricle and extend into lateral parts of the parabrachial nucleus (Atlas, level 13–14). According to early reports the nucleus locus ceruleus contains NT-positive cells (Uhl et al. 1979; Jennes et al. 1982). However, recent studies could not confirm this finding, the reason for this discrepancy probably consisting in exactly defining the boundaries of the locus ceruleus; it has been noted that cells in the central gray lateral to the locus ceruleus could easily be classified as belonging to the locus ceruleus (Minagawa et al. 1983; Hökfelt et al. 1984).

Within the caudal medullary nuclei the main groups of NT cells are found in the nucleus of the solitary tract, the nucleus ambiguus and in the area postrema (Atlas, level 15 and Fig. 11A,B). There are NT-positive cells throughout the latter nucleus, but they are particularly concentrated in the caudal and dorsolateral part below the area postrema. It is this dorsolateral group of cells which also stains for tyrosine hydroxylase (Hökfelt et al. 1984) (Fig. 11A,B) and these cells, which are found in the same area as those staining for phenylethanolamine-N-methyltransferase form part of the so-called C_2 cell group (Fuxe et al. 1980). More medially, tyrosine hydroxylase and NT-positive cells are found; these cells are larger (20–25 μm in diameter) and they extend caudally into the commissural nucleus. Rostrally, other large cells are also found in the ventral and medial parts of the solitary tract nucleus (Hökfelt et al. 1984).

Caudal to the C_2 cell group, where NT and adrenaline co-exist, the main group of NT-positive cells is found in the substantia gelatinosa (primarily in the inner part of layer II/layer III) of the spinal trigeminal nucleus. The substantia gelatinosa of the rat spinal cord (Atlas, level 15–18), is characterized by the presence of NT cells in layers I/II at all levels of the cord from cervical to sacral (Hunt et al. 1981; Seybold and Elde 1982). The majority of cells is found in the inner half of layer II, while an occasional cell body is found in layer I, or in the outer part of layer II. The morphology of the cells in the inner part of layer II resembles the islet cells of Gobel (1978). However, not all mammals possess NT interneurons in the substantia gelatinosa. The axons of these cells make asymmetric synaptic connections particularly with the dendrite of other gelatinosa cells (Fig. 18). For instance, the substantia gelatinosa of the cat does not contain NT cells, although a few scattered NT fibers can be seen around the central canal.

NT-positive fibers in the pons-medulla are particularly concentrated in the trigeminal nucleus, the parabrachial nucleus and the surrounding pontine and medullary cell groups. Projections from the medullary A_2/C_2 cell group have been demonstrated to a number of regions rich in NT-LI, such as the paraventricular nucleus, supraoptic nucleus, median eminence, arcuate nucleus, septum, amygdala and parabrachial nucleus (Mantyh and Hunt 1984). It therefore seems likely that at least some of the NT-positive nerve fibers in the solitary tract nucleus, the parabrachial and raphe areas may be ascending NT fibers projecting to regions such as the hypothalamus and amygdala. Re-

388

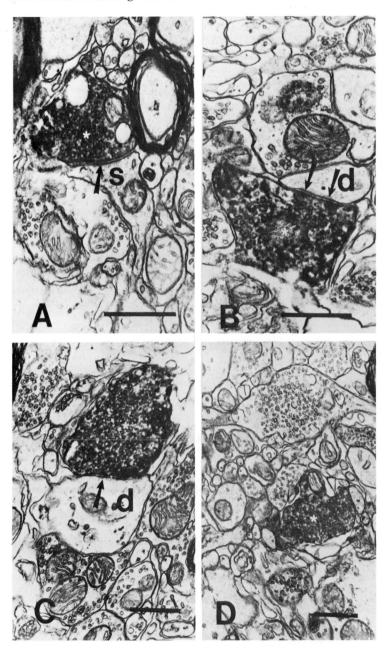

Fig. 18. Electron microscopic immunohistochemical localization of NT-containing axon terminals in layer III of the dorsal horn of the spinal cord. Arrows, synapse. s, spine; d, dendrite. Bar = A, 0.45 μm; B, 0.50 μm. C,D, 0.45 μm.

cently, NT-positive cells have been described that project from the solitary tract nucleus to the parabrachial nucleus, and from the latter to the thalamus, providing a series of ascending NT-containing projections, presumably conveying vagal sensory information to higher centers.

The distribution of specific NT binding sites in the rat pons-medulla and spinal cord correlates well with the distribution of NT-positive cell bodies and nerve fibers (Fig. 2d–f) (Hunt et al. 1981; Seybold and Elde 1982). High concentrations of specific NT binding sites are found in the substantia gelatinosa of the spinal trigeminal nucleus and the spinal cord and these NT binding sites are intrinsic to the substantia gelatinosa, being unaffected by dorsal rhizotomy (Ninkovic et al. 1981) (Fig. 19). Other regions with elevated levels of specific binding sites include the nucleus ambiguus, the solitary tract nucleus (Fig. 2d), the commissural nucleus and the central gray surrounding the fourth ventricle (Fig. 2d). Regions with moderate levels of specific binding sites include the medial vestibular and cochlear nuclei (Young and Kuhar 1981) and the lateral cuneate nucleus, the lateral reticular nucleus and the spinothalamic tract (Quirion et al. 1982).

The presence of NT-positive cells and receptors in the substantia gelatinosa of the rat led several groups to consider the possible role of these cells in antinociception. Initial experiments using intrathecal injections of NT suggested an antinociceptive action in tail flick, hot plate and writhing tests, consistent with a spinal site of action (Yaksh et al. 1982). However, a systematic study (Clineschmidt et al. 1982) could not confirm this result and doses up to 80 μg NT administered intrathecally were without an effect, indicating that the antinociceptive effect of NT is produced at supraspinal sites, possibly at the level of the brainstem. In this regard, Beitz (1982) has recently demonstrated that NT cells in the periaqueductal gray, nucleus solitarius and parabrachial nuclei project to the nucleus raphe magnus. As the nucleus raphe magnus is the origin for some of the descending serotonergic projections believed to be involved in antinociception

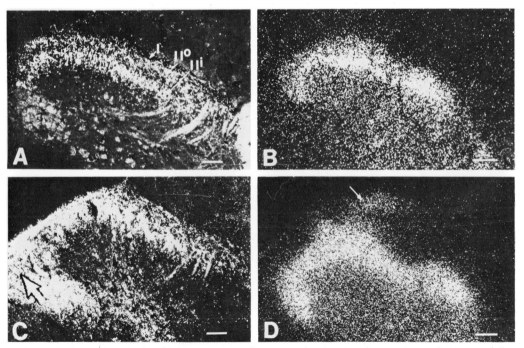

Fig. 19. Correspondence between the distribution of neuropeptides and their receptors in the superficial layers of the rat dorsal horn of the spinal cord. NT-LI (A) and Met-enkephalin-LI (C) were localized by immunoperoxidase staining. The autoradiographic distributions of ³H-NT and opiate (³H-etorphine) binding sites are shown in *B* and *D*, respectively. *C.* Arrow indicates presence of Met-enkephalin-LI within the dorsal white matter – an area that does not show a corresponding density of opiate receptors. *D.* Arrow shows the presence of opiate receptors on incoming dorsal root fibers. Bar = 100 μm.

(Fields and Basbaum 1978) an excitatory NT projection to this nucleus may be involved in central 'pain' control.

4. NEUROTENSIN IN PERIPHERAL TISSUES

Outside the CNS, the majority of NT-LI is found in the gastrointestinal tract, where it is present in substantial amounts in the ileum. High concentrations are also present in the anterior pituitary gland of various mammalian species and in the adrenal medulla of some species, especially the cat. Low concentrations of NT-LI are found in most peripheral tissues, where it is present in autonomic nerve fibers (Table 5). Current evidence suggests that NT may play a hormonal role in endocrine tissues and may function as a neurotransmitter in the peripheral nervous system.

TABLE 5. *Regional distribution of NT-LI in peripheral tissues of the rat (expressed as pmol/g tissue)*

Tissue	NT-LI
Esophagus	2.9 ± 0.3
Stomach	1.2 ± 0.1
Duodenum	0.5 ± 0.03
Jejunum	14.4 ± 0.9
Ileum	81.1 ± 5.4
Colon	5.5 ± 0.3
Pancreas	1.1 ± 0.08
Liver	1.6 ± 0.1
Spleen	0.7 ± 0.03
Kidney	0.9 ± 0.06
Ureter	<0.1
Bladder	0.2 ± 0.005
Penis	1.5 ± 0.1
Testis	1.6 ± 0.2
Epididymis	0.6 ± 0.02
Vas deferens	<0.1
Seminal vesicles	0.6 ± 0.04
Prostate gland	0.5 ± 0.06
Vagina	0.5 ± 0.03
Uterus	0.3 ± 0.01
Ovaries	0.4 ± 0.01
Fallopian tubes	0.5 ± 0.01
Heart auricle	1.8 ± 0.2
Heart ventricle	2.3 ± 0.3
Trachea	0.7 ± 0.1
Lung	1.4 ± 0.2
Thyroid gland	0.3 ± 0.005
Adrenal gland	1.4 ± 0.2
Submandibular gland	0.8 ± 0.1
Lacrimal gland	0.3 ± 0.005
Brown fat	<0.1
Skin	<0.1
Dorsal root ganglion	<0.1
Trigeminal ganglion	<0.1
Superior cervical ganglion	<0.1

Adult Sprague-Dawley rats were used and the values are expressed as means ± SEM (n = 8). Xenopsin-LI could not be detected in any of the tissues listed above (<0.1 pmol/g tissue).

4.1. GASTROINTESTINAL TRACT

By RIA, low concentrations of NT-LI are present in stomach and duodenum, medium amounts in jejunum and colon and high concentrations in the ileum of various mammalian species (Carraway and Leeman 1976; Holzer et al. 1982; Goedert and Emson 1983; Goedert et al. 1984e). By immunohistochemistry, NT-LI is found in nerve fibers throughout the gastrointestinal tract and in both nerve fibers and mucosal endocrine-like cells in the ileum and to a lesser extent in the jejunum (Helmstaedter et al. 1977b; Sundler et al. 1977b; Schultzberg et al. 1980; Reinecke et al. 1983) (Fig. 20A). NT receptors are found in the ileum, where they are heavily concentrated over the circular smooth muscle layer (Fig. 21).

The NT-containing cells are not identical with either enterochromaffin cells or other peptide-containing cells. Ultrastructurally, they are of the open type, reaching the gut lumen via an apical process with microvilli (Fig. 20A). The basal portion of the cell contains large electron-dense NT-containing secretory granules with a diameter of about 300 nm (Frigerio et al. 1977; Polak et al. 1977; Sundler et al. 1977a; Helmstaedter et al. 1977a). Interestingly, some intestinal NT cells seem to contract neighboring cells by way of a slender process (Sundler et al. 1982), suggesting a possible paracrine mode of action. Whereas there exists no functional evidence for the latter, several reports indicate a possible hormonal role for gastrointestinal NT (Rosell 1983). The ingestion of a mixed meal leads to an increase in plasma NT-LI (Mashford et al. 1978) and lipids are responsible for this effect, whereas amino acids and glucose do not produce a significant change in plasma NT-LI (Rosell and Rökaeus 1979). The intravenous infusion of NT leads to an inhibition of gastric motility and gastric acid secretion, as well as to a reduction in the pressure of the lower esophageal sphincter (Andersson et al. 1976,1977; Rosell et al. 1980). Moreover, the plasma NT-LI levels reached after a mixed meal are sufficient to elicit the effects on stomach and esophagus (Rosell et al. 1980; Rosell 1982). Thus, gastrointestinal NT appears to act like a classical hormone, being released into the circulation following a physiological stimulus at concentrations sufficient to act at a distant target site. However, the molecular nature of the plasma NT-LI present increased amounts following a mixed meal is somewhat controversial. Some results suggest that the immunoreactive material does correspond to intact NT, whereas other evidence indicates that it may be entirely due to biologically inactive amino-terminal NT fragments (Rosell et al. 1980; Theodorsson-Norheim and Rosell 1983). The interpretation of such results is further complicated by the fact that the plasma half-life of amino-terminal NT fragments is much longer than the half-life of the intact molecule (Aronin et al. 1982). At present, it therefore cannot be decided whether gastrointestinal NT acts as a classical hormone or whether it merely has paracrine actions.

As mentioned above, NT-LI is also present in nerve fibers in the gastrointestinal tract and intestinal smooth muscle preparations constitute a simple and sensitive biological assay system for NT (Kitabgi 1982). NT exerts both contractile and relaxant action on the guinea-pig ileum longitudinal smooth muscle. Whereas the relaxant effect is tetrodotoxin-resistant, the contractile effect is tetrodotoxin-sensitive and mediated through the release of acetylcholine and substance P (Kitagbi and Freychet 1978; Kitabgi and Freychet 1979b; Monier and Kitabgi 1980; Yau et al. 1983). The stimulatory effect of NT on anion secretion across the guinea-pig ileal mucosa is also indirect and probably mediated through the release of substance P (Kachur et al. 1982). Although the presence of NT-LI and of NT receptors (Fig. 21), as well as the potent effects of exogenous NT on intestinal smooth muscle preparations, suggest that NT may be a physiological regu-

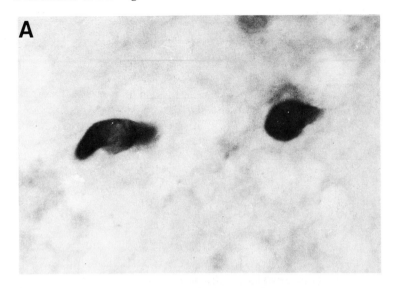

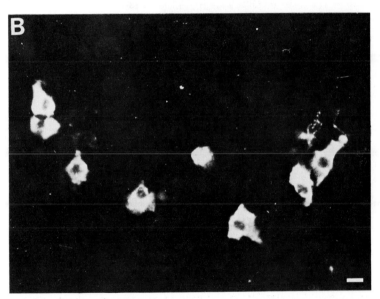

Fig. 20. A. NT-immunoreactive cells in the rat ileum (× 800), as demonstrated by the peroxidase–antiperoxi-dase technique. *B.* Cells in the rat anterior pituitary gland containing NT-LI demonstrated by immunofluorescence. Bar = 10 μm.

lator of bowel motility, they do constitute insufficient grounds for establishing such a function.

Nerve stimulation of the guinea-pig ileum circular smooth muscle produces a non-cholinergic, non-adrenergic relaxation of the muscle tone (Bauer and Kuriyama 1982); this response is abolished in the presence of the calcium-dependent potassium channel blocker apamin, as is the relaxing effect of NT (Kitabgi and Vincent 1981; Huidobro-Toro and Yoshimura 1983). In view of the localization of NT receptors over the circular smooth muscle layer and in the absence of specific NT receptor antagonists we studied

Fig. 21. Autoradiographic localization of specific ³H-NT binding sites in the guinea-pig ileum. Note 2 bands of silver grains over the longitudinal (L) and the circular (C) muscle layers, respectively.

the effects of transmural nerve stimulation on the tone of a guinea-pig ileum circular smooth muscle preparation incubated in the presence of a carboxy-terminus directed NT antiserum. Preimmune serum did not influence the nerve stimulation-induced muscle relaxation, whereas the latter was prevented in the presence of NT antiserum. Similarly, the effect of exogenous NT was prevented in the presence of NT antiserum but unchanged in the presence of preimmune serum. The nerve stimulation-induced relaxation was tetrodotoxin-sensitive, while the effect of NT was tetrodotoxin-resistant. It thus appears that the NT-LI present in intestinal nerve fibers acts like a classical neurotransmitter and that NT constitutes a non-adrenergic, non-cholinergic inhibitory neurotransmitter in the circular smooth muscle layer of the guinea-pig ileum.

TABLE 6. *Concentration of NT-LI in the anterior pituitary gland of various mammalian species*

Species	NT-LI (pmol/g)
Rat	92 ± 3.2 (20)
Guinea pig	24 ± 2.8 (6)
Rabbit	102 ± 8.4 (5)
Cat	42 ± 1.3 (8)
Pig	<0.2 (5)
Cow	4 ± 0.3 (7)
Human	9 ± 1.6 (4)

Each value represents the mean ± SEM of the number of determinations shown in parentheses.

4.2. ANTERIOR PITUITARY GLAND

High levels of NT-LI are found in the anterior pituitary gland of the rat, where it is present in cells (Fig. 20B) (Carraway and Leeman 1976; Uhl et al. 1977a,b; Goedert et al. 1982). The anterior pituitary itself contains only a moderate density of ^{3}H-NT binding sites which are primarily concentrated over the intermediate lobe (Fig. 22). The immunoreactive material is indistinguishable from synthetic NT, as judged by gel chromatography and HPLC and NT-LI is found in the anterior pituitary gland of a variety of mammalian species, including man (Goedert et al. 1982,1984a) (Table 6). The rat NT-containing cells have a diameter of about 10 μm and they are of an elongated shape; at present, it is not known whether NT co-exists with any of the known anterior pituitary hormones. The levels of anterior pituitary gland NT-LI are drastically reduced by surgical and chemical thyroidectomy, whereas adrenalectomy and gonadectomy are without a significant effect (Goedert et al. 1982,1984a; Sheppard and Shennan 1983). The effect of hypothyroidism is reversed by L-triiodothyronine and it is probably due to an inhibitory influence of thyrotropin-releasing hormone (TRH) on NT synthesis, since the administration of TRH to normal animals mimics the effect of hypothyroidism (Goedert et al. 1982). In this line, it has been reported that NT reduces basal thyroid-stimulating hormone (TSH) levels, the cold-induced TSH rise, the elevated plasma TSH levels following thyroidectomy and the TSH response to TRH (Maeda and Frohman 1978; Nemeroff et al. 1980; McCann et al. 1982). Therefore, a functional relationship seems to exist between anterior pituitary gland NT-LI and the hypothalamus/pituitary/thyroid axis.

At present, it is unknown whether NT is synthesized in the anterior pituitary gland or whether it originates in the hypothalamus and reaches the pituitary gland by the portal blood system. In the rat, indirect evidence argues against a hypothalamic origin (Goedert et al. 1984a). The levels of NT-LI in the anterior pituitary gland represent 60% of the median eminence values, assuming that 50% of the hypothalamic NT-LI is present in that region. In addition, hypothyroidism leads to a very large reduction in anterior pituitary gland NT-LI with no concomitant change in the hypothalamus and pituitary stalk transection does not affect anterior pituitary NT-LI levels. A possible physiological role of anterior pituitary NT is unknown at present. It probably plays no role as a peripheral hormone, since hypophysectomy does not change plasma NT-LI levels (Goedert et al. 1984a). It is tempting to speculate that NT may be involved in the paracrine interactions that have been described in the rat anterior pituitary gland (Denef and Andries 1983).

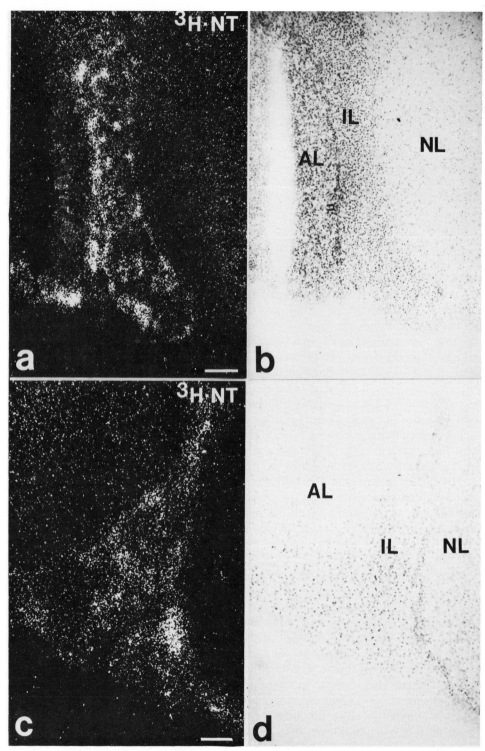

Fig. 22. Autoradiography of ^{3}H-NT in the rat pituitary. Note the patchy distribution of binding sites (a,c) primarily concentrated over the intermediate lobe (IL) and the paucity of ^{3}H-NT binding sites over the anterior lobe (AL) and neural lobe (NL). *b,d.* Nissl-stained sections to show localization of tissue boundaries. Bar = 100 μm.

396

4.3. ADRENAL GLAND

NT-LI has been measured by RIA in variable amounts in the adrenal gland of various mammalian species, as well as in the splanchnic nerve of the cat (Lundberg et al. 1982; Goedert and Emson 1983; Goedert et al. 1983b; Terenghi et al. 1983). The adrenal medulla contains more than 90% of the adrenal gland NT-LI and the immunoreactive material concentrates in a manner identical to catecholamines in a chromaffin granule preparation from the adrenal medulla of the cow (Goedert et al. 1983b). Morphologically, NT-LI is found in noradrenaline-containing cells in the cat adrenal medulla, where it is present in spherical, electron-dense granules with a diameter of 200 nm (Terenghi et al. 1983). NT receptors are heavily localized over the zona reticularis of the rat adrenal cortex with lower amounts in the adrenal medulla and only background labeling in the outer cortical layers (Goedert et al. 1984f). A possible function for adrenal medullary NT-LI is unknown at present. The demonstration of its calcium-dependent release from the cat adrenal medulla (Corder et al. 1982) is compatible with a role as an adrenomedullary hormone. However, nothing is known about possible peripheral target tissues. Alternatively, adrenal medullary NT-LI may have a local influence on the adrenal cortex and influence steroid production through its receptors in the zona reticularis. In this respect, it is interesting to notice that NT-LI has been reported to occur in close proximity to blood vessels in the cat adrenal medulla (Terenghi et al. 1983).

4.4. OTHER TISSUES

RIA studies have indicated that low concentrations of NT-LI are present throughout most peripheral tissues of various mammalian species (Goedert and Emson 1983; Goedert et al. 1984e) and that the immunoreactive material co-elutes with synthetic NT in the limited number of cases where it has been characterized (Reinecke et al. 1982; Goedert and Emson 1983; Goedert et al. 1984e). Immunohistochemically, NT-LI has been detected in nerve fibers in autonomic ganglia of the cat (Lundberg et al. 1982) and in the heart of several mammalian species (Weihe and Reinecke 1981; Reinecke et al. 1982), as well as in cells in the intermediolateral column of the guinea-pig spinal cord (Reinecke et al. 1983). NT thus appears to be present in preganglionic autonomic nerve fibers. In the cat, it is found in both sympathetic and parasympathetic ganglia, whereas in the rat it is probably present in preganglionic parasympathetic nerve fibers (Goedert and Emson 1983; Goedert et al. 1984e).

In the heart, NT-immunoreactive nerve fibers are found in association with the sinu-atrial and the atrio-ventricular nodes, the coronary vasculature and both atrial and ventricular muscle cells (Weihe and Reinecke 1981; Reinecke et al. 1982). Moreover, NT has been shown to exert a strong positive inotropic and chronotropic effect on spontaneously beating rat and guinea-pig auricles, as well as to cause a dose-dependent constriction of rat coronary blood vessels (Quirion et al. 1978, 1979). The structure–activity profile of these responses is consistent with the presence of cardiac NT receptors, although they have not yet been demonstrated using ligand binding techniques. Similarly, the existence of bronchial NT receptors has been inferred from the fact that rat bronchial smooth muscle responds to NT with a concentration-dependent increase in contractile tension (Aas and Helle 1982). In general, much remains to be learned about the distribution of NT-LI and of NT receptors in peripheral tissues.

NT exerts a variety of vascular effects following intravenous injection, some of which are mediated through histamine release, and NT has been shown to be very potent in releasing histamine from mast cell preparations 'in vitro' (Rioux et al. 1982; Carraway et al. 1982b; Rossie and Miller 1982; Krüger et al. 1982). The physiological significance of these findings is unclear at present, since the plasma NT-LI concentrations circulating under normal conditions are too low to have significant vascular effects. It is, however, conceivable that in certain situations the local NT-LI concentrations may be high enough to induce histamine release from mast cells. In this respect, it is interesting to notice that NT-LI has been demonstrated in bacteria and that NT increases the phagocytic ability of both macrophages and neutrophil granulocytes (Bhatnagar and Carraway 1981; Bar-Shavit et al. 1982; Goldman et al. 1983), suggesting that it may be a physiological mediator of inflammation.

5. DISCUSSION

Like most neuropeptides, NT is present in cells of the central and peripheral nervous system, as well as of the neuroendocrine and the endocrine system, implying that it may function as a neurotransmitter or neuromodulator, a neuroendocrine regulator and a peripheral hormone, depending on its location. It seems to arise early in evolution, since material immunoreactive with the carboxy-terminal end of mammalian NT has been found in bacteria and in the nerve cells of primitive invertebrates, such as Hydra (Bhatnagar and Carraway 1981; Grimmelikhuijzen et al. 1981).

There are 4 major groups of NT-positive cells in the rat CNS: those in the spinal cord (substantia gelatinosa), those in the brainstem-medulla (which are continuous with the catecholamine-containing NT cells which are found around the ventricles up to A12), those in the hypothalamus and finally the 'limbic' group of NT cells present particularly in the amygdala, septum and bed nucleus. With the exception of the substantia gelatinosa cell group, all the other NT cells are closely related to the catecholamine system containing either dopamine or adrenaline. In some cell groups, this association is due to co-existence of NT with the catecholamine, but in other areas the distribution of non-catecholamine-containing NT cells, their processes and receptors also seem to reflect an association with the catecholamines (especially dopamine). This close apposition of NT and dopamine seems also to be reflected pharmacologically, as shown by the fact that dopamine receptor blocking drugs elevate NT-LI content in dopamine-innervated areas, such as the striatum, nucleus accumbens, frontal cortex, and olfactory tubercle (Govoni et al. 1980; our unpublished observations) and that in these regions dopamine release is also potentiated by NT (De Quidt and Emson 1983; Okuma et al. 1983); this would be consistent with the presence of some presynaptic NT receptors on the dopamine terminals, as suggested by receptor binding studies (Palacios and Kuhar 1981; Goedert et al. 1984c). It is, of course, not known if NT normally acts in this 'feed forward' fashion to potentiate dopamine release, but it would be of interest to determine if local application of NT 'in vivo' potentiates dopamine release, as it does 'in vitro'. If NT does potentiate dopamine release 'in vivo' this would be difficult to reconcile with the numerous observations suggesting that NT possesses neuroleptic-like actions, such as hypothermia, blockade of amphetamine-induced locomotor activity, muscle relaxation and catalepsy (Nemeroff et al. 1979,1980; Nemeroff and Prange 1982). The behavioral effects of intraventricular NT seem to be particularly related to the ventral tegmental area/A10 dopamine system, where the majority of dopamine/NT-containing cells is localized (Kalivas et al. 1981, 1983). A puzzling observation is that the increase in locomotor activity effected by microinjection of NT into the ventral tegmental area can be antagonized by injecting NT into the nucleus accumbens (Kalivas et al. 1981,1983; Nemeroff et al. 1980). Thus, NT injected into the cell body region activates the neuron whilst injected into the terminal area of the same neurons, the peptide has the opposite effect (Kalivas et al. 1982a,b). If we assume that in both regions NT is excitatory on dopaminergic cell bodies and nerve fibers, then the explanation must lie in the response of the neurons distal to the dopamine receptor in the nucleus accumbens region (McCarthy et al. 1979). It may be of therapeutic value, if the relationship between NT and dopamine systems can be unravelled, as NT-related compounds may provide novel neuroleptics and anti-Parkinsonian drugs.

The co-existence of NT with dopamine in the tuberoinfundibular dopamine system (A12) suggests that in addition to any direct effects NT may have at the level of the median eminence, it may also act in a 'feed forward' fashion to potentiate dopamine release. As discussed before, this would be consistent with the ability of intraventricularly administered NT to potentiate prolactin secretion. It is also likely that an important site of action of NT may be the intermediate lobe of the pituitary gland, where NT receptors are heavily concentrated.

Apart from the possible role of the tuberal NT/dopamine cells in neuroendocrine regulation, NT cells in the paraventricular and supraoptic nuclei may be able to modulate the release of vasopressin and oxytocin. The presence of NT cell bodies in the medial preoptic and septal regions may allow NT to influence gonadotropin release and local injections of NT into these areas (which also contain gonadotropin-releasing hormone-positive neurons) potentiate luteinizing hormone release in the anesthetized rat in vivo (Ferris et al. 1982). The medial preoptic area also contains the highest density of sites for NT-induced hypothermia (Clineschmidt et al. 1982; Bissette et al. 1982), the positive sites matching closely with the distribution of NT-containing cell bodies in this area. Outside the medial preoptic region the central gray is rich in sites in which hypothermia and antinociception can be induced by NT (Clineschmidt et al. 1982; Bissette et al. 1982) and their localization correlates well with the known distribution of NT cells and receptors (Clineschmidt et al. 1982). In contrast to the opiate systems, where both central and spinal sites of action can be demonstrated (Yaksh et al. 1982), NT is only antinociceptive when given centrally (Clineschmidt et al. 1982; Yaksh et al. 1982). Given its potency, a stable and biologically active NT analogue with the ability to cross the blood–brain barrier could form the basis of a new class of analgesic drugs.

In peripheral tissues, the NT-LI present in gastrointestinal nerve fibers seems to play a role as a neurotransmitter and the same may be true for the immunoreactive material found in autonomic fibers. There exists some evidence for a hormonal role of the NT-LI found in mucosal cells of the small intestine, although a paracrine function cannot be excluded. Similarly, adrenal medullary NT-LI could serve either as a peripheral hormone or exert a local influence, whereas a paracrine action seems to be more likely for the NT-LI present in cells of the anterior lobe of the pituitary gland.

Hopefully, specific NT antagonists will be developed in a near future, so that the possible physiological functions of NT in both central and peripheral tissues can be put on a firmer basis.

6. ACKNOWLEDGMENTS

We are grateful to Dr B. Everitt, Dr T. Hökfelt, Dr S.P. Hunt, Dr S. Ibata, Dr S. Inagaki and Dr M. Toyamaha for the provision of figures used in this chapter. Dr M. Goedert was a British Council scholar and Dr P. Mantyh an NINCDS postdoctoral fellow. Thanks are especially due to Mrs. M. Wynn for her careful correction and typing of the manuscript.

7. REFERENCES

Aas P, Helle KB (1982): Neurotensin receptors in the rat bronchi. *Regul. Peptides, 3,* 405–413.

Andrade R, Aghajanian, GK (1981): Neurotensin selectively activates dopaminergic neurons in the substantia nigra. *Soc. Neurosci. Abstracts, 7,* 573.

Andersson S, Chang D, Folkers K, Rosell S (1976): Inhibition of gastric acid secretion in dogs by neurotensin. *Life Sci., 19,* 367–370.

Andersson S, Rosell S, Hjelmquist, D, Chang D, Folkers K (1977): Inhibition of gastric and intestinal motor activity in dogs by (Gln⁴)-neurotensin. *Acta Physiol. Scand., 100,* 231–235.

Araki K, Tachibara S, Nakajima T, Yasuhara T (1973): Isolation and structure of a new active peptide 'Xenopsin'. *Chem. Pharm. Bull. (Tokyo), 21,* 2801–2804.

Aronin N, Carraway RE, Ferris CF, Hammer RA, Leeman SE (1982): The stability and metabolism of intravenously administered neurotensin in the rat. *Peptides, 3,* 637–643.

Bar-Shavit Z, Terry S, Blumberg S, Goldman R (1982): Neurotensin–macrophage interaction: specific binding and augmentation of phagocytosis. *Neuropeptides, 2,* 325–331.

Bauer V, Kuriyama H (1982): The nature of non-cholinergic, non-adrenergic transmission in longitudinal and circular muscles of the guinea-pig ileum. *J. Physiol. (London), 332,* 375–391.

Beitz AJ (1982): The sites of origin of brain stem neurotensin and serotonin projections to the rodent nucleus raphe magnus. *J. Neurosci., 2,* 829.

Bhatnagar YM, Carraway R (1981): Bacterial peptides with C-terminal similarities to bovine neurotensin. *Peptides, 2,* 51–59.

Bissette G, Luttinger D, Mason GA, Hernandez DE, Loosen PT (1982): Neurotensin and thermoregulation. *Ann. NY Acad. Sci., 400,* 268–282.

Brecha N, Karten HJ, Schenker C (1981): Neurotensin-like and somatostatin-like immunoreactivity within amacrine cells of the retina. *Neuroscience, 6,* 1329–1340.

Carraway R (1982): A critical analysis of three approaches to radioimmunoassay of peptides: applications to the study of the neurotensin family. *Ann. NY Acad. Sci., 400,* 17–35.

Carraway R, Bhatnagar YM (1980): Isolation, structure and biological activity of chicken intestinal neurotensin. *Peptides, 1,* 167–174.

Carraway R, Ferris CF (1983): Isolation, biological and chemical characterization, and synthesis of a neurotensin-related hexapeptide from chicken intestine. *J. Biol. Chem., 258,* 2475–2479.

Carraway R, Leeman SE (1973): The isolation of a new hypotensive peptide, neurotensin, from bovine hypothalami. *J. Biol. Chem., 248,* 6854–6861.

Carraway R, Leeman SE (1974): The amino acid sequence, chemical synthesis and radioimmunoassay of neurotensin. *Fed. Proc., 33,* 548–552.

Carraway R, Leeman SE (1975a): The amino acid sequence of a hypothalamic peptide, neurotensin. *J. Biol. Chem., 250,* 1907–1911.

Carraway R, Leeman SE (1975b): The synthesis of neurotensin. *J. Biol. Chem., 250,* 1912–1918.

Carraway R, Leeman SE (1976): Characterization of radioimmunoassayable neurotensin in the rat. Its distribution in the central nervous system, small intestine and stomach. *J. Biol. Chem., 251,* 7045–7052.

Carraway R, Kitabgi P, Leeman S (1978): The amino acid sequence of radioimmunoassayable neurotensin from bovine intestine. *J. Biol. Chem., 253,* 7996–7998.

Carraway R, Ruane S, Feurle G, Taylor S (1982a): Amphibian neurotensin (NT) is not xenopsin (XP), dual presence of NT-like and XP-like peptides in various amphibia. *Endocrinology, 110,* 1094–1101.

Carraway R, Cochrane DE, Lansman JB, Leeman SE, Paterson BM, Welch HJ (1982b): Neurotensin stimulates exocytotic histamine secretion from rat mast cells and elevates plasma histamine levels. *J. Physiol. (London), 323,* 403–414.

Carraway R, Ruane SE, Ritsema RS (1983): Radioimmunoassay for Lys⁸,Asn⁹,Neurotensin 8–13: tissue and subcellular distribution of immunoreactivity in chickens. *Peptides, 4,* 111–116.

Checler F, Labbé C, Granier G, Van Rietschoten J, Kitabgi P, Vincent JP (1982): [Trp¹¹]-neurotensin and xenopsin discriminate between rat and guinea-pig neurotensin receptors. *Life Sci., 31,* 1145–1150.

Clineschmidt BV, McGuffin J (1977): Neurotensin administered intracisternally inhibits responsiveness of mice to noxious stimuli. *Eur. J. Pharmacol., 46,* 395–396.

Clineschmidt BV, Martin GE, Veber DF (1982): Antinocisponsive effects of neurotensin and neurotensin-related peptides. *Ann. NY Acad. Sci., 400,* 283–304.

Cooper PE, Fernstrom MH, Rorstad OP, Leeman SE, Martin JB (1981): The regional distribution of somatostatin, substance P and neurotensin in human brain. *Brain Res., 218,* 219–232.

Corder R, Mason DFJ, Perrett D, Lowry PJ, Clement-Jones V, Linton EA, Besser GM, Rees LH (1982): Simultaneous release of neurotensin, somatostatin, enkephalins and catecholamines from perfused cat adrenal glands. *Neuropeptides, 3,* 9–17.

Cuello AC, Del Fiacco-Lampis M, Paxinos G (1983): Combined immunohistochemistry with stereotaxic lesions. In: Cuello AC (Ed.), *Immunohistochemistry*, pp. 477–496. J. Wiley, New York.

Denef C, Andries M (1983): Evidence for paracrine interactions between gonadotrophs and lactotrophs in pituitary cell aggregates. *Endocrinology, 112*, 813–822.

De Quidt ME, Emson PC (1983): Neurotensin facilitates dopamine release in vitro from rat striatal slices. *Brain Res., 274*, 376–380.

Enjalbert A, Arancibia S, Priam M, Bluet-Pajot MT, Kordon C (1982): Neurotensin stimulation of prolactin secretion in vitro. *Neuroendocrinology, 34*, 95–98.

Emson PC, Goedert M, Horsfield P, Rioux F, St Pierre S (1982): The regional distribution of chromatographic characterisation of neurotensin-like immunoreactivity in the rat central nervous system. *J. Neurochem., 38*, 992–999.

Emson PC, Horsfield PM, Goedert M, Rossor MN, Hawkes CH (1985): Neurotensin in human brain. Regional distribution and effects of neurological illness. *Brain Res.*, in press.

Ferris CF, Pau JX, Singer EA, Boyd ND, Leeman SE (1982): Role of neurotensin in the central regulation of luteinizing hormone release. *Ann. NY Acad. Sci., 400*, 379–380.

Fields HL, Basbaum AI (1978): Brainstem control of spinal pain-transmission neurons. *Annu. Rev. Physiol., 40*, 217–248.

Frigerio B, Ravazola M, Ito S, Buffa R, Capella C, Solcia E, Orci L (1977): Histochemical and ultrastructural identification of neurotensin cells in the dog ileum. *Histochemistry, 54*, 123–131.

Fuxe K, Bolme P, Agnati LF, Jonsson G, Anderson K, Kohler C, Hökfelt T (1980): Central adrenaline neurones. In: Fuxe K, Goldstein M, Hökfelt B, Hökfelt T (Eds), *Vol. 33, Werner-Gren. Int. Symp. Ser.*, pp. 161–172. Pergamon Press, Oxford.

Gilbert RFT, Emson PC (1981): Neuronal coexistence of peptides with other putative transmitters. In: Iversen LL, Iversen SD, Snyder SH (Eds), *Handbook of Psychopharmacology, Vol. 16*, pp. 509–556. Plenum, New York.

Gobel S (1978): Golgi studies of the neurons in layer II of the medulla (trigeminal nucleus caudalis). *J. Comp. Neurol., 180*, 395–412.

Goedert M, Emson PC (1983): The regional distribution of neurotensin-like immunoreactivity in central and peripheral tissues of the cat. *Brain Res., 272*, 291–297.

Goedert M, Lightman SL, Nagy JI, Marley PD, Emson PC (1982): Neurotensin in the rat anterior pituitary gland. *Nature (London), 298*, 163–165.

Goedert M, Mantyh PW, Hunt SP, Emson PC (1983a): Mosaic distribution of neurotensin-like immunoreactivity in the cat striatum. *Brain Res., 274*, 176–179.

Goedert M, Reynolds GP, Emson PC (1983b): Neurotensin in the adrenal medulla. *Neurosci. Lett., 35*, 155–160.

Goedert M, Lightman SL, Emson PC (1984a): Neurotensin in the rat anterior pituitary gland: effects of endocrinological manipulations. *Brain Res., 299*, 160–163.

Goedert M, Mantyh PW, Emson PC, Hunt SP (1984b): Inverse relationship between neurotensin receptors and neurotensin-like immunoreactivity in the cat striatum. *Nature (London), 307*, 543–546.

Goedert M, Pittaway K, Emson PC (1984c): Neurotensin receptors in the rat striatum: lesion studies. *Brain Res., 299*, 164–168.

Goedert M, Pittaway K, Williams BJ, Emson PC (1984d): Specific binding of tritiated neurotensin to rat brain membranes: characterisation and regional distribution. *Brain Res., 304*, 71–81.

Goedert M, Sturmey N, Williams BJ, Emson PC (1984e): The comparative distribution of neurotensin- and xenopsin-like immunoreactivity in *Xenopus laevis* and rat tissues. *Brain Res., 308*, 273–280.

Goedert M, Mantyh PW, Hunt SP, Emson PC (1984f): Localisation of specific neurotensin binding sites in the rat adrenal gland. *Brain Res., 299*, 389–392.

Goldman R, Bar-Shavit Z, Romeo D (1983): Neurotensin modulates human neutrophil locomotion and phagocytic capability. *FEBS Lett., 159*, 63–67.

Govoni S, Hong JS, Yang HY, Costa E (1980): Increase of neurotensin content elicited by neuroleptics in nucleus accumbens. *J. Pharmacol. Exp. Ther., 215*, 413–417.

Graybiel AM (1982): Correlative studies of histochemistry and fiber connections in the central nervous system. In: Chan-Palay V, Palay SL (Eds), *Cytochemical Methods in Neuroanatomy*, pp. 45–67. Alan R. Liss, New York.

Graybiel AM, Ragsdale CW (1978): Histochemically distinct compartments in the striatum of human, monkey and cat demonstrated by acetylthiocholinesterase stain. *Proc. Natl Acad. Sci. USA, 57*, 5723–5726.

Graybiel AM, Ragsdale CW, Moon Edley S (1979): Compartments in the striatum of the cat observed by retrograde cell labeling. *Exp. Brain Res., 34*, 189–195.

Graybiel AM, Ragsdale CW, Yoneoka ES, Elde RP (1981): An immunohistochemical study of enkephalins and other neuropeptides in the striatum of the cat with evidence that the opiate peptides are arranged to form mosaic patterns in register with the striosomal compartments visible by acetylcholinesterase staining. *Neuroscience, 6*, 377–397.

Grimmelikhuijzen CP, Carraway RE, Rökaeus Å, Sundler F (1981): Neurotensin-like immunoreactivity in the nervous system of Hydra. *Histochemistry, 72*, 199–209.

Hammer RA, Leeman SE, Carraway R, Williams RH (1980): Isolation of human intestinal neurotensin. *J. Biol. Chem., 255*, 2476–2480.

Hara Y, Shiosaka S, Seraba E, Sakanaka M, Inagaki S, Takagi H, Kawai Y, Takatsuki K, Matsuzaki T, Tohyama M (1982): Ontogeny of the neurotensin containing neuron system of the rat: immunohisto-chemical analysis I. Forebrain and diencephalon. *J. Comp. Neurol., 208*, 177–195.

Haubrich DR, Martin GE, Pflueger AB, Williams M (1982): Neurotensin effects on brain dopaminergic sys-tems. *Brain Res., 231*, 216–221.

Heimer L (1972): The olfactory connections of the diencephalon in the rat: an experimental, light and electron-microscopic study with special emphasis on the problem of terminal degeneration. *Brain Behav. Evol., 6*, 484–523.

Helmstaedter V, Feurle GE, Forssman WG (1977a): Ultrastructural identification of a new cell type – the N-cell as a source of neurotensin in the gut mucosa. *Cell Tissue Res., 184*, 445–452.

Helmstaedter V, Taugner C, Feurle GE, Forssman WG (1977b): Localization of neurotensin-immunoreactive cells in the small intestine of man and various mammals. *Histochemistry, 53*, 35–41.

Henry JL (1982): Electrophysiological studies on the neuroactive properties of neurotensin. *Ann. NY Acad. Sci., 400*, 216–226.

Herkenham M, Pert CB (1981): Mosaic distribution of opiate receptors, parafascicular projections and acetyl-cholinesterase in rat striatum. *Nature (London), 291*, 415–418.

Hökfelt T, Rehfeld J, Skirboll L, Ivemark B, Goldstein M, Markey K (1980a): Evidence for the coexistence of dopamine and CCK in mesolimbic neurones. *Nature (London), 285*, 476–477.

Hökfelt T, Skirboll L, Rehfeld JF, Goldstein M, Markey K, Dann O (1980b): A subpopulation of mesence-phalic dopamine neurons projecting to limbic areas contains a cholecystokinin-like peptide: evidence from immunohistochemistry combined with retrograde tracing. *Neuroscience, 5*, 2093–2124.

Hökfelt T, Everitt BJ, Theodorsson-Norheim E, Goldstein M (1984): Occurrence of neurotensin-like immuno-reactivity in subpopulations of hypothalamic, mesencephalic and medullary catecholamine neurons. *J. Comp. Neurol., 222*, 543–560.

Holzer P, Bucsics A, Saria A, Lembeck F (1982): A study of the concentrations of substance P and neurotensin in the gastrointestinal tract of various mammals. *Neuroscience, 7*, 2919–2924.

Huidobro-Toro JP, Yoshimura K (1983): Pharmacological characterization of the inhibitory effects of neu-rotensin on the rabbit ileum myenteric plexus preparation. *Br. J. Pharmacol., 80*, 645–653.

Hunt SP, Kelly JS, Emson PC, Kimmel JR, Miller RJ, Wu JY (1981): An immunohistochemical study of neuronal populations containing neuropeptides and γ-aminobutyric acid within the superficial layers of the dorsal horn. *Neuroscience, 6*, 1883–1898.

Ibata Y, Jukui K, Okamura H, Kawakami T, Tanaka M, Obata HL, Tsuto T, Terubayashi H, Yanaihara C, Yanaihara N (1983): Coexistence of dopamine and neurotensin in hypothalamic arcuate and periven-tricular neurons. *Brain Res., 269*, 177–179.

Inagaki S, Kubota Y, Shinoda K, Kawai Y, Tohyama M (1983a): Neurotensin-containing pathway from the endopiriform nucleus and the adjacent prepiriform cortex to the dorsomedial thalamic nucleus in the rat. *Brain Res., 260*, 143–146.

Inagaki S, Shinoda K, Kubota Y, Shiosaka S, Matsuzaki T, Tohyama M (1983b): Evidence for the existence of a neurotensin-containing pathway from the endopiriform nucleus and the adjacent prepiriform cortex to the anterior olfactory nucleus and nucleus of diagonal band (Broca) of the rat. *Neuroscience, 8*, 487–493.

Inagaki S, Yamano M, Shiosaka S, Takagi H, Tohyama M (1983c): Distribution and origins of neurotensin-containing fibers in the nucleus ventromedialis hypothalami of the rat: an experimental immunohisto-chemical study. *Brain Res., 273*, 229–235.

Iversen LL, Iversen SK, Bloom FE, Douglas C, Brown M, Vale W (1978): Calcium-dependent release of so-matostatin and neurotensin from rat brain in vitro. *Nature (London), 273*, 161–163.

Jennes L, Stumpf WE, Kalivas PW (1982): Neurotensin: topographical distribution in rat brain by immuno-histochemistry. *J. Comp. Neurol., 210*, 211–224.

Kachur JF, Miller RJ, Field M, Rivier J (1982): Neurohumoral control of ileal electrolyte transport. II. Neu-rotensin and substance P. *J. Pharmacol. Exp. Ther., 220*, 456–463.

Kahn D, Abrams G, Zimmerman EA, Carraway R, Leeman SE (1981): Neurotensin neurons in the rat hypo-thalamus: an immunocytochemical study. *Endocrinology, 107*, 47–53.

Kahn D, Hou-Yu A, Zimmerman EA (1982): Localization of neurotensin in the hypothalamus. *Ann. NY Acad. Sci., 400*, 117–130.

Kalivas PW, Nemeroff CB, Prange AJ Jr (1981): Increase in spontaneous motor activity following infusion of neurotensin into the ventral tegmental area. *Brain Res., 229*, 255–259.

Kalivas PW, Jennes L, Nemeroff CB, Prange AJ Jr (1982a): Neurotensin: topographical distribution of brain sites involved in hypothermia and antinociception. *J. Comp. Neurol. 210*, 225–238.

Kalivas PW, Nemeroff CB, Prange AJ (1982b): Neuroanatomical sites of action of neurotensin. *Ann. NY Acad. Sci., 400*, 307–316.

Kalivas PW, Burgess SK, Nemeroff CB, Prange AJ Jr (1983): Behavioral and neurochemical effects of neurotensin microinjection into the ventral tegmental area of the rat. *Neuroscience, 8*, 495–505.

Kataoka K, Mizuno N, Frohman LA (1979): Regional distribution of immunoreactive neurotensin in monkey brain. *Brain Res. Bull., 4*, 57–60.

Kitabgi P (1982): Effects of neurotensin on intestinal smooth muscle: application to the study of structure–activity relationships. *Ann. NY Acad. Sci., 400*, 37–53.

Kitabgi P, Freychet P (1978): Effects of neurotensin on isolated intestinal smooth muscles. *Eur. J. Pharmacol., 50*, 349–357.

Kitabgi P, Freychet P (1979a): Neurotensin: contractile activity, specific binding and lack of effect on cyclic nucleotides in intestinal smooth muscle. *Eur. J. Pharmacol., 55*, 35–42.

Kitabgi P, Freychet P (1979b): Neurotensin contracts the guinea-pig longitudinal intestinal smooth muscle by inducing acetylcholine release. *Eur. J. Pharmacol., 56*, 403–407.

Kitabgi P, Vincent JP (1981): Neurotensin is a potent inhibitor of guinea-pig colon contractile activity. *Eur. J. Pharmacol., 74*, 311–318.

Kitabgi P, Carraway R, Van Rietschoten J, Granier C, Morgat JL, Menez A, Leeman SE, Freychet P (1977): Neurotensin: specific binding to synaptic membranes from rat brain. *Proc. Natl Acad. Sci. USA, 74*, 1846–1850.

Kitabgi P, Poustis C, Granier C, Van Rietschoten J, Morgat JL, Freychet P (1980): Neurotensin binding to extraneural and neural receptors: comparison with biological activity and structure–activity relationships. *Mol. Pharmacol., 18*, 11–19.

Kobayashi RM, Brown M, Vale W (1977): Regional distribution of neurotensin and somatostatin in rat brain. *Brain Res., 126*, 584–588.

Krüger PG, Aas P, Onarheim J, Helle KB (1982): Neurotensin-induced release of histamine from mast cells in vitro. *Acta Physiol. Scand., 114*, 467–468.

Langevin H, Emson PC (1982): Distribution of substance P, somatostatin and neurotensin in the human hypothalamus. *Brain Res., 246*, 65–69.

Lazarus LH, Brown MR, Perrin MH (1977): Distribution, localization and characteristics of neurotensin binding sites in the rat brain. *Neuropharmacology, 16*, 625–629.

Loosen PT, Nemeroff CB, Bissette G, Burnett GB, Prange AJ, Lipton MA (1978): Neurotensin-induced hypothermia in the rat: structure–activity studies. *Neuropharmacology, 17*, 109–113.

Lundberg JM, Rökaeus Å, Hökfelt T, Rosell S, Brown M, Goldstein M (1982): Neurotensin-like immunoreactivity in the preganglionic nerves and in the adrenal medulla of the cat. *Acta Physiol. Scand., 114*, 153–155.

Maeda K, Frohman LA (1978): Dissociation of systemic and central effects of neurotensin on the secretion of growth hormone, prolactin, and thyrotropin. *Endocrinology, 103*, 1903–1908.

Maeda K, Frohman LA (1981): Neurotensin release by rat hypothalamic fragments in vitro. *Brain Res., 210*, 261–269.

Manberg PJ, Youngblood WW, Nemeroff CB, Rossor M, Iversen LL, Prange AJ, Kiger JS (1982): Regional distribution of neurotensin in human brain. *J. Neurochem., 38*, 1777–1780.

Mantyh PW, Hunt SP (1984): Neuropeptides are present in projection neurons at all levels in visceral and taste pathways: from periphery to sensory cortex. *Brain Res., 299*, 297–331.

Marley PD, Emson PC, Rehfeld J (1982): Effect of 6-hydroxydopamine lesions of medial forebrain bundle on the distribution of cholecystokinin in rat fore-brain. *Brain Res., 252*, 382–385.

Mashford ML, Nilsson G, Rökaeus Å, Rosell S (1978): The effect of food injection on circulating neurotensin-like immunoreactivity in the human. *Acta Physiol. Scand., 104*, 244–246.

Mazella J, Poustis C, Labbé C, Checler F, Kitabgi P, Granier C, Van Rietschoten J, Vincent JP (1983): Mono-iodo[Trp¹¹]neurotensin, a highly radioactive ligand for neurotensin receptors. *J. Biol. Chem., 258*, 3476–3481.

McCann SM, Vijayan E, Koenig J, Krulich L (1982): The effects of neurotensin on anterior pituitary hormone secretion. *Ann. NY Acad. Sci., 400*, 160–170.

McCarthy PS, Walker RJ, Yajima K, Kitagawa K, Woodruff GN (1979): The action of neurotensin on neurons in the nucleus accumbens and cerebellum of the rat. *Gen. Pharmacol., 10*, 331–333.

Michell RH (Ed.) (1982): Inositol phospholipids and cell calcium. *Cell Calcium, 3*, 285–502.

Miletic V, Randic M (1979): Neurotensin excites cat spinal neurones in laminae I–III. *Brain Res., 169*, 600–604.

Minagawa H, Shiosaka S, Inagaki S, Sakanaka M, Takatsuki K, Ishimoto I, Senba E, Kawai Y, Hara Y, Mitsuzaki T, Tohyama M (1983): Ontogeny of neurotensin-containing neuron system of the rat: immunohistochemical analysis. II. Lower brain stem. *Neuroscience, 8,* 467–486.

Monier S, Kitabgi P (1980): Substance P-induced autodesensitization inhibits atropine-resistant neurotensin-stimulated contractions in guinea-pig ileum. *Eur. J. Pharmacol., 65,* 461–463.

Nemeroff C, Prange AJ Jr (1982): Neurotensin. *Ann. NY Acad. Sci., 400,* 1–444.

Nemeroff CB, Osbahr AJ III, Manberg PJ, Ervin GN, Prange AJ Jr (1979): Alterations in nociception and body temperature after intracisternal administration of neurotensin, β-endorphin, other endogenous peptides and morphine. *Proc. Natl Acad. Sci. USA, 76,* 5368–5376.

Nemeroff CB, Bissette G, Manberg PG, Osbahr AG, Breese GR, Prange AJ (1980): Neurotensin-induced hypothermia: evidence for an interaction with dopaminergic systems and the hypothalamic-pituitary-thyroid axis. *Brain Res., 195,* 69–84.

Ninkovic M, Hunt SP, Kelly JS (1981): Effect of dorsal rhizotomy on the autoradiographic distribution of opiate and neurotensin receptors and neurotensin-like immunoreactivity within the rat spinal cord. *Brain Res., 230,* 111–119.

Okuma Y, Fukuda Y, Osumi Y (1983): Neurotensin potentiates the potassium-induced release of endogenous dopamine from rat striatal slices. *Eur. J. Pharmacol., 93,* 27–33.

Palacios JM, Kuhar MJ (1981): Neurotensin receptors are located on dopamine-containing neurons in rat midbrain. *Nature (London), 294,* 587–589.

Polak JM, Sullivan SM, Bloom SR, Buchan AMJ, Facer P, Brown MR, Pearse AGE (1977): Specific localisation of neurotensin in human intestine by radioimmunoassay and immunocytochemistry. *Nature (London), 270,* 183–184.

Quirion R, Rioux F, Regoli D (1978): Chronotropic and inotropic effects of neurotensin on spontaneously beating auricles. *Can. J. Physiol. Pharmacol., 56,* 671–673.

Quirion R, Rioux F, Regoli D, St Pierre S (1979): Neurotensin-induced coronary vessel constriction in perfused rat hearts. *Eur. J. Pharmacol., 55,* 221–223.

Quirion R, Gaudreau P, St Pierre S, Rioux F, Pert CB (1982): Autoradiographic distribution of ³H-neurotensin receptors in rat brain: visualization by tritium sensitive film. *Peptides, 3,* 757–763.

Reinecke M, Weihe E, Carraway R, Leeman SE, Forssman WG (1982): Localization of neurotensin immunoreactive nerve fibers in the guinea-pig heart: evidence derived by immunohistochemistry, radioimmunoassay and chromatography. *Neuroscience, 7,* 1785–1795.

Reinecke M, Forssmann WG, Thiekötter G, Triepel J (1983): Localization of neurotensin-immunoreactivity in the spinal cord and peripheral nervous system of the guinea-pig. *Neurosci. Lett., 37,* 37–42.

Rioux F, Quirion R, St Pierre S, Regoli D, Jolicoeur F, Belanger F, Barbeau A (1981): The hypotensive effect of centrally administered neurotensin in rats. *Eur. J. Pharmacol., 69,* 241–247.

Rioux F, Kerouac R, Quirion R, St Pierre S (1982): Mechanisms of the cardiovascular effects of neurotensin. *Ann. NY Acad. Sci., 400,* 56–72.

Rivier C, Brown M, Vale W (1977): Effect of neurotensin, substance P and morphine sulphate on the secretion of prolactin and growth hormone in the rat. *Endocrinology, 100,* 751–754.

Roberts GW, Crow TJ, Polak JM (1981): Neurotensin: first report of a cortical pathway. *Peptides 2, Suppl. 1,* 37.

Roberts GW, Woodhams PL, Polak JM, Crow TJ (1982): Distribution of neuropeptides in the limbic system of the rat: the amygdaloid complex. *Neuroscience, 7,* 99–131.

Rosell S (1983): The role of neurotensin in the uptake and distribution of fat. *Ann. NY Acad. Sci., 400,* 183–195.

Rosell S, Rökaeus Å (1979): The effect of ingestion of amino acids, glucose and fat on circulating neurotensin-like immunoreactivity in the human. *Acta Physiol. Scand., 107,* 263–267.

Rosell S, Thor K, Rökaeus Å, Nyqvist O, Levenhaupt A, Kager L, Folkers K (1980): Plasma concentration of neurotensin-like immunoreactivity and lower oesophageal sphincter pressure in man following infusion of neurotensin. *Acta Physiol. Scand., 109,* 369–375.

Rossie SS, Miller RJ (1982): Regulation of mast cell histamine release by neurotensin. *Life Sci., 31,* 509–516.

Schultzberg M, Hökfelt T, Nilsson G, Terenius L, Rehfeld JF, Brown M, Elde R, Goldstein M, Said S (1980): Distribution of peptide- and catecholamine-containing neurons in the gastrointestinal tract of rat and guinea-pig: immunohistochemical studies with antisera to substance P, vasoactive intestinal polypeptide, enkephalins, somatostatin, gastrin/cholecystokinin, neurotensin and dopamine β-hydroxylase. *Neuroscience, 5,* 689–744.

Seybold VS, Elde RP (1982): Neurotensin immunoreactivity in the superficial laminae of the dorsal horn of the rat: light microscopic studies of cell bodies and proximal dendrites. *J. Comp. Neurol., 205,* 89–100.

Sheppard MC, Shennon KI (1983): The effect of thyroid hormones in vitro and in vivo on hypothalamic neurotensin release and content. *Endocrinology, 112,* 1966–1968.

404

Stanzione P, Zieglgänsberger W (1983): Action of neurotensin on spinal cord neurons in the rat. *Brain Res.*, *268*, 111–118.

Sundler F, Alumets J, Håkanson R, Carraway R, Leeman SE (1977a): Ultrastructure of the gut neurotensin cells. *Histochemistry, 53*, 25–34.

Sundler F, Håkanson R, Hammer RA, Alumets J, Carraway R, Leeman SE, Zimmerman EA (1977b): Immunohistochemical localisation of neurotensin in endocrine cells of the gut. *Cell Tissue Res., 178*, 313–321.

Sundler F, Håkanson R, Leander S, Uddman R (1982): Light and electron microscopic localization of neurotensin in the gastrointestinal tract. *Ann. NY Acad. Sci., 400*, 94–103.

Terenghi G, Polak JM, Varndell IM, Lee YC, Wharton J, Bloom SR (1983): Neurotensin-like immunoreactivity in a subpopulation of noradrenaline-containing cells of the cat adrenal gland. *Endocrinology, 112*, 226–233.

Theodorsson-Norheim E, Rosell S (1983): Characterization of human plasma neurotensin-like immunoreactivity after fat ingestion. *Regul. Peptides, 6*, 207–219.

Uhl G, Snyder SH (1976): Regional and subcellular distribution of brain neurotensin. *Life Sci., 19*, 1827–1832.

Uhl GR, Snyder S (1977): Neurotensin receptor binding, regional and subcellular distribution favour transmitter role. *Eur. J. Pharmacol., 41*, 89–91.

Uhl GR, Kuhar M, Snyder SH (1977a): Neurotensin: immunohistochemical localization in rat central nervous system. *Proc. Natl Acad. Sci. USA, 74*, 4059–4063.

Uhl GR, Bennett JP, Snyder SH (1977b): Neurotensin, a central nervous system peptide: apparent receptor binding in brain membranes. *Brain Res., 130*, 299–313.

Uhl GR, Goodman RR, Snyder SH (1979): Neurotensin-containing cell bodies, fibers and nerve terminals in the brain stem of the rat: immunohistochemical mapping. *Brain Res., 167*, 77–91.

Vijayan E, McCann SM (1979): In vivo and in vitro effects of substance P and neurotensin on gonadotropin and prolactin release. *Endocrinology, 105*, 64–68.

Weihe E, Reinecke M (1981): Peptidergic innervation of the mammalian sinus nodes: vasoactive intestinal polypeptide, neurotensin, substance P. *Neurosci. Lett., 26*, 283–288.

Yaksh TL, Schmauss C, Micevych PE, Abay EO, Go VLW (1982): Pharmacological studies of the application, disposition and release of neurotensin in the spinal cord. *Ann. NY Acad. Sci., 400*, 228–242.

Yau WM, Verdun PR, Youther ML (1983): Neurotensin: a modulator of enteric cholinergic neurons in the guinea-pig small intestine. *Eur. J. Pharmacol., 95*, 253–258.

Young WS, Kuhar MJ (1981): Neurotensin receptor localization by light microscopic autoradiography in rat brain. *Brain Res., 206*, 273–285.

Zieglgänsberger W, Siggins G, Brown M, Vale W, Bloom F (1978): Actions of neurotensin upon single neurones activity in different regions of rat brain. In: *Proceedings 7th International Congress of Pharmacology, Paris*, p. 126. Pergamon Press, London.

CHAPTER IX

Neuronal cholecystokinin*

J.J. VANDERHAEGHEN

1. INTRODUCTION

Early in this century, neurons with features of glandular cells were reported in the spinal cord (Speidel 1919) and in the hypothalamus (Scharrer 1928). The presence of peptide hormones in the hypophysis, hypothalamus, digestive system and amphibian skin has been established for many years. Substance P, a peptide material common to brain and gut, was identified in the early thirties (Von Euler and Gaddum 1931), and the idea that endocrine-polypeptide producing cells are of neural origin was expressed in the middle of the sixties (Pearse 1966).

The first demonstration that peptides previously found only in the digestive tract were also present in the central nervous system (CNS) was realized by the discovery of the gastrin-cholecystokinin family (G-CCK) peptide in the CNS of several vertebrates (Vanderhaeghen et al. 1975). It was later shown that G-CCK peptides are mainly present in the CNS as the carboxy terminal octapeptide of cholecystokinin (CCK-8) (Dockray 1976; Müller et al. 1977; Robberecht et al. 1978; Rehfeld 1978b; Beinfeld 1981), in its biologically active sulfated form (CCK-8(s)) (Robberecht et al. 1978). Other molecular forms of CCK are also present in the brain (Dockray 1976; Müller et al. 1977; Robberecht et al. 1978; Rehfeld 1978b; Beinfeld 1981), including CCK tetrapeptide (Rehfeld and Golterman 1979) and CCK-39 (Jansen and Lamers 1983). CCK-8(s) has been shown to be synthesized in the brain and to share properties with neurotransmitters and releasing factors. It has been reported to be involved in various pathological and behavioral conditions (Vanderhaeghen 1981; Morley 1982; Williams 1982; Emson and Marley 1983).

In this chapter we describe the distribution of CCK in the nervous system of the rat together with some reference to man and several other mammals. An attempt is made to report anatomical findings in relation to what is known about their functional significance.

2. MATERIALS AND METHODS

The distribution of G-CCK immunoreactivities is given in the brain, spinal cord and

*This work was partly supported by grants from the Belgian National Fund for Medical Scientific Research (FRSM 3.4521.82–85) and for Scientific Research (FNRS 78–84), the Queen Elisabeth Medical Foundation (1981–84) and the ANAH Rotary Belgium (1982).

Handbook of Chemical Neuroanatomy. Vol. 4: GABA and Neuropeptides in the CNS, Part I.
A. Björklund and T. Hökfelt, editors.
© Elsevier Science Publishers B.V., 1985.

hypophysis of the rat employing immunohistochemistry and radioimmunoassay (RIA). Additional studies have been performed in man, monkey, dog, cat, ox and pig. Only CCKs and not gastrins have been reported in the brain. (For practical reasons, we use the abbreviation CCK for the observed G-CCK immunoreactivities in the brain. In the hypophysis, both gastrins and cholecystokinins have been reported. Therefore we use the abbreviation G-CCK.)

2.1. PRODUCTION OF ANTISERA

CCK-8(s) antiserum 2330/6/1/a was obtained in Dendermond rabbits. CCK-8(s) (Squibb) was conjugated to thyroglobulin (Sigma) using the carbodiimide (Sigma) coupling procedures (Skowsky and Fischer 1972). After dialysis against water at room temperature for 24 hr, 1 mg of conjugate, diluted in 1 ml of 0.15 M sodium chloride, was emulsified with an equal volume of Freund's complete adjuvant and injected subcutaneously at monthly intervals into the back at multiple sites. The animal was bled from the ear veins 8 days after the 6th injection.

2.2. PREPARATION OF THE TISSUE EXTRACTS

Different regions of the human CNS were studied using autopsy material obtained less than 24 hr after death. Hypophysis and various brain areas were obtained from Wistar rats weighing between 200–300 g. Animals were killed by decapitation and the tissues were immediately dissected. For extraction of the immunoassayable material, a 10% weight/volume suspension of fresh tissue in 0.05 M potassium phosphate buffer, 0.15 M saline, pH 7.4 was prepared using a glass homogenizer and a motor-driven Teflon pestle at 4°C. The homogenate was boiled for 15 min and then centrifuged at 100,000 × **g** for 15 min. Samples of the supernatant were taken for RIA.

2.3. RADIOIMMUNOASSAY PROCEDURE

The CCK peptides in tissue extracts were measured with CCK-8(s) antiserum 2330/6/1/ a, using synthetic CCK-8(s) (Squibb) as standard and ^{125}I-labeled human synthetic gastrin hexadecapeptide (G2-17) (Imperial Chemical Industries, Cheshire) as tracer. G2-17 was radioiodinated using the chloramine-T method (Hunter and Greenwood 1967; Gonguli and Hunter 1971). The monoiodinated form was separated using DEAE-Sephadex (Brown et al. 1976). 200 μl of sample in serial dilutions were mixed with 50 μl of tracer containing 5000 c.p.m. of ^{125}I G2-17 and 50 μl of CCK antiserum used at a final dilution of 1/1,300,000 and incubated for 2 days at 4°C. Potassium phosphate buffer 0.1 M, pH 7.4, with 1 g/100 ml bovine albumin RIA grade IV (Sigma) was used as diluent. The tissue extracts were assayed in triplicate. Bound and free tracer were separated using charcoal coated with human serum (Herbert et al. 1965; Donald 1968). Antibody-bound and unbound tracers were separated by centrifugation after the addition of 20 mg of charcoal. The results were expressed in pmoles of CCK-8(s) equivalents/g wet weight of original tissue.

2.4. SPECIFICITY OF ANTISERA

The rabbit antiserum to CCK-8(s) (2330/6/1/a) cross-reacts with gastrin on an approximately equimolar basis. The sensitivity of the RIA is 5 pmoles CCK-8(s)/L or 5 pmoles

G2-17/L. Serial dilutions of brain extracts give displacement curves parallel to those obtained with the 2 synthetic peptides. The antiserum does not recognize Met-enkephalin, Leu-enkephalin, β-endorphin, ACTH(18–39), α-MSH, bombesin, neurotensin, angiotensin I and II, oxytocin, Arg-vasopressin, mesotocin, bovine neurophysin I and II, growth hormone (UCB), ACTH(1–17) (Organon), rat prolactin, rat thyrotropin stimulating hormone (TSH), rat follicle stimulating hormone (FSH) (NIH, Bethesda, MD), luteinizing releasing hormone (LH-RH) (Ayerst, Montreal), thyroglobulin, bovine insulin (Sigma) and human calcitonin (CIBA) at concentrations up to 10^{-7} M.

2.5. IMMUNOHISTOCHEMICAL STAINING PROCEDURES

Experimental animals

Three-month-old Wistar rats were used. Forty-eight hours before killing, some rats were injected intraventricularly with 20 μl colchicine (10 mg/ml, Sigma) dissolved in 0.017 M NaCl. Some animals received 1–3 μl colchicine (1 mg/ml, 0.017 M NaCl) injected directly into the cerebral hemispheres or into the spinal cord either at the cervical, thoracic or lumbar level 48 hr before killing. In some animals, the corpus callosum was neurosurgically sectioned 8 days before decapitation.

Tissue preparation

Rats were anesthetized with chloral hydrate. A group of rats was perfused with the fixative 'Bouin Hollande Sublimé' (Ganter and Jolles 1969) through the heart for 30 min after a 15-sec wash with 0.15 M NaCl. Brains and spinal cords were removed together with the hypophysis, post-fixed overnight in 'Bouin Hollande Sublimé' and embedded in paraffin. Sagittal and coronal sections 7 μm thick were made at 100-μm intervals and used for immunohistochemical study. Other groups of rats were perfused through the heart with 0.15 M NaCl for 1 min followed by 4% paraformaldehyde in 0.1 M potassium phosphate buffer, pH 7.4, for 30 min. Brains and spinal cords were removed immediately and post-fixed overnight. Thick frozen sections (60 μm) were obtained after incubation of the tissue blocks in a sucrose solution (30 g/100 ml) for 24 hr at 4°C. Hypophyses from rat, dog, pig, monkey, ox and humans were removed, fixed overnight in 'Bouin Hollande Sublimé', embedded in paraffin, sectioned at 7 μm thickness and deparaffinized prior to immunohistochemical staining.

Staining methods

G-CCK peptides were visualized in the nervous system and hypophysis by the peroxidase–antiperoxidase (PAP) technique (Sternberger 1979). The staining of frozen tissues with the PAP technique was made on floating sections. The CCK-8(s) antiserum 2330/6/1/a was used at a final dilution between 1/5,000 and 1/10,000 for deparaffinized sections and 1/10,000 and 1/20,000 for floating sections.

Controls

Controls were performed on adjacent sections by using solid-phase absorption (Vandesande et al. 1977) of the antiserum with the peptides cited above for RIA coupled to activated Sepharose-4B (Pharmacia) or by liquid phase absorption at concentrations up to 100 μg of peptide per ml of serum. To eliminate nonspecific immunoglobulin binding by ionic interactions, additional specificity controls were also performed (Buffa et al. 1979; Grube 1980; Grube and Weber 1980).

3. DISTRIBUTION OF GASTRIN AND CHOLECYSTOKININ IN THE CENTRAL NERVOUS SYSTEM AND HYPOPHYSIS STUDIED BY RADIOIMMUNO-ASSAY – RESULTS AND DISCUSSION

3.1. CCK IN THE NERVOUS SYSTEM OF VERTEBRATES AND INVERTEBRATES

CCK has been detected by RIA in the CNS of various vertebrates including fishes, amphibians, birds and mammals (Vanderhaeghen et al. 1975). These results indicated that the distribution of CCK in the brain was established relatively early in vertebrate evolution. In addition, reports have appeared on the presence of G-CCK in the neuroendocrine systems of invertebrates (Larson and Vigna 1983), such as insects (Kramer et al. 1977) and celenterates (Grimmelikhuijzen et al. 1980).

3.2. CCK IN THE DEVELOPING NERVOUS SYSTEM

The level of CCK increases continuously and markedly from birth to the 25th day of age, when it reaches the adult value. CCK is already present at birth and reaches half of its maximal value around the 15th day after birth (Fig. 1). Newly synthesized CCK-8(s) and CCK-4-like material has been demonstrated in the synaptosomes of different parts of the rat brain, and high molecular weight forms of CCK have been shown to

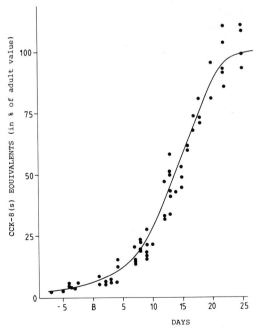

Fig. 1. Study of the CCK in rat cerebral hemispheres during development. B: Birth.

be precursors of CCK-8(s) (Goltermann et al. 1980a,b). The ratio of large to small CCK peptides is constant throughout postnatal development except for the period around birth, where the larger molecular forms are more abundant and it has been speculated that the proteolytic cleavage of precursors may be less active during this period (Goltermann et al. 1981).

3.3. CCK DISTRIBUTION IN RAT BRAIN

In the rat, CCK is widely distributed in the CNS (Table 1). Several other publications

TABLE 1. *CCK (pmoles $\pm$ SEM CCK-8(s)/g w.w.) in the central nervous system and hypophysis of rat and man*

	Rat			Man		
Olfactory bulb	50	$\pm$	2	32	$\pm$	8
Olfactory tract				32	$\pm$	6
Cerebral cortex						
Frontal	222	$\pm$	9	241	$\pm$	15
Parietal				256	$\pm$	24
Temporal				288	$\pm$	47
Occipital				149	$\pm$	3
Hippocampal	67	$\pm$	7	113	$\pm$	15
Basal ganglia						
Accumbens	141	$\pm$	5			
Caudate-putamen	153	$\pm$	11			
Caudate				63	$\pm$	13
Putamen				58	$\pm$	5
Globus pallidus				22	$\pm$	4
Olfactory tubercle	95	$\pm$	3			
Amygdala	165	$\pm$	14			
Thalamus				4	$\pm$	1
Hypothalamus				66	$\pm$	5
Mammillary bodies				5	$\pm$	2
Dorsal hypothalamus	74	$\pm$	23			
Ventral hypothalamus	126	$\pm$	17			
Hypophysis						
Anterior lobe	1					
Postero-intermediate lobe	171	$\pm$	37			
Mesencephalon						
Total	28	$\pm$	4			
Superior colliculi	63	$\pm$	9	14	$\pm$	2
Inferior colliculi	171	$\pm$	23	20	$\pm$	2
Metencephalon						
Rostral	5	$\pm$	1			
Caudal	5	$\pm$	1			
Locus ceruleus				32	$\pm$	6
Pons				7	$\pm$	1
Medulla						
Total	8	$\pm$	1			
Inferior oliva				44	$\pm$	1
Tegmentum				16	$\pm$	3
Pyramidal tracts				10	$\pm$	2
Spinal cord						
Cervical	13	$\pm$	1	5	$\pm$	1
Dorsal	11	$\pm$	2	3	$\pm$	1
Lumbo-sacral	11	$\pm$	2	16	$\pm$	2

are in agreement with the values in Table 1 (Schneider et al. 1979; Emson et al. 1980a; Beinfeld et al. 1981). The highest levels are observed in the cerebral cortex, caudate-putamen, nucleus accumbens, amygdala and ventral hypothalamus. In the brainstem, the pons and medulla have relatively low CCK levels while the mesencephalon is particularly rich in CCK. The spinal cord has substantial CCK concentrations, particularly in the lumbo-sacral region (Vanderhaeghen 1981). The quantitative distribution of CCK in rat brain is comparable to the distribution in guinea pig (Larsson and Rehfeld 1979), pig (Rehfeld 1978b; Rehfeld and Goltermann 1979) and human brain. Also in the human brain the highest concentration of CCK is observed in the cerebral cortex (Table 1). As with many neuropeptides, CCK material is not observed in the cerebellum but is present in the retina (Eskay and Beinfeld 1982). No difference in the levels of CCK was observed in the brain of genetically obese and non-obese rats (Finkelstein et al. 1981). More precise determinations of brain CCK will be found in papers using microdissection or punch techniques (Barden et al. 1981; Beinfeld and Palkovits 1981, 1982).

3.4. G-CCK IN POSTERIOR HYPOPHYSIS

G-CCK-like material is present in the rat postero-intermediate lobe (Table 1), where it is present in a concentration similar to that found in the cerebral cortex. In the rat, this material consists mainly of CCK-8(s) since it co-eluted with the synthetic peptide on Sephadex G-50 and in 2 high pressure liquid chromatographic systems (Beinfeld et al. 1980). Nearly all of the CCK in the posterior pituitary has an extrapituitary origin since it becomes undetectable 1 week after stalk sectioning (Beinfeld et al. 1980). High levels of G-CCK are also present in the posterior lobe of the bovine hypophysis (Beinfeld 1982; Lotstra and Vanderhaeghen, unpublished data). In contrast, much lower levels are present in the posterior lobes of the pig (Beinfeld 1982; Lotstra and Vanderhaeghen, unpublished data), dog, human and monkey hypophysis (Lotstra and Vanderhaeghen, unpublished data 1983). The rat male hypophyseal neural lobe contains twice as much CCK as the female one (Deschepper et al. 1983).

3.5. G-CCK IN ADENOHYPOPHYSIS

In carefully dissected bovine or rat hypophysis free of posterior lobe only low levels of G-CCK are detectable. In rat, pig, monkey, dog or human only low levels of G-CCK are detectable in the whole hypophysis (Lotstra and Vanderhaeghen, unpublished data). It has been reported that the porcine and rat hypophyses contain mainly gastrins (Rehfeld 1978a). Later, detailed studies on rat and bovine pituitary extracts revealed that they contain mainly CCK-8(s) and no detectable gastrins contrary to porcine pituitary which contain low level of both types of peptides (Beinfeld 1982).

3.6. CCK DISTRIBUTION IN HUMAN BRAIN

CCK is widely distributed in the human CNS (Vanderhaeghen et al. 1975; Vanderhaeghen 1981; Emson et al. 1982). The cerebral cortex and the hippocampus have the highest concentration of CCK in the brain. The striatum and the hypothalamus also have considerable levels of CCK (Table 1). Immunoreactive material is present in the brainstem including the substantia nigra, locus ceruleus, the colliculi, olivary complex and tegmentum medullae. The lumbar spinal cord has substantial CCK concentrations while the cervical and thoracic spinal cord have lower levels of CCK (Vanderhaeghen

1981). No material is detected in the cerebellum. Recently, normal cortical concentrations of CCK have been reported together with reduced choline acetyltransferase activity in patients with Alzheimer type senile dementia (Rossor et al. 1981). In the brain of patients with Huntington's disease there is a substantial decrease (50–60%) of CCK content in the globus pallidus and substantia nigra compared to control patients. No significant change of CCK content is observed in the frontal cortical areas, in the caudate or the putamen in Huntington's disease (Emson et al. 1980b). CCK is diminished in substantia nigra of parkinsonian patients (Studler et al. 1982). Those results indicate the possible implication of CCK in the pathology of several neurological conditions.

4. DISTRIBUTION OF GASTRIN AND CHOLECYSTOKININ IN THE CENTRAL NERVOUS SYSTEM AND HYPOPHYSIS STUDIED BY IMMUNOHISTO-CHEMISTRY – RESULTS AND DISCUSSION

CCK distribution in the rat brain and hypophysis is illustrated in Figures 2–8; schematically in the Atlas on pp. 428–431. CCK-positively stained material is present only in neuronal cell bodies and fibers and has never been found in glial elements (Lorén et al. 1979; Innis et al. 1979; Larsson and Rehfeld 1979; Vanderhaeghen et al. 1980a). The atlas by König and Klippel (1963) and the book by Hamilton (1976) have been used for identification of cerebral structures.

4.1. RETINA

We and others have observed in the rat retina, rare thick beaded CCK-positive nerve fibers at the innermost aspect of the inner plexiform layer close to the ganglion cell layer (Eriksen and Larsson 1981). The distribution is more complex in reptile, amphibian and chick retina, with CCK-positive neurons in the lower region of the frog inner nuclear layer (Osborne et al. 1982).

4.2. OLFACTORY BULBS, NUCLEI AND TRACTS

Nuclei olfactorii *(Fig. 2A and Atlas, 1, 2)*

Rare CCK-containing thick beaded nerve fibers and neuronal soma are present in the pars dorsalis, lateralis and medialis (Atlas, 1) of the nucleus olfactorius anterior (Fig. 2A, and Atlas, 1) and in its posterior part (Atlas, 2). Evidence has been presented that CCK is a neurotransmitter involved in olfaction in the nucleus olfactorius anterior (Dupont et al. 1982).

Main olfactory bulbs *(Fig. 2B, C and Atlas, 1)*

After direct injection of colchicine in the nearby frontal pole, CCK is observed in several nerve cells of the tufted type in the internal and external part of the external plexiform layer (Fig. 2B, C and Atlas, 1). CCK-positive dendrites coming from the nerve cells in the external part are seen intermingled with the glomerular soma.

412

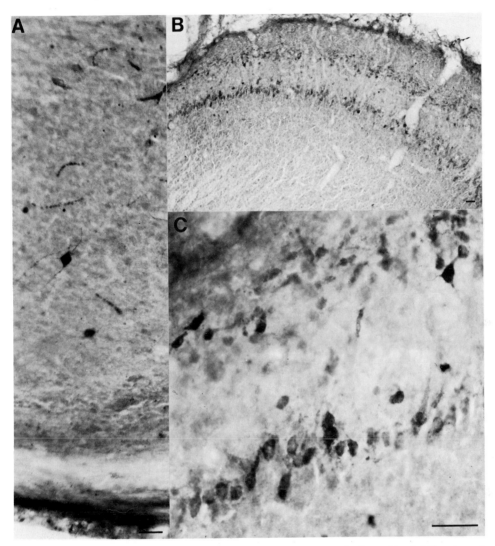

Fig. 2. Sagittal section of the rat olfactory bulb. CCK-positive neuronal cell bodies and beaded fibers in nucleus olfactorius anterior (A) and in the external plexiform layer of the main olfactory bulb (B, C). Colchicine injected directly in the cerebral frontal pole, paraformaldehyde fixation 60 μm thick sections, PAP technique. Bars, 50 μm.

Lamina medullaris interna bulbi olfactorii *(Atlas, 1)*

Rare beaded CCK-positive nerve fibers are present in the central region (Atlas, 1).

4.3. CEREBRAL CORTEX *(Figs 3 and 4, Atlas, 1–11)*

Neocortex *(Figs 3 and 4, Atlas 1–11)*

CCK-containing neuronal cell bodies are present in all cortical layers (Fig 3A) (Lorén et al. 1979; Innis et al. 1979; Vanderhaeghen 1981), especially in the superficial layers

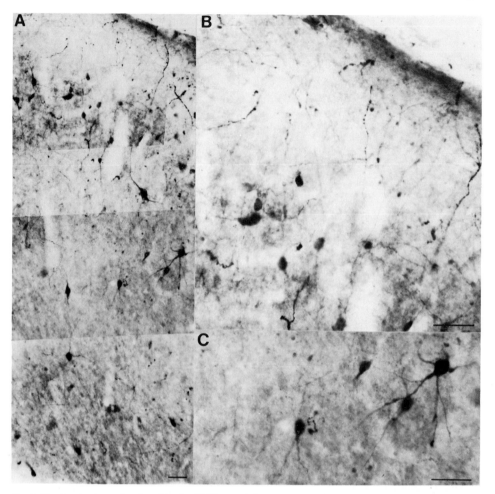

Fig. 3. Bipolar, horizontal and multipolar CCK-containing neuronal cell bodies (A, C). CCK-positive beaded nerve fibers, especially numerous in the superficial part of the cortex (B). Frontal section of the posterior part of the rat cerebral cortex. Colchicine injected directly in the cerebral cortex, paraformaldehyde fixation, 60 μm thick sections, PAP technique. Bars, 50 μm.

II and III (Fig. 3B). Bipolar, multipolar and bitufted CCK-containing neurons are observed especially in layer II and III (McDonald et al. 1982; Peters et al. 1983). The bipolar type (Fig. 3A) consists mainly of elongated cells with long dendrites oriented radially (Fig. 3B) below the border between layer III and IV throughout the depth of the cortex (Peters et al. 1983). In layer I, horizontal CCK-containing nerve cells with spindle shape or conical cell bodies and multipolar neurons are present (Peters et al. 1983). Only a few CCK-containing neurons of various shapes are present in layers IV to VI (Fig. 3A) (Peters et al. 1983). The elongated CCK-containing cells have been suggested to correspond to the interneuronal excitatory cell type termed 'non spiny bipolar neurons' (Emson and Marley 1983). Bitufted and multipolar neurons (Fig. 3C) are thought to be inhibitory neurons (Peters et al. 1983). CCK is therefore present in different types of neurons, some known to be excitatory and others, inhibitory neurons. Electron microscopy does not favor the existence of CCK-containing pyramidal cells (Peters et al.

414

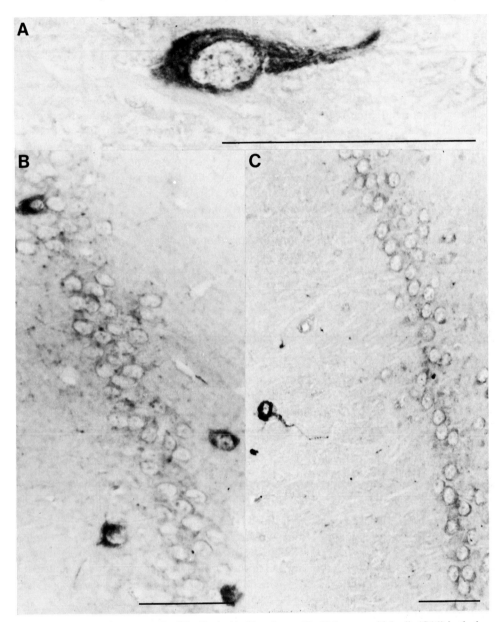

Fig. 4. CCK-containing neuronal cell bodies in (A, B) and near (B, C) the pyramidal cells (CA1) in the horn of Ammon. Transverse section of the rat hippocampus. 'Bouin Hollande sublimé' fixation, paraffin embedding, 5 μm thick sections, PAP technique. Bars, 50 μm.

1983). Study of development of occipital cortical neurons has also been reported (McDonald et al. 1982).

Cingulate gyri, prepyriform, periamygdaloid and entorhinal cortex *(Atlas, 2–11)*

CCK-containing neuronal cell bodies are more numerous in these paleocortical regions of the cerebral cortex than in the neocortical regions. Numerous CCK-containing nerve terminals are present around the neuronal cell bodies present in these regions.

Hippocampus *(Fig. 4, and Atlas, 2, 3, 8–11)*

In the hippocampal complex, CCK-containing neuronal cell bodies and terminals (Fig. 4A) are present in different regions including the anterior region (Atlas, 2, 3), the dentate gyrus, the pyramidal layer CA1–4 (Fig. 4B) and the stratum radiatum (Fig. 4C). CCK nerve soma and terminals are also numerous in the presubiculum and the subiculum. In the pyramidal layers of cornu ammonis, thin CCK-positive nerve fibers are visible forming a delicate network around nerve cell bodies. The response of pyramidal neurons to applications of CCK-8(s) and its structural analogs have been determined using an in vitro hippocampal slice preparation and intracellular recording techniques (Kelly and Dodd 1981; Dodd and Kelly 1981). The rate of onset of the CCK-evoked response is similar to that of the response evoked by glutamate.

4.4. CLAUSTRUM *(Atlas, 3–9)*

Numerous CCK-containing neuronal cell bodies (Atlas, 3–9) are present in this region.

4.5. AMYGDALOID COMPLEX *(Atlas, 6–9)*

Numerous CCK-containing neurons are present in the nucleus amygdaloideus corticalis and fewer in the other amygdaloid nuclei. A high concentration of thick and thin CCK-positive nerve terminals are present in the nuclei amygdaloideus medialis, centralis, corticalis and lateralis and in the massa intercalata. They are frequently arranged in a network surrounding cell bodies.

4.6. BASAL GANGLIA *(Atlas, 2–9)*

Caudate-putamen *(Atlas, 4–8)*

Thin CCK-positive fibers are present in the internal and ventral parts of the middle and caudal portions of the caudate-putamen (Atlas, 4–8). It has been shown that dopamine modulates CCK release in the rat neostratum (Meyer and Krauss 1983). We were unable to find neuronal cell bodies, even after direct injection of colchicine in the nucleus caudate-putamen (Vanderhaeghen 1981; Gilles et al. 1983).

Nucleus accumbens *(Atlas, 2, 3)*

CCK-containing nerve soma have not been observed even after direct injection of colchicine into the striatum (Vanderhaeghen et al. 1981b; Gilles et al. 1983). CCK-positive nerve terminals are concentrated in the caudal, medial portion of the nucleus (Atlas, 2, 3).

Nucleus interstitialis stria terminalis *(Atlas, 4, 5)*

Numerous CCK-positive nerve terminals are observed in the different parts of the nucleus (Atlas, 4, 5). Numerous CCK-containing neuronal cell bodies are observed in the different parts of the nucleus after direct colchicine injection in the nearby striatum (Atlas, 5) (Vanderhaeghen et al. 1981b; Gilles et al. 1983).

Nucleus septi lateralis *(Atlas, 3, 4)*

CCK-positive nerve terminals are present in the ventral and lateral parts of the nucleus (Atlas, 3, 4). A few CCK-containing nerve soma can be demonstrated after direct injection of colchicine in the nearby striatum (Atlas, 4) (Vanderhaeghen et al. 1981b).

4.7. THALAMUS *(Atlas, 6–9)*

No CCK-positive nerve soma was detected in this region. A network of CCK-positive nerve fibers surrounding cell bodies is present in the nucleus periventricularis and in the nuclei dorsalis and ventralis corporis geniculati lateralis (Atlas, 6–9).

4.8. PREHYPOTHALAMIC STRUCTURES *(Atlas, 4, 5)*

After intraventricular colchicine injection, soma as well as thick and thin CCK-positive nerve fibers are present in moderate numbers in the nucleus preopticus, especially in the suprachiasmatic and periventricular areas (Atlas, 4, 5). After direct injection of colchicine in the caudate-putamen, numerous CCK-containing neuronal cell bodies are observed in the nucleus preopticus medialis (Atlas, 4, 5) (Vanderhaeghen et al. 1981b). CCK-containing nerve fibers, but no CCK-containing cell bodies, are detected in the tuberculum olfactorium.

4.9. HYPOTHALAMUS *(Atlas, 5–9)*

Magnocellular neurons *(Atlas, 5–7)*

CCK-positive somas are present in the peripheral part of the paraventricular nucleus (Atlas, 7), in the supraoptic accessory nuclei and the dorsal part of the main supraoptic nucleus (Atlas, 5, 6). The distribution of CCK neuronal cells has suggested the possibility of coexistence of CCK and oxytocin in the same neurons (Vanderhaeghen et al. 1980a). Recently, in the rat, after intracisternal colchicine injection, and in the ox, without colchicine injection, a direct demonstration of co-localization of CCK and oxytocin-neurophysin I was obtained in the supraoptic and paraventricular nuclei, using double staining procedures and serial sections (Vanderhaeghen et al. 1981a). Recently, in the same bovine nuclei, co-localization of Met- and Syn-enkephalin (Liston et al. 1983) with oxytocin has been reported (Vanderhaeghen et al. 1983). In neurohypophyseal nerve fibers, co-localization of CCK, Met-enkephalin and oxytocin has been reported (Martin et al. 1983).

Median eminence

CCK-positive nerve fibers are present both in the internal and external zones, although more numerous in the external part, in man, dog, ox, monkey, pig and rat (Fig. 5), (Lotstra and Vanderhaeghen, unpublished data). In the rat external zone, but not in the posterior hypophysis, CCK terminals visualized by immunohistochemistry disappear 21 days after bilateral adrenalectomy (Fig. 5) (Vanderhaeghen et al. 1980b; De-

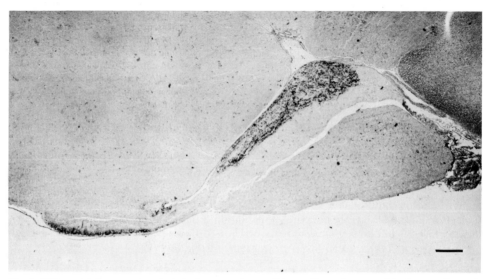

Fig. 5. CCK-containing nerve terminals in the external part of the median eminence and in the neurohypophysis. Sagittal section of the rat hypothalamo-hypophyseal region. 'Bouin Hollande sublimé' fixation, paraffin embedding, 5 μm thick sections, PAP technique.

schepper et al. 1983). In contrast, vasopressin and to a lesser extent oxytocin, increase in the same situation. Using RIA under the same conditions, the content of CCK in the mediobasal hypothalamus but not in the neuro-intermediate hypophyseal lobe is reduced, and this effect can be reversed by dexamethasone treatment (Anhut et al. 1983). CCK and gastrin have been shown to exert various direct or indirect actions on hypophyseal secretions. At microgram doses, gastrin, which possesses a carboxy terminal pentapeptide similar to CCK, has similar actions on pituitary hormone release; however, its action on prolactin is opposite to that of CCK (Vijayan et al. 1979). It was shown that pentagastrin at microgram doses has a suppressive effect on the pituitary-adrenocortical system of the rat, lowering the level of plasma corticosterone after intraperitoneal and intraventricular injections in the morning. After intracerebroventricular injection, an inhibitory effect of CCK on vasoactive intestinal polypeptide-induced-stimulation of adrenocortical secretion has been reported (Itoh and Hirota 1983). The potassium-stimulated release of CCK from hypothalamic slices is profoundly depressed by 10^{-7} M morphine (Micevych et al. 1982).

Gastrin reduces the release of ACTH from incubated pituitary tissue in vitro (Vijayan et al. 1978). CCK-8(s) produces a marked increase in GH release from incubated rat anterior pituitary and from cultured GH-3 pituitary tumor cells at 10^{-6} to 10^{-8} M (Itoh et al. 1979). CCK-8(s) was also noted to significantly increase prolactin release in normal rat pituitary monolayer cultures (Malarkey et al. 1981). CCK-8(s) does not promote prolactin release from either normal or tumor-bearing human pituitary (Morley et al. 1979).

Periventricular nucleus

CCK-positive somas are observed regularly in the rostral two-thirds of the hypothalamus (Atlas, 4–8).

Dorsomedial and ventromedial nuclei

A few CCK-positive somas are present in the nucleus dorsomedialis (Atlas, 8). A dense network of CCK-positive thin fibers are present in these 2 nuclei (Atlas, 8, 9), giving a butterfly-wing appearance to the section (Atlas, 8).

Suprachiasmatic nuclei

A few positive neuronal cell bodies are present in the suprachiasmatic nucleus (Atlas, 6).

Other hypothalamic nuclei

CCK is completely absent from the corpus mamillaris (Atlas, 9). Only occasional CCK-positive nerve cell bodies and fibers are present in the remaining hypothalamic nuclei.

4.10. HYPOPHYSIS

Large species differences have been observed in the hypophysis. G-CCK has been observed in neural lobe nerve terminals (Fig. 5) in all species studied, although they are present in much greater number in the rat and ox. G-CCK is also present in anterior and intermediate adenohypophyseal cells of various species but not in the rat (Lotstra et al. 1980)

Posterior hypophysis

Numerous CCK-positive nerve fibers have been observed only in the rat (Fig. 5) and the ox posterior hypophysis. It is only in those 2 species that high levels of CCK have been measured by RIA (Beinfeld 1982; Lotstra and Vanderhaeghen, unpublished data). In the dog, pig, monkey and man, only a few fibers are observed using immunohistochemistry, especially near the intermediate lobe (Lotstra et al. 1980; Lotstra and Vanderhaeghen, unpublished data). In addition to the species differences, a sex difference has been reported in the rat (Deschepper et al. 1983). As measured by RIA, CCK in the male rat neurohypophysis is twice that of the female and is reduced to female levels by castration or estrogen treatment (Deschepper et al. 1983).

Gastrin in the adenohypophysis

No G-CCK-containing cells have been detected in the adenohypophysis of the rat (Vanderhaeghen et al. 1980a). In the ox, monkey, pig, and dog, G-CCK-positive cell bodies are numerous in the adenohypophysis, particularly in the intermediate lobe, but also in the anterior lobe (Lotstra et al. 1980). A few CCK-positive cells are present in the human anterior hypophysis (Lotstra and Vanderhaeghen, unpublished data). Using serial sections, it has been demonstrated in the dog that some α-MSH-containing cells and ACTH-containing cells also contain G-CCK (Lotstra et al. 1980). These results have been confirmed 1 year later in the cat hypophysis (Larsson and Rehfeld 1981). The role of gastrin-containing cells in the adenohypophysis and the physiological significance of the presence of both gastrin and α-MSH or ACTH in some cells remain to be studied. The absence of G-CCK cells in the rat hypophysis agrees with the absence of gastrin reported in the rat hypophysis (Beinfeld 1982). The presence of gastrin in the porcine hypophysis (Rehfeld 1978a; Beinfeld 1982) may be explained by the numerous G-CCK cells observed in this species. These results favor the view that in the hypophysis, the G-CCK cells contain gastrins and the G-CCK nerve terminals cholecystokinins.

4.11. BRAINSTEM *(Figs 6A,B,C and 7A, Atlas, 10–13)*

Mesencephalon *(Fig. 6B,C, Atlas, 10, 11)*

After intraventricular injection of colchicine, CCK-positive neuronal cell bodies are observed in the mesencephalon, in the nucleus linearis rostralis (Fig. 6B,C, Atlas, 10, 11), in cells located immediately around the aqueduct of Sylvius (Atlas, 10, 11), and in the A10, A9 medial part and A8 regions (Atlas, 10, 11) of Dahlström and Fuxe (1964). Scarce CCK-positive nerve fibers are also observed in these regions. A dense network of CCK-positive nerve fibers is also present in the nucleus interpeduncularis (Atlas, 11) and in the superior (Atlas, 10, 11) and inferior colliculi. The large number of CCK-containing neuronal cell bodies in dopamine A10, A9, A8 regions of Dahlström and Fuxe (Vanderhaeghen et al. 1979, 1980a) has suggested that CCK and dopamine may coexist in some of these cells (Vanderhaeghen et al. 1980a). This has been indirectly confirmed by the homolateral decrease of CCK-radioimmunoassayable material in the mesencephalon after stereotaxic injection of 6-OH dopamine into the ventral mesencephalon of the rat and by the associated decrease of G-CCK in known rostral projections of mesencephalic dopamine cells, i.e. the frontal pole, the pyriform cortex and the nucleus accumbens (Vanderhaeghen 1981; Gilles et al. 1983). The coexistence of dopamine and CCK has been proved more directly by the observation that tyrosine-hydroxylase and CCK are sometimes present in the same mesencephalic neurons (Hökfelt et al. 1980a–c). CCK peptides can reduce the dopamine turnover in some telencephalic nuclei (Kovacs et al. 1981; Katsuura et al. 1980; Fuxe et al. 1980). The finding of CCK in mesolimbic dopamine neurons is interesting in view of the suggested involvement of CCK in the etiology of schizophrenia. It is possible that hyperactivity of the dopaminergic system is involved in this disease and that the beneficial effects of neuroleptic drugs are related to the blocking of dopamine receptors (Snyder 1980). Recently, a decrease in CCK levels has been observed in the CSF of schizophrenic patients (Verbanck et al. 1984). If a defect in the metabolism of CCK is related to the etiopathogeny of schizophrenia, then CCK may play a role in the treatment of this mental disease. The occurrence of CCK and dopamine in some mesencephalic neurons suggests that CCK could be implicated in some diseases of the nigrostriatal system, such as Parkinson's disease. A diminution of CCK has been recently reported in substantia nigra of parkinsonian brains (Studler et al. 1982), and CCK has been shown to effect tremor induced in the rat by harmine and ibogaine (Zetler 1983).

Metencephalon *(Fig. 6A, Atlas, 12)*

After intracisternal colchicine injection, a few CCK-positive neuronal cell bodies are present in the nucleus parabrachialis dorsalis (Atlas, 12) and in the caudal part of the nucleus raphe dorsalis (Fig. 6A, Atlas, 12). CCK-positive nerve fibers are detected in the nucleus raphe dorsalis, in the nuclei dorsalis and ventralis lemniscus lateralis and in the nucleus raphe magnus.

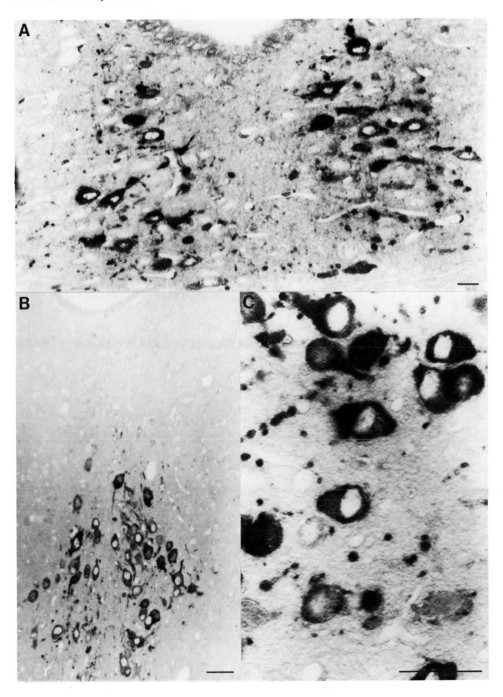

Fig. 6. CCK-positive neuronal cell bodies in the caudal part of the nucleus raphes dorsalis, near the 4th ventricle (A) and in the nucleus linearis rostralis (B, C). Transverse section of the rat brainstem. 'Bouin Hollande sublimé' fixation, paraffin embedding, 5 μm thick sections, PAP technique. Bars, 50 μm.

421

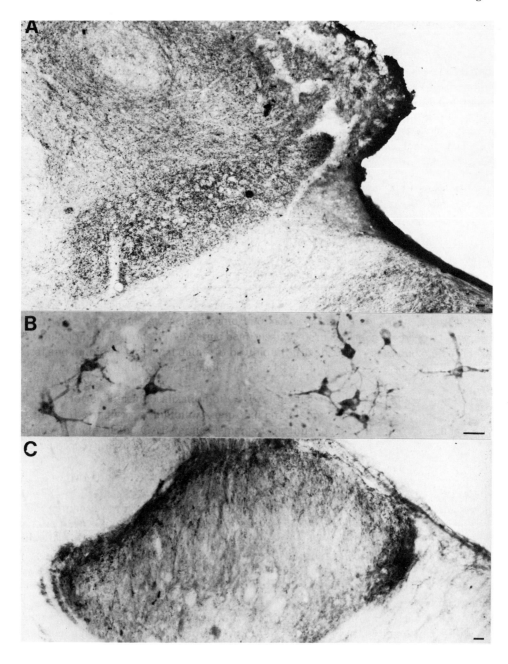

Fig. 7. Numerous CCK-containing nerve terminals in the cat nucleus tractus solitarii (A). CCK neuronal cell bodies in lamina X of Rexed of the spinal cord (B). Numerous CCK-containing terminals, especially in the superficial part of the dorsal horn (C). Transverse section of the cat medulla (A). Transverse section of rat lumbar spinal cord locally injected with colchicine (B). Transverse section of the rat lumbar spinal cord (C). Paraformaldehyde fixation, 60 μm thick sections, PAP technique. Bars, 50 μm.

Medulla oblongata *(Fig. 7A, Atlas, 13)*

Positive CCK nerve fibers are present in the tractus spinalis of the trigeminal nerve, in the area postrema (Atlas, 13) and in the inferior olivary complex (Atlas, 13). CCK-positive neuronal cells are present in the nucleus gracilis (Atlas, 13) and in the nucleus reticularis medullae, pars paramedianus and ventralis (Atlas, 12, 13). A rich network of CCK-positive thin nerve fibers is present in the nucleus tractus solitarii (Fig. 7A, Atlas, 13) and in the nucleus commissuralis. G-CCK immunoreactivity has been reported in the vagus nerve (Uvnäs-Wallensten et al. 1977). Using iontophoresis, an inhibitory effect of CCK on neurons in the nucleus tractus solitarii has been reported (Morin et al. 1983).

4.12. CEREBELLUM

No CCK-positive nerve cell bodies or fibers have been detected in the cerebellum.

4.13. SPINAL CORD *(Fig. 7BC, Atlas, 14–16)*

Numerous CCK-positive nerve fibers are concentrated in layers I–II of Rexed (1964) (Fig. 7C, Atlas, 14–16), and are less abundant in the remaining parts of the dorsal horn and in the posterior gray commissure (Vanderhaeghen et al. 1980a; Vanderhaeghen 1981). In addition, a few CCK-positive nerve fibers are observed in the anterior and intermedio-lateral horns. In rats treated with colchicine, CCK-positive neuronal cell bodies are present in 2 groups of symmetrically located neurons near the central canal in the intermedio-medial nucleus of area X of Rexed (Fig. 7B, Atlas, 16). These CCK neuronal perikarya are observed only in the lumbosacral cord forming a discontinuous column (Vanderhaeghen et al. 1982). No positive-reacting perikarya were observed in the cervical and thoracic regions (Atlas, 14, 15). The presence of CCK neuronal cell bodies exclusively in the lumbosacral region can be tentatively correlated with the higher levels of CCK material measured by RIA in this region, as compared to those measured at cervical and thoracic levels (Table 1).

4.14. SPINAL SENSORY GANGLIA

The existence of CCK has been reported in small neuronal cell bodies in rat primary sensory neurons (Dalsgaard et al. 1982; Otten and Lorez 1983). Co-localization of CCK with substance P has been reported in these cells (Dalsgaard et al. 1982).

5. CHOLECYSTOKININ PATHWAYS AND TRACTS

5.1. ANTERIOR COMMISSURA *(Fig. 8C)*

Beaded CCK-positive nerve fibers are present in the anterior commissure (Fig. 8C) at the level of its posterior arm (Vanderhaeghen et al. 1981b).

5.2. CORPUS CALLOSUM *(Fig. 8B)*

Thick beaded CCK-positive nerve fibers are observed in corpus callosum (Fig. 8B). Numerous fibers, some of them having an onion-bulb appearance, are seen in animals after transection of the corpus callosum (Vanderhaeghen et al. 1981b). In the corpus callo-

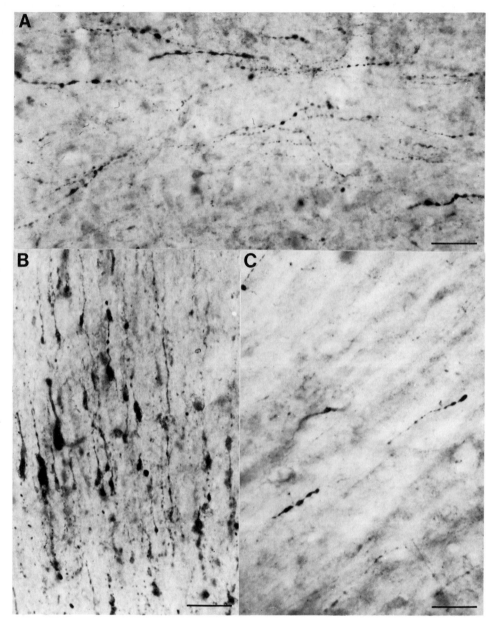

Fig. 8. Numerous CCK-positive beaded nerve fibers in the medial forebrain bundle (A), the surgically sectioned corpus callosum with onion bulb formations (B) and in the anterior commissure (C). Paraformaldehyde fixation, 60 μm thick section (B). 'Bouin Hollande sublimé' fixation, paraffin embedding, 5 μm thick sections (A, C). PAP technique. Bars, 50 μm.

sum, the presence of these fibers suggests that at least some of the CCK-positive cortical neuronal cell bodies project to the other cerebral hemisphere in addition to the local projections already described (Emson et al. 1980a). Corpus callosum lesions increase CCK concentrations in cortical areas with homeotopic connections (Meyer et al. 1982b).

5.3. MEDIAL FOREBRAIN BUNDLE *(Fig. 8A)*

Numerous thick beaded CCK-positive nerve fibers are present in the bundle in its various parts from the brainstem to the olfactory tract (Fig. 8A) (Vanderhaeghen et al. 1980a).

5.4. THE PATHWAY FROM A10 DOPAMINE MESENCEPHALIC REGION TO NUCLEUS ACCUMBENS

Unilateral injection of 6-OH dopamine into the vicinity of the ventral tegmental area and the substantia nigra reduces CCK content of the nucleus accumbens ipsilateral to the injection by 20–70% (Vanderhaeghen 1981; Gilles et al. 1983; Studler et al. 1982). By combining immunohistochemistry and retrograde tracing techniques, CCK-dopamine-containing cell bodies in A10 were shown to project to the caudal part of the medial nucleus accumbens (Hökfelt et al. 1980c).

5.5. PATHWAYS FROM A10 DOPAMINE MESENCEPHALIC REGION TO FRONTAL POLE, OLFACTORY TUBERCLE AND INTERSTITIAL NUCLEUS OF THE STRIA TERMINALIS

Unilateral electrolytic lesion of the medial forebrain bundle is followed by an increase of CCK in the homolateral ventral tegmental area and a fall of CCK in the ipsilateral olfactory tubercle and the interstitial nucleus of the stria terminalis (Williams et al. 1981). Unilateral injection of 6-OH dopamine in the vicinity of the ventral tegmental area and the substantia nigra lowered the CCK concentration in the frontal poles but not in the more caudal part of the frontal lobe (Vanderhaeghen 1981; Gilles et al. 1983).

5.6. PATHWAYS FROM AMYGDALA, CLAUSTRUM AND PYRIFORM CORTEX TO CAUDATE-PUTAMEN

The origin of CCK nerve terminals in the caudate-putamen has been investigated. Unilateral injection of 6-OH dopamine in the vicinity of the ventral tegmental area and the substantia nigra lowered the dopamine concentration in the caudate-putamen ipsilateral to the injection, but did not decrease its CCK content (Vanderhaeghen 1981: Gilles et al. 1983). Unilateral electrolytic lesion of the medial forebrain bundle or unilateral knife-cut of the upper brainstem is followed by an increase of CCK in the homolateral ventral tegmental area but not by a fall of CCK in the caudate-putamen (Williams et al. 1981: Gilles et al. 1983). These results indicate that neurons in the substantia nigra or in ventral tegmental area are not responsible for the presence of CCK in the caudate-putamen. The caudate-putamen receives afferents from the neocortex, the amygdala, the thalamus, the substantia nigra, the ventral tegmental area and the raphe nucleus. Apart from the thalamus, all of these structures contain CCK-positive neuronal cell bodies. Recent results indicate that a knife-cut which severes the afferents from the amygdala reduces CCK content of the caudate-putamen by about 30% (Meyer et al. 1982a). Another cut severing the claustrum and the pyriform cortex from the caudate-putamen decreases CCK content in the caudate by about 70% (Meyer et al. 1982a). These results suggest that the caudate-putamen receives its CCK-containing afferents from the pyriform cortex, the claustrum and the amygdala.

5.7. PATHWAY FROM THE HYPOTHALAMUS TO THE POSTERIOR HYPOPHYSIS

CCK is undetectable in the posterior hypophysis 1 week after stalk sectioning. Paraventricular nucleus lesion reduces the CCK content of the posterior pituitary by 60% (Beinfeld et al. 1980). The CCK content of the posterior pituitary is dramatically decreased by physiological changes which stimulate the release of vasopressin and oxytocin (Beinfeld et al. 1980; Deschepper et al. 1983). Studies have shown that in lactating animals with an elevated release of oxytocin, the CCK content of the posterior pituitary is reduced to 17% of the levels present in control animals (Beinfeld et al. 1980). In rats given a 2% saline solution to drink for 5 days, a treatment which is known to reduce vasopressin by 80%, the pituitary CCK content was about 20% of control (Beinfeld et al. 1980; Deschepper et al. 1983).

5.8. PATHWAYS FROM SPINAL SENSORY GANGLIA TO POSTERIOR HORN

CCK is released from the spinal cord in various conditions, including bilateral electrical stimulation of sciatic nerves. A significant although incomplete depletion of CCK is observed in dorsal horns after unilateral rhizotomy (Yaksh et al. 1982). These results suggest that the primary sensory neurons are a source of CCK-positive nerve fibers in the dorsal horns. The incomplete disappearance (Yaksh et al. 1982), or absence of disappearance of CCK (Marley et al. 1982) from the dorsal horn following rhizotomy is not consistent with this hypothesis. This discrepancy may result from the existence of an intraspinal source of CCK, such as CCK-positive neuronal cell bodies of the lumbosacral spinal cord (Vanderhaeghen et al. 1982) and from imperfect dissection of the posterior horn. It has been shown that the application of CCK to the isolated hemisected toad spinal cord causes a tetrodotoxin-sensitive depolarization of both roots (Phillis and Kirkpatrick 1979). On both intact and slice preparations of rat spinal cord, iontophoretically applied CCK-8(s) causes a moderate to strong excitation of about half of all tested dorsal horn neurons. In the rat spinal cord slice preparation, the excitatory response to CCK is not altered when the superfusing solution (Krebs-Ringer buffer) is replaced with Ca^{2+}-free, high Mg^{2+} Krebs solution. This latter finding indicates that CCK-8(s) might act directly on the postsynaptic sites of dorsal horn units, which is consistent with the possibility that CCK-8(s) acts on postsynaptic sites in the dorsal horn of the spinal cord as a neurotransmitter or a modulator (Jeftinija et al. 1981).

Numerous pharmacological data support the hypothesis that CCK-8(s) plays a role in the regulation of nociceptive activity in the CNS by acting at both spinal and supraspinal levels, probably by an opiate-independent mechanism (Zetler 1980). Recently, however, perispinally administered CCK-8(s) has been reported to antagonize opiate mediated analgesia (Faris and Komisaruk 1982).

6. CONCLUSIONS

CCK is widely distributed in the rat cerebral cortex, the striatum, the limbic system, the hypothalamus, the dorsal and ventral mesencephalic tegmental area, the substantia nigra, the medulla oblongata and the spinal cord.

In the rat, it has been demonstrated that CCK and dopamine coexist in some mesencephalic neurons projecting to some limbic areas but not to the caudate-putamen.

CCK is present in the magnocellular neuronal cell bodies of the paraventricular and supraoptic nuclei and in nerve fibers of the internal and external zones of the median eminence and of the posterior hypophysis. Immunocytochemistry shows coexistence of CCK as well as Met- and Syn-enkephalin with oxytocin-neurophysin I in some magnocellular neurons of the supraoptic and paraventricular nuclei and in posterior lobe nerve fibers, both in rat and bovine hypothalamus. CCK acts directly or indirectly via the hypothalamus on the pituitary gland and may therefore be considered to act as releasing factor or may participate in modulation of releasing factor(s).

G-CCK immunoreactivity has been demonstrated in adenohypophyseal cells of several mammals but not in the rat. G-CCK immunoreactivity coexists in some of these cells with α-MSH in the intermediate lobe and with ACTH in the anterior lobe.

CCK has been implicated in a variety of neurological (Parkinson, Huntington, epilepsia) and psychiatric disorders (bipolar depression, schizophrenia).

The neuroanatomy of CCK combined with a large body of neuropharmacological, behavioral and electrophysiological data, indicate that CCK may be involved in several neurobiological functions related to for example pain perception, regulation of feeding, lactation, control of water balance, stress, thermoregulation, some emotional behaviors, motor function and the hypothalamo-hypophyseal axis.

Atlas. Frontal diagrams of the rat brain at various levels. CCK-containing nerve cells are represented by black dots, CCK-containing nerve terminals by 4 different intensities of gray, from pale to deep gray, and CCK-containing neurites by oblique dotted lines.

For abbreviations, see the General Abbreviations List, p. 609.

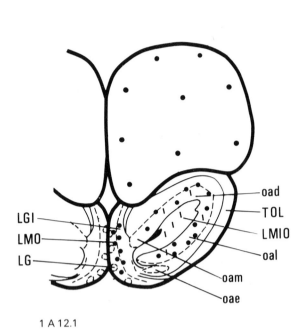

1 A 12.1

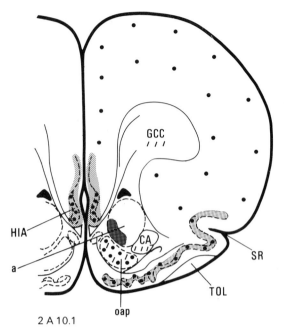

2 A 10.1

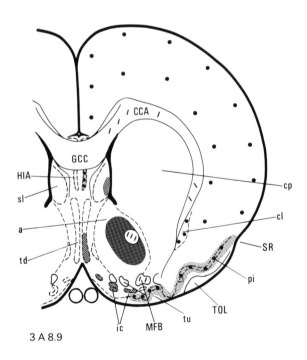

3 A 8.9

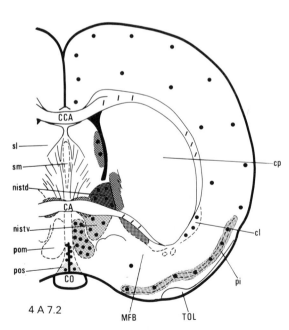

4 A 7.2

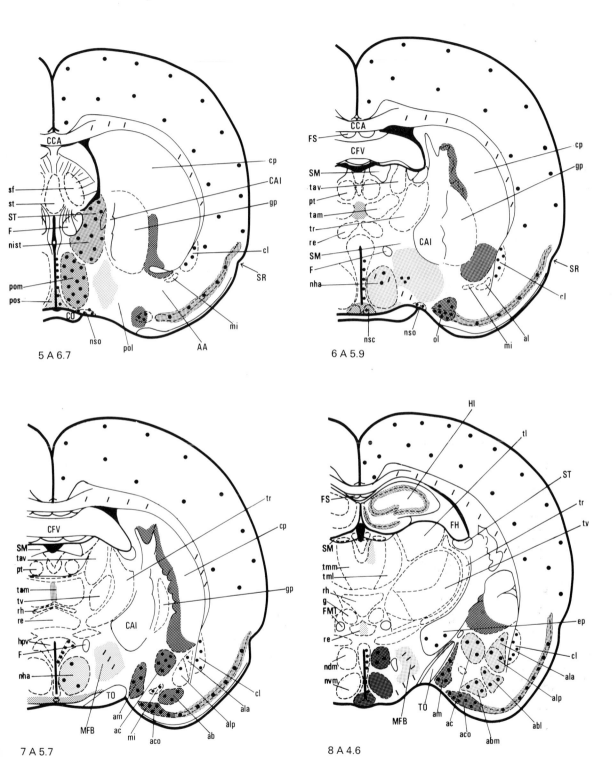

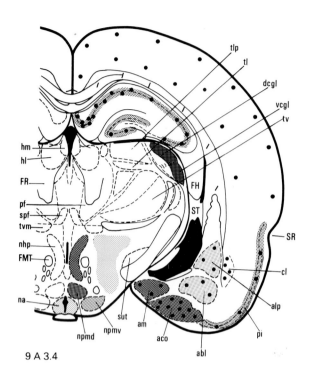

9 A 3.4

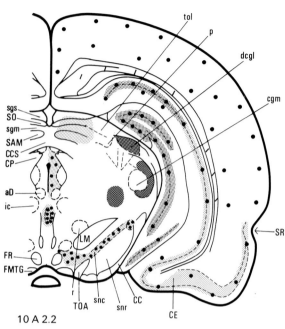

10 A 2.2

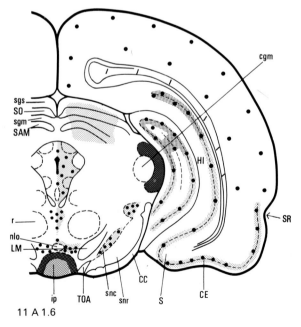

11 A 1.6

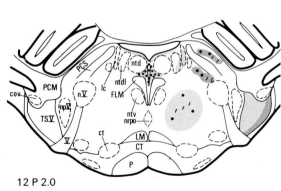

12 P 2.0

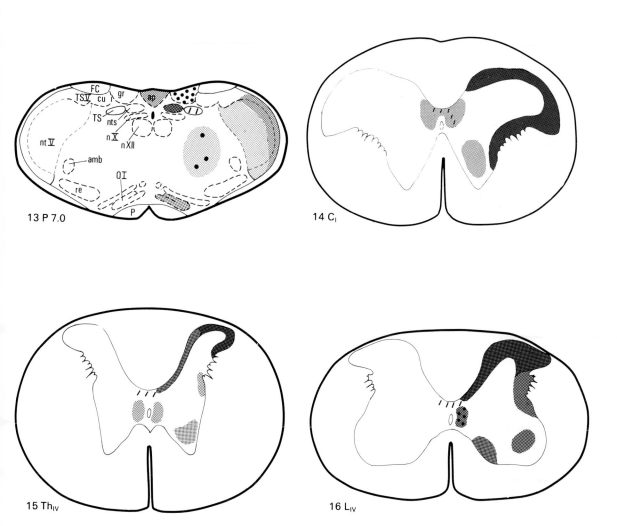

7. ACKNOWLEDGMENTS

The author acknowledges the expert assistance of G. Vierendeels and G. Nanson.

8. REFERENCES

Anhut H, Meyer DK, Knepel W (1983): Cholecystokinin-like immunoreactivity of rat medio-basal hypothalamus: investigation of a possible hypophysiotropic function. *Neuroendocrinology, 36*, 119–124.

Barden N, Merand Y, Rouleau D, Moore S, Dockray GJ, Dupont A (1981): Regional distribution of somatostatin and cholecystokinin-like immunoreactivities in rat and bovine brain. *Peptides, 2*, 299–302.

Beinfeld MC (1981): An HPLC and RIA analysis of the cholecystokinin peptide in rat brain. *Neuropeptides, 1*, 203–209.

Beinfeld MC (1982): Chromatographic characterization of gastrin/cholecystokinin peptides in bovine and porcine pituitary. *Peptides, 3*, 531–534.

Beinfeld MC, Palkovits M (1981): Distribution of cholecystokinin (CCK) in the hypothalamus and limbic system of the rat. *Neuropeptides, 2*, 123–129.

Beinfeld MC, Palkovits M (1982): Distribution of cholecystokinin (CCK) in the rat lower brain stem nuclei. *Brain Res., 238*, 260–265.

Beinfeld MC, Meyer DK, Brownstein MJ (1980): Cholecystokinin octapeptide in the rat hypothalamo-neurohypophyseal system. *Nature (London), 288*, 376–378.

Beinfeld MC, Meyer DK, Eskay RL, Jensen RT, Brownstein MJ (1981): The distribution of cholecystokinin in the central nervous system of the rat as determined by RIA. *Brain Res., 212*, 51–57.

Brown TR, Bacchi N, Mack RE, Booth E, Jones DP (1976): Isolation of monoiodinated gastrin using DEAE-sephadex and its characteristics in the gastrin radioimmunoassay. *Clin. Chim. Acta, 67*, 321–323.

Buffa R, Crivelli O, Fiocca R, Fontana P, Solcia E (1979): Complement-mediated unspecific binding of immunoglobulins to some endocrine cells. *Histochemistry, 63*, 15–21.

Dahlström A, Fuxe K (1964): Evidence for the existence of monoamine containing neurons in the central nervous system. I. Demonstration of monoamines in the cell bodies of brain stem neurons. *Acta Physiol. Scand., 62, Suppl. 232*, 1–80.

Dalsgaard C-J, Vincent SR, Hökfelt T, Lundberg JM, Dahlström A, Schultzberg M, Dockray GJ, Cuello AC (1982): Coexistence of cholecystokinin- and substance P-like peptides in neurons of the dorsal root ganglia of the rat. *Neurosci. Lett. 33*, 159–163.

Deschepper C, Lotstra F, Vandesande F, Vanderhaeghen JJ (1983): Cholecystokinin varies in the posterior pituitary and external median eminence of the rat according to factors affecting vasopressin and oxytocin. *Life Sci., 32*, 2571–2577.

Dockray GJ (1976): Immunochemical evidence of cholecystokinin-like peptides in brain. *Nature (London), 264*, 568–570.

Dodd PR, and Kelly JS (1981): The actions of cholecystokinin and related peptides on pyramidal neurones of mammalian hippocampus. *Brain Res., 205*, 337–350.

Donald RA (1968): Application of the coated charcoal separation to the radioimmunoassay of plasma corticotropin. *J. Endocrinol., 41*, 499–508.

Dupont A, Mérand Y, Savard P, Leblanc J, Dockray GJ (1982): Evidence that cholecystokinin is a neurotransmitter of olfaction in nucleus olfactorius anterior. *Brain Res., 250*, 386–390.

Emson PC, Marley PD (1983): Cholecystokinin and vasoactive intestinal polypeptide. In: Iversen L, Iversen SD, Snyder SH (Eds), *Handbook of Psychopharmacology, Vol. 16*, pp. 255–305. Plenum Publishing Corporation, New York.

Emson PC, Hunt SP, Rehfeld JF, Golterman N, Fahrenkrug J (1980a): Cholecystokinin and vasoactive intestinal polypeptide in the mammalian CNS: distribution and possible physiological roles. In: Costa E, Trabucchi M (Eds), *Neural Peptides and Neuronal Communication*, pp. 63–74. Raven Press, New York.

Emson PC, Rehfeld JF, Langevin H, Rossor M (1980b): Reduction in cholecystokinin-like immunoreactivity in the basal ganglia in Huntington's disease. *Brain Res., 198*, 497–500.

Emson PC, Rehfeld JF, Rossor MN (1982): Distribution of cholecystokinin-like peptides in the human brain. *J. Neurochem., 38*, 1177–1179.

Eriksen EF, Larsson LI (1981) Neuropeptides in the retina: evidence for differential topographical localization. *Peptides, 2*, 153–157.

Eskay RL, Beinfeld MC (1982): HPLC and RIA of cholecystokinin peptides in the vertebrate neural retina. *Brain Res., 246*, 315–318.

Faris P, Komisaruk BR (1982): Evidence for the neuropeptide cholecystokinin as an antagonist of opiate analgesia. *Science, 219*, 310–311.

Finkelstein JA, Steggles AW, Lotstra F, Vanderhaeghen JJ (1981): Levels of gastrin-cholecystokinin like immunoreactivity in the brain of genetically obese and non-obese rats. *Peptides, 2*, 19–21.

Fuxe K, Andersson K, Locatelli V, Agnati LF, Hökfelt T, Skirboll L, Mutt V (1980): Cholecystokinin peptides produce marked reduction of dopamine turn-over in discrete areas in the rat brain following intraventricular injection. *Eur. J. Pharmacol., 67*, 329–331.

Ganter P, Jolles G (1969): In: *Histochimie Normale et Pathologique, Vol. 2*, p. 1395. Gauthier-Villars, Paris.

Gilles C, Lotstra F, Vanderhaeghen JJ (1983): CCK nerve terminals in the rat striatal and limbic areas originate partly in the brain stem and partly in telencephalic structures. *Life Sci., 32*, 1683–1690.

Goltermann NR, Rehfeld JF, Petersen HR (1980a): In vivo biosynthesis of cholecystokinin in rat cerebral cortex. *J. Biol. Chem., 255*, 6181–6185.

Goltermann NR, Rehfeld JF, Petersen HR (1980b): Concentration and in vivo synthesis of cholecystokinin in subcortical regions of the rat brain. *J. Neurochem., 35*, 479–483.

Goltermann NR, Stengaard-Pedersen K, Rehfeld JF, Christensen NJ (1981): Newly synthesized cholecystokinin in subcellular fractions of the rat brain. *J. Neurochem., 36*, 959–965.

432

Gonguli PC, Hunter WM (1971): In: Kirkhan KE, Hunter WM (Eds), *Radioimmunoassay Methods*, p. 54. Churchill/Livingstone, Edinburgh.

Grimmelikhuijzen CJP, Sundler F, Rehfeld JF (1980): Gastrin/CCK-like immunoreactivity in the nervous system of coelenterates. *Histochemistry, 69*, 61–68.

Grube D (1980): Immunoreactivities of gastrin (G-) cells. Non-specific binding of immunoglobulins to G-cells by ionic interactions. *Histochemistry, 66*, 149–167.

Grube D, Weber E (1980): Immunoreactivities of gastrin (G-) cells. I. Dilution dependent staining of G-cells by antisera and non-immune sera. *Histochemistry, 65*, 223–237.

Hamilton LW (1976): *Basic Limbic System Anatomy of the Rat*. Plenum Press, New York.

Herbert V, Lon KS, Gottlieb CW, Bleicher SJ (1965): Coated charcoal assay of insulin. *J. Clin. Endocrinol., 25*, 1375–1384.

Hökfelt T, Johansson O, Ljundahl A, Lundberg JM, Schultzberg M (1980a): Peptidergic neurones. *Nature (London), 284*, 515–521.

Hökfelt T, Rehfeld JF, Skirboll L, Ivemark B, Goldstein M, Markey K (1980b): Evidence for coexistence of dopamine and cholecystokinin in mesolimbic neurones. *Nature (London), 285*, 476–478.

Hökfelt T, Skirboll L, Rehfeld JF, Goldstein M, Markey K, Dann O (1980c): A subpopulation of mesencephalic dopamine neurones projecting to limbic areas contains a cholecystokinin-like peptide: evidence from immunohistochemistry combined with retrograde tracing. *Neuroscience, 5*, 2093–2124.

Hunter WM, Greenwood FC (1967): Preparation of 131 iodine labelled human growth hormone of high specific activity. *Nature (London), 194*, 495–496.

Innis RB, Correa FMA, Uhl GR, Schneider B, Snyder SH (1979): Cholecystokinin octapeptide-like immunoreactivity: histochemical localization in rat brain. *Proc. Natl Acad. Sci. USA, 76*, 521–525.

Itoh S, Hirota R (1983): Inhibitory effect of cholecystokinin octapeptide on vasoactive intestinal peptide-induced stimulation of adrenocortical secretion. *Jpn. J. Physiol., 33*, 301–304.

Itoh S, Hirota R, Katsuura G, Odaguchi K (1979): Adrenocortical stimulation by a cholecystokinin preparation in the rat. *Life Sci., 25*, 1725–1730.

Jansen JBJ, Lamers CBHW (1983): Immunological evidences of cholecystokinin-39 in porcine brain. *Life Sci., 32*, 911–913.

Jeftinija S, Miletic V, Randic M (1981): Cholecystokinin octapeptide excites dorsal horn neurons both in vivo and in vitro. *Brain Res., 213*, 231–236.

Katsuura G, Hirota R, Itoh S (1980): Effect of a cholecystokinin preparation on brain monoamines in the rat. *Jpn. J. Physiol., 30*, 811–814.

Kelly JS, Dodd J (1981): Cholecystokinin and gastrin as transmitters in the mammalian central nervous system. In: Martin JB, Reichlin S, Bick KL (Eds), *Neurosecretion and Brain Peptides*, p. 133. Raven Press, New York.

König JF, Klippel RA (1963): *The rat brain. A Stereotaxic Atlas of Forebrain and Lower Parts of the Brain Stem*. Williams and Wilkins Comp., Baltimore.

Kovacs GL, Szabo G, Penke B, Telegdy G (1981): Effects of cholecystokinin octapeptide on striatal dopamine metabolism and on apomorphine-induced stereotyped cage-climbing in mice. *Eur. J. Pharmacol., 69*, 313–319.

Kramer KJ, Speirs RD, Childs CN (1977): Immunochemical evidence for a gastrin-like peptide in insect neuroendocrine system. *Gen. Comp. Endocrinol., 32*, 423–426.

Larson BA, Vigna SR (1983): Species and tissue distribution of cholecystokinin/gastrin-like substances in some invertebrates. *Gen. Comp. Endocrinol., 50*, 469–475.

Larsson LI, Rehfeld JF (1979): Localization and molecular heterogeneity of cholecystokinin in the central and peripheral nervous system. *Brain Res., 165*, 201–218.

Larsson LI, Rehfeld JF (1981): Pituitary gastrins occur in corticotrophs and melanotrophs. *Science, 213*, 768–770.

Liston R, Vanderhaeghen JJ, Rossier J (1983): Presence in brain of synenkephalin, a proenkephalin-immunoreactive protein which does not contain enkephalin. *Nature (London), 302*, 62–65.

Lorén I, Alumets J, Håkanson RH, Sundler F (1979): Distribution of gastrin and cholecystokinin-like peptides in rat brain. *Histochemistry, 59*, 249–257.

Lotstra F, Vanderhaeghen JJ, Gilles C (1980): Gastrin-like peptides in anterior and intermediate lobe cells of the hypophysis: relationship with alpha-MSH and ACTH cells. *Neuroendocrinol. Lett., 6*, 333–338.

McDonald JK, Parnavelas JG, Karamanlidis AN, Rosenquist G, Brecha N (1982): The morphology and distribution of peptide-containing neurons in the adult and developing visual cortex of the rat. III. Cholecystokinin. *J. Neurocytol., 11*, 881–895.

Malarkey WB, O'Dorisio TM, Kennedy M, Cataland S (1981): The influence of vasoactive intestinal polypeptide and cholecystokinin on prolactin release in rat and human monolayer cultures. *Life Sci., 28*, 2489–2495.

Marley PD, Nagy JI, Emson PC, Rehfeld JF (1982): Cholecystokinin in the rat spinal cord: distribution and lack of effect of neonatal capsaicin treatment and rhizotomy. *Brain Res., 238*, 494–498.

Martin R, Geis R, Holl R, Schäfer M, Voigt KH (1983): Co-existence of unrelated peptides in oxytocin and vasopressin terminals of rat neurohypophysis: immunoreactive methionine⁵-enkephalin-, leucine⁵-enkephalin- and cholecystokinin-like substances. *Neuroscience, 8*, 213–227.

Meyer DK, Beinfeld MC, Oertel WH, Brownstein MJ (1982a): Origin of the cholecystokinin-containing fibers in the rat caudatoputamen. *Science, 215*, 187–188.

Meyer DK, Beinfeld MC, Brownstein MJ (1982b): Corpus callosum lesions increase cholecystokinin concentrations in cortical areas with homeotopic connections. *Brain Res., 240*, 151–153.

Meyer DK, Krauss J (1983): Dopamine modulates cholecystokinin release in neostriatum. *Nature (London), 301*, 338–340.

Micevych PE, Yaksh TL, Go VLW (1982): Opiate-mediated inhibition of the release of cholecystokinin and substance P, but not neurotensin from cat hypothalamic slices. *Brain Res., 250*, 283–289.

Morin MP, De Marchi P, Champagnat J, Vanderhaeghen JJ, Rossier J, Denavit-Saubie M (1983): Inhibitory effect of cholecystokinin octapeptide on neurons in the nucleus tractus solitarius. *Brain Res., 265*, 333–339.

Morley JE (1982): Minireview: the ascent of cholecystokinin (CCK) from gut to brain. *Life Sci., 30*, 479–493.

Morley JE, Melmed S, Briggs J, Carlson HE, Hershman JM, Solomon TE, Lamers C, Damassa DA (1979): Cholecystokinin octapeptide releases growth hormone from the pituitary in vitro. *Life Sci., 25*, 1201–1206.

Müller JE, Straus E, Yalow RS (1977): Cholecystokinin and its COOH-terminal octapeptide in the pig brain. *Proc. Natl Acad. Sci. USA, 74*, 3035–3037.

Osborne NN, Nicholas DA, Dockray GJ, Cuello AC (1982): Cholecystokinin and substance P immunoreactivity in retinas of rats, frogs, lizards and chicks. *Exp. Eye Res., 34*, 639–649.

Otten U, Lorez HP (1983): Nerve growth factor increases substance P, cholecystokinin and vasoactive intestinal polypeptide immunoreactivities in primary sensory neurones of newborn rats. *Neurosci. Lett., 34*, 153–158.

Pearse AGE (1966): 5-Hydroxy-tryptophan uptake by dog thyroid C cells and its possible significance in polypeptide hormone production. *Nature (London), 211*, 598–600.

Peters A, Miller M, Kimerer LM (1983): Cholecystokinin-like immunoreactive neurons in rat cerebral cortex. *Neuroscience, 8*, 431–448.

Phillis JW, Kirkpatrick JR (1979): Actions of various gastrointestinal peptides on the isolated amphibian spinal cord. *Can. J. Physiol. Pharmacol., 57*, 887–899.

Rehfeld JF (1978a): Localization of gastrins to neuro- and adenohypophysis. *Nature (London), 271*, 771–773.

Rehfeld JF (1978b): Immunohistochemical studies on cholecystokinin. II. Distribution and molecular heterogeneity in the central nervous system and small intestine of man and hog. *J. Biol. Chem., 253*, 4022–4030.

Rehfeld JF, Golterman NR (1979): Immunochemical evidence of cholecystokinin tetrapeptide in hog brain. *J. Neurochem., 32*, 1339–1341.

Rexed B (1964): Some aspects of the cytoarchitectonics and synaptology of the spinal cord. In: Eccles JC, Schade JP (Eds), Organization of the spinal cord. *Prog. Brain Res., 11*, 58–90. Elsevier Pub., Amsterdam.

Robberecht P, Deschodt-Lanckman M, Vanderhaeghen JJ (1978): Demonstration of biological activity of brain gastrin-like peptidic material in the human: its relationship with the COOH-terminal octapeptide of cholecystokinin. *Proc. Natl Acad. Sci. USA, 75*, 524–528.

Rossor MN, Rehfeld JF, Emson PC, Mountjoy CQ, Roth M, Iversen LL (1981): Normal cortical concentration of cholecystokinin-like immunoreactivity with reduced choline acetyltransferase activity in senile dementia of Alzheimer type. *Life Sci., 29*, 405–410.

Scharrer E (1928): Die Lichtempfindlichkeit blinder Elritzen. I. Untersuchungen über das Zwischenhirn der Fische. *Z. Vergleich. Physiol., 7*, 1–38.

Schneider DS, Monahan JW, Hirsch J (1979): Brain cholecystokinin and nutritional status in rats and mice. *J. Clin. Invest., 64*, 1348–1356.

Skowsky WR, Fischer DA (1972): The use of thyroglobulin to induce antigenicity to small molecules. *J. Lab. Clin. Med., 80*, 134–144.

Snyder SH (1980): Schizophrenia: etiology and treatment. In: *Biological Aspects of Mental Disorder*, pp. 58–68. Oxford University Press, Oxford.

Speidel CC (1919): Gland cells of internal secretion in the spinal cord of the skates. *Carnegie Inst. Washington Publ., 13*, 1–31.

Sternberger LA (1979): The unlabelled antibody peroxidase-antiperoxidase (PAP) method. In: Wiley J (Ed.), *Immunocytochemistry, 2nd Ed.*, pp. 104–109. John Wiley and Sons, New York.

Studler JM, Javoy-Agid F, Cesselin F, Legrand JC, Agid Y (1982): CCK-8-immunoreactivity distribution in human brain: selective decrease in the substantia nigra from parkinsonian patients. *Brain Res., 243*, 176–179.

Uvnäs-Wallensten K, Rehfeld JF, Larsson LI, and Uvnäs B (1977): Heptadecapeptide gastrin in the vagal nerve. *Proc. Natl Acad. Sci. USA, 74*, 5707–5710.

Vanderhaeghen JJ (1981): Gastrins and cholecystokinins in central nervous system and hypophysis. In: Dumont JE, Nunez J (Eds), *Hormone and Cell Regulation, European Symposium, 1st Ed., Vol. 5*, pp. 149–168. Elsevier/North-Holland Pub., Amsterdam.

Vanderhaeghen JJ, Signeau JC, Gepts W (1975): New peptide in the vertebrate CNS reacting with antigastrin antibodies. *Nature (London), 257*, 604–605.

Vanderhaeghen JJ, De Mey J, Lotstra F, Gilles C (1979): Localization of gastrin-cholecystokinin-like peptides in the brain and hypophysis of the rat. *Acta Neurol. Belg., 79*, 62–63.

Vanderhaeghen JJ, Lotstra F, De Mey J, Gilles C (1980a): Immunohistochemical localization of cholecystokinin- and gastrin-like peptides in the brain and hypophysis of the rat. *Proc. Natl Acad. Sci. USA, 77*, 1190–1194.

Vanderhaeghen JJ, Lotstra F, Gilles C (1980b): Gastrin(s) and cholecystokinin(s) in central nervous system and pituitary: relationship with dopamine, oxytocin and alpha MSH containing cells and with limbic and nigrostriatal systems. *Horm. Res., 12*, 182–183.

Vanderhaeghen JJ, Lotstra F, Vandesande F, Dierickx K (1981a): Coexistence of cholecystokinin and oxytocin-neurophysin in some magnocellular hypothalamo-hypophyseal neurones. *Cell Tissue Res., 221*, 227–231.

Vanderhaeghen JJ, Lotstra F, Vierendeels G, Gilles C, Deschepper C, Verbanck P (1981b): Cholecystokinin in the central nervous. *Peptides, 2, Suppl. 2*, 81–88.

Vanderhaeghen JJ, Deschepper C, Lotstra F, Vierendeels G, Schoenen J (1982): Immunohistochemical evidence for cholecystokinin-like peptides in neuronal cell bodies of the rat spinal cord. *Cell Tissue Res., 223*, 463–467.

Vanderhaeghen JJ, Lotstra F, Liston DR, Rossier J (1983): Proenkephalin, met-enkephalin and oxytocin immunoreactivities are co-localized in bovine hypothalamic magnocellular neurons. *Proc. Natl Acad. Sci., USA, 80*, 5139–5143.

Vandesande F, Dierickx K, De Mey J (1977): The origin of vasopressinergic and oxytocinergic fibres of the external region of the median eminence of the rat hypophysis. *Cell Tissue Res., 180*, 443–452.

Verbanck PMP, Lotstra F, Gilles C, Linkowski P, Mendlewicz J, Vanderhaeghen JJ (1984): Reduced cholecystokinin immunoreactivity in the cerebrospinal fluid of patients with psychiatric disorders. *Life Sci., 34*, 67–72.

Vijayan E, Samson WK, McCann SM (1978): Effects of intraventricular injection of gastrin on release of LH, prolactin, TSH and GH in conscious ovarietomized rats. *Life Sci., 23*, 2225–2232.

Vijayan E, Samson WK, McCann SM (1979): In vivo and in vitro effects of cholecystokinin on gonadotropin, prolactin, growth hormone and thyrotropin release in the rat. *Brain Res., 172*, 295–301.

Von Euler US, Gaddum JH (1931): An unidentified depressor substance in certain tissue extracts. *J. Physiol. (London), 72*, 74–87.

Williams JA (1982): Cholecystokinin: a hormone and a neurotransmitter. *Biomed. Res., 3*, 107–121.

Williams RG, Gayton RG, Zhu W-Y, Dockray G (1981): Changes in brain cholecystokinin octapeptide following lesions of the medial forebrain bundle. *Brain Res., 213*, 227–230.

Yaksh TL, Abay EO II, Go VLW (1982): Studies on the location and release of cholecystokinin and vasoactive intestinal peptide in rat and cat spinal cord. *Brain Res., 242*, 279–290.

Zetler G (1980): Analgesia caused by caerulein and cholecystokinin octapeptide (CCK-8). *Neuropharmacology, 19*, 415–422.

Zetler G (1983): Cholecystokinin octapeptide (CCK-8), ceruletide and analogues of ceruletide: effects on tremors induced by oxotremorine, harmine and ibogaine. A comparison with prolyl-leucylglycine amide (MIF), anti-parkinsonian drugs and clonazepam. *Neuropharmacology, 22*, 757–766.

CHAPTER X

An atlas of the distribution of GABAergic neurons and terminals in the rat CNS as revealed by GAD immunohistochemistry*

ENRICO MUGNAINI AND WOLFGANG H. OERTEL

1. SUMMARY

This atlas of GAD-immunoreactive nerve cell bodies and nerve terminals demonstrates:
- the ubiquitous distribution of GAD-immunoreactive neuronal profiles in the central nervous system (CNS) with a wide range of variation in density
- the prominence of GABAergic elements throughout the CNS and thus the prominence of inhibition in nervous system function
- the prominence of *disinhibition* (inhibition of a GABAergic neuron by another GABAergic neuron) in certain systems
- the extraordinary *variation* of GABAergic cell types
- the notion that GABAergic neurons represent not only *interneurons,* but also *projection* neurons; there appear to exist more numerous and, in part, vast populations of GABAergic *projection neurons* than previously thought
- brain regions with a high proportion or a low proportion of GABAergic nerve cell bodies
- the existence of brain regions that do not correspond to a specifically named nucleus, but contain a high density of GABAergic cell bodies and/or nerve terminals
- brain regions with a high density or a low density of GABAergic nerve terminals
- the presence of special *patterns* of GABAergic innervation in various CNS regions
- the possible *coexistence* of *glutamic acid decarboxylase* (GAD), i.e. the biosynthetic enzyme for GABA, with different *neuropeptides* in neurons of various brain regions.

2. INTRODUCTION

GABA, a 4 carbon amino acid, was discovered in brain tissue in 1950 (Awapara et al. 1950; Roberts and Frankel 1950; Udenfriend 1950). GABA is produced mainly through enzymatic decarboxylation of glutamic acid by glutamic acid decarboxylase (GAD). Neurons which synthesize GABA are usually referred to as 'GABA neurons' or 'GABA-ergic neurons'. Both the amino acid GABA and the enzyme GAD are found highly concentrated in axon terminals (Salganikoff and De Robertis 1965). Electrophysiological and pharmacological investigations indicate that GABA is an inhibitory neurotrans-

*Supported by US-PHS grant 09904-15 (E.M.) and DFG grant Oe-95/2-1 (W.H.O.).

Handbook of Chemical Neuroanatomy. Vol. 4: GABA and Neuropeptides in the CNS, Part I.
A. Björklund and T. Hökfelt, editors.
© Elsevier Science Publishers B.V., 1985.

mitter in the mammalian CNS (Ito and Yoshida 1964; Krnjévic and Schwartz 1966; Obata and Takeda 1969).

2.1. BIOCHEMISTRY

Biochemical assays of microdissected samples of various nervous tissues have shown that GABA and GAD are ubiquitously, although unevenly, distributed in the CNS (Tappaz et al. 1976), but such methods lack the resolution for their localization at the cellular level. Thus, morphological analysis with a method to *visualize* GABAergic neuronal profiles is necessary (Roberts 1979).

2.2. GAD IMMUNOHISTOCHEMISTRY

GAD is considered a reliable endogenous marker protein for GABAergic neurons. Due to its large size (ca. 120,000 daltons (Wu et al. 1973; Oertel et al. 1981b)) it hardly leaks from the neurons after the tissue has been adequately fixed (Section 4.3), unless the tissue sections are treated with strong detergents.

In 1973, the group of Dr Eugene Roberts purified GAD (Wu et al. 1973; Wu 1976) and produced a specific GAD antiserum in the rabbit. This antiserum allowed for the first time to visualize unequivocally GABAergic axon terminals and nerve cell bodies by light- and electron microscopic immunocytochemistry (Saito et al. 1974; McLaughlin et al. 1974; Wood et al. 1976; Roberts 1979). Fortunately, neurons that use neurotransmitters different from GABA do not contain significant amounts of GAD and remain, therefore, unlabeled or contain a signal indistinguishable from background. Other GAD antisera have successively been produced in various laboratories (Maitre et al. 1978; Perez de la Mora et al. 1981; Oertel et al. 1981b; Brandon 1983). A detailed comparison of the biochemical, immunological and immunohistochemical properties of the different GAD antisera is given elsewhere (Oertel et al. 1983b).

2.3. GABA AUTORADIOGRAPHY

Uptake of GABA is a property not only of many types of GABA neurons (Hökfelt and Ljungdahl 1972) but also of glial cells (Beart et al. 1974; Iversen and Bloom 1972) and probably even of some non-GABAergic neurons (Belin et al. 1980). Autoradiographic localization of exogenous radioactive GABA, although generally helpful for the anatomical localization of GABA neurons (Chronwall and Wolff 1980; Cuénod et al. 1982; Neale et al. 1983; Ottersen and Storm-Mathisen 1984b), often engenders problems of interpretation (see also Oertel et al. 1983b; see Fig. 40 legend: nucleus subthalamicus on page 509).

2.4. GABA IMMUNOHISTOCHEMISTRY

Recently, antibodies to GABA itself have been produced (Storm-Mathisen et al. 1983; Seguela et al. 1984; Anderson et al. 1984; Hodgson et al. 1985; Wenthold, personal communication). Glutaraldehyde-containing fixatives retain GABA, a small molecule, in the tissue during the histological preparative procedures. With the standard techniques presently available, antibodies to GABA reveal clearly the GABAergic axon terminals (and processes) and also reliably demonstrate GABA-containing neurons in some brain areas such as the neocortex, hippocampus, thalamus and cerebellar cortex (Ottersen and

Storm-Mathisen 1984a,b,c; Somogyi et al. 1985a). Advances in methodology may further improve the sensitivity of the technique.

In *Volume 3* of This Series a mouse brain atlas of GABAergic elements was produced, based on radioactive GABA uptake and on the use of a rabbit antiserum to GABA (Ottersen and Storm-Mathisen 1984b). Homologous structures are usually correspondingly labeled in the present atlas, based on GAD immunohistochemistry, and the atlas by Ottersen and Storm-Mathisen (1984b). The two maps agree in numerous respects. Most of the differences may be accountable to the fact that GAD antisera have been available for a longer period and, therefore, the methodology for GAD immunohistochemistry has substantially been improved (Mugnaini and Dahl 1983).

3. QUICK ORIENTATION GUIDE

3.1 WHY AN ATLAS OF GABAERGIC NEURONS?

γ-Aminobutyric acid (GABA) is the most widespread inhibitory amino acid transmitter in the mammalian nervous system. Quantitatively, the 'GABA system' is probably as important for inhibitory mechanisms as glutamic acid is for excitatory processes. Whereas monoaminergic neurons and cholinergic neurons constitute relatively small populations of neurons, GABAergic neurons have been considered – based on biochemical and autoradiographical data – to be ubiquitously distributed, to make up a substantial proportion of all nerve cell bodies (Olsen 1980), and even more so of all axon terminals (McGeer et al. 1978).

The morphological localization of GABAergic nerve cell bodies and terminals is crucial for the analysis of inhibitory neuronal circuits involved in the various brain functions. A map of the GABAergic elements will, thus, help to define neurochemically a large proportion of all central neurons.

3.2. COMMENTS

The emphasis of this atlas is placed on the presentation of the available data in diagrammatic form: Drawings of coronal serial sections of the CNS are used as templates for the distribution of GABAergic cell bodies and (axon) terminals. Accompanying photographs furnish examples of the actual basis for scoring the distribution of GABAergic cell bodies and (axon) terminals and illustrate principal aspects of the 'GABAergic systems' in selected brain areas.

The two main goals of this chapter are: to present a first attempt at producing a general map of GABAergic elements in the rat CNS; and to highlight some special regional and subregional *patterns* of the distribution of GABAergic axon terminals and cell bodies.

These patterns may help to clarify general principles in the typology of GABAergic neurons and their relations to other classes of neurons.
A systematic study of specific details in individual regions of the central nervous system is in progress and remains outside the scope of this account.

3.3. HOW TO USE THE ATLAS

Most of the information is presented in figures, tables and schemes. The atlas consists of 6 main parts: Figures 1–3 (pp. 441–444), Figures 4–24 (pp. 449–465), schematic drawings of coronal serial sections (pp. 466–485), Table 1 (brain areas) (pp. 487–501), Figures 25–149 (pp. 502–568), and discussion (pp. 569–594).

Figures 1–3 demonstrate the results of the different fixation techniques for axon terminal staining, cell body staining and a combination of axon terminal and cell body staining.

Figures 4–24 demonstrate the distribution of terminals at low magnification at 16 different frontal planes in the rostrocaudal direction (Figs 4–19) and give examples of the distribution of cell bodies at low magnification in sagittal, horizontal and frontal planes (Figs 20–24).

The *Schematic atlas drawings of coronal serial sections* demonstrate with different symbols: the density of nerve cell bodies on the left side and the density of nerve terminals (and fibers) on the right side. The scoring system is identical to the one used in Table 1 (Grades from 0–5).

Table 1 lists in alphabetical order:
– abbreviation and corresponding denomination of the individual brain regions
– density of GABAergic nerve cell bodies (grades 0–5, 5 being the highest grade; asterisk denotes that reliable cell body staining requires pretreatment with colchicine)
– density of GABAergic nerve terminals (grades 0–5, 5 being the highest grade)
– level of appearance of the brain structure in the rostrocaudal direction (stereotaxic plane) relative to the interaural axis
– list of references concerning the area under consideration obtained with GABA immunohistochemistry, GAD immunohistochemistry or [³H] GABA autoradiography
– number of the half-tone figures on which the respective brain area is depicted

Figures 25–149 illustrate selected brain areas.

Discussion: General features of the GABAergic system(s) are outlined. The discussion includes paragraphs and tables dealing with: GABAergic cell types; GABAergic interneurons and GABAergic projection neurons; brain areas with high or low proportions of GABAergic cell bodies; brain areas with high or low density of GABAergic nerve terminals; inhibition and disinhibition; coexistence of GABA (i.e. GAD) and neuropeptides.

4. METHODS

Techniques used for the localization of GAD immunoreactivity are outlined. For technical details, the reader is asked to consult the references given.

4.1. EXPERIMENTAL ANIMALS

Male and female albino rats (Sprague Dawley, body weight 150–300 g) were obtained from local suppliers. Half of the animals received a stereotaxic injection of 10–20 μg colchicine (Sigma) dissolved in 0.9% NaCl (10 μg colchicine/1 μl NaCl) directly into the brain area of interest or in its immediate vicinity. In particular, 'topical colchicine injection' was used in the striatum and 'striatum-like' areas (Table 4) and in several brain areas with a low content of GAD immunoreactive cell bodies (Table 5), as indicated in Tables 1 and 4 with an asterisk). (See also Sections 4.4 and 4.6).

4.2. PREPARATION OF SHEEP GAD ANTISERUM S3

GAD antiserum S3 (fourth bleed) – hereafter termed antiserum S3 – was raised in sheep and characterized by enzyme precipitation and immunoelectrophoresis as detailed elsewhere (Oertel et al. 1981b). In short, a polyvalent antiserum S1 against GAD was produced in sheep by intradermal injection of a protein band containing GAD enzyme activity, obtained in polyacrylamide gel electrophoresis under non-denaturing conditions. This polyvalent antiserum S1 precipitated GAD activity to 100% in brain homogenate supernatant and detected 3 precipitin lines in crossed immunoelectrophoresis against 150-fold purified GAD. One of the antigen–antibody precipitin arcs was radioactively labeled by means of the irreversible GAD inhibitor [2-^{3}H]γ-acetylenic GABA (Oertel et al. 1980). Injection of these pooled antigen–antibody precipitin lines into an unimmunized sheep yielded a GAD antiserum S3. GAD antiserum S3 precipitated 85% of the GAD activity in brain homogenate supernatant. It detected one antigen in crossed immunoelectrophoresis in a 150-fold purified GAD preparation and altered the mobility of one antigen in brain homogenate supernatant in crossed immunoelectrophoresis with intermediate gel. Besides GAD activity, antiserum S3 immunoprecipitates the enzyme activity of cysteine sulfinic acid decarboxylase (brain form II) (CSD II). GAD activity and CSD II activity are considered to reside on the same enzyme (Oertel et al. 1981c; Wu 1982). In agreement with Wu (1982), GAD is different from CSD I (Oertel et al. 1981c; Legay et al. 1985). CSD I may be the biosynthetic enzyme for taurine. Finally, GAD antiserum S3 fails to immunoprecipitate GABA transaminase enzyme activity (Oertel et al. 1983b), like the rabbit GAD antiserum (Saito 1976i; Wu 1976).

Although improbable, it cannot be excluded that part of the immunoreactive material dealt with may be a protein structurally very similar to GAD. The revealed material, therefore, should be correctly described as GAD-*like* immunoreactivity, but for the sake of simplicity the terms 'GAD immunoreactivity' or 'GAD positivity' will be used herein.

4.3. FIXATION AND TISSUE PREPARATION

Rats were anesthetized with sodium pentobarbitone (Nembutal 40 mg/kg i.p.) and perfused transcardially via the ascending aorta. The blood was flushed out of the system with 100–150 ml saline (0.9% NaCl), followed by 500–750 ml of one of the following fixatives at room temperature (Mugnaini and Dahl 1983):

4.3.1. Axon terminal staining

10% commercial formalin and 0.5% zinc salicylate in half strength saline, pH 4.0 at 18–20°C. The sections were immunoreacted with the single (Sternberger 1979) or double (Ordronneau et al. 1981) PAP procedure, with (or without) detergent pretreatment (Fig. 1).

Fig. 1. Motor area of cortex frontoparietalis from a coronal section in a rat processed for *immunostaining of terminals*. At the top of the micrograph the high density of terminals in the outer portion of layer 1 is a commonly observed feature (see also Figs 3, 5–11). To exclude definitely that it represents a surface artefact, however, quantitative immunoelectron microscopy and/or microassay of GAD enzyme activity is required. A lower density of GAD-positive punctates and fibers is seen in the inner part of layer 1. Layers 2 and 3 are characterized by a medium to high density of mainly perisomatic and peridendritic axon terminals. In layer 5b, pyramidal shaped cells are outlined by GAD immunoreactive terminals (see Inset). Within layer 6 sublaminae are distinguishable.
Inset: Pyramidal cell bodies in layer 5b, outlined by GAD immunoreactive boutons. wm: white matter. × 106; Inset × 367.

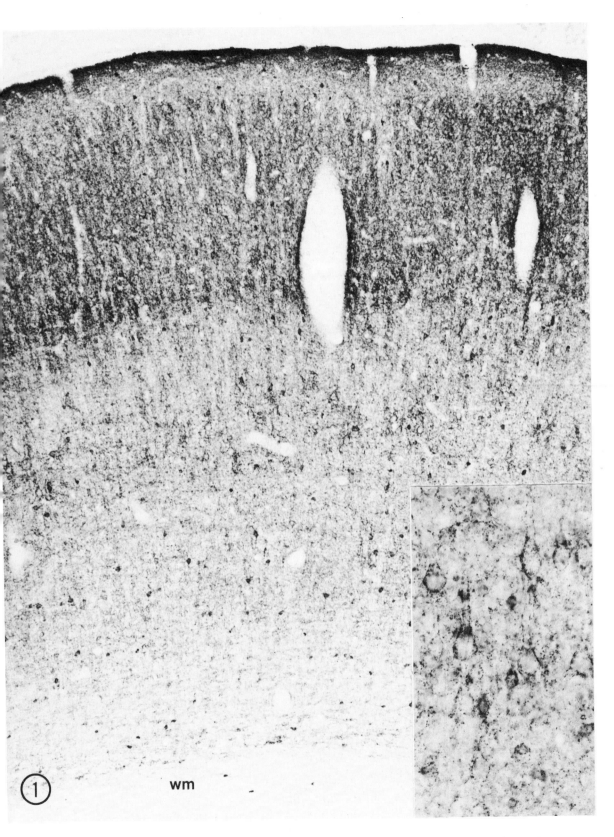

①   wm

4.3.2. Cell body staining

Same composition as above, but at pH 6.5. The sections were immunoreacted with the single or double PAP procedure without detergent pretreatment (Fig. 2). Increased sensitivity and reliability of cell body staining was obtained when 0.5% zinc dichromate was used instead of zinc salicylate at pH 4.0. The mordent zinc dichromate allowed cell body staining not only in cortical (Fig. 2), hippocampal (Fig. 34) or cerebellar (Fig. 126) regions, but also in areas such as the hypothalamus (Figs 73–75) or in the reticular formation. The question of colchicine pretreatment is discussed in Section 4.4.

4.3.3. Combined staining of axon terminals and cell bodies

Zinc salicylate/formalin fixative or zinc dichromate/formalin fixative as outlined above, but at pH 5.0. The sections were immunoreacted with the *double* PAP procedure, without detergent pretreatment (Fig. 3).

4.3.4. Colchicine pretreated animals

4% (w/v) freshly depolymerized formaldehyde in 0.1 M phosphate buffer pH 7.3 or any of the above fixatives. The sections were immunoreacted with the single or double PAP procedure.

For Vibratome® sectioning brain and spinal cord were removed 30–60 min after perfusion. Sections were cut at 25 μm on a Vibratome in 0.5 M Tris buffer, pH 7.6 at 4–6°C.

For cutting on a freezing microtome, animals were additionally perfused with a 5% sucrose solution in saline. The brain and spinal cord were dissected and placed in 30% sucrose in saline. After the tissue block(s) had sunk, the tissue was quickly frozen on dry ice and cut at 25 μm. Examples of sections prepared according to the first 3 fixative schedules as outlined above are shown in *Figures 1–3*.

4.4. COLCHICINE PRETREATMENT

Neuronal cell bodies in certain brain regions appear to contain GAD at concentrations that are barely at the threshold or definitely below the detection level of standard immunohistochemical procedures. It has therefore been customary in the past few years to use topical or intraventricular injections of colchicine. Colchicine, a blocker of axonal transport, prevents the enzyme from moving down the axon. Hence, by continued synthesis, GAD reaches somatal levels detectable by sensitive procedures (Ribak et al. 1978), such as the peroxidase–antiperoxidase (PAP) method of Sternberger (1979) or the avidin–biotin–peroxidase complex (ABC) technique (Hsu et al. 1981). This approach is not without problems. Colchicine treatment may decrease staining of the axon terminals and may not diffuse sufficiently to affect all the neuronal cell bodies in a given area. Furthermore, depolymerization of the microtubules caused by this drug may alter neuronal shape. Also, the size of the cells may increase substantially, especially after survival times longer than 24 hours. Many experimental animals become therefore necessary even for analysis of small brain regions.

Due to improvement of fixation techniques, fixation parameters can now be selected

---

→

Fig. 2. Cortex frontoparietalis from a coronal section in a rat processed for *immunostaining of cell bodies.* Note the varying size and orientation of GABAergic cell bodies present in all layers. Staining of terminals in this section is barely discernible in the background. Note the scattered GAD immunoreactive neurons (arrows) in the subcortical white matter (wm). × 103.

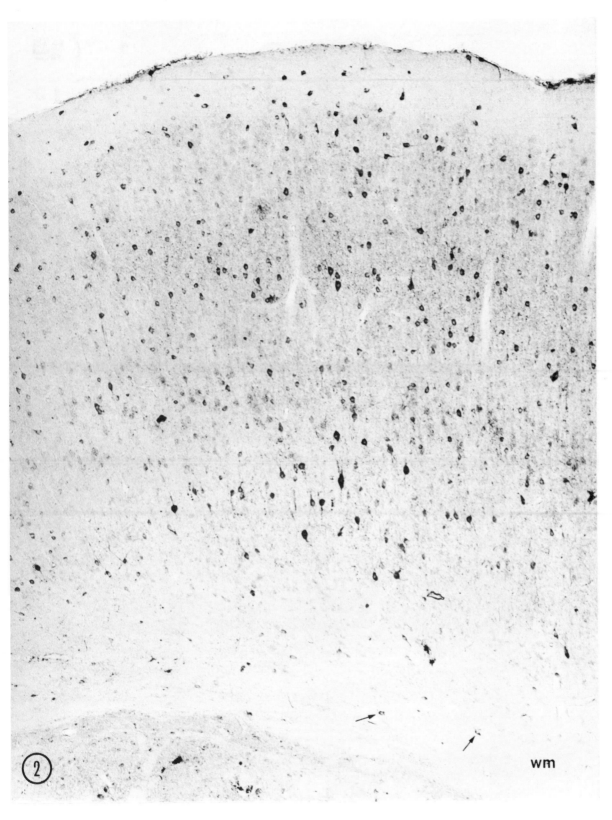

2

wm

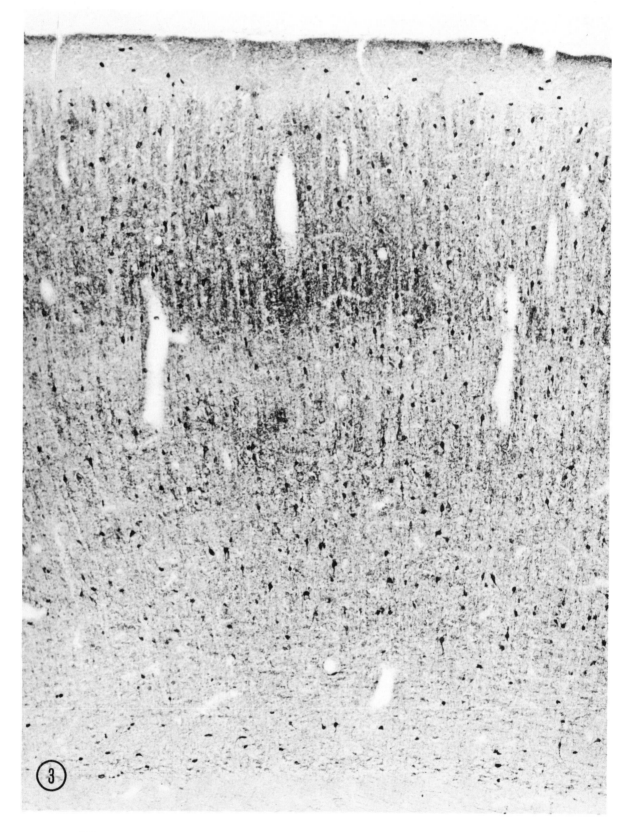

for optimal visualization of either the axon terminals or the cell bodies. In many cases, good visualization of both structures at the same time was obtained without the use of colchicine injections in the brain, or of detergent treatment of the sections. Especially, combination of the mordating action of zinc salts (zinc salicylate, zinc dichromate) with the moderate cross-linking properties of formalin at acidic pH (Mugnaini and Dahl 1983) (Section 4.3) have made the pretreatment of animals with colchicine obsolete for the demonstration of cell body staining in most regions of the rat CNS.

Only the so-called striatum and striatum-like regions and few other areas may require colchicine injections in order to evaluate GABA nerve cell body density, as the fixative (Section 4.3) alone can result in inconsistent cell body staining in untreated animals. These 'colchicine-dependent areas' are indicated by an asterisk in Tables 1 and 4.

In nearly all other areas, specimens of topically colchicine pretreated animals were very similar to specimens of normal animals in respect to cell body distribution.

4.5. PAP PROCEDURE – GAD IMMUNOHISTOCHEMISTRY

GAD immunoreactivity was localized by the indirect antibody–enzyme method (PAP technique) of Sternberger (Sternberger 1979) in a single or double sequence. These standard procedures are detailed elsewhere (Ordronneau et al. 1981; Oertel et al. 1981d, 1982b; Mugnaini and Dahl 1983). Tris buffer (0.5 M, pH 7.6) was used as diluent. Floating freezing microtome sections or Vibratome sections were incubated in sheep GAD antiserum S3 in dilution 1:2000. Rabbit-anti sheep immunoglobulin 1:50 (Miles Lab.) and goat peroxidase–antiperoxidase complex (goat PAP) 1:100 (Sternberger-Meyer, Garretsville, MD, USA) were employed as secondary and tertiary antisera. 3′,3′-Diaminobenzidine (DAB) (Sigma) was used as chromogen. Some of the sections were postfixed for 30 sec in 0.005% OsO_4 in phosphate buffered saline. Sections were either wet-mounted or dry-mounted. Wet-mounted Vibratome sections are preferable for detailed analysis with high-power lenses, since they afford a better preservation of tissue and cell structure.

4.6. PREPARATION OF BRAIN SERIES

Separate and/or combined brain series were produced (Section 4.3.1 to 4.3.3) for the distribution of axon terminals and the distribution of nerve cell bodies. Brain series were prepared in the frontal, sagittal and horizontal planes. Two different approaches were used: (1) Six consecutive sections of 25 μm thickness, each series 250 μm apart were collected. Five sections were stained for GAD immunoreactivity with slightly different protocols and one stained for cresyl violet. (2) Alternatively, series of two consecutive 25-μm sections spaced were stained for GAD immunoreactivity with the same protocol. The first was slightly osmicated and the second was counterstained with cresyl violet.

The atlas drawings are mainly based on 4 of our best series of frontal sections produced for visualization of axon terminals or of cell bodies *without colchicine pretreatment*. In critical areas, where the signal was unclear for unknown reasons, scoring of the labeling was controlled in additional series, produced with the use of colchicine or with variants of the basic procedure. Such areas are indicated in Tables 1 and 4 by an asterisk (see Section 4.4).

Fig. 3. Motor area of cortex frontoparietalis from a coronal section in a rat processed for *simultaneous immunostaining of terminals and cell bodies.* Albeit slightly underdeveloped with respect to the patterns seen with the 'specific' fixation protocols, both the patterns for immunostaining of terminals and the pattern for immunostaining of cell bodies show up with sufficient clarity. × 106.

4.7. LOW-POWER HALF-TONES

Counterstaining of the sections after the incubations and the diaminobenzidine reaction is usually of unsatisfactory quality and the immunolabeling becomes obscured at low magnification. The photographs shown therefore were taken from bins of immunoreacted sections that were not counterstained. A number of low-power photographs of representative sections are shown in Figures 4–24. Axon terminal distribution is illustrated in the frontal plane in Figures 4–19 and in the horizontal plane in Figure 22. Cell body distribution is exemplified in sagittal planes in Figures 20 and 21, in a horizontal plane in Figure 22 and in frontal planes in Figures 23 and 24. The approximate stereotaxic level is given at the top or bottom of the individual illustrations. The photographs (Figures 4–19) of the 'axon terminal' series and the Figures 23 and 24 (examples of cell body distribution in the frontal plane) *are unlabeled,* as the corresponding schematic atlas drawings can easily be used as a guide. The remaining photographs (Figures 20–22) of the 'cell body' series have been sparingly labeled as they can be compared to standard sections in a rat brain atlas such as the one of Paxinos and Watson (1982).

4.8. EVALUATION OF THE SECTIONS AND SCORING

For the sake of simplicity, the frequency of occurrence (density) of GABAergic boutons and cell bodies is scored on a scale of 0 to 5, 5 being the maximal density. Scoring based on only 5 gradations was often difficult, as the true representation of differences in the densities of both boutons and cell bodies would have required a larger scale in some brain regions. In such cases we have chosen to *overscore* or *underscore* with the aim to emphasize noteworthy differences in neighboring areas in the schematic atlas drawings and give an intermediate score in Table 1.

4.8.1. Axon terminal density

In general, axon terminal density is scored as *overall density per unit area.* This rule was also applied to regions where gray and white matter intermingle creating a reticulate or striped pattern (exception, see under Grade 5). In such regions, the density of boutons around neuronal processes or cell bodies was sometimes high (at high power), but the overall density of immunostaining appeared low under a low-power objective lens. In these instances, we have tended towards *underscoring* such regions in the drawings. This drawback is partially rectified in some cases by the accompanying half-tones (Figs 25–149). Another problem in scoring was faced in the areas with a high density of GAD-negative neuronal cell bodies such as seen in the hippocampal pyramidal cell layer or layer 3 of the primary olfactory cortex. These areas contain a high density of GABAergic terminals (around the soma, the axon hillock or dendrites) with respect to the neuropil, as known from ultrastructural studies (Freund et al. 1983; Somogyi et al. 1983c). In respect to overall density per unit area or volume the density of terminals is, however, intermediate (Grade 3).

   In areas where white fiber bundles are clearly demarcated from the neuropil, the white matter is not considered, e.g. in the nucleus caudatus. A density of Grade 5 for the axon terminals usually means that they appear highly concentrated per unit area. It is known from electron microscopic immunocytochemistry, however, that even in such areas there are non-GABAergic boutons intermingled with the labeled ones (Ribak et al. 1976, 1981; Oertel et al. 1981d; Somogyi et al. 1983c).

Examples for scoring axon terminal density

Grade 0: white matter, including scarcely distributed punctate profiles

| | *example:* | fornix (F) |

Grade 1: very low density   *example:*   n.gelatinosus thalami (g), cranial motor nuclei

Grade 1 (Variant)   used to characterize an area of very low axon terminal density (Grade 1) *plus* nerve fibers with GAD-immunoreactive varicosities

           example: n.ventroposterioris lateralis thalami (tvpl)

Grade 2: low density   *example:*   n.amygdaloideus lateralis (al)

The density of GAD-immunoreactive nerve terminals of the *cortical areas including the hippocampus* is exemplified in a few schematic drawings (BO and A 3.4). For the sake of simplicity, in most of the schematic drawings a uniform score of Grade 2 has been employed for the density of GAD-immunoreactive nerve terminals, although laminar and sublaminar differences are present. (For details, see Figs 1, 3, 5–11.)

Grade 2 (Variant)   used to characterize areas with a higher axon terminal density in the neuropil (Grade 3–4) when fiber tracts are heavily intermingled

           example: fasciculus medialis prosencephali (MFB)

Grade 3: medium density   *example:*   n. caudatus/putamen (excluding white fiber bundles) (cp)

Grade 4: high density   *example:*   n.septi lateralis (sl)

Grade 5: very high density   *example:*   pallidum ventrale (vp)

The terminal density of the globus pallidus, the nucleus entopeduncularis and the substantia nigra pars reticulata are also scored with density Grade 5. This is justified by the extreme similarity in ultrastructural features between the pallidum ventrale and the above 3 areas, although inconsistent with the rating of overall density per unit area for brain regions with reticulate appearance (Section 4.8.1).

Fibers   GAD-immunoreactive fibers are indicated without a score

           example: pedunculus corporis mammillaris (PCMA)

4.8.2. Cell body density

Cell body density is indicated by 5 different types of symbols.

Grade 0: no symbol   no cell bodies

           example: organum subcommissurale (sco)

Grade 1:   very few cells (you have to search for them); less than 5% of the total neuronal population

           example: n.reticularis tegmenti pontis (rtp)

Grade 2:   few cell bodies; between 5% and 15% of the total neuronal population

           example: n.amygdaloideus lateralis (al)

Grade 3:	many cell bodies; between 15% and 50% of the total neuronal population
	example: colliculus inferior (CI)
Grade 4:	majority; between 50% and 90% of the total neuronal population
	example: lamina glomerulosa bulbi olfactorii (LG), n.septi lateralis (sl)
Grade 5:	vast majority; more than 90% of the neuronal population or nearly all cell bodies
	example: n.caudatus/putamen (cp), lamina cellularum Purkinje cerebelli (pcl)
Grade 5 (Variant):	the vast majority of scattered neurons in a cell-poor area are GAD immunoreactive
	example: lamina moleculare (I) of the neocortex

Density of GAD-immunoreactive nerve cell bodies of the *cortical areas including the hippocampus* have been uniformly scored throughout the atlas and are only indicated in a few schematic drawings (BO, A 10.5 to A 8.6 and A 3.4). For details, see Figures 2, 21, 23, 33 and 34 and the quoted references in Table 1.

The present atlas and the scoring system should be considered preliminary. More satisfactory results await further improvements of the immunocytochemical procedures and the use of objective scoring methods, such as ultrastructural quantitation.

4.9. THE ATLAS

The atlas drawings (adapted from König and Klippel 1963) are the same as used by most authors in This Series. Occasionally, however, we have felt it necessary to slightly alter the borders and the terminology furnished to us by the editors, using either the atlas of Paxinos and Watson (1982) or our own judgement. We wish to point out that on several occasions the boundaries of zones of given density of immunostaining do not follow the boundaries of the nuclei as shown in the atlas or as indicated by the cell densities in Nissl-stained sections. This is both fortunate and unfortunate. It is unfortunate as it makes the student's task more difficult. When barely evident, such incongruences have been ignored; but when conspicuous they have been noted in the atlas. It is fortunate, as the GAD immunostaining appears often to offer a new perspective on brain structure.

Figs. 4–24. Low-magnification half-tones.

Figs. 4–19. Distribution of GAD-immunoreactive terminals. These low-magnification photographs are taken from 16 coronal sections through the brain and spinal cord. Sections were immunostained for GAD-immunoreactive nerve terminals. The half-tones illustrate the basis for scoring the density of GAD-immunoreactive terminals in individual nuclei as shown on the right-hand side of the schematic atlas drawings. Anterior and posterior levels in respect to the interaural axis correspond to the levels used in the schematic atlas drawings on pages 466-485. Figures 4–13: ×19; Figures 14–19: ×40.

Figs. 20–24. Distribution of GAD-immunoreactive cell bodies. These low-power photographs of selected sagittal, horizontal and coronal sections illustrate the basis for scoring the distribution of GABAergic cell bodies in individual nuclei as shown on the left-hand side of the schematic atlas drawings.
For abbreviations, see the General Abbreviations List, p. 609 and Table 1 pp. 487-501.

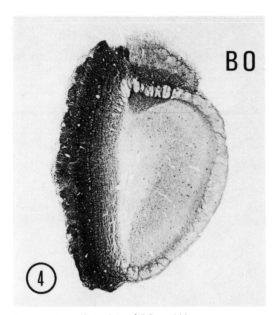

Fig. 4. Bulbus olfactorius, *cf.* BO, p. 466.

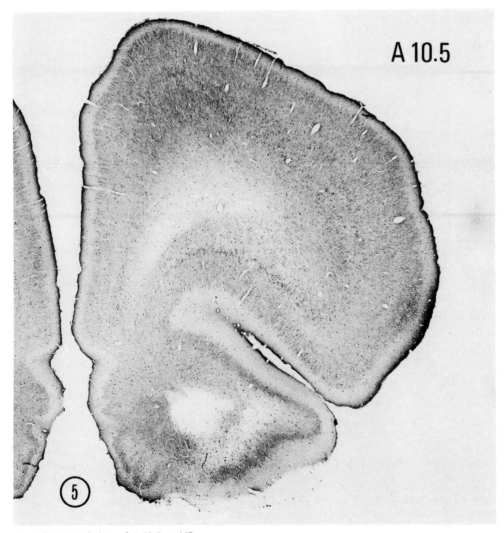

Fig. 5. Prosencephalon, *cf.* A 10.5, p. 467.

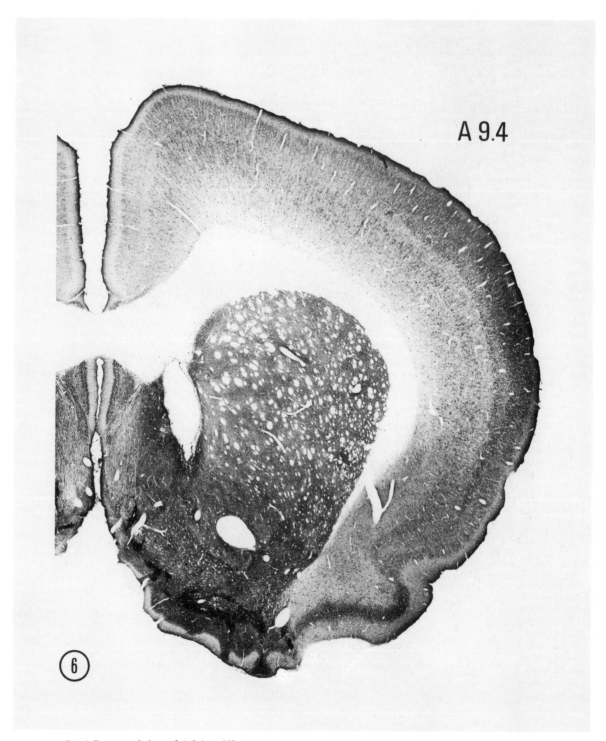

Fig. 6. Prosencephalon, cf. A 9.4, p. 468.

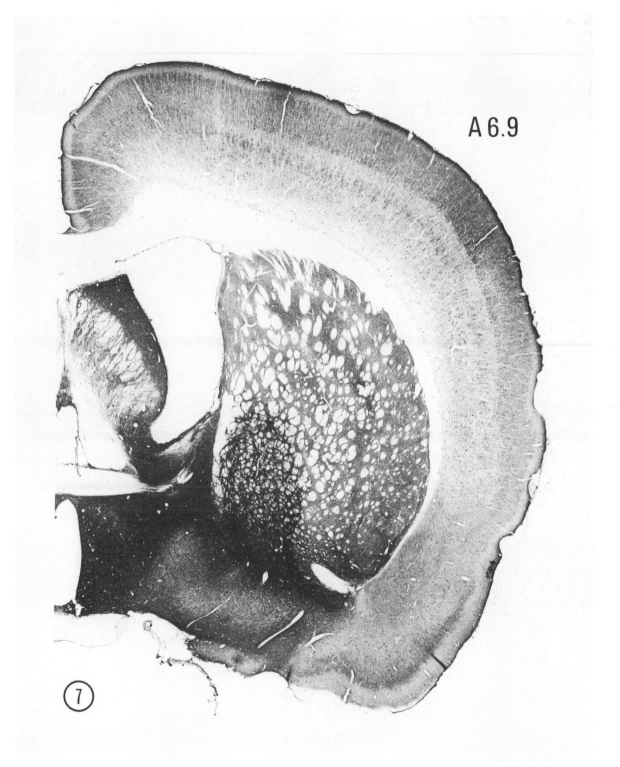

A 6.9

⑦

Fig. 7. Level of commissura anterior, *cf.* A 6.9, p. 470.

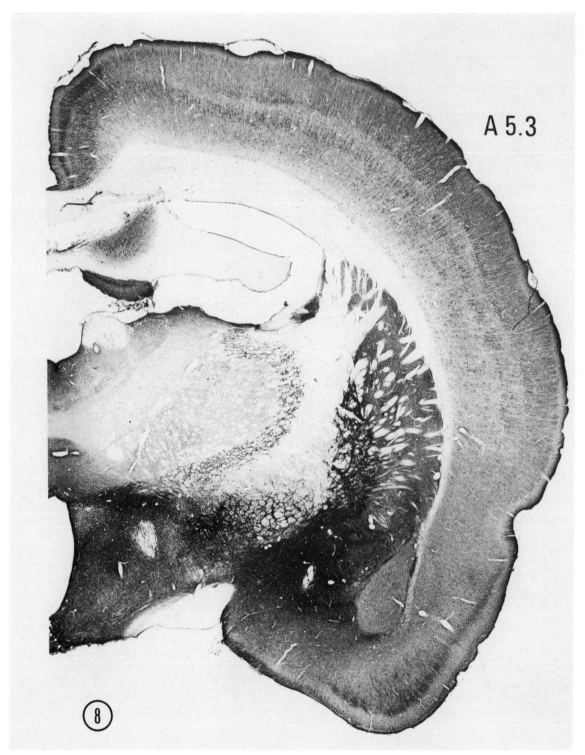

A 5.3

⑧

Fig. 8. Retrochiasmatic level, *cf.* A 5.3, p. 472.

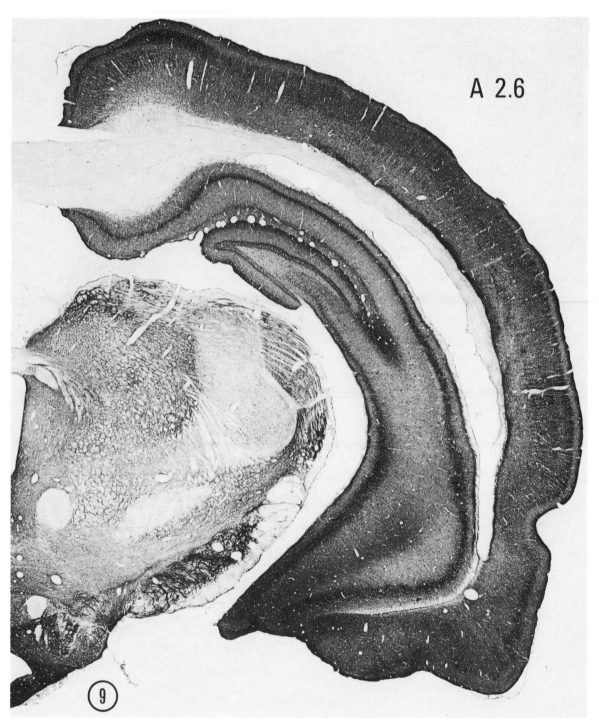

Fig. 9. Level of commissura posterior, *cf.* A 2.6, p. 476.

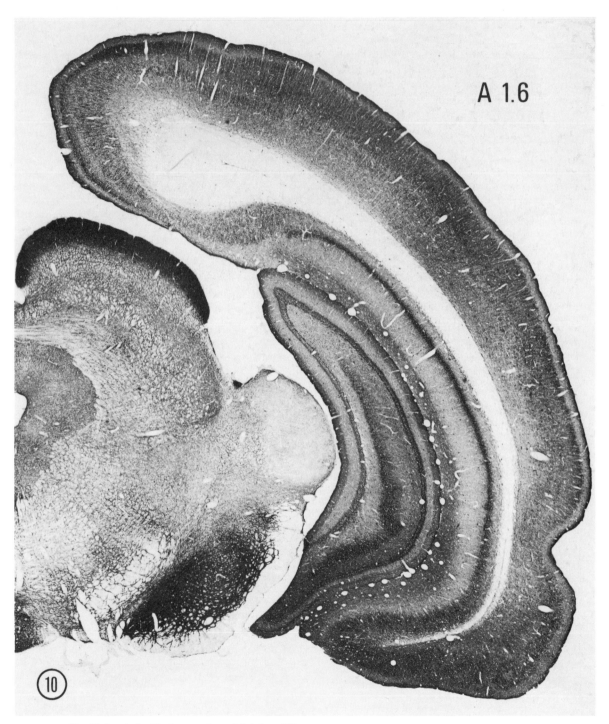

Fig. 10. Level of colliculus superior, *cf.* A 1.6, p. 477.

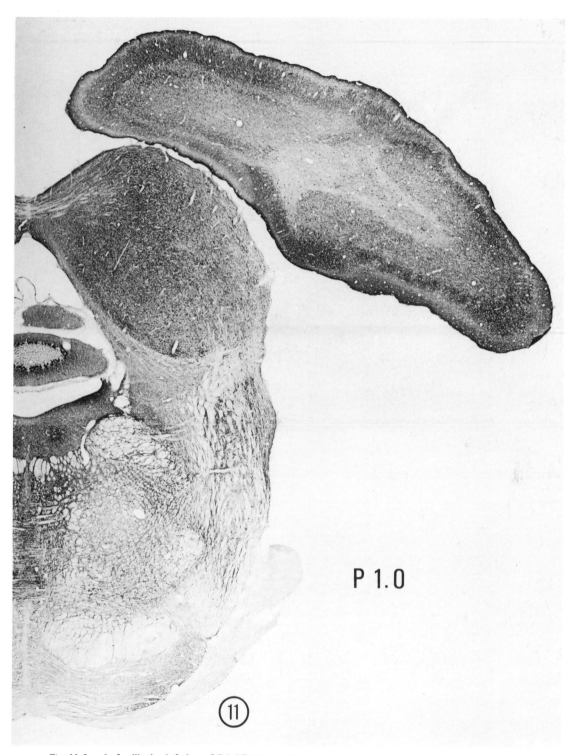

Fig. 11. Level of colliculus inferior, *cf.* P 0.5/P 1.5, p. 480.

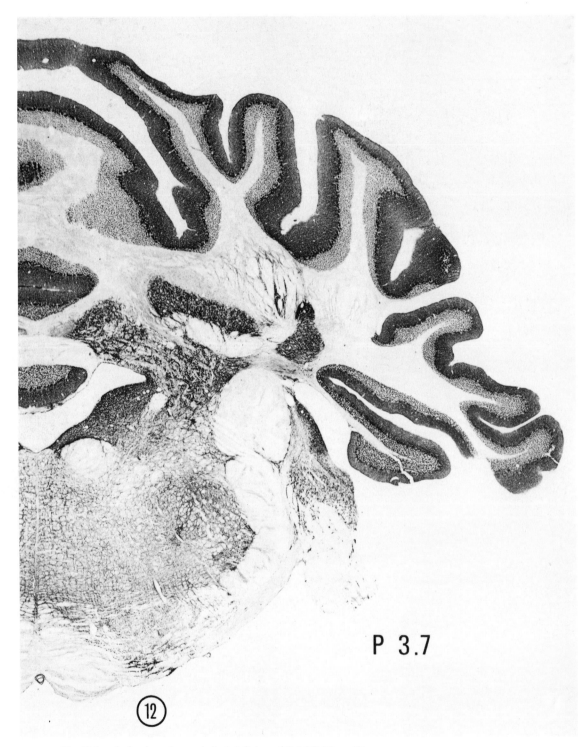

P 3.7

⑫

Fig. 12. Level of pedunculus cerebellaris inferior, *cf.* P 3.4/P 3.9, p. 481.

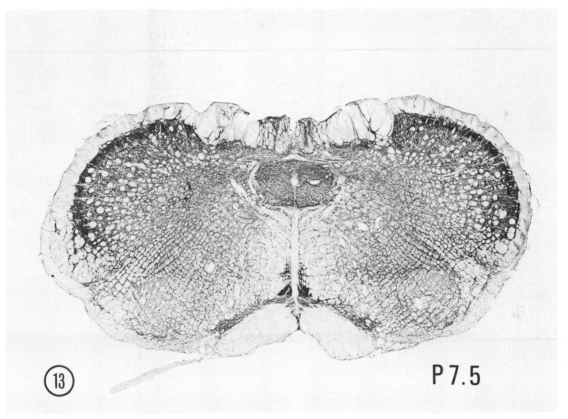

Fig. 13. Lower medullary level, *cf.* P 7.0/P 8.0, p. 483.

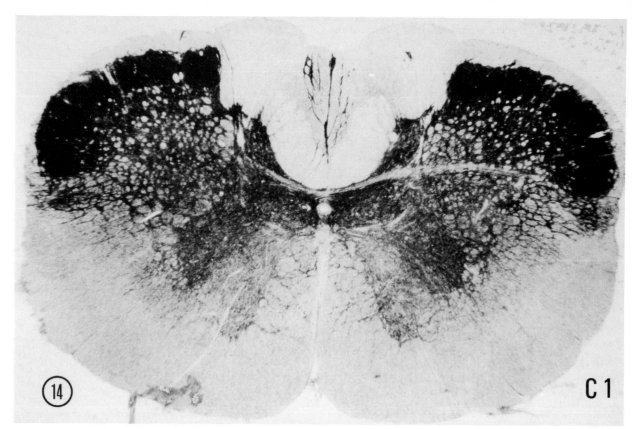

Fig. 14. Medulla spinalis, *cf*. C1, p. 484.

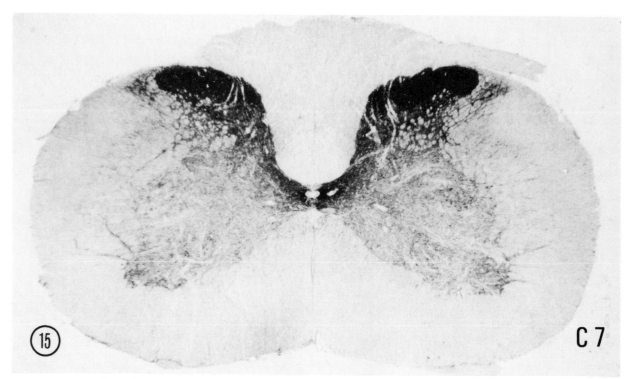

Fig. 15. Medulla spinalis, *cf*. C5, p. 484.

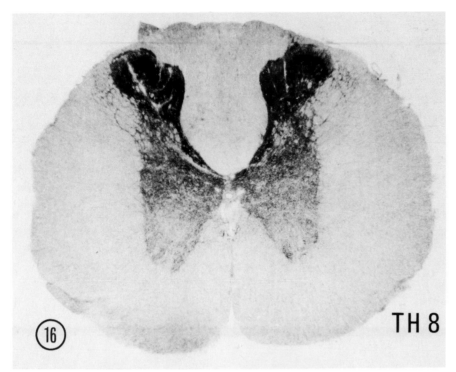

Fig. 16. Medulla spinalis, *cf.* Th8, p. 485.

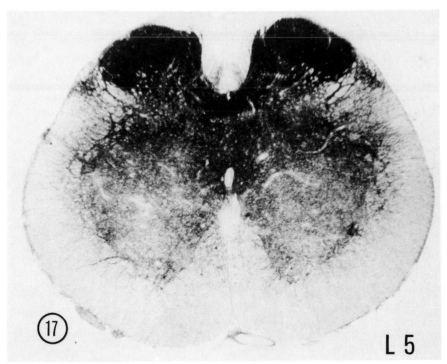

Fig. 17. Medulla spinalis, *cf.* L5, p. 485.

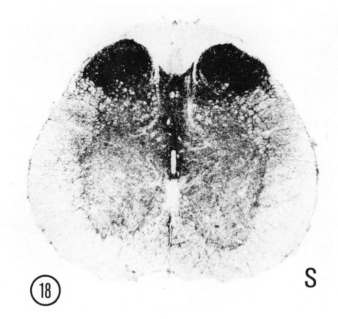

Fig. 18. Medulla spinalis.

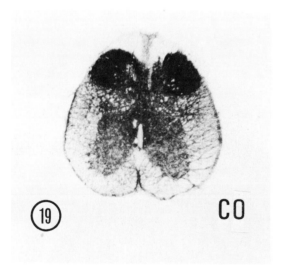

Fig. 19. Medulla spinalis.

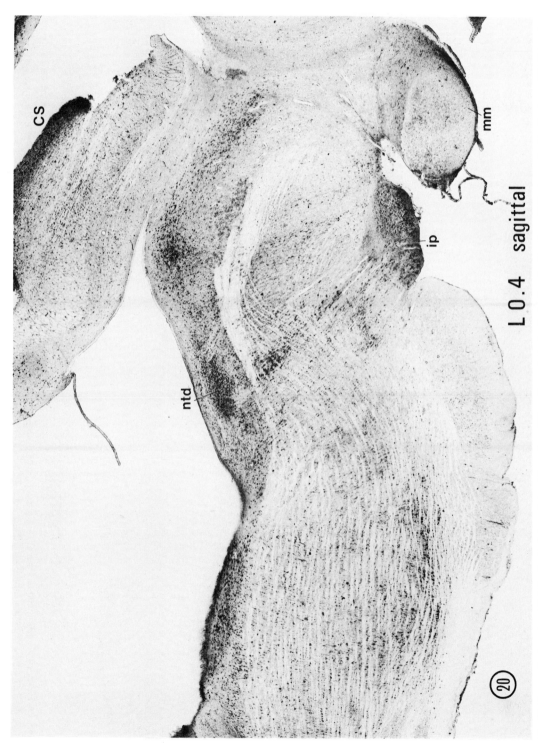

Fig. 20. Parasagittal section (slightly tilted), 0.4 mm lateral from the midline, through the fasciculus longitudinalis medialis shows the distribution of GABAergic cell bodies in the brainstem from upper medullary to diencephalic levels. × 19.3.

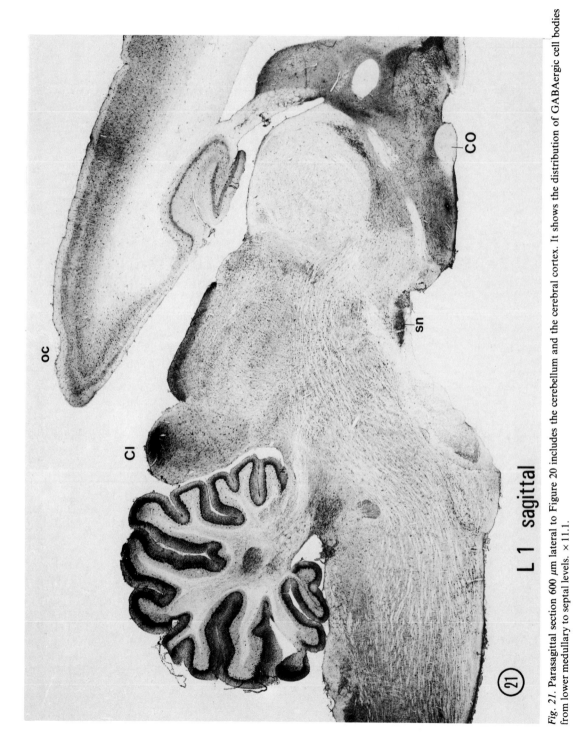

L 1 sagittal

Fig. 21. Parasagittal section 600 μm lateral to Figure 20 includes the cerebellum and the cerebral cortex. It shows the distribution of GABAergic cell bodies from lower medullary to septal levels. × 11.1.

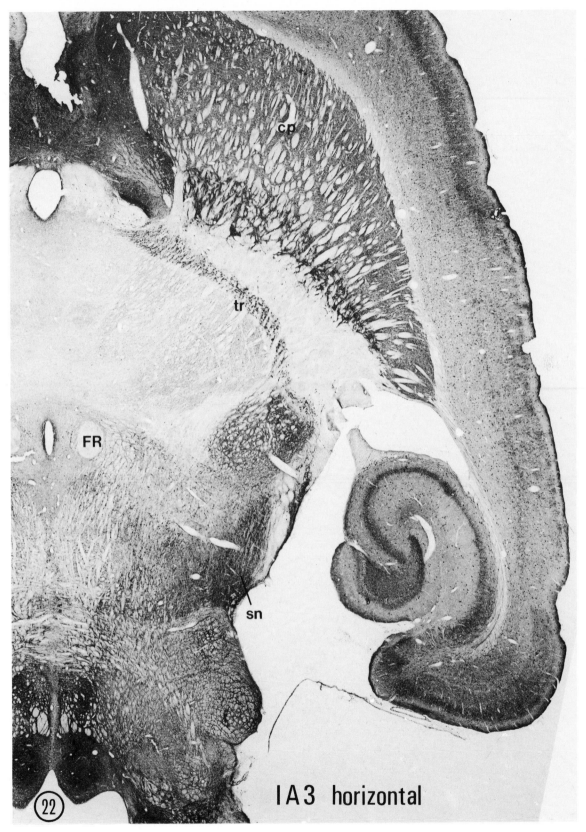

Fig. 22. Horizontal section through the decussatio pedunculorum cerebellarium superiorum shows distribution of GAD-immunoreactive cell bodies and terminals from mesencephalic to septal levels. × 16.

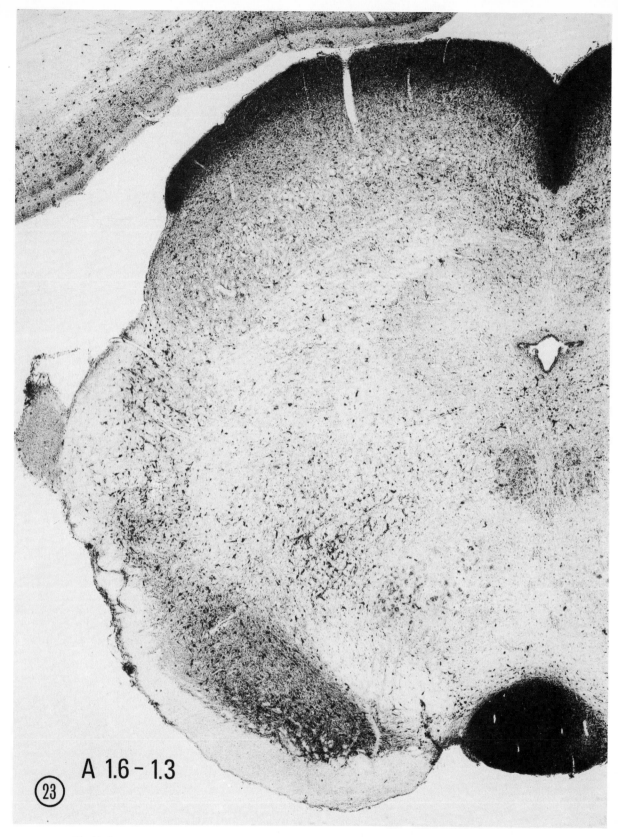

A 1.6 - 1.3

(23)

Fig. 23. Coronal section at the level of colliculus superior demonstrates the distribution of cell bodies. Staining of terminals is also evident, especially in colliculus superior, nucleus interpeduncularis and around the neurons of nucleus originis nervi oculomotorii and of nucleus ruber. ×37. *cf.* schematic drawings A 1.3–A 1.6, pp. 477-478.

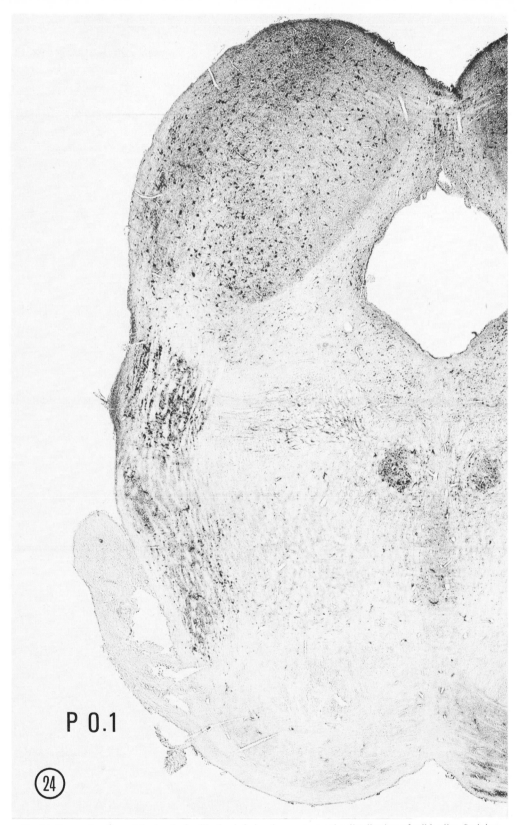

P 0.1

(24)

Fig. 24. Coronal section at the level of colliculus inferior demonstrates the distribution of cell bodies. Staining of terminals is barely higher than background in the tegmentum, but is more evident in colliculus inferior and along the border of the section, where penetration of immunoreagents has been enhanced by sectioning artefacts. × 27. *cf.* schematic drawing P 0.1, p. 479.

5. SCHEMATIC DRAWINGS

The Atlas: Scoring of bouton densities is presented on the right-hand side of the section drawing and scoring of cell body densities on the left-hand side using the different scale symbols as presented below. *For abbreviations,* see the General Abbreviations List.

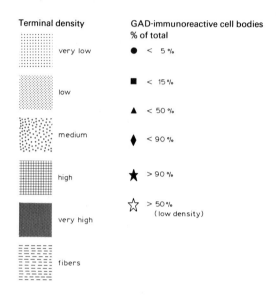

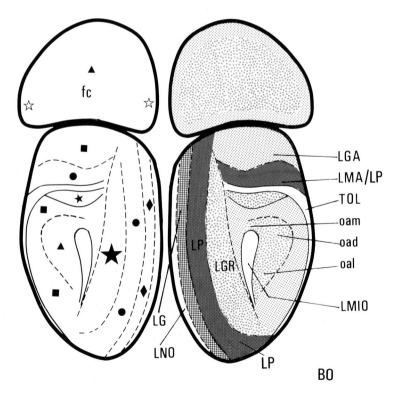

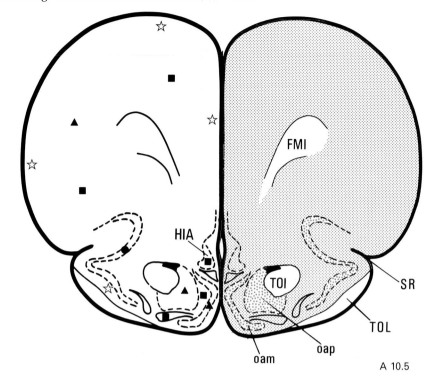

A 10.5

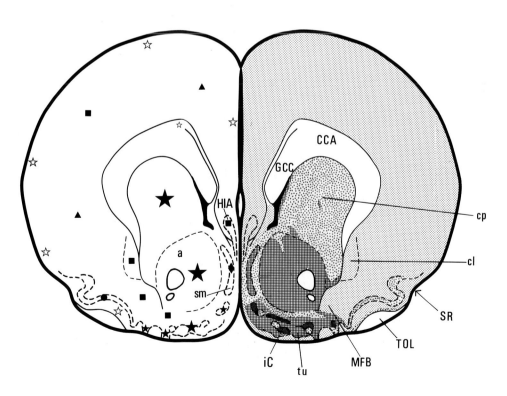

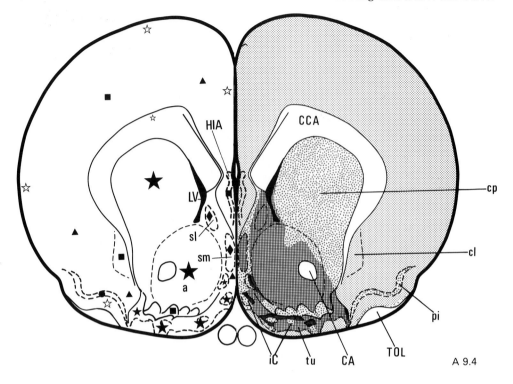

A 9.4

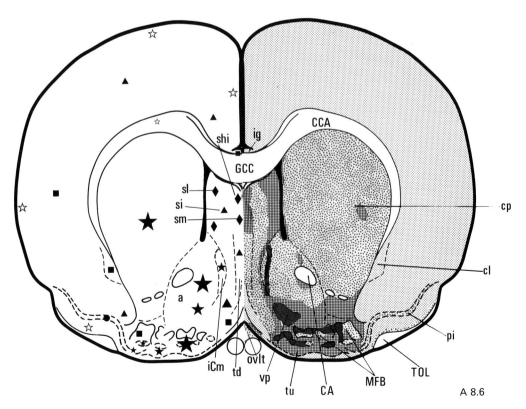

A 8.6

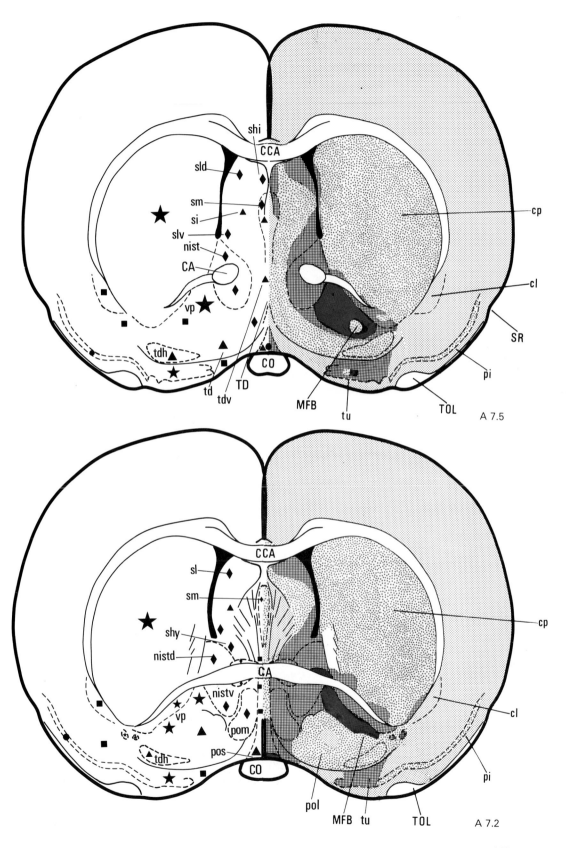

A 7.5

A 7.2

469

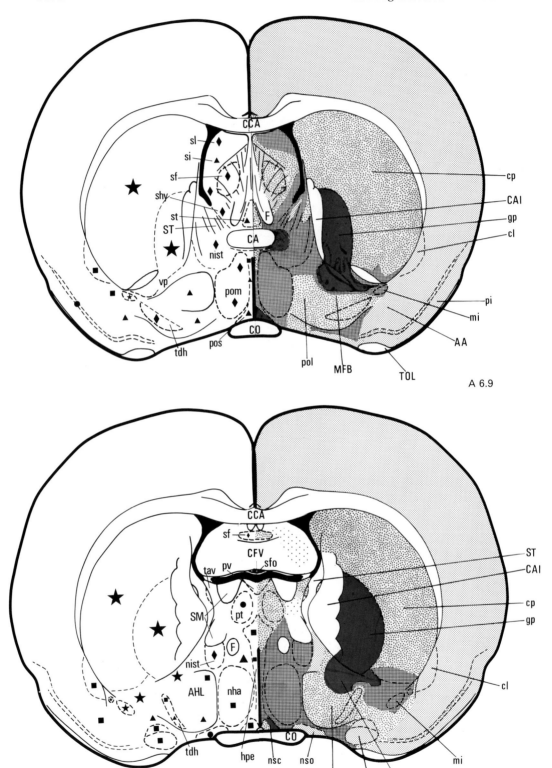

A 6.9

A 6.3

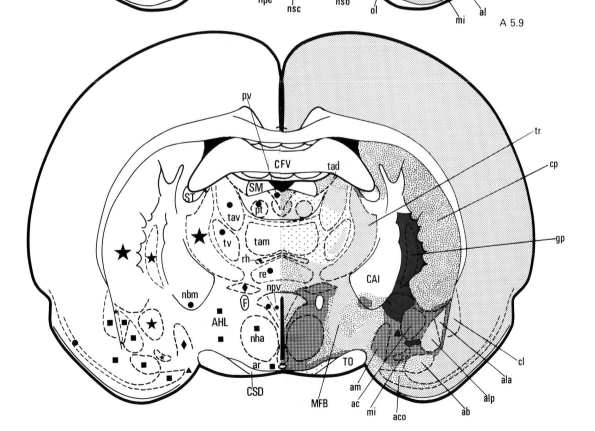

A 5.9

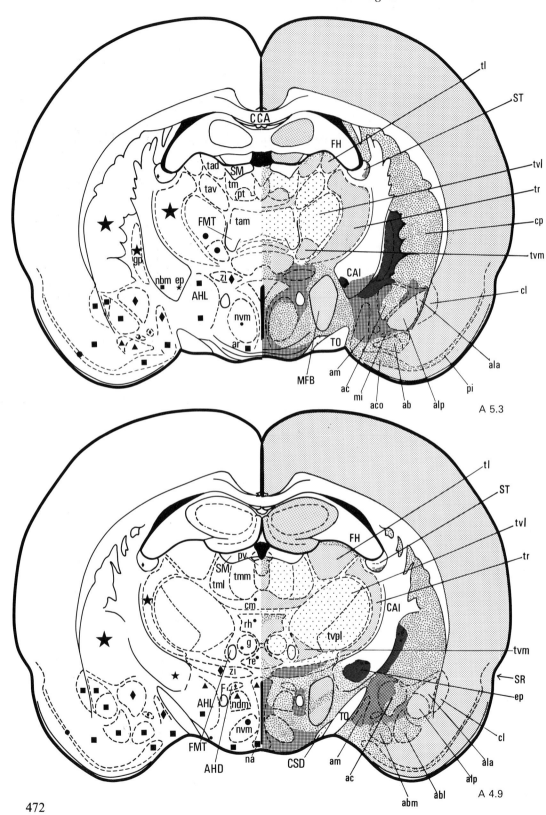

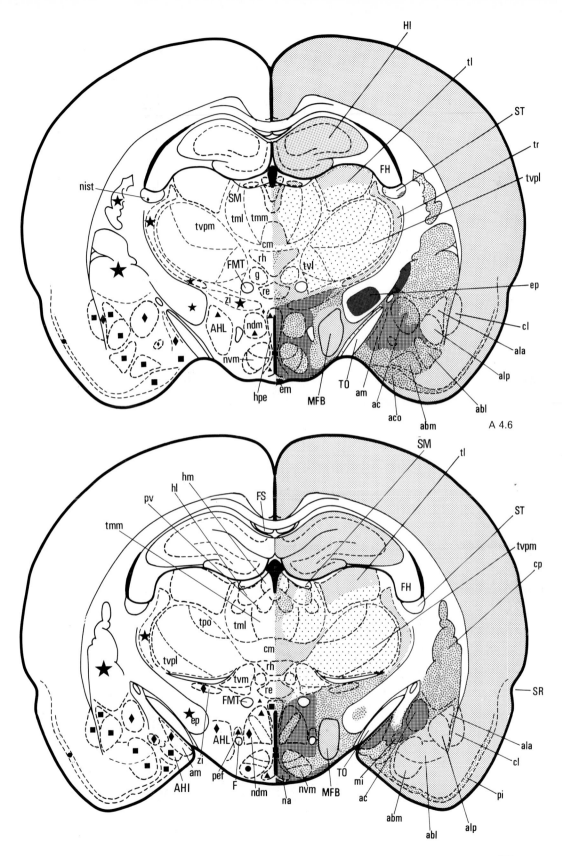

A 4.6

473

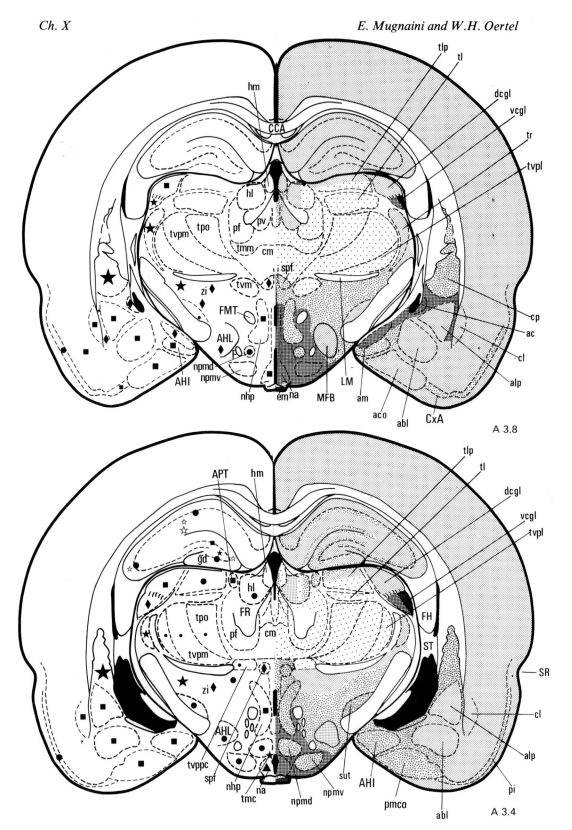

A 3.8

A 3.4

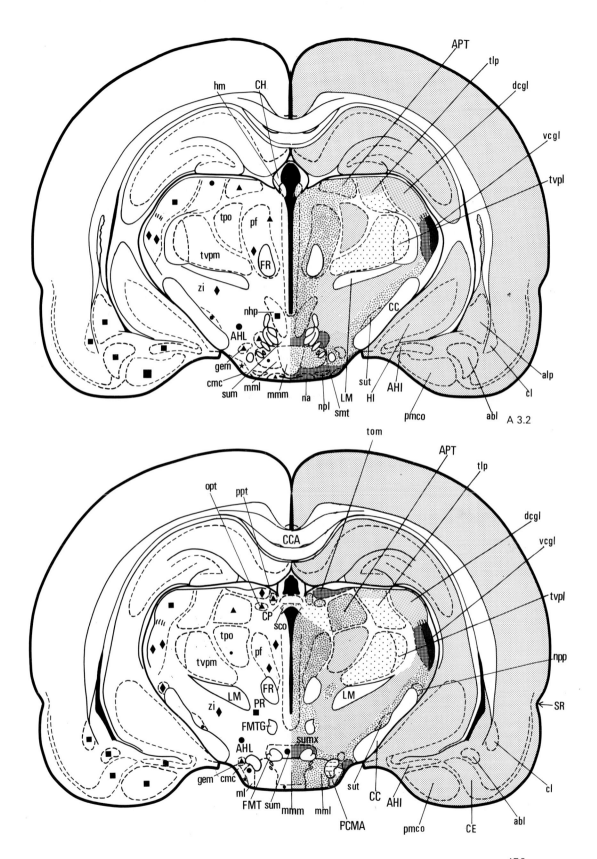

A 3.2

475

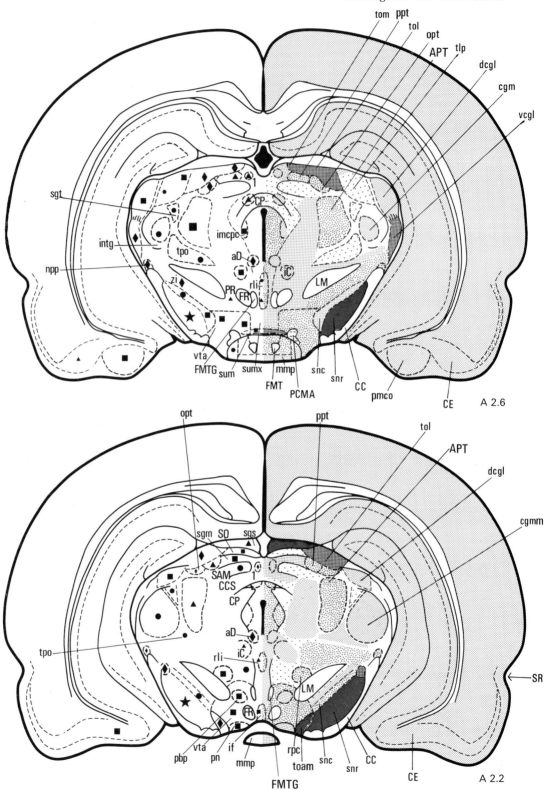

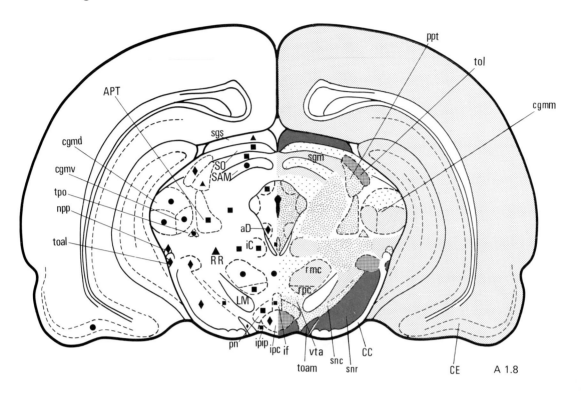

A 1.8

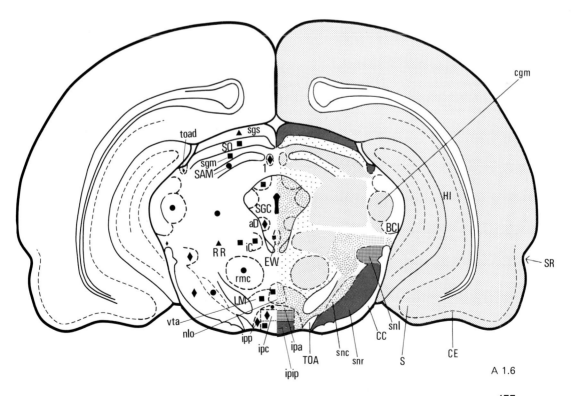

A 1.6

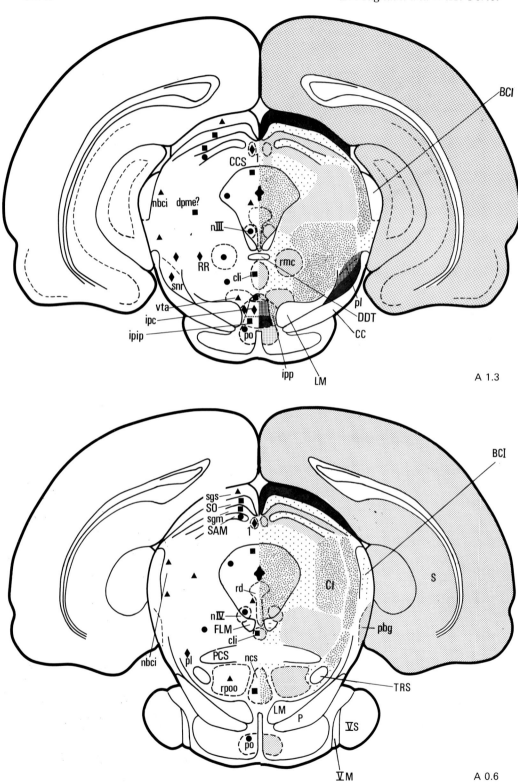

BCl

CCS
nbci   dpme?
nⅢ
RR   rmc
cli
snr
vta   pl
ipc   DDT
ipip   po   CC
        ipp   LM

A 1.3

BCl

sgs
SO
sgm
SAM
rd   Cf   S
nⅣ
FLM
cli
nbci   pl   PCS   ncs
rpoo   pbg
                        TRS
        LM   P
        ⅤS
po
ⅤM

A 0.6

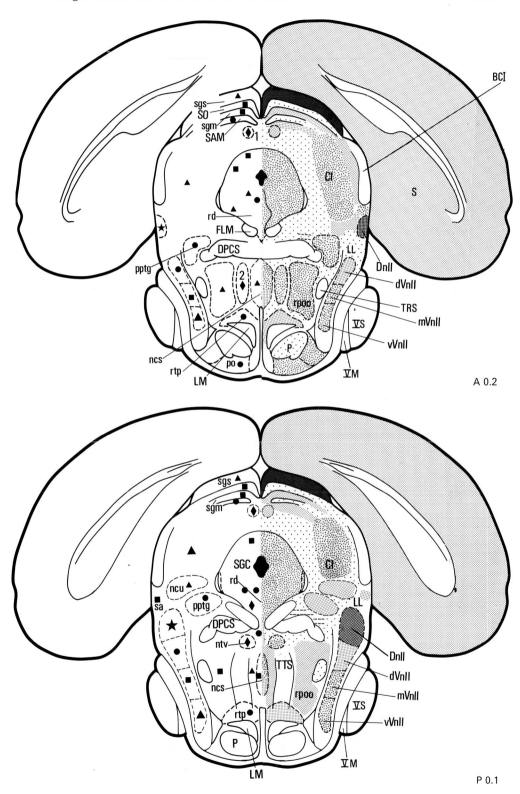

A 0.2

P 0.1

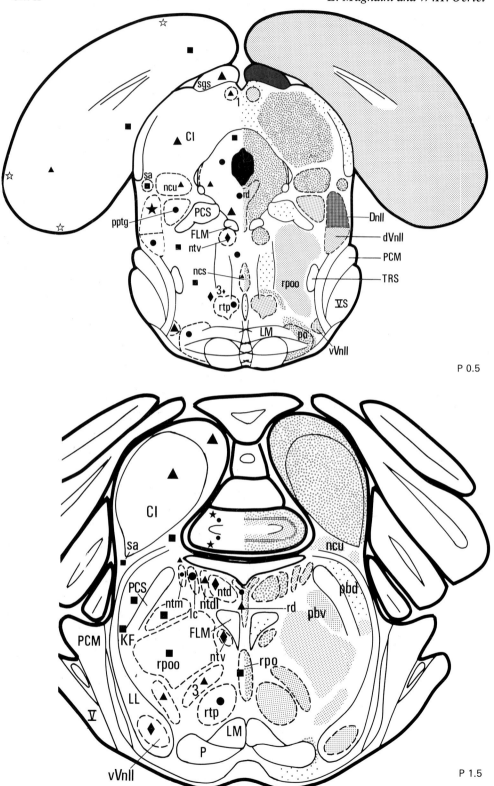

P 0.5

P 1.5

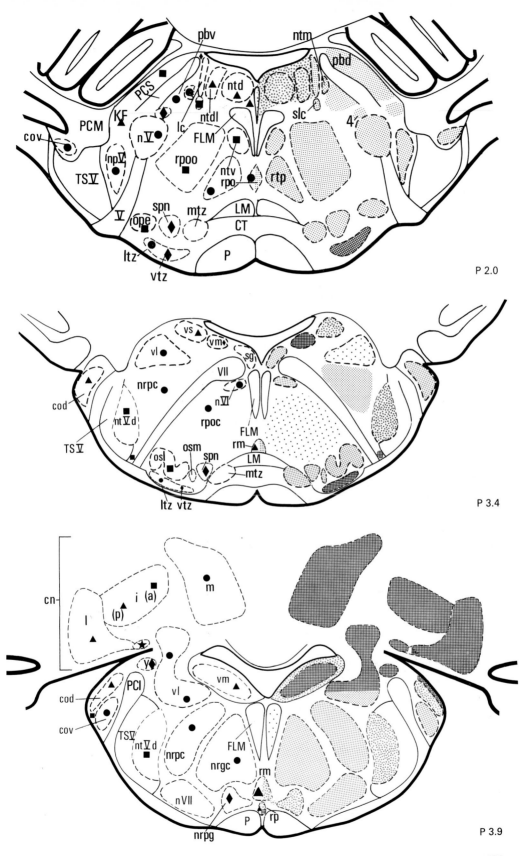

P 2.0

P 3.4

P 3.9

481

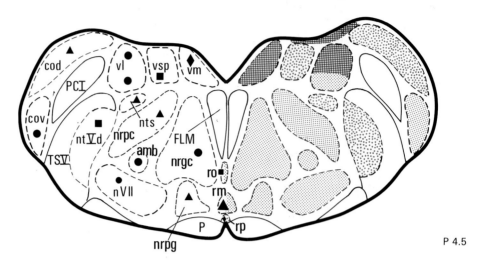

P 4.5

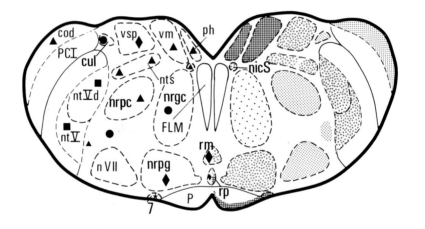

P 5.0

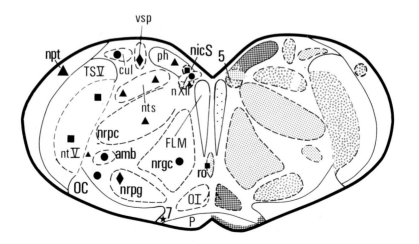

P 5.5

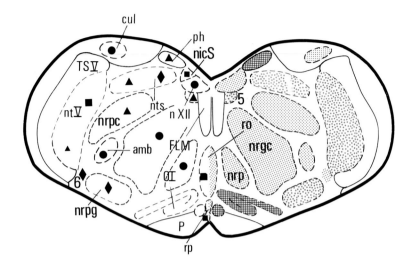

P 6.0

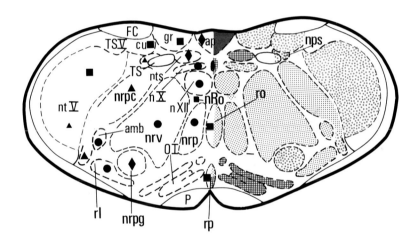

P 7.0

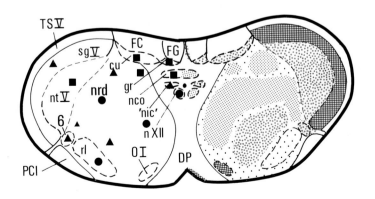

P 8.0

483

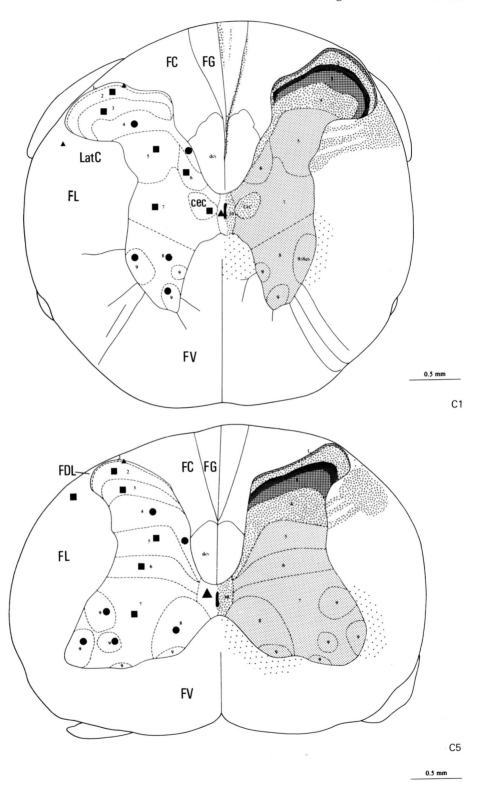

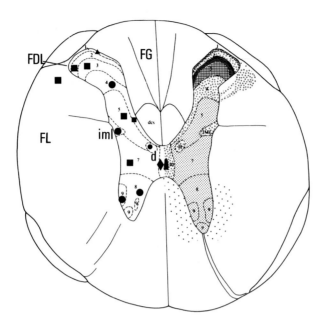

TH8

0.5 mm

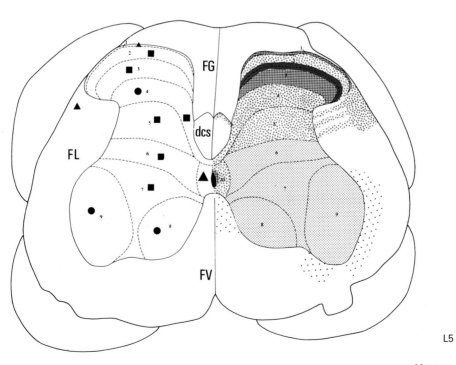

L5

0.5 mm

6. BRAIN AREAS

Table 1 lists abbreviation and corresponding denomination of the individual brain regions in alphabetical order.

Respective density of GAD-positive cell bodies is graded according to the following density score:

0 = none; 1 = less than 5% of total neurons; 2 = less than 15%; 3 = less than 50%; 4 = less than 90%; 5 = more than 90% of total neurons.

Respective density of GAD-positive axon terminals is graded according to the following density score:

0 = none or hardly any; 1 = very few; 2 = few; 3 = medium; 4 = high; 5 = very high.

To facilitate the use of TABLE 1, its organization is explained by an example:

Abbrevia-tion[1]	Brain region	Density of		Level of appearance in frontal plane[2]	References of techniques used[3,4]	Figure number[5]
		Cell bodies	Axon terminals		GAD IHC GABA IHC [³H]GABA AR	
Dnll	N. dorsalis lemnisci lateralis	5	3–4	A0.2–P0.5	1	103, *110, 111*

Dnll is the abbreviation for: *N. dorsalis lemnisci lateralis.* More than *90% of all neurons* in the n. dorsalis lemnisci lateralis are GAD-immunoreactive, as indicated by the numeral *5* in the column Density of cell bodies. Furthermore, the n. dorsalis lemnisci lateralis has a *medium to high density of GAD-immunoreactive nerve terminals,* as indicated by the numeral *3–4* in the column Density of axon terminals. The n. dorsalis lemnisci lateralis is found in the schematic atlas drawings 0.2 mm anterior to 0.5 mm posterior of the interaural axis (König and Klippel 1963) (A0.2–P0.5 in the column Level of appearance in frontal plane).

According to the column References only one study has so far been performed with GAD immunohistochemistry on the n. dorsalis lemnisci lateralis. This is reference number *1* in the list of References (Section 11).

The column Figure number indicates that the n. dorsalis lemnisci lateralis is illustrated in Figures 103, *110* and *111*. In the Figures with italicized number the n. dorsalis lemnisci lateralis is shown at higher magnification.

Notes to Table 1 →

[1]Brain regions with neurons labeled by the GAD antiserum but not corresponding to a specifically named nucleus are indicated by arabic numerals and tentatively given a topographically qualifying name as listed at the end of the alphabetical list (p.501).
[2]See schematic atlas drawings (pp. 466–485) according to König and Klippel (1963). A = anterior, P = posterior.
[3]Reference numbers indicate publication on GAD immunohistochemistry (GAD IHC), GABA immunohistochemistry (GABA INC) and [³H]GABA autoradiography ([³H]GABA AR).
[4]Reference numbers in square brackets indicate publication on tissue culture.
[5]Number of half-tone plate where brain region is illustrated. Numbers in brackets indicate very low power areas. Italicized numbers indicate half-tone at higher magnification.
* = cell body density scored after topical colchicine pretreatment of the animal.

TABLE 1. *List of brain areas*

Abbrevia-tion[1]	Brain region	Density of		Level of appearance in frontal plane[2]	References of techniques used[3,4] GAD IHC GABA IHC [³H]GABA AR	Figure number[5]
		Cell bodies	Axon terminals			
a*	Nucleus accumbens					
	medialis	5	4	A9.7–A8.6	126a, 166	(6), 39, 40,
	lateralis	5	3–4		175	52, *55*
A	Aquaeductus cerebri	/	/	A2.8–P0.5		
AA	Area amygdala anterior	(2–)3	(2–)3–4	A6.9 (?)		68
ab	*Nucleus amygdaloideus basalis*	2	(2–)3	A5.7–A5.3		56
abl	pars lateralis	2	(2–)3	A4.9–A2.8	127	
abm	pars medialis	2(–3)	(2–)3	A4.9–A4.1		
ac*	Nucleus amygdaloideus centralis	4–5	3–4	A5.7–A3.8	165, 167a	(8), 56, 57, 58,*59*, 72
aco	Nucleus amygdaloideus corticalis	2(–3)	3	A5.7–A4.6 see *pmco*		68
ACU = *ncu*	Area cuneiformis			see *ncu*		
aD	Nucleus accessorius Darkschewitsch	4	2	A2.6–A1.6	180	*62*, 92, *119*
AHD	Area hypothalamica dorsalis	3–4	(3–)4	A4.9–A4.6	49a	69
AHI	Area amygdalo-hippocampalis	2–3	3	A4.1–A2.8		72
AHL	Area hypothalamica lateralis					
	pars rostralis	2–3	3	A6.3–A4.6	49a, 239	*71*,
		(3–)4	2–3	A4.1–A3.8		75
	pars caudalis	1(–2)	2(–3)	A3.4–A2.8		
al	*Nucleus amygdaloideus lateralis*	2	2	A5.9		(8), 56, 58
ala	pars anterior	2	2	A5.7–A4.1		*59*, 68
alp	pars posterior	2	2	A5.7–A3.2		
am	Nucleus amygdaloideus medialis	4(–5)	4	A5.7–A3.8	167a	(8), *56*, 57, 69, *72*
amb	Nucleus ambiguus	1	2	P4.5–P7.0		
ap	Area postrema	4	5	P7.0		99, 122, 139
APT	Area pretectalis (anterior)	2–3	3	A3.4–A1.8	174	(9), 60, *61*, 63, 64, 92
AR	Area retrochiasmatica	2	4	A5.7–A5.3		(8)
AVT = *vta*	Area ventralis tegmenti (Tsai)			see *vta*		
bac	Nucleus commissurae anterioris (bed nucleus)	1–2	3	not shown A6.0		
BCI	Brachium colliculi inferioris	0	0(–1)	A1.6–P0.5		23
BIN = *nbci*	Nucleus brachii conjunctivi inferioris			see *nbci*		
BO	Bulbus olfactorius			BO	71, 72, 139, 140, 189	4, 25, *27*, *28–31*
BOA	Bulbus olfactorius accessorius			BO	139	28
C I,VII	Medulla spinalis, pars cervicalis segmenta I et VII			C1, C7 see *sc*		14, 15
CA	Commissura anterior	0	0(–1)	A9.7–A6.9		(6, 7, 21), 35, 36, 40, 73, 74, 75
CAI	Capsula interna	0	0(–1)	A7.2–A4.1		(7, 8, 22), 40, 56, 60, 68, 72
CC	Crus cerebri	0	0(–1)	A3.2–A1.3		(9, 10, 23), 64, 86
CCA	Corpus callosum	4–5	0(–1)	A9.7–A2.8		(6–9), 42

TABLE 1 (*continued*)

Abbreviation[1]	Brain region	Density of		Level of appearance in frontal plane[2]	References of techniques used[3,4] GAD IHC GABA IHC [^{3}H]GABA AR	Figure number[5]
		Cell bodies	Axon terminals			
ccgm = *cgm*	Nucleus centralis corporis geniculati medialis			see *cgm*		
CCS	Commissura colliculorum superiorum	0	0–1	A2.2–A0.6		(10, 20, 23), 100
ce	Cortex entorhinalis	2–3	2–3	A2.8–A1.6	260	32, 33
cec	Nucleus centralis cervicalis	1–2	2–3	C1		
CFV	Commissura fornicis ventralis (Comm. hippocampi ventralis)	0	0–1	A6.3–A5.7		(21)
cgm (=ccgm)	*Nucleus centralis corporis geniculati medialis*	1	2	A2.6–A1.6	5	(10), 60, 63, 82, 109
cgmd	pars dorsalis	1	1	A2.2–A1.8	174	
cgmm	pars medialis	1	2	A1.8		
cgmv	pars ventralis	1	2	A1.8		
CH	Commissura habenularum			A3.2 not scored		
ci	Cortex cingularis	2–3	2–3	A9.4–A2.8 not indicated		(6–9)
CI	Colliculus inferior	3	3	A0.6–P1.5	203, 244	(11, 24), 63, 103, *105, 108*
cl	Claustrum	2–3	2–3	A9.7–A2.8		(6, 7), 26
cli	Nucleus raphe caudalis linearis	(1–)2	2	A1.3–A0.6		93
cm	Nucleus centromedianus thalami	0–1	1–2	A4.9–A3.4	179, 224	69
cmc	Nucleus caudalis magnocellularis hypothalami posterioris	5	4	A3.2–A2.8	49a, 233, 247, 250	73, 74, *80, 84*
cn	Nuclei cerebellares	1–5	4–5	see *i(a) i(p) m l*	137, 138, 150, 159	12, 127
CO I–III	Medulla spinalis, pars coccygis, segmenta I–III			not shown, see *sc*		19
CO	Chiasma opticum	0	0(–1)	A7.5–A5.9		(7), 40, 73, 74, 75
cod	Nucleus cochlearis dorsalis	3	2–3	P3.4–P5.0	141	114, 116
cov	Nucleus cochlearis ventralis	1	2	P2.0–P4.5	2, 3	114, 117
cp(*)	Nucleus caudatus/putamen	5	3	A9.7–A3.4	6, 11, 26, 136, 165, 166, [174a], 193	(6, 7, 8, 22), 25, 26, 35, 36, 40, *42, 43,* 47, 56
CP	Commissura posterior	0	0–1	A2.8–A2.2		(9), 63, *98*
CS	Colliculus superior	1–3	1–5	see *sgs SO sgm SAM*	90, 133, 134	(10, 23), *100, 101,* 102
CSD	Commissura supraoptica dorsalis	0	1	A5.7–A4.6		(56, 72)
ct	Nucleus corporis trapezoidei			see *ltz mtz vtz*		

TABLE 1 (*continued*)

Abbreviation[1]	Brain region	Density of		Level of appearance in frontal plane[2]	References of techniques used[3,4] GAD IHC GABA IHC [3H]GABA AR	Figure number[5]
		Cell bodies	Axon terminals			
CT	Corpus trapezoideum	0	0–1	P2.0		
cu	Nucleus cuneatus	2	3	P7.0–P8.0		139, 140, 141, 142
cul	Nucleus cuneatus lateralis	1	2	P5.0–P6.0		
CV	Cornu ventrale (medullae spinalis)			see *sc*, lamina Rexed 7–9		(14–19)
CxA	Area cortico-amygdaloidea (cortex-amygdala transition zone)	2–3	3	A3.8		(8)
d	Nucleus dorsalis (medullae spinalis)	1	2–3	TH8		
dcgl	Nucleus dorsalis corporis geniculati lateralis	2	2	A3.8–A2.2	50, 80, 168, 180, 228	(9), 60, 63, 64, *66*, 109
dcs	Tractus corticospinalis dorsalis	0	0–1	C1–L5		(14–17)
DDT	Decussatio dorsalis tegmentalis	0	0	A1.3		93
Dnll	N. dorsalis lemnisci lateralis	5	3–4	A0.2–P0.5	1	11, 24, 103, 110, *111*
DP	Decussatio pyramidis	0	0	P8.0		
DPCS	Decussatio pedunculorum cerebellarium superiorum	0	0 fibers	A0.2–P0.1		87
dpme	N. mesencephalicus profundus	(1–)2	2(–3)	A1.8–A1.3		(10)
dtn = *toad*	Dorsal terminal nucleus of the optical accessory tract			see *toad*		
dVnll	Nucleus ventralis lemnisci lateralis, pars dorsalis	1	2	A0.2–P0.5	4	11, 24, 110
em	Eminentia mediana	0	3/5	A4.6–A3.8	23, 237, 238, 239	70, 76
ep	Nucleus entopeduncularis	5	5	A5.3–A4.1	167, 193	40, *48*, 56, 70, 72
(epV)	Ependyma ventricularis	0	0(–1)		21 (?)	
EW	Nucleus Edinger-Westphal	2	3	A1.6		(92)
F	Fornix	0	0	A6.9–A3.8		(7, 8), 73, 74
fc	Cortex frontalis	2–3	2–3	BO–A10.5		(5)
FC	Fasciculus cuneatus	0	0	P7.0–C5		(13), 139, 140, 142
FD	Funiculus dorsalis (medullae spinalis)			see *FC* *FG*		
FDL	Fasciculus dorsalis lateralis (medullae spinalis)	0	1–2	C5, TH8		(15, 16)
FG	Fasciculus gracilis	0	0	P8.0–L5		142
FH	Fimbria hippocampi	0	0	A5.3–A3.4		(8), 32, 33, 40, 64
FL	Funiculus lateralis (medullae spinalis)	0	0–1	C1–L5		(14–19)
FLM	Fasciculus longitudinalis medialis	0	0(–1) fibers	A1.8–P6.0		(10, 11, 20, 22, 24), *93, 121*
FMI	Forceps minor	0	0(–1)	A10.5		39
FMT	Fasciculus mamillothalamicus	0	0	A5.3–A2.8		80
FMTG	Fasciculus mamillotegmentalis	0	0	A2.8–A2.2		
FR	Fasciculus retroflexus	0	0	A3.4–A2.2		(22), 62, 92, 94

489

TABLE 1 (*continued*)

Abbreviation[1]	Brain region	Density of		Level of appearance in frontal plane[2]	References of techniques used[3,4]	Figure number[5]
		Cell bodies	Axon terminals		GAD IHC GABA IHC [³H]GABA AR	
FS	Fornix superior	0	0	A4.9–A3.4		
FV	Funiculus ventralis (medullae spinalis)	0	0–1	C1–L5		(14–19)
g	Nucleus gelatinosus thalami	0–1	1	A4.9–A4.1		(69)
GCC	Genu corporis callosi	5	0(–1)	A9.7–A8.6		
gcl	Lamina granularis cerebelli	1–2	2(–3)	P1.5–P2.0	159, 191, 205	123, 124, 125, *126*
gd (see *HI*)	Gyrus dentatus			see *HI*		
gem	Nuclei gemini	3	2	A3.2–A2.8		80
gp	Globus pallidus	5	5	A6.9–A4.6	167, 193	(7, 8, 22), 40, *44*, 47, 68, 72
gr	Nucleus gracilis	2	3	P7.0–P8.0		122, 139, 140–142
H	Cerebellum (hemispheres)			P1.5–P2.0 see *gcl* *mol* *pcl*	32, 33, 84, 85, 129, 131, 135, 159, 161, 191	123, 124, *125*
h	Habenula			see *hl* *hm*	7,65	
HI	Hippocampus	2–3	2–3	A5.3–A1.3	99, 15, 58, [100] 110, 161, 182, 191, 209, 213, 218, 221	(9, 10, 21, 22), *32, 33, 34*, 64
	stratum lacunosum-moleculare	4–5	2–3			
	stratum pyramidale	1–2	3			
	stratum oriens	4	2–3			
	stratum radiatum	4–5	2–3			
– gd	gyrus dentatus			A4.1–A2.2		
	hilus	4–5	2–3		27a, 63, 114, 209, 213, 221 252	(9, 21, 22), *32, 33, 34*
	stratum granulosum	1–2	3			
	stratum moleculare	4	2–3	see *ig*		
HIA	Hippocampus, pars anterior	2–3	2–3	A10.5–A9.4		38
hl	Nucleus habenulae lateralis	1	1–3	A4.6–A3.4	7	63, 69
hm	Nucleus habenulae medialis	0	1–2	A4.6–A3.2	7	(63)
hpe	Nucleus periventricularis hypothalami	2(–3)	3–4	A6.9–A3.8	49a, 239, 239a	68, 69
hpv = *npv*	Nucleus paraventricularis hypothalami			see *npv*		
hy	*Hypophysis*				160, 247	
hy,pd	lobus anterior, pars distalis	0	0	not shown		
hy,im	lobus anterior, pars intermedia	0	2–3	not shown		*77, 78*
hy,n	lobus posterior (pars nervosa)	0	2	not shown		*78*
i	Nucleus interpositus cerebelli					127, 129, 132
i(a)	pars anterior	2(–3)	4–5	P3.9		
i(p)	pars posterior	3	4–5	P3.9		
ic	Nucleus interstitialis Cajal	2(–3)	2	P2.6–P1.6		62, 92, 94, 119
iC	Insula Callejae				48, 118, 167a	51, 52, 53
	granule cell cluster ('striatal')	5	3	A9.4–A7.5		*54*
	cap region ('pallidal')	5	5	A9.4–A7.5		*54*

490

TABLE 1 (*continued*)

Abbreviation[1]	Brain region	Density of		Level of appearance in frontal plane[2]	References of techniques used[3,4]	Figure number[5]
		Cell bodies	Axon terminals		GAD IHC GABA IHC [³H]GABA AR	
iCM	Insula Callejae magna			see *iC* A8.6		
if	Nucleus interfascicularis	2	3	A2.2–A1.8		86
ig	Induseum griseum	2–3	2–3	*A8.6*–A2.8 see *HI*		38
imcpc	N. interstitialis magnocellularis commissurae posterioris	2	2	A2.6		
iml	Columna cellularis intermedio-lateralis (medullae spinalis)	1	(2–)3	TH8		*148*
inc	Cortex insularis	2–3	2–3	not indicated		
inf = *l*	Subnucleus parvocellularis nuclei lateralis cerebelli			see *l*		
intg	Nucleus intermedialis corporis geniculati (intermediate geniculate nucleus)	0	1	A2.6		
io = *OI*	Nucleus olivaris inferior			see *OI*		
ip	*Nucleus interpeduncularis*					20, 23, 86, 87, 93, *121*
ipa	pars apicalis	1–2	2–3	A1.6		88,
ipc	pars centralis	4	4	A1.8–A1.3		88, *89*
ipip	pars inferior posterior	2	5	A1.8–A1.3		89
ipp	pars paramediana (=lateralis)	4	2	A1.6–A1.3		88, *89*
KF	Nucleus Köllike-Fuse	(2–)3	2	P1.5–P2.0		
l	Nucleus lateralis cerebelli	3	4–5	P3.9	137, 138, 159, 205	127, *130*
	Subnucleus parvocellularis nuclei lateralis cerebelli (inf)	5	4–5	P3.9		135
L V	Medulla spinalis, pars lumbalis, segmentum L V			L5 see *sc*, Lamina Rexed		17
latC	Nucleus cervicalis lateralis	2–3	3	C1		
lc	Locus ceruleus	0–1	2–3	P1.5–P2.0	23	146
LG	Lamina glomerulosa bulbi olfactorii	4	4	BO	140, 189	27, 29, 30
LGA	Lamina glomerulosa bulbi olfactorii accessorii	2	2	BO		28
LGI = *LGR*	Lamina granularis interna			see *LGR*		
LGR	Lamina granularis bulbi olfactorii	5	3	BO	140, 189	27, 29, 31
LL	Lemniscus lateralis	0	0 fibers	A0.2–P1.5		
lld	N. lemnisci lateralis dorsalis			see *Dnll*		
llv	N. lemnisci lateralis ventralis			see *dVnll* *mVnll* *vVnll*		
llr = *Dnll*	N. lemnisci lateralis rostralis			A0.2 see *Dnll*		
LM	Lemniscus medialis	0	0	A4.1–P3.4		(9, 10), 64 90, 93

491

TABLE 1 (*continued*)

Abbrevia-tion[1]	Brain region	Density of		Level of appearance in frontal plane[2]	References of techniques used[3,4] GAD IHC GABA IHC [³H]GABA AR	Figure number[5]
		Cell bodies	Axon terminals			
LMA	Lamina cellularum mitralium bulbi olfactorii accessorii	1	5	BO		28
LMIO	Lamina medullaris interna bulbi olfactorii	0	0	BO		
LMO	Lamina molecularis bulbi olfactorii			see *LP*		
LNO	Lamina nervi olfactorii	0	0(−1)	BO		29
LP(= LPE)	Lamina plexiformis externa bulbi olfactorii	1 superfic. profund. 4–5	5	BO	140, 189	27, 29
ltn = *toal*	Lateral terminal nucleus of optic accessory tract			see *toal*		
ltz(= ct)	Nucleus lateralis corporis trapezoidei	1	4	P2.0	3	112
LV	Ventriculum laterale	/	/	A9.7–A6.3		
m	Nucleus medialis cerebelli	1	4	P3.9		(124), 127, 131
MFB	Fasciculus medialis pros-encephali	(2)	2–3	A9.7–A2.8		(8), 35, 68
mi*	Massae intercalatae	4–5	4	A7.2–A4.1	167a	(8), 58, *59*
mm	*Nucleus mamillaris medialis*				239, 247	(20), 80,
mml	pars lateralis	0–1	3	A3.2–A2.8		73, 121
mmm	pars medialis	0	3	A3.2–A2.6		79
mmn	pars mediana	0	2–3	not shown		
mmp (= nmp)	pars posterior	0–1	2–3	A2.8–A2.2		81
ml	*Nucleus mamillaris lateralis*					79
	dorsalis	1	1	A2.8–A2.6		
	ventralis	1	2–3	A2.8–A2.6		
mol	Lamina molecularis cerebelli	5	3	P1.5–P2.0	138, 159, 191, 205	123, 124, *125*, *126*
mp = *PCMA*	Pedunculus corporis mamillaris	0	0 fibers	A2.8–A2.6		
mr = *ncs*	Nucleus raphe medianus			see *ncs*		
mtn = *toam*	Medial terminal nucleus of the optic accessory tract			see *toam*		
mtz(= ct)	N. medialis corporis trapezoidei	0	2	P2.0–P3.4	3	112
mVnll	Nucleus ventralis lemnisci lateralis, pars medialis	2	2–3	A0.2–P0.1	4	(11, 24)
na	Nucleus arcuatus	2–3	4	A4.9–A3.2	49a, 122a, 239, 239a, 247	69, 70, 76, 80
nbci(= BIN)	N. brachii conjunctivi inferioris	3	3	A1.3–A0.6		23
nbm	Nucleus basalis magnocellularis (Meynert)	(1–)2	3–4	A5.9–A5.3		(8), 56, 68, 72
nco	Nucleus commissuralis	2	2	P8.0		
ncs(= mr)	Nucleus centralis superior					
	dorsalis	3	3	A0.6–P0.5		97
	ventralis (nucleus raphe medianus)	2–3	2			
ncu(= ACU)	Nucleus cuneiformis	3	2–3	P0.1–P0.5		(11, 24), 103

TABLE 1 (*continued*)

Abbrevia-tion[1]	Brain region	Density of		Level of appearance in frontal plane[2]	References of techniques used[3,4] GAD IHC GABA IHC [³H]GABA AR	Figure number[5]
		Cell bodies	Axon terminals			
ndm	*Nucleus dorsomedialis hypothalami*				241a	69, 70, 73
ndmc	pars compacta	0–1	3	A4.1		
ndmd	pars dorsalis	(2–)3	3–4	A4.9–A4.1		
ndmv	pars ventralis	4	4	A4.9–A4.1		
nha	Nucleus hypothalamicus anterior	2	4	A6.3–A5.7		(8), 68, 73
nhp	Nucleus hypothalamicus posterior	2	3	A3.8–A3.2		(9)
'nic'	Nucleus intercalatus	(2–)3	2–3	P8.0		
nicS	Nucleus intercalatus Staderini	2–3	2–3	P5.0–P6.0		122
nist*	*Nucleus interstitialis striae terminalis*	4(–5)	4–5	A7.5–A6.3		(7), 35, *36*, (68)
nistd*	pars dorsalis	4(–5)	4	A7.2		
nistv*	pars ventralis (including 'bed of the stria terminalis' (101))	4(–5)	4	A7.2		
nlo	Nucleus linearis oralis	2–3	2–3	A1.6		(88?)
nmp = *mmp*	Nucleus mamillaris medialis pars posterior			see *mmp*		
np = *pbv*	Nucleus parabrachialis ventralis			see *pbv*		
np V	Nucleus sensorius principalis nervi trigemini	1	2	P2.0		
npd = *pbd*	Nucleus parabrachialis dorsalis			see *pdb*		
npe = *hpe*	Nucleus periventricularis hypothalami			see *hpe*		
npf = *pef*	Nucleus perifornicalis			see *pef*		
npl	Nucleus mamillaris prelateralis	?	4	A3.2		
npmd	Nucleus premamillaris dorsalis	1	2–3	A3.8–A3.4		
npmv	Nucleus premamillaris ventralis	0–1	3–4	A3.8–A3.4		73
npp	Nucleus peripeduncularis	4	3–4	A2.8–A1.6	180	*50*, 64
nps	Nucleus parasolitarius	3	3	P7.0		
npt	Nucleus paratrigeminalis	3	3	P5.5		144
npv(= hpv)	*Nucleus paraventricularis hypothalami*	1	2	A5.7–A5.3	241a	(8)
npvm	pars magnocellularis	0–1	2	A5.7–A5.3		
npvp	pars parvocellularis	1	2–3	A5.7–A5.3		
nrd	Nucleus reticularis medullae oblongatae, pars dorsalis	1	2	P8.0		
nrgc(= rgi)	Nucleus reticularis gigantocellularis	1(–2)	(1–)2	P3.9–P6.0		
nrm = *rm*	Nucleus raphe magnus			see *rm*		
nRo	Nucleus of Roller	(1–)2	2	P7.0		
nro = *ro*	Nucleus raphe obscurus			see *ro*		
nrp	Nucleus reticularis paramedianus	1(–2)	2	P6.0–P7.0		137, 138
nrpc = 'rpc'	Nucleus reticularis parvocellularis	1	2	P3.4–P3.9		
		3	2	P4.5–P7.0		

TABLE 1 (*continued*)

Abbreviation[1]	Brain region	Density of		Level of appearance in frontal plane[2]	References of techniques used[3,4] GAD IHC GABA IHC [³H]GABA AR	Figure number[5]
		Cell bodies	Axon terminals			
nrpg	Nucleus reticularis paragiganto-cellularis	4 3 4	3 2 3	P5.0–P7.0 P4.5 P3.9	105 (?)	96, 138, 144
nrpo = rpo	Nucleus raphe pontis			see *rpo*		
nrv	Nucleus reticularis medullae oblongatae, pars ventralis	1(–2)	2	P7.0		(137)
nsc	Nucleus suprachiasmaticus	2–3	3–5	A6.3–A5.9	49a, 239	68
nso	Nucleus supraopticus	0–1	2	A6.3–A5.9	49a	68, 75
nt V	Nucleus tractus spinalis nervi trigemini, pars interposita pars caudalis	2(–3)	3	P5.0–P8.0		(13), 143, 144
nt Vd	Nucleus tractus spinalis nervi trigemini, pars dorsomedialis (= pars oralis)	1(–2)	3	P3.4–P5.0		
ntd	Nucleus tegmenti dorsalis (Gudden)	4(–5) 3	3 3	P1.5 P2.0		20, 22, *121*
ntdl	Nucleus tegmenti dorsalis lateralis	2–3	3	P1.5–P2.0		20, 92, *121*
ntm	Nucleus tractus mesencephali	0–1	2	P1.5–P2.0		
nts	Nucleus tractus solitarii	3–4	(3–)4	P4.5–P7.0	24, 94, 183	122, 139, 140–142
ntv	Nucleus tegmenti ventralis	4(–5) 2	3 2	P0.1–P1.5 P2.0		20, 97, *121*
nvm	Nucleus ventromedialis hypothalami	1	3(–4)	A5.3–A4.1	49a, 239, 247	69, 70, 73, 76
n III	Nucleus originis nervi oculomotorii	1	2	A1.3	120	92, 121
n IV	Nucleus originis nervi trochlearis	1	2	A0.6	120	92, 121
n V	Nucleus originis nervi trigemini	1	2	P2.0		145, 146
n VI	Nucleus originis nervi abducentis	1	2	P3.4		
n VII	Nucleus originis nervi facialis	0–1	2	P3.9–P5.0		
n X	Nucleus originis nervi vagi (dorsal motor nucleus N X)	1	2–3	P7.0		122, 139
n XII	Nucleus originis nervi hypoglossi	1	(1–)2	P5.5–P8.0		122, 139, 140–142
oa	*Nucleus olfactorius anterior*	3	3	BO, A10.5		25
oad	pars dorsalis	3	3	BO		
oae	pars externa	3	3	not shown (A12.1)		
oal	pars lateralis	3	3	BO		
oam	pars medialis	3	3	BO, A10.5		
oap	pars posterior	3	3	A10.5		

TABLE 1 (*continued*)

Abbreviation[1]	Brain region	Density of		Level of appearance in frontal plane[2]	References of techniques used[3,4] GAD IHC GABA IHC [³H]GABA AR	Figure number[5]
		Cell bodies	Axon terminals			
oc	Cortex occipitalis (striate cortex)	2–3	2–3	A1.8–P0.5 not indic.	19, 37, 38, 56, 74, 79, 82, [149], 190, 195a, 196, 196a, 209, 214, 215, 216, 220, 221, 223, 256, 257	(10, 11, 21)
OC	Tractus olivocerebellaris	0	0	P5.5		
OI(=io)	*Oliva inferior*	0	4	P5.5–P8.0	137a, 150	(13), 137, 138
	β-subnucleus	0	5			
	dao: oliva accessoria dorsalis	0	4			
	mao: oliva accessoria medialis	0	4			
	po: oliva principalis	0	4			
ol	Nucleus tractus olfactorii lateralis	2	2	A6.3–A5.9		68
ope	Nucleus preolivaris externus	2	2	P2.0		
opt	Nucleus olivaris pretectalis	3–4	3	A2.8–A2.6		65
OS=sfo	Organum subfornicale			see *sfo*		
os	*Nucleus olivaris superior*	2	2	P3.4		
osl	pars lateralis	2–3	2	P3.4		112
osm	pars medialis	0	2	P3.4 see *ltz* see *mtz* see *spn* see *vtz*	3	112
ovlt (=OVLT)	Organum vasculosum laminae terminalis	0	1–3	A8.6		(35)
P	Tractus corticospinalis	0	0(−1)	A0.6–P7.0		96
p=ppt	Nucleus pretectalis (posterior)			see *ppt*		
PaS	Parasubiculum					(11), 32, 33
pbd (=npd, pbl)	Nucleus parabrachialis dorsalis (lateralis)	2	(1–)2	P1.5–P2.0		
pbg	Nucleus parabigeminalis	0	2	A0.6		
pbl=pbd	Nucleus parabrachialis dorsalis (lateralis)			see *pbd*		
pbm=pbv	Nucleus parabrachialis ventralis (medialis)			see *pbv*		
pbp	N. parabrachialis pigmentatus	2	2	A2.2		
pbv (=pbm)	Nucleus parabrachialis ventralis (medialis)	1–2	2	P1.5–P2.0		
pc	Cortex parietalis (frontoparietalis)	2–3	2–3	A9.7–A2.6 not indicated		(1–3)
PCI	Pedunculus cerebellaris inferior	0	0	P3.9–P5.0		114, 116, 117
pcl	Lamina cellularum Purkinje cerebelli	5	4	P1.5–P2.0	32, 33, 138, 159, 161, 191, 205	123, 124, *125, 126*
PCM	Pedunculus cerebellaris medialis	0	0	P0.5–P2.0		

TABLE 1 (*continued*)

Abbreviation[1]	Brain region	Density of		Level of appearance in frontal plane[2]	References of techniques used[3,4] GAD IHC GABA IHC [³H]GABA AR	Figure number[5]
		Cell bodies	Axon terminals			
PCMA (=mp)	Pedunculus corporis mamillaris	0	0 fibers	A2.8–A2.6		73
pcmc = cmc	Nucleus caudalis magnocellularis hypothalami posterioris (pars postmamillaris)			see cmc	233, 247, 250	
PCS	Pedunculus cerebellaris superior	0	0	A0.6–P2.0		92
pef(=npf)	Nucleus perifornicalis	3(–4)	4	A4.1	239, 247	70
PEG = SGC	Periaqueductal gray			see SGC		
pf	Nucleus parafascicularis thalami					
	pars rostralis pars caudalis (=posterior to FR)	0	1	A3.8–A3.4	179, 180, 224	62, 92
	(dorso-medialis)	2	3–4	A3.2–A2.8		
	(ventro-lateralis)	3–4	3–4			
ph	Nucleus prepositus hypoglossi	3–4	4	P5.0–A6.0		122
pi	cortex piriformis (primary olfactory cortex)	2	2–3	A10.5–A2.6		(5–8), 25 26, 35
pin	Corpus pineale	0	0	not shown		
pl(=rr)	Nucleus paralemniscalis	4	3–4	A1.3–A0.6		110
pmco	Nucleus amygdaloideus corticalis posteromedianus	2–3	2–3	A3.4–A2.6		(9)
po	Nuclei pontis	1(–2)	2–3	A1.3–P0.5		20, 121
pol	Nucleus preopticus lateralis	3	3	A7.2–A6.9	49a	(7), 75
pom	Nucleus preopticus medialis	4	4	A7.2–A6.9	49a, 122	(7), 73, 74
pos	Nucleus preopticus suprachiasmaticus	3–4	4–5	A7.2–A6.9		35
ppt(=p)	Nucleus pretectalis (posterior)	3	3	A2.8–A1.8	174, 180	65
pptg	Nucleus pedunculopontinus tegmentalis	1	2–3	A0.2–P0.5		(24)
PR	Area prerubralis (prerubral field)	2–3	2(–3)	A2.8–A2.6		
PrS	Praesubiculum					32,33
pt	Nucleus paratenialis	0–1	2–3	A6.3–A5.7		68
pv	Nucleus paraventricularis thalami	0–1	3(–4)	A6.3–A3.4		68, 69
r	Nucleus ruber	1–2	2	see rmc see rpc		(10, 22, 23) 94
rd	Nucleus raphe dorsalis	1	2(–3)	A0.6–P1.5	20, 59, 145	(22, 24), 92, 93, 97
re	Nucleus reuniens	0–1	2–3	A5.9–A4.1		(8), 68, 69
rgi =nrgc	Nucleus reticularis gigantocellularis			see nrgc		
rh	Nucleus rhomboideus	0–1	2–3	A5.7–A4.1		(8,68)
rl	Nucleus reticularis lateralis	1	1–2	P7.0–P8.0		
rli	Nucleus raphe linearis	1–3	2–3	A2.6–A2.2		94, 119
rm(=nrm)	Nucleus raphe magnus	3–4	2	P3.4–P4.5		118
		4	3	P5.0		

TABLE 1 (*continued*)

Abbreviation[1]	Brain region	Density of		Level of appearance in frontal plane[2]	References of techniques used[3,4]	Figure number[5]
		Cell bodies	Axon terminals		GAD IHC GABA IHC [³H]GABA AR	
rmc	Nucleus ruber pars magnocellularis	1(–2)	2	A1.8–A1.3		90, 91
ro(=nro)	Nucleus raphe obscurus	2	2	P4.5–P7.0		
rp(=rpa)	Nucleus raphe pallidus					96, 120
	pars rostralis	3–4	3dors. 4ventr.	P3.9–P5.0		
	pars caudalis	2	2dors. 4ventr.	P6.0–P7.0		
rpa=rp	Nucleus raphe pallidus			see *rp*		
rpc	Nucleus ruber pars parvocellularis	2	2	A2.2–A1.8		91
'rpc' =nrpc	Nucleus reticularis parvocellularis			see *nrpc*		
rpo (=nrpo)	Nucleus raphe pontis	1–2	2–3	P1.5–P2.0		
rpoc	Nucleus reticularis pontis caudalis	1	1–2	P3.4		
rpoo	Nucleus reticularis pontis oralis	3 2	2–3 2	A0.2 P0.1–P2.0		
RR	Area retrorubralis (retrorubral field)	3–4	3	A1.8–A1.3		90, 93, 94
rr=pl	Nucleus paralemniscalis (nucleus retrorubralis)			see *pl*		
rtp	Nucleus reticularis tegmenti pontis	1	2	A0.2–P2.0		96
S	Subiculum	2	2–3	A0.6–A0.2		32, 33
S(II-IV)	Medulla spinalis, pars sacralis segmenta II-IV			not shown see *L 5*, see *sc*		18
sa	Sagulum	(1–)2	2–3	P0.1–P0.5		(24)
SAM	Stratum album mediale colliculi superioris	1	1	A2.2–P0.1		100
sc	Medulla spinalis (spinal cord)			C1, C7, TH8, L5, CO	15, 16, 17, [17a], 18, 93, 130, 197	14–19, 143, 147
	Laminae Rexed					
	I	3	3–4			149
	IIa	2	3			149
	b	2	5			149
	IIIa	2	5			149
	b	2	4			
	IV	1(2–3)	3			147
	V	2	2–3			
	VI	2	2(–3)			
	VII	2	(1–)2			
	VIII	1	1–2			
	IX	1	1–2			
	X	3	3–4			143, 147
scl	Nucleus subceruleus	2	2	P1.5–P2.0		

TABLE 1 (continued)

Abbreviation[1]	Brain region	Density of		Level of appearance in frontal plane[2]	References of techniques used[3,4] GAD IHC GABA IHC [^{3}H]GABA AR	Figure number[5]
		Cell bodies	Axon terminals			
sco	Organum subcommissurale (subcommissural organ) terminals only in hypependymal layer	0	1–2	A2.8	60	63, 98
sf	Nucleus septalis fimbrialis	4	3	A6.9–A6.3		(7)
sfo(=OS)	Organum subfornicale	1–2	5	A6.3–A5.9		
sg	Nucleus suprageniculatus facialis	0	1–2	P3.4		136
sg V	Nucleus tractus spinalis nervi trigemini, substantia gelatinosa	3	4	P8.0		(13, 143)
SGC (=PEG,SGPV)	*Substantia grisea centralis*	2–3	3	A2.6–P0.5	20, 180	(10, 23), 63, 93, 97,
SGCD	pars dorsalis	2	3	A1.8–P0.5		100, *121*
sgm	Stratum griseum mediale colliculi superioris	2	2	A2.2–P0.1		100
SGPV=SGC	Substantia grisea periventricularis			see *SGC*		
sgs	Stratum griseum superficiale colliculi superioris	3	5	A2.2–P0.5		100, 101
sgt	Nucleus suprageniculatus thalami	0–1	1	A2.6		109
shi	Nucleus septohippocampalis	4	4	A8.6–A7.5		39
shy	Nucleus septohypothalamicus	4	4	A7.2–A6.9	98	(7)
si	Nucleus septi intermedius	3	3	A8.6–A6.9	111, 175	(35)
sin	Substantia innominata			terminology not used see *a* (*AA*) *nbm!* *nist* *tdh* *VP*		
sl*	Nucleus septi lateralis	4	4	A9.4–A6.9	111, 175 [186a]	(6, 7) 35, 39
sm	Nucleus septi medialis	(3–)4	3–4	A9.7–A6.9	111, 175	35, 38
SM	Stria medullaris thalami	0	0 fibers	A6.3–A4.1		60, 63, 68, 75
smc	Cortex sensomotorica	3	2–3	A9.7–A2.8	75, 81, 89, 192	
smt	Nucleus submamillothalamicus	2–3	3–4	A3.2		
sn	*Substantia nigra*				23, 156,	40, *45, 49*
snc	Substantia nigra pars compacta	1–2	(2–)3	A2.6–A1.6	161, 162,	50, 64, 81,
snl	Substantia nigra pars lateralis	3–4	4	A2.2–A1.6	[174b],	85, 86, 94,
snr	Substantia nigra pars reticulata (terminals more numerous at the medial aspect)	4–5	5	A2.6–A1.3	188, 194	110
SO	Stratum opticum colliculi superioris	2	1–2	A2.2–P0.1		100
sor	Nucleus supraopticus retrochiasmaticus	0–1	2			75

498

TABLE 1 (*continued*)

Abbreviation[1]	Brain region	Density of		Level of appearance in frontal plane[2]	References of techniques used[3,4] GAD IHC GABA IHC [^{3}H]GABA AR	Figure number[5]
		Cell bodies	Axon terminals			
spf	Nucleus subparafascicularis	4	3	A3.8–A3.4		62
spn	Nucleus paraolivaris superior	4	2	P2.0–P3.4		112
SR	Sulcus rhinalis	/	/	A10.5–A0.6		
st	Nucleus triangularis septi	3	3	A6.9		(7)
ST	Stria terminalis	0–1	0–1 fibers	A6.9–A3.4		57, 60, 69
sum	Nucleus supramamillaris	1–2	4	A3.2–A2.6	49a	80
sumx	Decussatio supramamillaris	0	2	A2.8–A2.6		
sut	Nucleus subthalamicus	1	3	A3.8–A2.8	166	40, 41, 69
tad	N. anterior dorsalis thalami	0	2(–3)	A5.3		60, 63, 68
tam	N. anterior medialis thalami	0	1	A5.9–A5.3		68
tav	Nucleus anterior ventralis thalami	0–1	1–2(–3) (tubercle like)	A5.9–A5.3	119a	60, 63, 68
tc	Cortex temporalis	2–3	2–3	A2.2–A0.6		(10)
TD	Tractus diagonalis (Broca)	3	3	A7.5		
td	*Nucleus tractus diagonalis* (Broca)	3–4	3	A8.6–A7.5	175	(7), *37*
tdh	pars horizontalis	3–4	3	A7.5–A6.3	111, 271	
tdv	pars verticalis	3–4	3	A8.6–A7.5	111	
TH I–XII	Medulla spinalis, pars thoracica, segmenta I–XII			TH8 see *sc*		16
tl	Nucleus lateralis thalami					
	rostralis	0	2(–3)	A5.3–A4.1		(69)
	caudalis	0	1 (tubercle like)	A3.8–A3.4		
tlp	Nucleus lateralis thalami, pars posterior	1–2	1–2(–3) (tubercle like)	A3.8–A2.6	174, 180	64
tm	Nucleus medialis thalami	0	1	A5.3		
tmc	Nucleus tuberalis magnocellularis hypothalami posterioris	5	4	A3.4	233, 247	
tml	Nucleus medialis thalami, pars lateralis	0	1	A4.9–A4.1		69
tmm	Nucleus medialis thalami, pars medialis	0	1	A4.9–A3.8		69
TO	Tractus opticus	0	0	A5.7–A3.2		56, 72
TOA	Tractus opticus basalis (accessorius)	0	0	A1.6		
toa	*Nucleus terminalis tractus optici accessorii*					63
toad(=dtn)	pars dorsalis	4	5	A1.6		82, 83
toal(=dtl)	pars lateralis	4	5	A1.8	180	
toam(=mtn)	pars medialis (basalis)	4	5	A2.2–A1.8	174, 180	74, 81, 84, 85, 86
TOI	Tractus olfactorius intermedius	0	0	A10.5		
TOL	Tractus olfactorius lateralis	0	0	A10.5–A5.9		25
tol	Nucleus tractus optici, pars lateralis	4	4	A2.6–A1.8	174, 180	65
tom	Nucleus tractus optici, pars medialis	4	4	A2.8–A2.6	180	

TABLE 1 (*continued*)

Abbreviation[1]	Brain region	Density of		Level of appearance in frontal plane[2]	References of techniques used[3,4] GAD IHC GABA IHC [³H]GABA AR	Figure number[5]
		Cell bodies	Axon terminals			
tpo	Nucleus posterior thalami					
	rostralis	0–1	1–2	A4.1–A2.8		(69)
	caudalis	1(–2)	1–2	A2.6–A2.2		
tr	Nucleus reticularis thalami	5	2	A5.9–A3.4	80, 88, 163	40, *56*, 60, 63, 68, 69, 70, 72
TRS	Tractus rubrospinalis	0	0(–1)	A0.6–P0.5		
TS	Tractus solitarii	0	0	P7.0		
TS V	Tractus spinalis nervi trigemini	0	0	P2.0–P8.0		
TTS	Tractus tectospinalis	0	0(–1)	P0.1–P0.5		
tu	Tuberculum olfactorium	5	4	A9.7–A7.2	118, 167a	35, 37, 39, 40, 51, 52, 53
tv	Nucleus ventralis thalami	0–1	1(–2)	A5.7–A2.8 see *tvl* *tvm*		
tvl	Nucleus ventrolateralis thalami	0	1–2	A5.3–A4.6	119a	
tvm	Nucleus ventralis medialis thalami, pars magnocellularis	0–1	1–2	A5.3–A3.8		(69)
tvpl	Nucleus ventroposterior lateralis thalami	0	1–2	A4.9–A3.2	179, 180, 224	64, 69
tvpm	Nucleus ventroposterior medialis thalami	0	1–2	A4.6–A2.8	179, 180	64, 69
tvppc	Nucleus ventroposterior thalami pars parvocellularis	0–1	1	A3.4		
vcgl	*Nucleus ventralis corporis geniculati lateralis*	4	4	A3.8–A2.6	80, 180	60
vcglmc	pars magnocellularis	4	4–5	A3.8–A2.8		64, 67
vcglpc	pars parvocellularis	4	3–4	A3.8–A2.8		64, 67
vl	Nucleus vestibularis	1	1	P3.4	91, 152	127, 128,
	lateralis	1	4–5dors 2ventr.	P3.9–P4.5 P3.9–P4.5		133, 135
vm	Nucleus vestibularis medialis					
	rostralis	4	4	P3.4	152	122, 127,
	caudalis	3–4	4	P3.9–P5.0		133, 134, 136
vp	Pallidum ventrale (ventral pallidum)	4–5	5	A7.5–A5.9	166, 268, 269, 270	40, 53, 55, 68
vs	Nucleus vestibularis superior	3	3	P3.4	152	133, 135
vsp	Nucleus vestibularis spinalis					
	rostralis	2	3	P4.5	152	133, 134
	caudalis	4	3	P5.0–P5.5		
vta	Area ventralis	2	3	A2.6–A1.6		93, 121
(=AVT)	tegmenti (Tsai)	2–3	2	A1.3		
vtz	N. ventralis corporis trapezoidei	4	4	P3.9		112, 113
vVnll	Nucleus ventralis lemnisci lateralis pars ventralis	3(–4)	2–3	A0.2–P1.5	4	(24)
y	Pars 'y' nucleorum vestibulorum	4	4	P3.9		127, 135
zi(=ZI)	Zona incerta (pars lateralis)	4(–5)	3	A5.3–A4.6	49a, 162,	(9), 40, *46*,
		4	3	A4.1–A2.6	247	64, 69, 70, 71, 74
V	Nervus trigeminus	0	0	P1.5–P2.0		

TABLE 1 (*continued*)

Abbreviation[1]	Brain region	Density of		Level of appearance in frontal plane[2]	References of techniques used[3,4]	Figure number[5]
		Cell bodies	Axon terminals		GAD IHC GABA IHC [^{3}H]GABA AR	
V M	Nervus trigeminus, radix motoria	0	0	A0.6–P0.1		
V S	Nervus trigeminus, radix sensoria	0	0	A0.6–P1.5		
VII	Nervus facialis	0	0	P3.4		136
VIII	Nervus acousticovestibularis	0	+	not shown		115

Tentative name of brain areas indicated by arabic numerals (see Note 1 on page 487)

1	Area commissuralis colliculi superioris et inferioris	3–4	2	A2.6–P0.5		(23), *102*, 106, 107
2	Area parvocellularis paramediana tegmentalis	3–4	(2–)3	A0.2(–P0.1)		(97)
3	Area parvocellularis parareticularis tegmentalis	3–4	2–3	P0.5–P1.5		20, 96, 121
4	Area supra/retrotrigeminalis nuclei motorii V (Nucleus supratrigeminalis of Lorente de Nó)	4	2	P2.0		145, 146
5	Area reticularis subhypoglossa	3(–4)	3	P5.5–P6.0		122
6	Area reticularis paratrigeminalis ventralis	3–4	2–3	P6.0–P8.0		(138, 144)
7	Area parapyramidalis (=corresponds to area 'B1 lateral' of serotonin-containing neurons)	5	4	P5.0–P5.5		96

Remaining parts of the nervous system and neuroendocrine system

Retina	Amacrine cells subpopulation	15, 28, 29, 55, 210, 242, 265, 272
Inner ear, spiral ganglion		49
Enteric system		99, 116
Adrenal medulla	Chromaffin cells	104
Pancreas	β-islet cells	46, 249

7. DETAILED MICROGRAPH SERIES

For abbreviations, consult the General Abbreviations List, p. 609, and Table 1, pp. 487-501.

Figs 25 and 26. These micrographs include bulbus olfactorius (BO), nucleus olfactorius anterior, primary olfactory cortex, nuclei septi, nucleus accumbens, nucleus caudatus/putamen (cp), claustrum, and nucleus endopiriformis. Some of the GAD distribution patterns are shown in the rostral forebrain in the horizontal plane from rats processed for immunostaining of both cell bodies and terminals. The planes of sections correspond approximately to Figures 58 and 59 in the atlas of Paxinos and Watson (1982).
Fig. 25. Conspicuous density of immunostained terminals is seen in bulbus olfactorius (BO). The arrow points to a band of stained boutons underneath the tractus olfactorius lateralis. × 31.
Fig. 26. Note the differences in immunostaining patterns in the nucleus caudatus/putamen (cp) *vs* the claustrum (cl) and the nucleus endopiriformis (star). These two latter nuclei appear similar as far as GAD staining patterns are concerned and this similarity continues at temporal levels. R indicates rostral direction. × 28.

BULBUS OLFACTORIUS (BO).

Fig. 27. Micrograph of the gradients of immunostaining in lamina plexiformis externa bulbi olfactorii (intensely stained zone) and lamina granularis bulbi olfactorii (LGR); note also the high density of GAD-positive periglomerular cells in lamina glomerulosa bulbi olfactorii (LG). Arrows point to GAD-immunoreactive deep short-axon cells. × 156.
Fig. 28. Bulbus olfactorius accessorius (BOA) contains scattered GAD-positive periglomerular cells (arrows). × 57.
Fig. 29. Granule cells (bottom) contain immunoreaction product in their thin cytoplasm and ascending dendrites. Mitral cells (star) are GAD-negative. Most of the puncta in outer and inner portions of lamina plexiformis externa bulbi olfactorii (LPE) correspond to gemmules of granule cell dendrites known to form dendro-dendritic synapses. Few, small GAD-positive neurons are present in LPE. Tufted cells are GAD-negative. An interglomerular region covered by the lamina nervi olfactorii at the top of the micrograph includes two populations of periglomerular cells: one population is GAD-positive and the other GAD-negative. × 390.
Fig. 30. Clustered GAD-positive profiles are contained in a glomerulus (gl). A lightly immunostained superficial short axon cell (arrow) and several GAD-negative periglomerular cells are present among numerous, densely stained GAD-positive periglomerular cells. × 910.
Fig. 31. This detail of the granule cell layer shows a deep short axon neuron (arrow) in contact with GAD-positive puncta. × 780.

HIPPOCAMPUS

Figs 32–34. Patterns of immunostaining in the hippocampal formation in horizontal (Figs 32 and 33) and sagittal (Fig. 34) sections. The plane of the sections in Figures 32 and 33 approximately corresponds to Figure 58 in the atlas of Paxinos and Watson (1982).
Fig. 32. This low-power micrograph represents a section processed for immunostaining of nerve terminals. Note that the cortical staining patterns vary substantially and permit identification of areas such as cortex entorhinalis (ce), subiculum (S) or the border between regio superior and regio inferior (arrow). Some of the cortical laminae and sublaminae (such as the superficial 4 layers of area entorhinalis, pars externa of stratum moleculare of the gyrus dentatus, and the stratum lacunosum-moleculare) are also evident. See also Figure 22. × 40.
Fig. 33. In this section processed for immunostaining of cell bodies, GABAergic neurons appear present in all hippocampal cortical layers, although they occur only sparsely in the stratum moleculare of the gyrus dentatus. × 40.
Fig. 34. A detail of the dorsal hippocampus in a sagittal section, processed for cell body staining, demonstrates the high density of GABAergic neurons in the subgranular zone and the hilus of gyrus dentatus at this level. Note also the rich complement of terminals in stratum pyramidale and stratum granulosum. × 112.

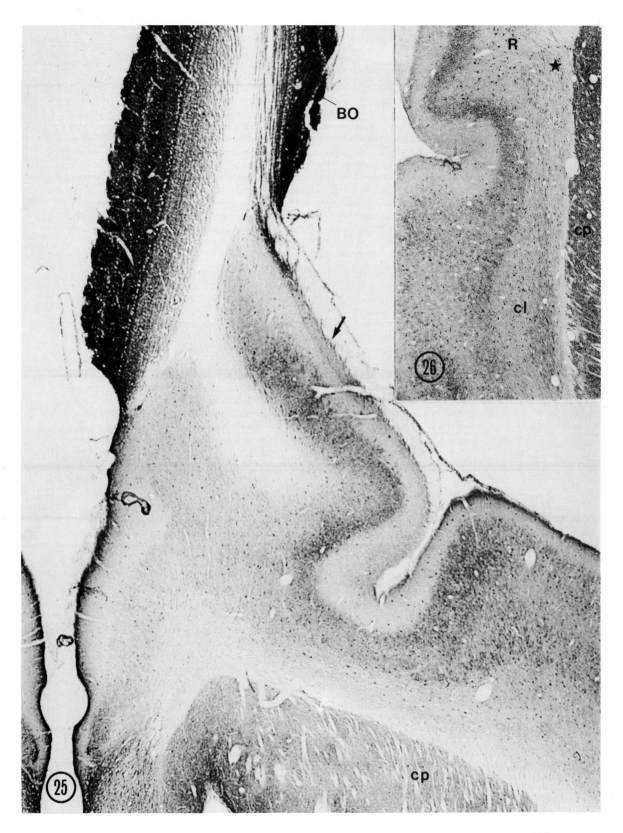

BO

cp

R

cl

cp

25

26

503

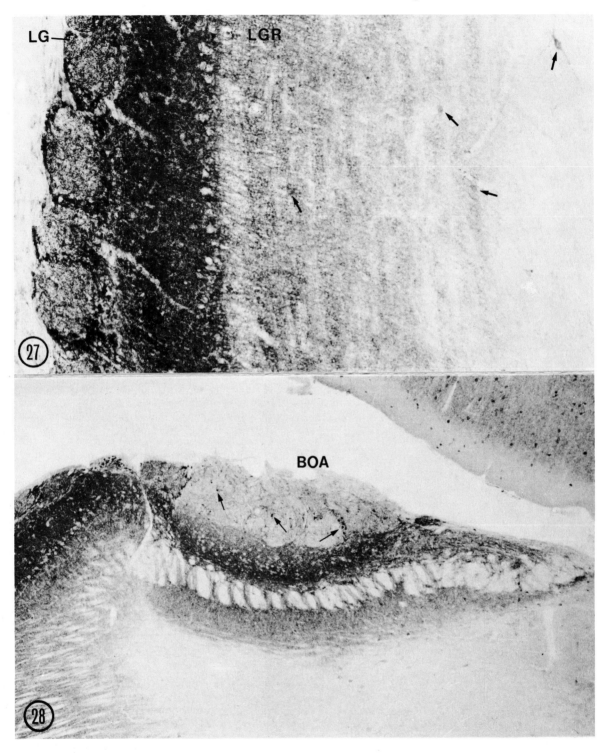

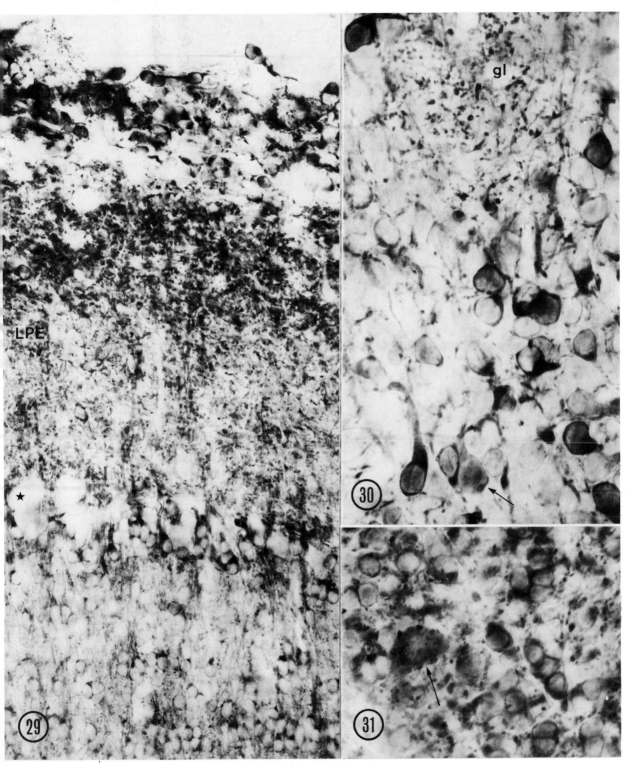

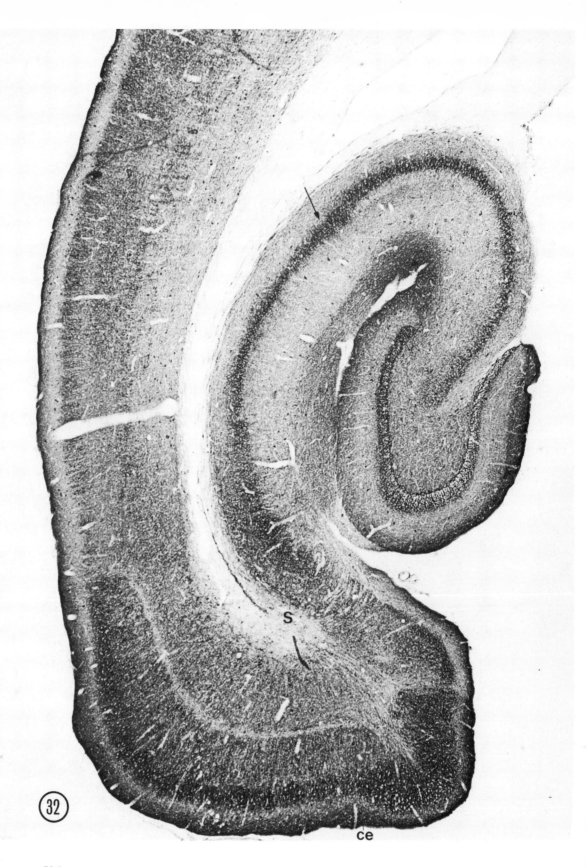

506

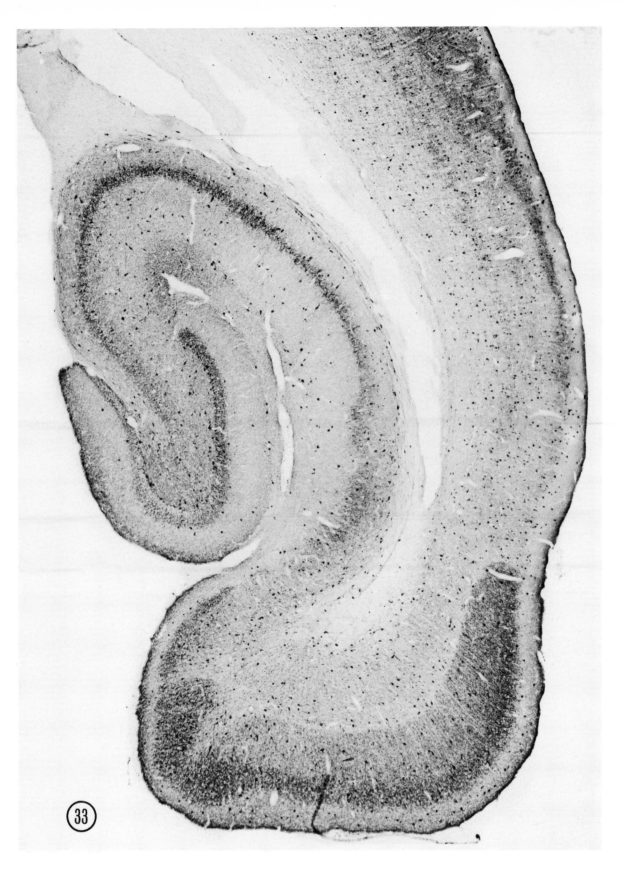

(33)

507

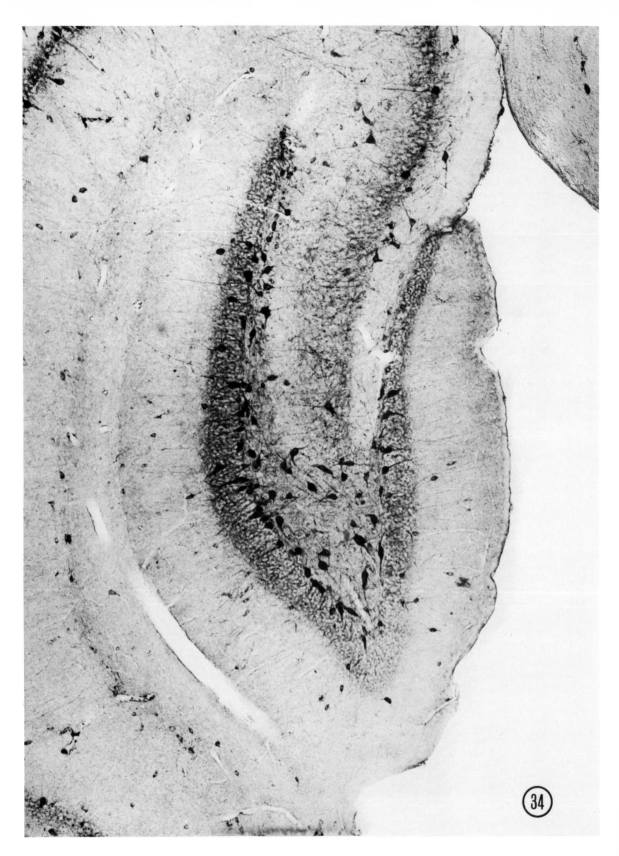

34

508

PROSENCEPHALON

Fig. 35. This detail of a coronal forebrain section shows the patterns of immunostaining of terminals in nucleus caudatus/putamen (including the fundus striati), the nucleus tractus diagonalis (Broca), the nucleus interstitialis striae terminalis, pallidum ventrale and tuberculum olfactorium. Organum vasculosum laminae terminalis (arrowhead) and nucleus preopticus suprachiasmaticus (pos) are also shown. Areas indicated by small and large arrows are shown in Figures 36 and 37 in corresponding sections immunostained for cell bodies. × 20.

Fig. 36. Cell body staining in the nucleus interstitialis striae terminalis (nist) after topical colchicine injection. × 53.

Fig. 37. Cell body staining in the nucleus tractus diagonalis (Broca) (td). Arrow indicates the midline. A portion of tuberculum olfactorium (tu) is visible on the right-hand side. The plane of this coronal section is anterior to that of Figure 35. × 200.

SEPTUM

Figs 38 and 39. Cell body staining in induseum griseum (ig), tenia tecta (arrow) (Fig. 38), and nuclei septi (Fig. 39) in coronal sections. Note the high density of GAD-immunoreactive cell bodies in nucleus septohippocampalis (shi) and nucleus septi lateralis (sl). Portions of the forceps minor of the corpus callosum, tuberculum olfactorium (tu) and nucleus accumbens (a) are included in both figures. Staining of GAD-immunoreactive terminals in corresponding regions are shown in Figure 6. Fig. 38 × 60. Fig. 39 × 74.

BASAL GANGLIA

Fig. 40. This parasagittal section processed for cell body staining shows the distribution of GABAergic neurons in the basal ganglia, the thalamus and the zona incerta. The plane of section approximately corresponds to Figure 50 in the atlas of Paxinos and Watson (1982). Note that the cell bodies in the globus pallidus (pallidum dorsale) (gp) and pallidum ventrale (vp), the nucleus entopeduncularis (ep), the nucleus reticularis thalami (tr), the substantia nigra pars reticulata (snr) and zona incerta (zi) are more densely stained than those in the nucleus caudatus/putamen (cp) and nucleus accumbens (a). At the ventral aspect the tuberculum olfactorium (tu) is seen below nucleus accumbens and pallidum ventrale. The prominence of immunostaining in the nucleus reticularis thalami is striking. The nucleus subthalamicus (sut) below the zona incerta, the substantia nigra pars compacta and most of the nuclei thalami are nearly free of GABAergic neurons, although they contain immunostained boutons. The low number of GAD-immunoreactive neurons in nucleus subthalamicus contrasts with the finding that [³H]GABA is retrogradely transported from globus pallidus to numerous neurons of the nucleus subthalamicus (Nauta and Cuénod 1982) (see section 2.3). × 20.

Fig. 41. This detail of the nucleus subthalamicus (sut) from a parasagittal section stained for terminals demonstrates that immunostained boutons are predominantly located in the neuropil. × 100.

Nucleus caudatus/putamen

Fig. 42. Nucleus caudatus/putamen (cp): scattered medium-size to large nerve cell bodies in the corpus striatum are densely labeled without topical colchicine injection. × 335.

Fig. 43. The vast majority of small to medium-size striatal neurons become distinctly immunoreactive after topical colchicine injection. × 222.

Pallidum

Figs 44–46. In globus pallidus (gp) (Fig. 44), nucleus entopeduncularis (not shown) and substantia nigra pars reticulata (snr) (Fig. 45) GAD-immunoreactive terminals are organized in parallel rows and ring-like arrays forming a characteristic peridendritic pattern among small-to-large GABAergic cell bodies. In the zona incerta (zi) (Fig. 46), on the contrary, terminals are scattered in the neuropil among small to medium-size neurons. GABAergic neurons in the zona incerta after topical colchicine injection are also shown in Figure 71. Figures 44, 45 and 46 are taken from specimens of colchicine pretreated rats. × 770.

Figs 47–50. GAD-immunoreactive cell bodies in globus pallidus (gp) (Fig. 47), nucleus entopeduncularis (ep) (Fig. 48), substantia nigra pars reticulata (snr) (Figs 49 and 50), and nucleus peripeduncularis (npp) (Fig. 50) after topical colchicine injections. Most neurons (small-to-large) are GAD-immunoreactive in these regions. Figure 50 shows the change in cell shape and size at the transition between substantia nigra pars reticulata (snr) (bottom left) and the nucleus peripeduncularis (npp) (top right). In Figure 47 (top), note also the abrupt change in staining pattern at the border between nucleus caudatus/putamen (cp) and globus pallidus. Figs 47, 48: × 108. Fig. 49: × 160. Fig. 50: × 108.

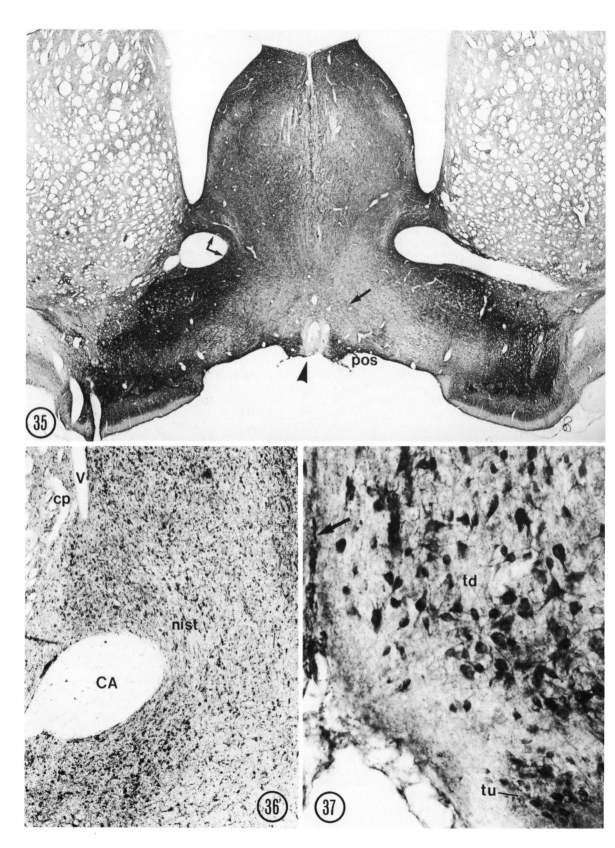

510

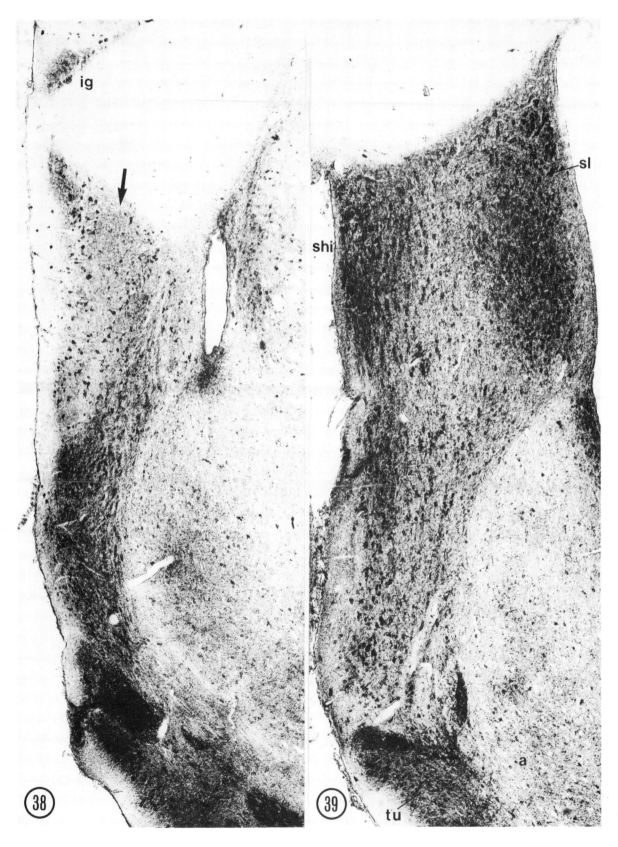

511

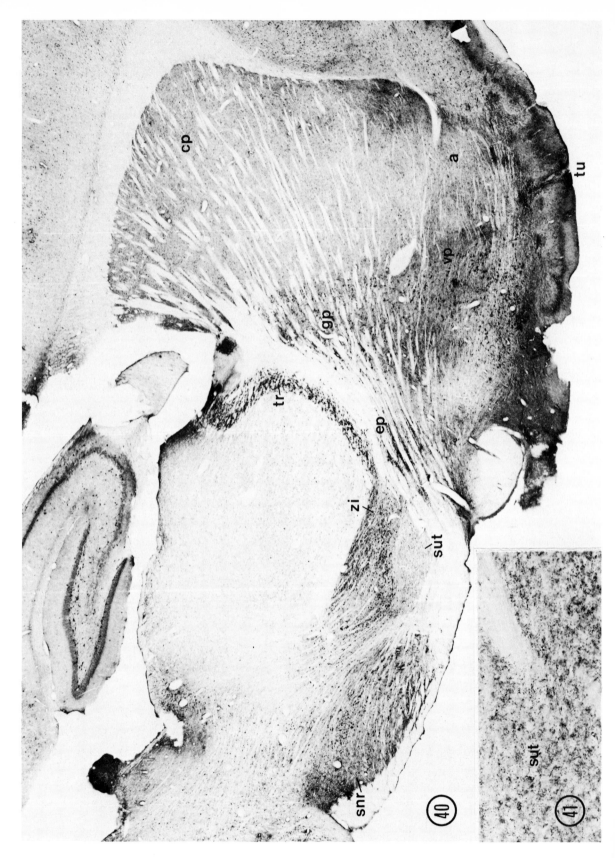

512

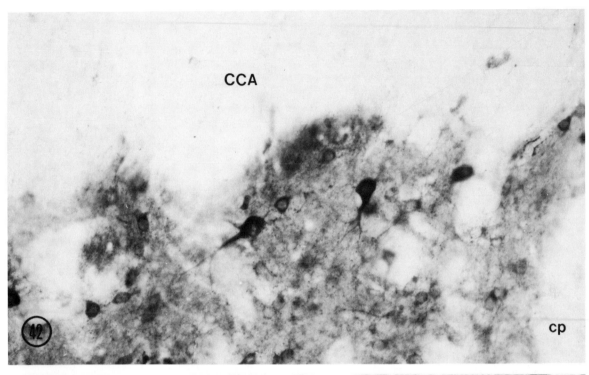

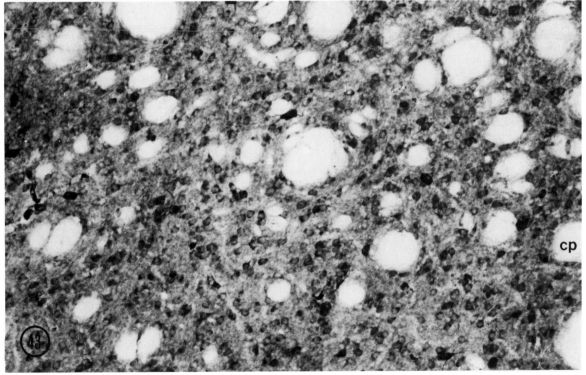

513

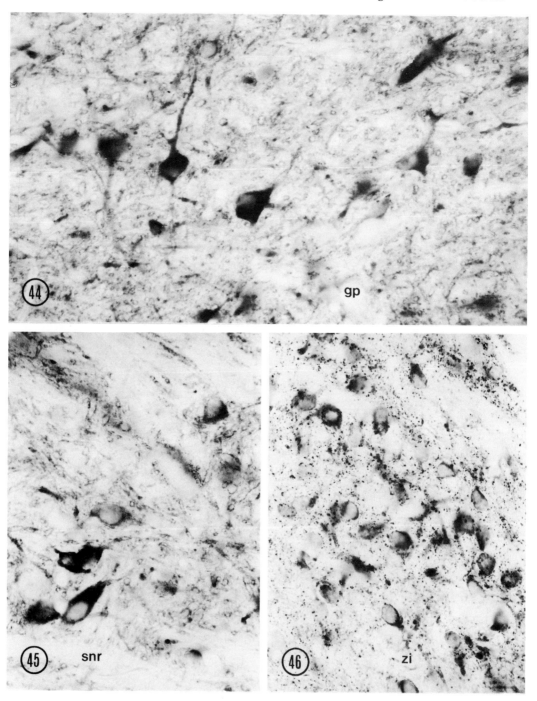

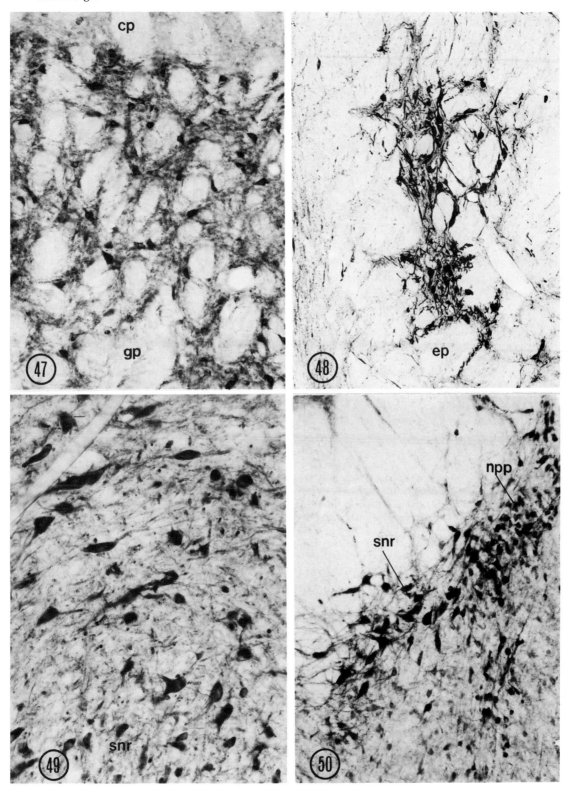

Tuberculum olfactorium

Fig. 51. Bouton staining in tuberculum olfactorium (tu) in horizontal section shows different patterns of immunoreaction in deep fibrocellular layer of pallidum ventrale (darkest regions) and striatal bridges (rounded clearer compartments). The islands of Calleja (arrows; iC) are barely visible at this magnification. × 30.

Fig. 52. Cell body staining in the tuberculum olfactorium (tu) in a sagittal section, after a colchicine injection into the preoptic area shows the predominant GABAergic nature of the neuronal populations in this region. The large neurons in the deep fibrocellular layer of the tuberculum olfactorium (a ventral stratum of the pallidum ventrale), the granular neurons in the islands of Calleja (iC), the medium-size neurons and the scattered medium-size to large neurons in nucleus accumbens (a), the fundus striati and the multiform (polymorph) layer and dense cell (pyramidal) layer of tuberculum olfactorium (tu) (Millhouse and Heimer 1984) appear GAD-positive (see also Fig. 53). × 100.

Pallidum ventrale

Fig. 53. The deep fibrocellular layer (vp) of the tuberculum olfactorium (tu), like the rest of the pallidum ventrale, contains a pallidal type of peridendritic bouton staining. The dense cell (pyramidal) layer of tuberculum olfactorium (Millhouse and Heimer 1984) with its very high density of GAD-immunoreactive nerve cells is illustrated just below the label *tu*. × 200.

Insula Callejae

Fig. 54. The granular cell bodies in the island of Calleja (iC) are GAD-positive. The cap region (top left), an extension of the deep fibrocellular layer of pallidum ventrale, contains a peridendritic bouton staining pattern, here partly obscured by the high density of the staining. × 333.

Nucleus accumbens

Fig. 55. In this micrograph of the nucleus accumbens septi (a), most neurons are small-to-medium and moderately GAD-immunoreactive. One medium-to-large neuron exhibits dense GAD positivity (upper right quadrant). The same types and distribution of GAD-positive neurons are observed in the striatal bridges leading to the tuberculum olfactorium and in the dense cell (pyramidal) layer (Fig. 53) and multiform (polymorph) layer of the tuberculum olfactorium. This pattern of cell body staining resembles that of the nucleus caudatus/putamen. *cf.* Figures 42 and 43. × 178.

BASAL GANGLIA AND AMYGDALA COMPLEX

Figs 56–59. Patterns of bouton staining (Fig. 56) and cell body staining (Figs 57–59) in parts of the basal ganglia and the amygdala complex.

Fig. 56. Note the striatal type pattern of bouton staining in the nucleus amygdaloideus centralis (ac) and nucleus amygdaloideus medialis (am). This pattern differs substantially from the lighter, definitely non-striatal pattern of the nucleus amygdaloideus lateralis (al) and nucleus amygdaloideus basalis lateralis. The density of immunostaining is higher in the nucleus amygdaloideus medialis than in the nucleus amygdaloideus centralis, but in both nuclei it is lower than that found in the globus pallidus (gp) and nucleus entopeduncularis (ep). Streaks of peridendritic terminal staining from the globus pallidus 'infiltrate' the fundus striati and the nucleus amygdaloideus centralis. These streaks presumably correspond to the met-enkephalin-positive 'woolly fibers' (Haber and Nauta 1983). Portion of the caudal continuation of the rodent equivalent of the 'nucleus basalis magnocellularis of Meynert' (arrow) is included. Coronal section. *cf.* Figure 8 on p. 452 for terminal staining and Figure 72 for cell body staining. × 64.

Fig. 57. Numerous small to medium-size neurons and scattered large neurons appear immunostained in nucleus amygdaloideus centralis (ac) and nucleus amygdaloideus medialis (am) after topical colchicine injection. This suggests that these nuclei have striatum-like cell body populations. Coronal section. *cf.* Figs. 58 and 59. × 69.

Figs 58 and 59. Relatively few GABAergic neurons are present in nucleus amygdaloideus lateralis (al) and nucleus amygdaloideus basalis lateralis.

Fig. 58. In the massae intercalatae (arrow) scattered medium-size to large neurons exhibit intense GAD immunoreactivity in sections without colchicine pretreatment. Note the continuity in the complement of GABAergic neurons at the transition between fundus striati (cp) (Fig. 58, right upper quadrant) and nucleus amygdaloideus centralis (ac) (Fig. 58, left upper quadrant). *R* and *C* indicate the rostral and caudal directions. This figure is taken from a sagittal section 4.5 mm from the midline. × 67.

Fig. 59. In the massae intercalatae (arrows), the vast majority of medium-size cells become GAD-positive after colchicine pretreatment (*cf.* Fig. 58). Thus, the massae intercalatae possess a 'striatum-like' pattern of cell body staining. This figure is taken from a coronal section at a level corresponding to Figure 19 from the atlas of Paxinos and Watson (1982). *L* and *M* indicate the lateral and medial directions. × 137.

516

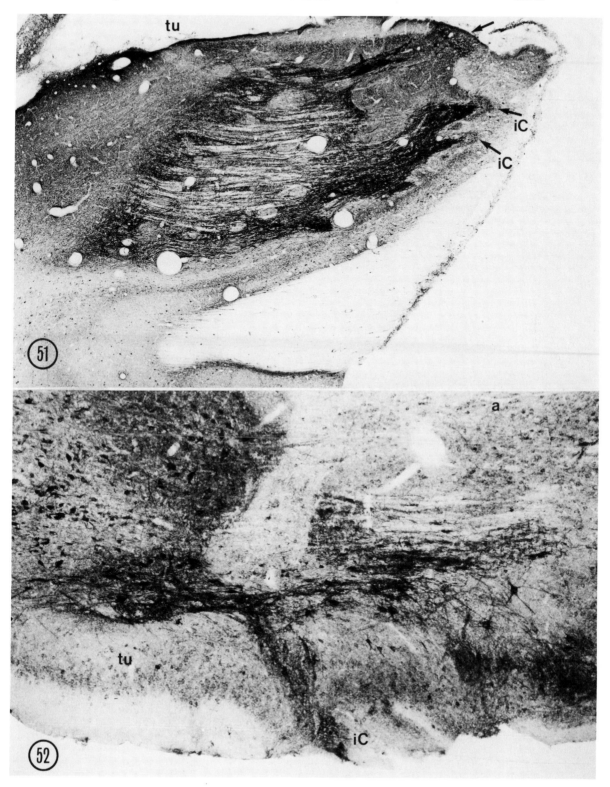

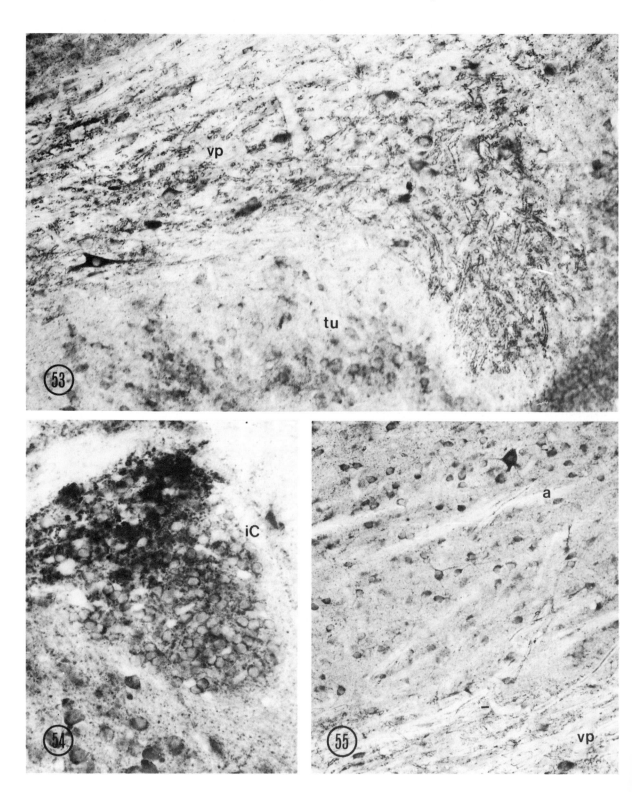

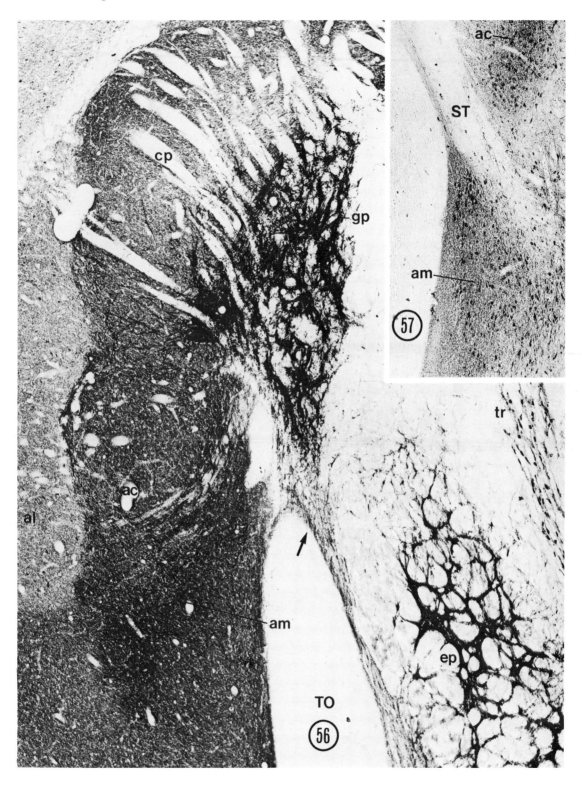

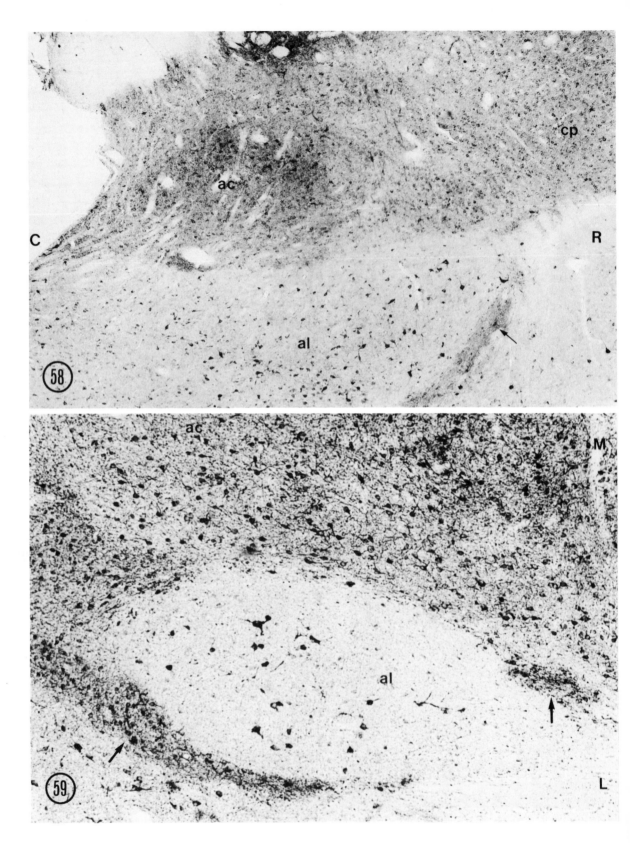

520

DIENCEPHALON

Fig. 60. Immunostaining of terminals shows varying degrees of density and patchy-to-diffuse modes of distribution in several thalamic subdivisions in horizontal section. Note that the GABAergic neurons of the nucleus reticularis thalami (tr) are definitely stained even after processing for bouton staining. Staining patterns of nucleus dorsalis corporis geniculati lateralis (dcgl), nucleus ventralis corporis geniculati lateralis (vcgl) and corpus geniculatum mediale (cgm) differ substantially from one another. See also Figure 63. × 25.

Fig. 61. Immunostaining for cell bodies sharply demarcates the border between thalamus (right) and area pretectalis anterior (APT) (left) in sagittal section. A part of colliculus superior is seen at the top left. × 72.

Fig. 62. Numerous small neurons in the nucleus parafascicularis (pf) and nucleus subparafascicularis (spf) of the thalamus are GABAergic. These neurons may be continuous with the band of GABAergic cells in the substantia grisea centralis, shown in Figure 20. Larger GABAergic neurons are present in the nucleus accessorius Darkschewitsch (aD) and the nucleus interstitialis of Cajal complex (lower left). × 78.

Fig. 63. Patterns of bouton staining in nuclei habenulae (top center), thalamus, area pretectalis anterior (APT), substantia grisea centralis and the ventral aspects of colliculus superior and in colliculus inferior (CI) are presented in this horizontal section. The organum subcommissurale (star) is shown at higher magnification in Figure 98. Note also the high density of staining lateral to the organum subcommissurale. The most densely stained region of the habenula, the nucleus habenulae lateralis (hl) apparently corresponds to the target area of the pallidal/entopeduncular projection. toad: pars dorsalis of nucleus terminalis tractus optici accessorii (see Figs 81–85). Level of Figure 63 is dorsal to Figure 60. × 17.

Fig. 64. Bouton staining in nucleus dorsalis corporis geniculati lateralis (dcgl) and nucleus ventralis corporis geniculati lateralis pars magnocellularis (vcglmc) and pars parvocellularis (vcglpc), nucleus peripeduncularis (npp) and zona incerta (zi). *cf.* Figure 69, which is caudal to Figure 64. × 40.

Fig. 65–67. Varying patterns of cell body staining in the pretectal region (Fig. 65), nucleus dorsalis corporis geniculati lateralis (dcgl) (Fig. 66), and nucleus ventralis corporis geniculati lateralis (Fig. 67).

Fig. 65. The nucleus olivaris pretectalis (opt) and nucleus pretectalis posterior (ppt) are rich in GABAergic neurons. The neurons in the nucleus olivaris pretectalis and neurons in the nucleus tractus optici (pars lateralis) (tol) have characteristic densely stained and interwoven dendrites. × 78.

Fig. 66. Note the thin, long GAD-immunoreactive dendrites in nucleus dorsalis corporis geniculati lateralis (dcgl). × 143.

Fig. 67. Note the difference in cell orientation and neuropil staining in nucleus ventralis corporis geniculati lateralis pars magnocellularis (vcglmc) (top) and nucleus ventralis corporis geniculati lateralis pars parvocellularis (vcglpc) (bottom). × 143.

Fig. 68. Patterns of bouton staining in the hypothalamus, thalamus, basal ganglia and amygdala complex at the level of the chiasma opticum. Note the higher density of staining in the medial *vs* the lateral hypothalamus and the higher density of staining in the nucleus suprachiasmaticus (arrowhead) *vs* the nucleus supraopticus (arrow). Besides the globus pallidus, the pallidum ventrale and area amygdaloidea anterior (AA), high density of staining is also seen in the nucleus interstitialis striae terminalis (nist). Note the high density of GAD-positive terminals in the dorsal aspect of nucleus anterior ventralis thalami (tav) and in the dorsal aspect of nucleus anterior dorsalis thalami (tad) at this level, when compared with their ventral aspects ('tubercule-like appearance'). *cf.* Figures 8 (p. 452), 60 and 63 and Schematic atlas drawing A 6.3–A 4.1. Nucleus anterior medialis thalami, nucleus amygdaloideus lateralis (al), nucleus amygdaloideus basalis lateralis and nucleus tractus olfactorii lateralis (ol) stand out as they are less densely stained than neighboring nuclei. Note also the continuity of nerve terminal staining in the nucleus paraventricularis thalami and nucleus paraventricularis hypothalami. *cf.* Figure 60. × 34.

Fig. 69. Patterns of bouton staining in the hypothalamus posterior, the habenula, the posterior thalamus, the zona incerta and nucleus subthalamicus. Note the relatively dense patches in some of the thalamic nuclei and the particularly high density of staining in the nucleus habenulae lateralis (hl) and in the medial regions of the hypothalamus. In the medial hypothalamus the nucleus ventromedialis hypothalami (nvm) exhibits a slightly lower density of GAD-immunoreactive terminals than the nucleus arcuatus (na). *cf.* Figure 70 for cell body density. At the lower left corner, the medial part of the nucleus amygdaloideus medialis (am) with its high terminal density is also shown. Star: GAD-immunoreactive fibers in stria terminalis. sut: nucleus subthalamicus, see Figures 40 and 41. *cf.* Figure 64 which is rostral to Figure 69. × 34.

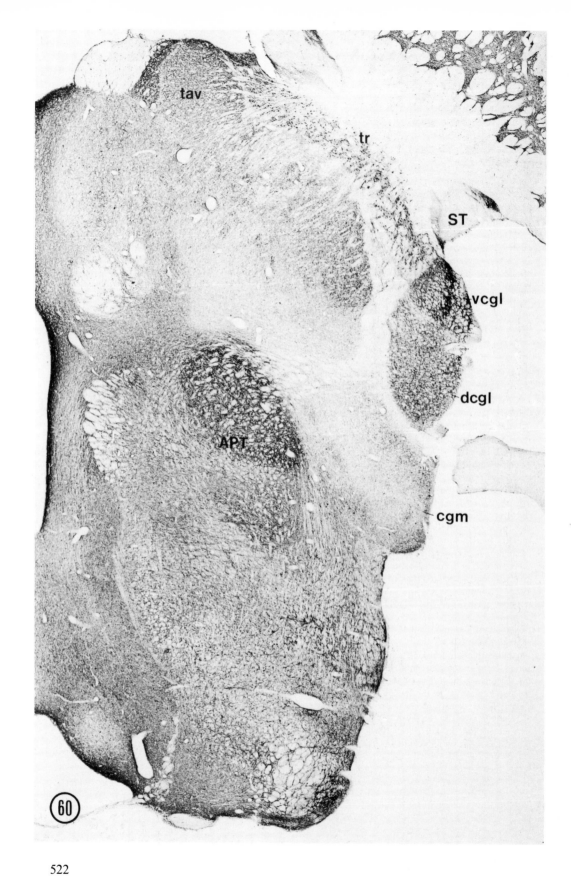

522

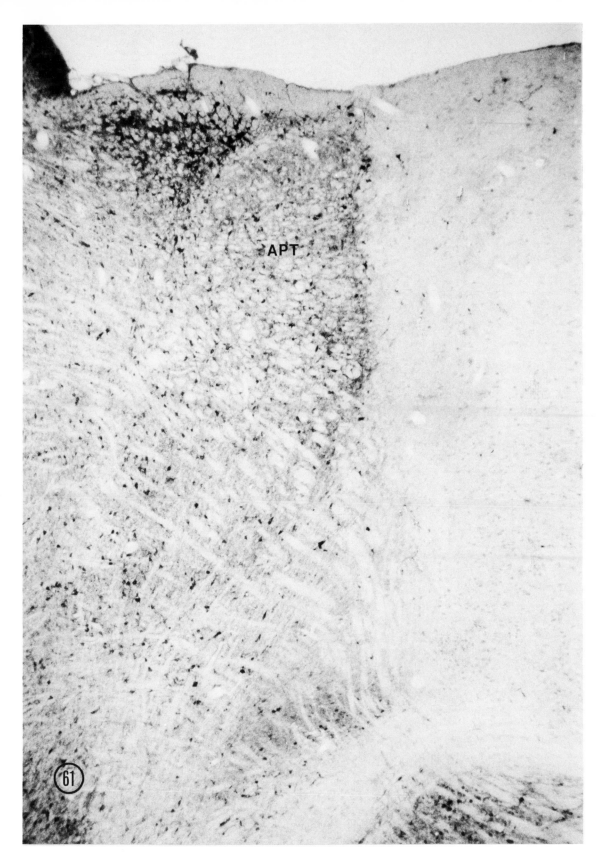

APT

61

523

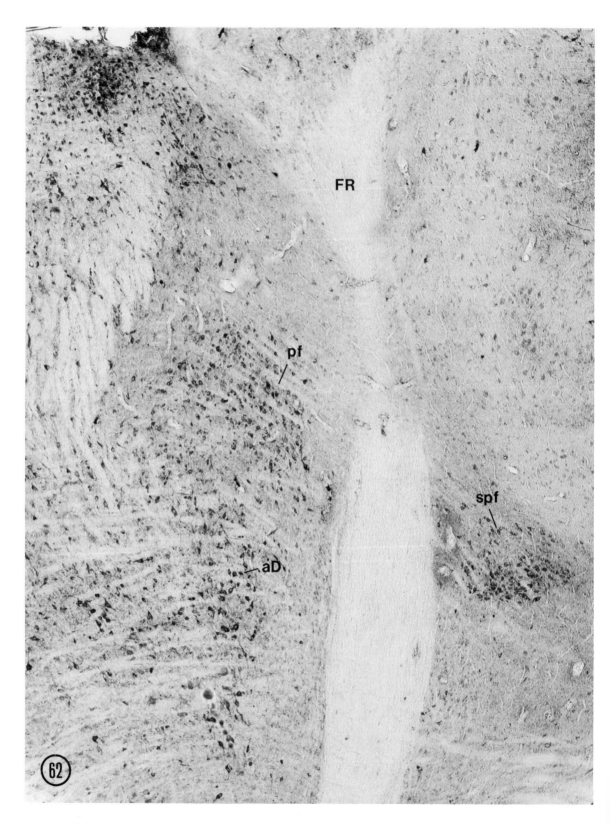

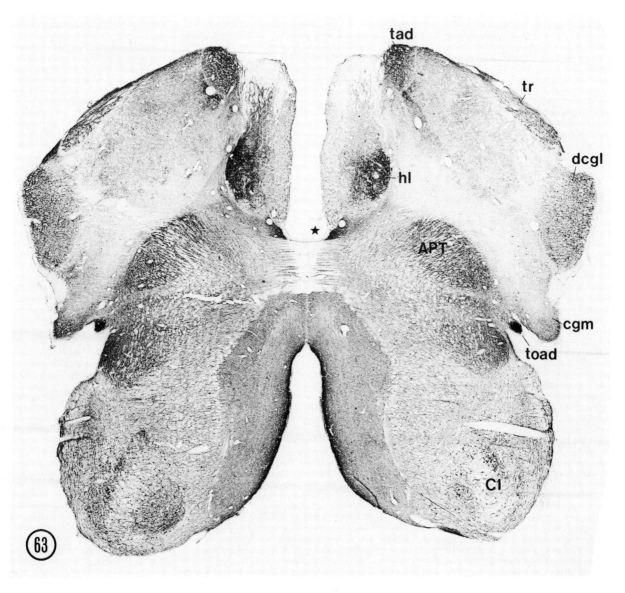

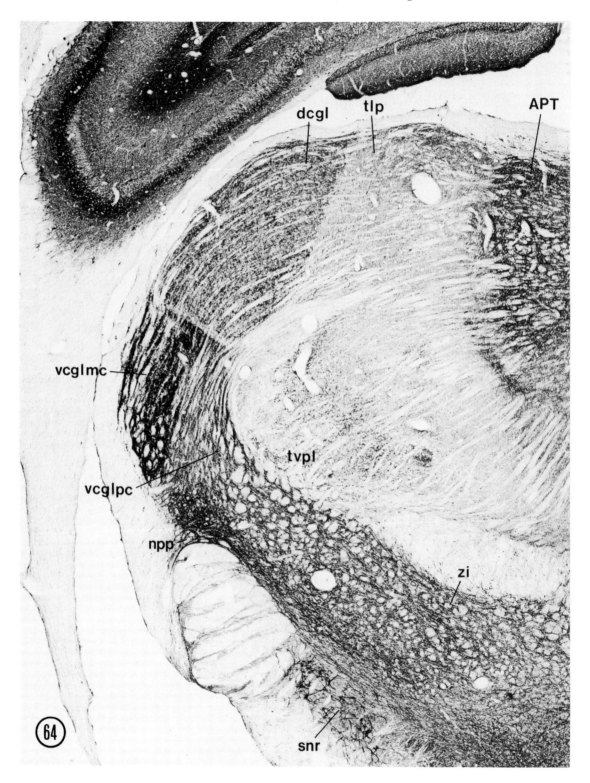

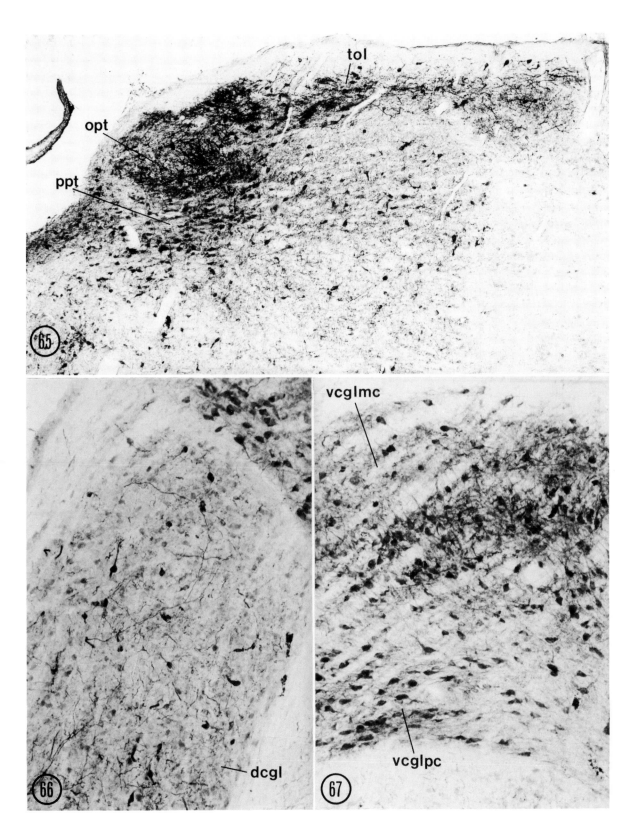

527

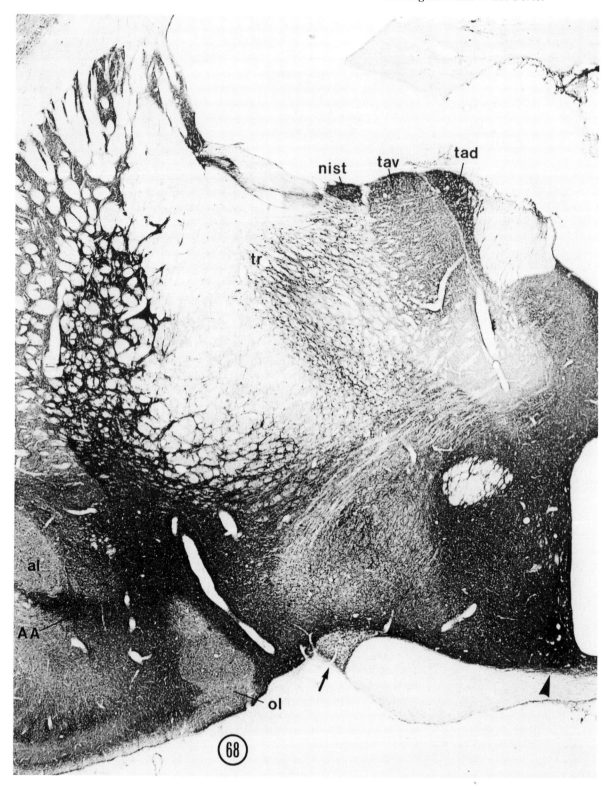

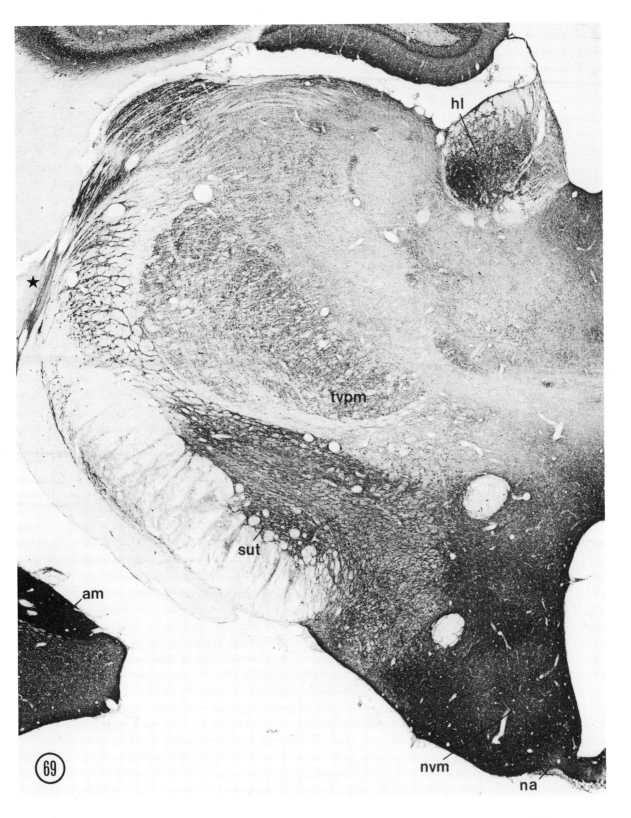

hl

★

tvpm

sut

am

nvm

na

⑥⑨

529

Fig. 70. Distribution of GABAergic neurons in the hypothalamic regions at the level of eminentia mediana (em) after topical colchicine injection. Nucleus ventromedialis hypothalami (nvm) has sparse GABAergic cell bodies, contrary to neighboring nuclei. The area indicated by an arrow is enlarged in Figure 71. GAD-positive cell bodies of the nucleus reticularis thalami (tr) are contiguous with GAD-immunoreactive neurons in zona incerta (zi). Compare for terminal staining with Figure 69. × 27.

Fig. 71. The transition between zona incerta (zi) (top) and the area hypothalamica lateralis (AHL) (bottom) is marked by an increase in somatal size of GABAergic neurons. This micrograph shows the region of area hypothalamica lateralis rich in GAD-immunoreactive nerve cell bodies (see for contrast Fig. 75 and Schematic atlas drawing A 3.2 (p. 475) for caudal aspect of AHL). × 70.

BASAL FOREBRAIN

Fig. 72. This detail from a coronal section shows cell body staining in the region lateral to Figure 70 – after topical colchicine injection, and includes parts of the nucleus reticularis thalami (tr; top), nucleus entopeduncularis (ep; center) and globus pallidus (gp; middle right). At the bottom, the nucleus amygdaloideus centralis (ac), the nucleus amygdaloideus medialis (am), and area amygdalohippocampalis (AHI) are illustrated. Portions of the caudal continuation of the rodent equivalent of the 'nucleus basalis magnocellularis of Meynert' (arrow) with scattered GABAergic neurons are visible along the optic tract (TO). Note the change in number of immunostained cell bodies at the transition between nucleus amygdaloideus medialis (am) and area amygdalohippocampalis (AHI). *D* and *V* indicate dorsal and ventral directions. *cf.* for GAD-positive terminal staining with Figure 56. × 49.

HYPOTHALAMUS

Figs 73–75. Changing densities of GABAergic cell bodies in hypothalamus in medial (top) to lateral (bottom) sagittal sections. The sections of Figures 73 and 74 are spaced 500 μm; those of Figures 74 and 75, 300 μm. Arrow in Figure 73 indicates pedunculus corporis mamillaris. Arrow in Figure 74 points to nucleus terminalis tractus optici accessorii, pars medialis. × 28.

Fig. 76. Detail from a specimen of a rat which received a topical colchicine injection into the basomedial hypothalamus. In the eminentia mediana immunoreactive terminals are concentrated in the external layer. The nucleus arcuatus (na) contains numerous immunoreactive terminals and cell bodies. In contrast, the neighboring nucleus ventromedialis hypothalami (nvm) is nearly free of GAD-immunoreactive cell bodies and has a medium density of terminal staining. In order to discern cytological details, this section was immunoreacted briefly. cf. Figures 69 and 70. × 112.

Hypophysis

Fig. 77. Numerous immunoreactive terminals occur among and within individual lobuli of lobus anterior, pars intermedia (im) of the hypophysis. × 302.

Fig. 78. Intralobular terminals are present in lobus anterior, pars intermedia (im), scattered terminals in lobus posterior (pars nervosa (n)), and a dense plexus of fibers and terminals at the border between these 2 subdivisions of the hypophysis. × 610.

Corpora mamillaria

Figs 79 and 80. Details of bouton staining (Fig. 79, horizontal section) and cell body staining (Fig. 80, coronal section) in the mammillary region.

Fig. 79. All mammillary subnuclei are richly provided with GABAergic terminals. × 51.

Fig. 80. The corpora mamillaria contain only very few GABAergic cell bodies. These are found, for the most part, in the region of nucleus supramamillaris (sum) and the nuclei gemini (gem). A very high density of GABAergic cell bodies is found in the nucleus caudalis magnocellularis hypothalami posterioris (cmc), where the GABAergic neurons form continuous bilateral sheets spanning from medial to lateral aspects. See Figures 73 and 74. Arrow indicates the midline. Fasciculus mamillothalamicus (FMT) is entirely GAD-negative. × 73.

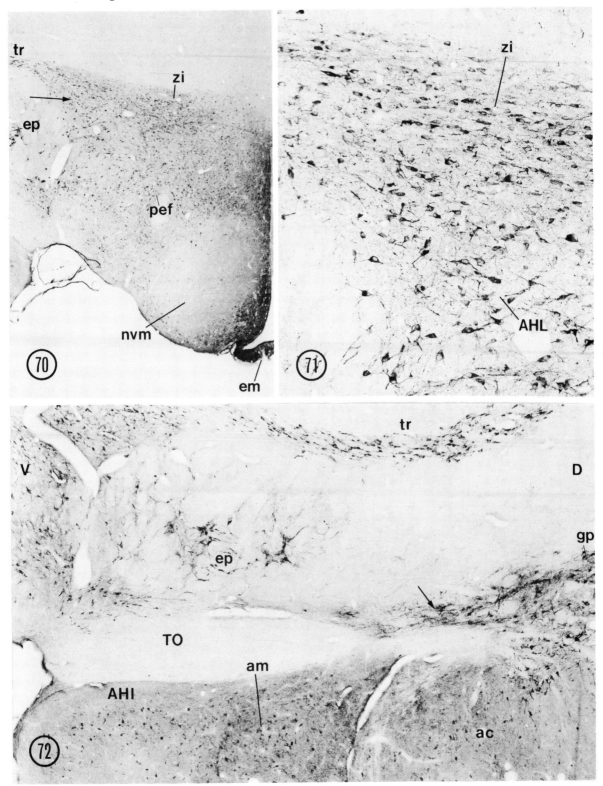

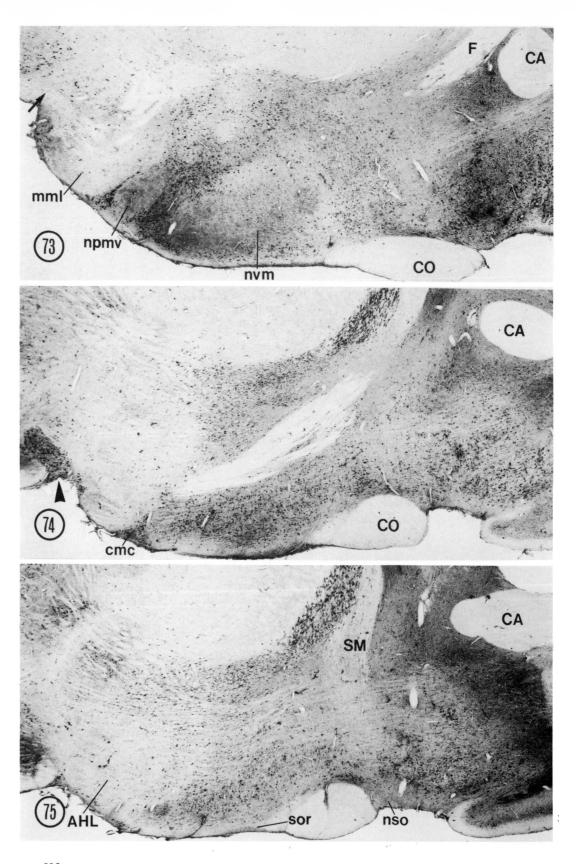

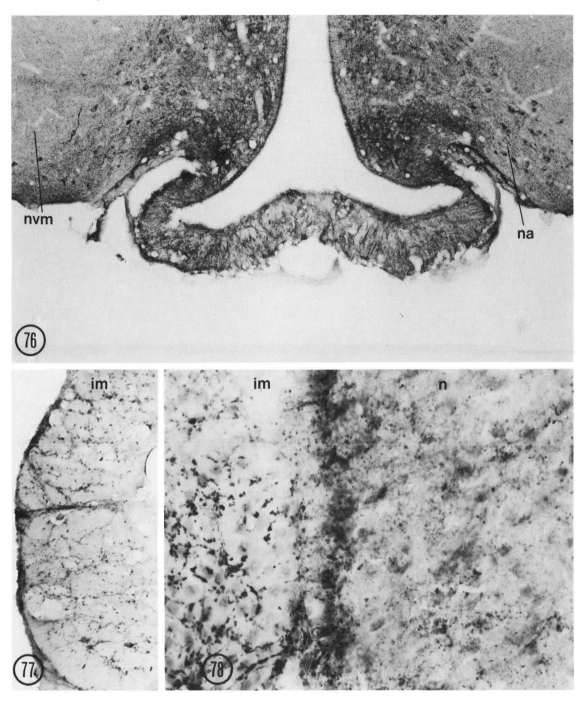

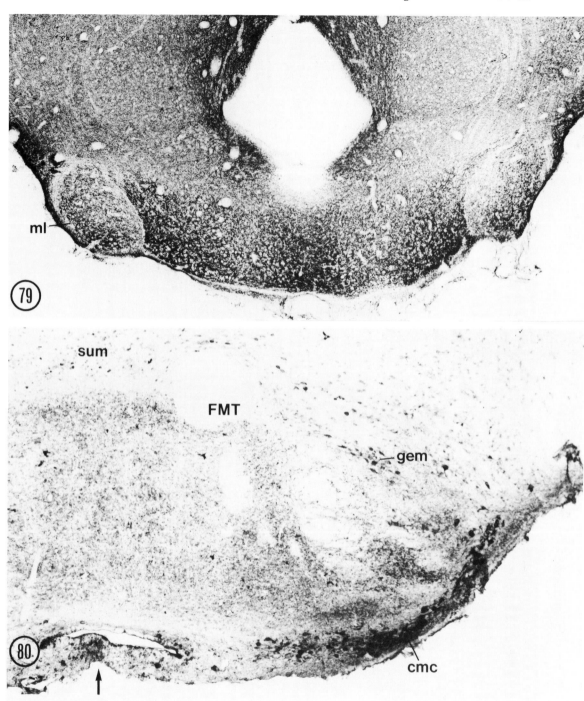

MESENCEPHALON

Nuclei terminales tractus optici accessorii

Figs 81–85. Nuclei terminales tractus optici accessorii in coronal sections processed for immunostaining of cell bodies. These nuclei are richly provided with GABAergic terminals and contain one of the highest densities of GAD-immunoreactive neurons observed in brain.

Fig. 81. Nucleus terminalis tractus optici accessorii pars medialis (toam). On the right side the medial aspect of the substantia nigra pars reticulata. × 72.

Figs 82 and 83. Nucleus terminalis tractus optici accessorii pars dorsalis (toad). Arrow indicates the area, which is enlarged in Figure 83. Fig. 82: × 50. Fig. 83: × 205.

Fig. 84. Note the difference in size and shape of GABAergic cell bodies in the nucleus caudalis magnocellularis hypothalami posterioris (cmc) and the nucleus terminalis tractus optici accessorii pars medialis (toam). GABAergic neurons are present also in regions of adjacent formatio reticularis. × 201.

Fig. 85. GAD-immunoreactive nerve cells in nucleus terminalis tractus optici accessorii pars medialis (toam) at higher magnification. The medial aspect of substantia nigra pars reticulata (snr) is seen on the upper right side. The nucleus terminalis tractus optici accessorii pars lateralis (not shown) expresses the same characteristics as pars medialis and pars dorsalis, but is inconspicuous in rat. × 205.

Nucleus interpeduncularis

Figs 86–89. The left-hand photographs show bouton staining; cell body staining in nucleus interpeduncularis on the right. Additional micrographs of the nucleus interpeduncularis in coronal sections are shown in Figures 23 and 93. The nucleus interpeduncularis pars paramediana (= lateralis) (ipp) is illustrated in sagittal view in Figures 20 and 121. Figure 86 is taken from a horizontal section and includes the nucleus interfascicularis (if). Figures 87, 88 and 89 are taken from coronal sections.

Figs 86 and 87. Medial portion of the nucleus interpeduncularis (pars centralis) contains more GABAergic terminals than the lateral subdivisions. Moreover, the nucleus interfascicularis (if) appears as an extension of the nucleus interpeduncularis rather than part of area ventralis tegmenti. Fig. 86: × 78. Fig. 87: × 75.

Figs 88 and 89. Most neurons in nucleus interpeduncularis pars paramediana (ipp) are GAD-immunoreactive. The nucleus interpeduncularis pars centralis (ipc) – with the exception of its most apical aspect (nucleus interpeduncularis pars apicalis; ipa?) – also contain a high density of GABAergic neurons. Fig. 88: × 80. Fig. 89: × 148.

Nucleus ruber

Figs 90 and 91. GABAergic cell bodies are rare in nucleus ruber pars magnocellularis (rmc) (Fig. 90, coronal section), whilst they make up the majority of the small neurons in nucleus ruber pars parvocellularis (rpc) (Fig. 91; sagittal section). Numerous GAD-positive cell bodies are present also in the area retrorubralis (RR) and the area perirubralis of the formatio reticularis. Portions of substantia nigra pars reticulata are included in Figure 90 (bottom right). R on the upper right in Fig. 91 indicates rostral direction. Fig. 90: × 135. Fig. 91: × 135.

FORMATIO RETICULARIS

Fig. 92. Cell body staining in formatio reticularis at the level of pons and mesencephalon and in the midline region as seen in this horizontal section. Note the high concentration of GAD-immunoreactive neurons in nucleus tegmenti dorsalis lateralis (ntdl), nucleus accessorius Darkschewitsch (aD), nucleus interstitialis Cajal (ic), nucleus subretrofascicularis and formatio reticularis perirubralis. Only scattered GABAergic neurons are present in the nuclei raphe. Portion of area pretectalis anterior (APT), also rich in GABAergic neurons, is included in the upper right-hand corner. The level of this micrograph approximately corresponds to Figure 58 in the atlas of Paxinos and Watson (1982). × 40.

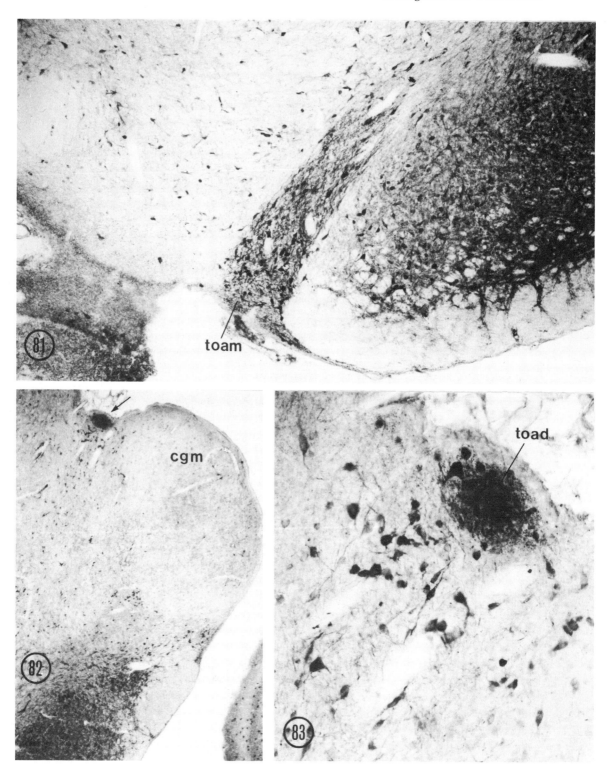

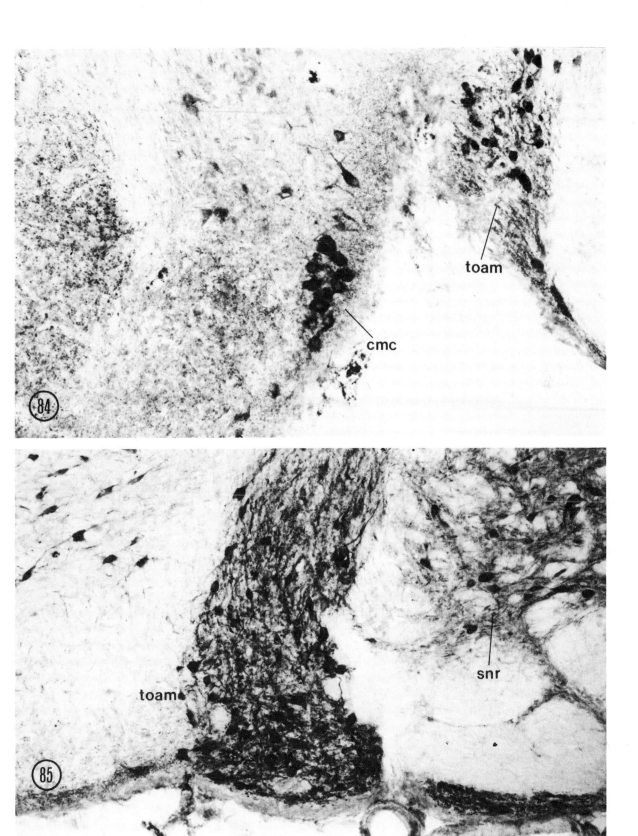

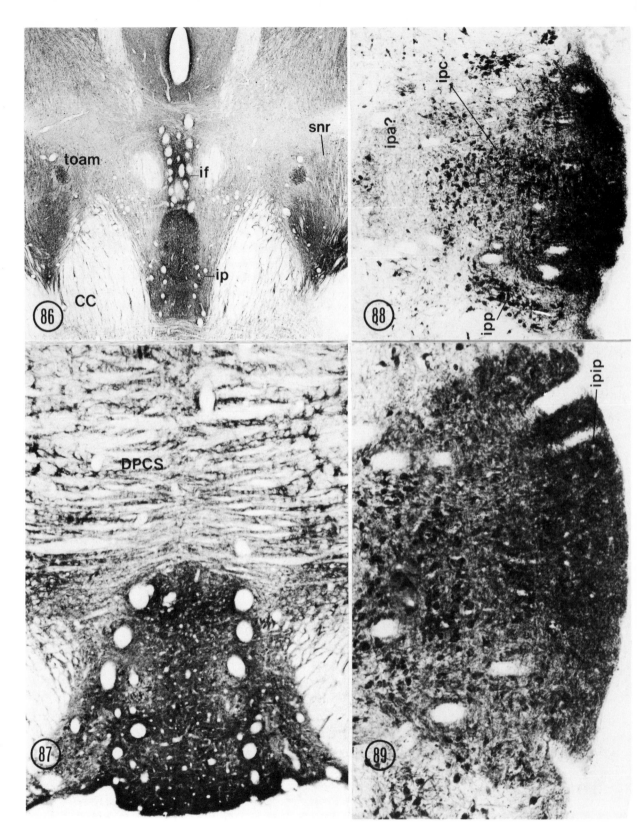

538

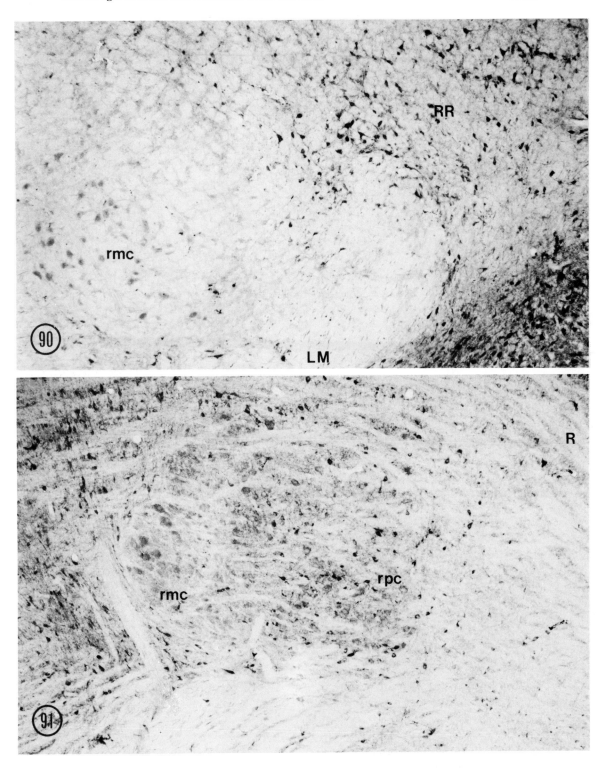

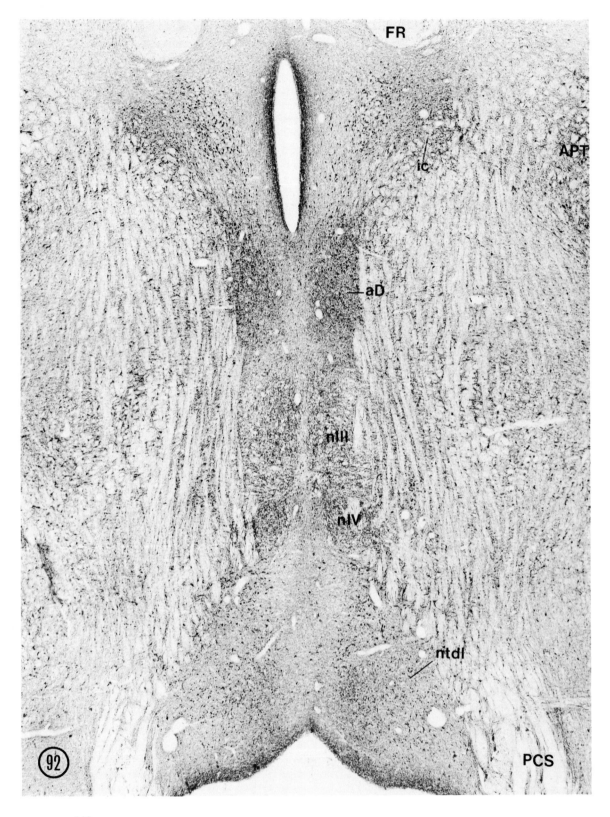

Fig. 93. Formatio reticularis of the central tegmental region at the level of decussatio dorsalis tegmentalis (DDT) is shown in a coronal section stained for cell bodies. Note the high concentration of GABAergic cell bodies in the region of the substantia grisea centralis (SGC) ventrolateralis located dorsally and laterally to nucleus raphe dorsalis (center top, below aquaeductus cerebri). Note the transversely cut GAD-positive fibers in the fasciculus longitudinalis medialis which is seen between nucleus raphe dorsalis and decussatio dorsalis tegmentalis (DDT). Numerous GAD-immunoreactive neurons are present in area retrorubralis (RR), area ventralis tegmenti (vta) and nucleus interpeduncularis (bottom). × 43.

Fig. 94. Formatio reticularis of the lateral tegmental region at the level of the fields of Forel (FF) is shown in a horizontal section stained for cell bodies. On the right, the substantia nigra pars reticulata (snr) is shown with its large complement of GABAergic neurons. On the left, nucleus raphe linearis (rli) is detected with scattered GABAergic cell bodies. The cell-poor area between nucleus raphe linearis and area retrorubralis (RR) is the periphery of nucleus ruber (r). × 41.

Figs 95 and 96. Discrete regions of the formatio reticularis pontis and medullaris, particularly rich in GABAergic neurons. Both photographs are from coronal sections processed for cell body staining with the midline included on the right-hand side.

Fig. 95. Note the small GABAergic cells forming an obliquely oriented neuronal pool rostral and lateral to nucleus reticularis tegmenti pontis (rtp). This region has been denominated with the arabic numeral *3. cf.* Figure 121. × 84.

Fig. 96. Note the accumulation of small to medium-size GABAergic neurons in nucleus reticularis paragigantocellularis (nrpg). A streak of intensely GAD-immunoreactive puncta (arrow) is observed at the ventral surface of the tractus corticospinalis (= pyramis; P) extending between the raphe pallidus (rp) and a discrete pool of GAD-immunoreactive nerve cells (7) at the lateral corner of the pyramis (*cf.* Figure 120). High density of GAD-positive terminals obscures these neuronal cell bodies at the illustrated magnification. This area has been denominated with the arabic numeral 7. Area 7 corresponds in location to the area 'B1 lateral' of serotonin-containing neurons (see Chapter III, *Vol. 3*, This Series). *cf.* Schematic atlas drawing P 5.0 and P 5.5. × 78.

Fig. 97. High density of GABAergic neurons in nucleus tegmenti ventralis (ntv). Scattered GABAergic neurons at this level are present in nucleus superioris centralis (ncs; = nucleus raphe medianus), the adjacent formatio reticularis, nucleus raphe dorsalis (rd), and the lateral aspect of substantia grisea centralis (SGC). Note the GAD-immunoreactive fibers lateral of the nucleus tegmenti ventralis. These fibers constitute the commissura Probst (arrowhead). Cell body staining. × 76.

ORGANA CIRCUMVENTRICULARIA

Fig. 98. Organum subcommissurale (sco): GAD-immunoreactive terminals are exclusively distributed as a thin band at the basis of the specialized epithelium and as bilateral accumulations at the lateral corners of organum subcommissurale. The cells of the epithelium are unstained (see also Fig. 63). Note the streaks of GAD-immunoreactive fibers in commissura posterior. Coronal section. × 184.

Fig. 99. In this coronal section of the area postrema (ap) stained for cell bodies the extremely numerous GABAergic cell bodies and terminals are evident. × 147.

For *Hypophysis* see Figures 77 and 78. Organum subfornicale and corpus pineale are not illustrated.

COLLICULUS SUPERIOR

Fig. 100. Stratum griseum superficiale colliculi superioris (sgs) including the stratum zonale, is particularly rich in GAD-immunoreactive boutons. The dorsal portion of substantia grisea centralis (lower left) is included in the photograph of this coronal section. Immunostaining of boutons is present in all layers of colliculus superior and is denser at points (patches) (arrows) in the layers beneath stratum opticum, particularly in stratum griseum mediale and stratum griseum profundum. Terminal staining. × 78.

Fig. 101. Stratum griseum superficiale colliculi superioris and stratum zonale are particularly rich in small-to-medium-size GABAergic neurons. Lower densities of such neurons are present in the other layers as seen in Figure 23. Cell body staining. × 125.

Fig. 102. A collection of medium-size and small GABAergic neurons characterizes the 'area commissuralis colliculi superioris' (arabic numeral *1*). This area forms a bilateral rostrocaudal band of cells which may bear some analogy to a correspondingly located area in the colliculus inferior. Cell body staining. *cf.* Schematic atlas drawing A 1.6–P. 0.5. × 68.

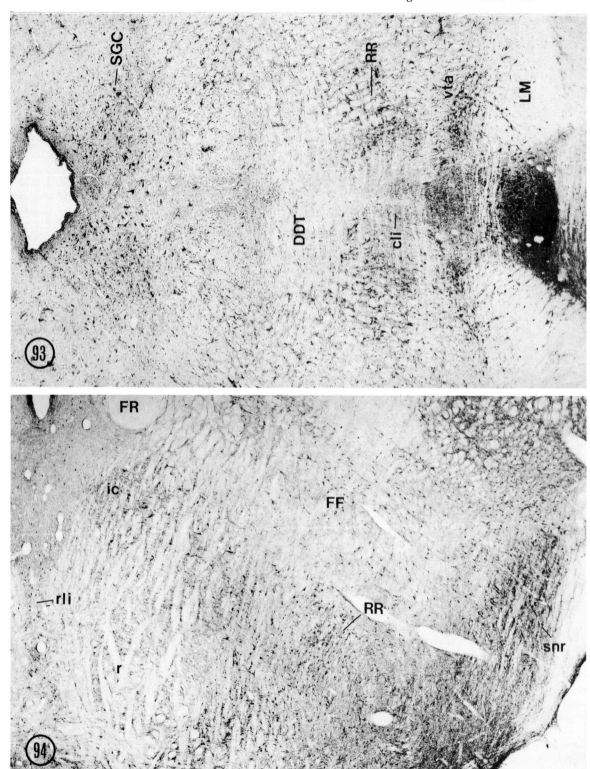

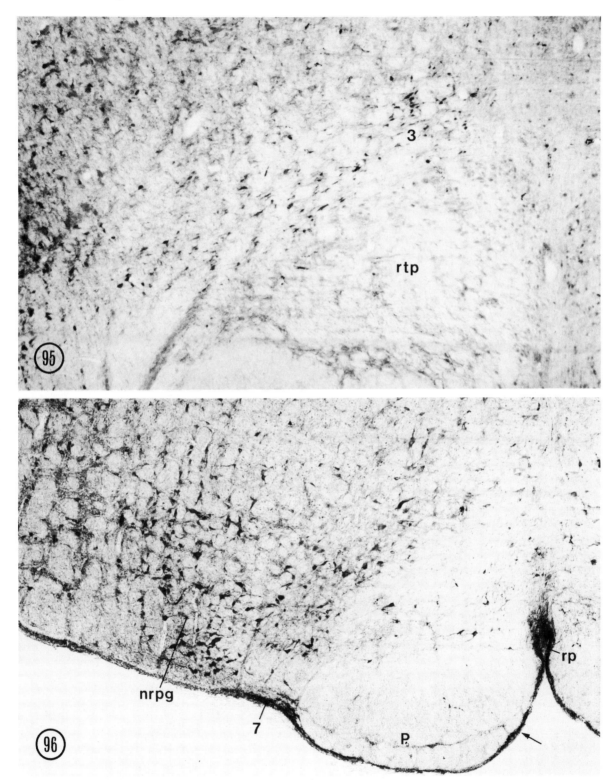

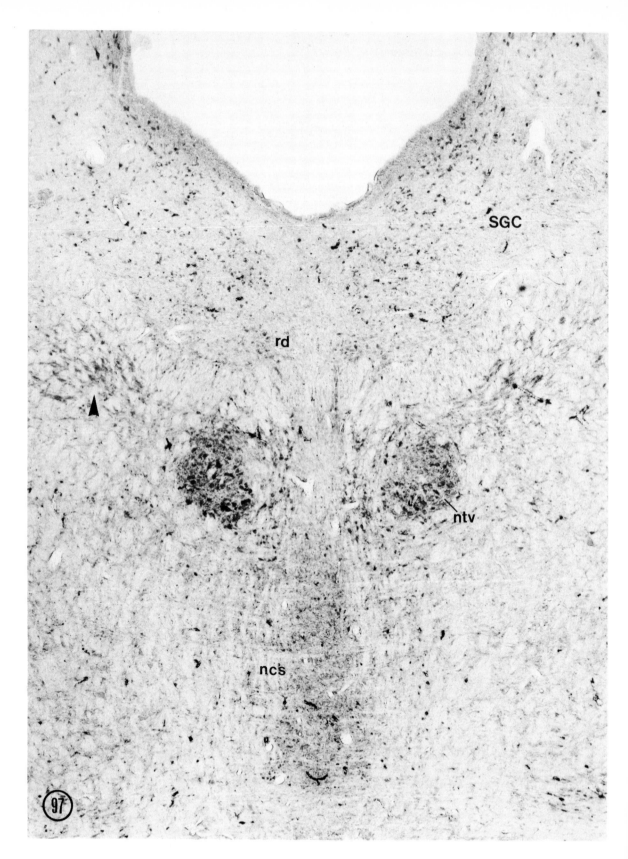

544

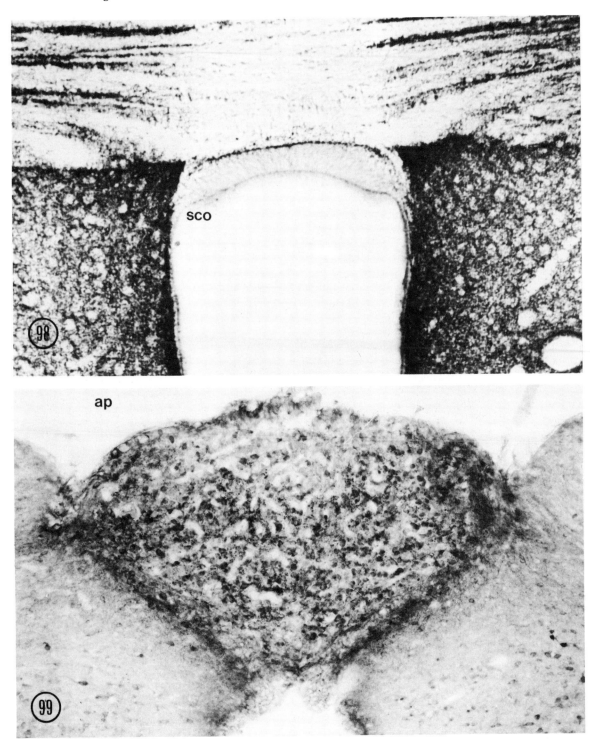

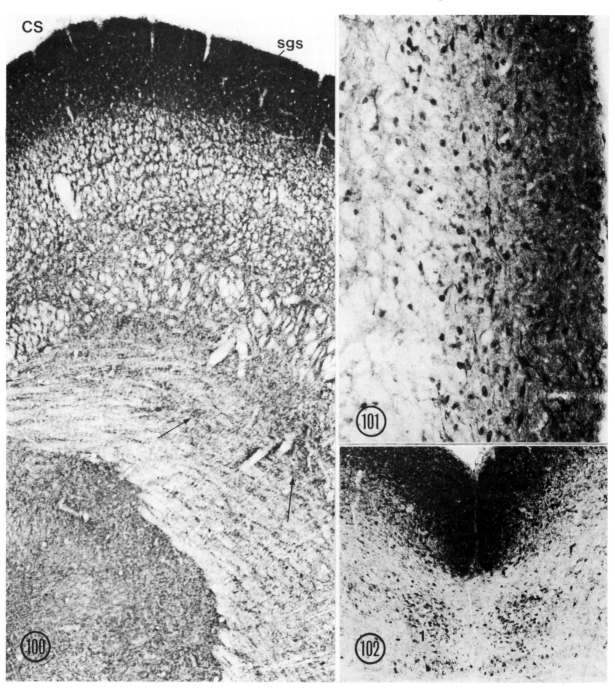

COLLICULUS INFERIOR – ACOUSTIC SYSTEM

Fig. 103. The external cortex of colliculus inferior (CI) contains patches of GABAergic terminals and cell bodies in layer 2 (arrow). Layer 3 of the external cortex (Faye-Lund and Osen (1985)) is characterized by very large GABAergic neurons (large arrowhead) as seen at higher magnification in Figure 105. Rather closely spaced medium-size neurons predominate in the nucleus centralis colliculi inferioris. Scattered, predominantly small neurons are present in nucleus cuneiformis (ncu). Portions of nucleus dorsalis lemnisci lateralis (Dnll) (lower right) and the lamina molecularis cerebelli (upper left) are included in the picture. A GAD-negative giant neuron covered with GABAergic terminals (*small arrowhead*) is seen enlarged in Figure 104. Full views of the distribution of GABAergic boutons and cell bodies in colliculus inferior are seen in Figures 11 (p. 455) and 24 (p.465). Cell body staining. × 53.

Fig. 104. Detail of Figure 103: A giant GAD-negative tegmental neuron at the basis of the colliculus inferior is densely innervated by GABAergic terminals around the cell body and main stem dendrite similar to large neurons in the nuclei cerebellares and nucleus vestibularis lateralis. × 477.

Fig. 105. High magnification photograph of the upper right-hand corner of Figure 103 illustrating a patch of GABAergic cell bodies and terminals in layer 2 of the external cortex of colliculus inferior (CI) and large GAD-immunoreactive neurons in layer 3. (Similar dense patches of acetylcholinesterase reaction product occur in layer 2 in the same region (personal observations), but a correspondence between the two remains to be established.) × 212.

Figs 106–108. Three partly overlapping photographs of 'area commissuralis colliculi inferioris' (arabic numeral *1*) in transverse section show changes in cell shape and size as well as in dendritic orientation of GAD-immunoreactive neurons from the midline to the dorsal aspect of the external cortex of the colliculus inferior (CI). Cell body staining. × 143.

Fig. 109. Nucleus centralis corporis geniculati medialis (cgm) and nucleus suprageniculatus thalami (sgt) contain few GABAergic neurons (*cf.* Fig. 82). The complement of immunostained puncta shows subtle variations in the various subdivisions of nucleus centralis corporis geniculati medialis, as also evident in Figures 9 (p. 453, 10 (454), 60 and 63. Portions of the nucleus dorsalis corporis geniculati lateralis (dcgl) and the nuclei pretectales (top middle and left) are included. Nucleus brachii conjunctivi colliculi inferioris, which is rich in GABAergic neurons, is shown in Figure 23. Cell body staining. × 67.

Fig. 110. Nucleus dorsalis lemnisci lateralis (Dnll), nucleus ventralis lemnisci lateralis, pars dorsalis (dVnll), rostral area paralemniscalis (pl) and adjacent regions of the formatio reticularis in a sagittal section. Unique among all these areas, dVnll contains few GABAergic neurons, whilst Dnll consists nearly exclusively of GABAergic neurons (*cf.* Fig. 111). Nucleus ventralis lemnisci lateralis pars medialis (mVnll) and pars ventralis (vVnll) are illustrated in Figure 24 (p. 465). Cell body staining. × 54.

Fig. 111. Many neurons in nucleus dorsalis lemnisci lateralis (Dnll) have dendrites oriented perpendicularly to the fibers of the lemniscus lateralis, as seen in this coronal section. The immunostained axons on the right-hand side are the axons (arrows) of neurons of nucleus dorsalis lemnisci lateralis that join to form the commissura Probst (see also Figs 24 and 97). Cell body staining. × 202.

Fig. 112. Nucleus olivaris superior in coronal section, processed for cell body staining. (Nomenclature according to Meessen and Olszewski 1949). Nucleus paraolivaris superior (spn) and nucleus olivaris superior pars lateralis (osl) contain numerous GABAergic neurons. Nucleus ventralis corporis trapezoidei (vtz) contains the highest concentration of GABAergic neurons and terminals in this region (*cf.* Fig. 113). Nucleus medialis corporis trapezoidei (mtz) and nucleus olivaris superior pars medialis (osm) are practically free of GAD-positive nerve cell bodies, although they are innervated by GABAergic terminals of unknown origin. ltz: nucleus lateralis corporis trapezoidei (= LVPO of Osen et al. 1984). Cell body staining. × 76.

Fig. 113. High magnification of the region of nucleus ventralis corporis trapezoidei (vtz) (= MVPO of Osen et al. 1984), containing numerous GABAergic neurons and terminals. Cell body staining. × 188.

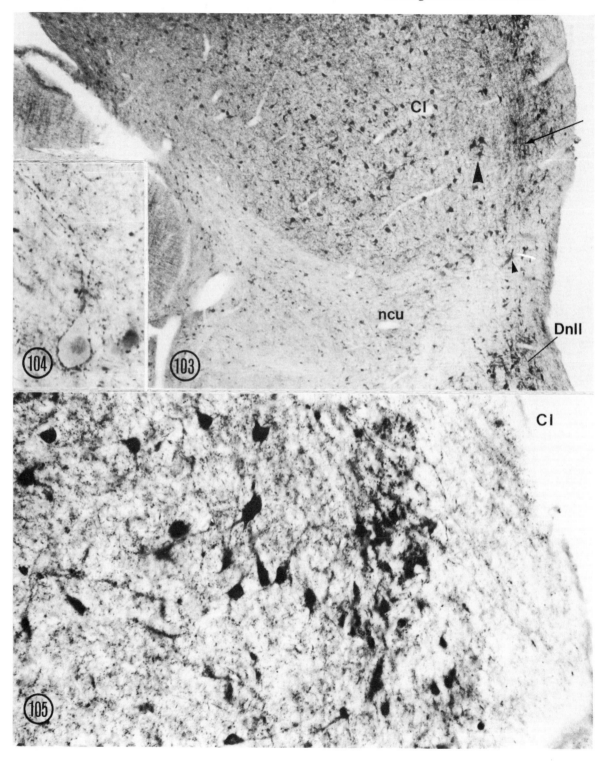

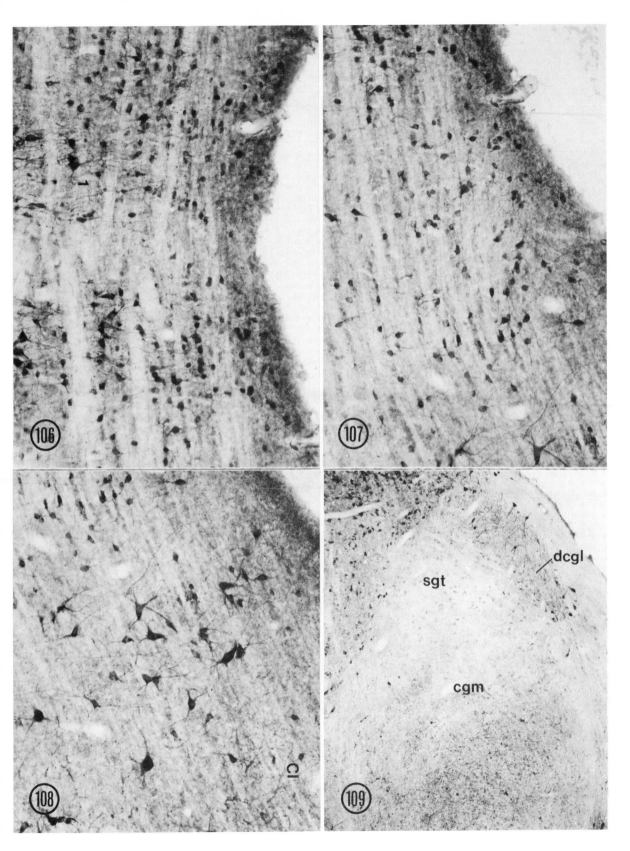

549

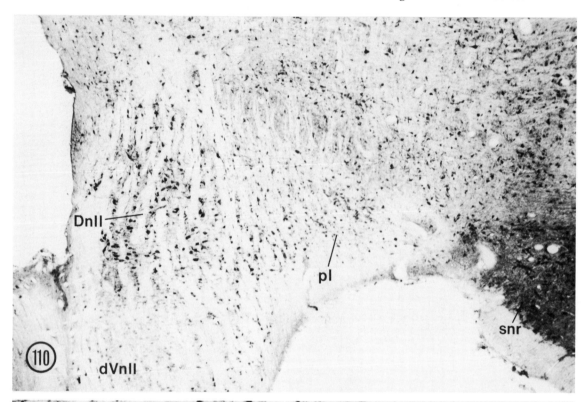

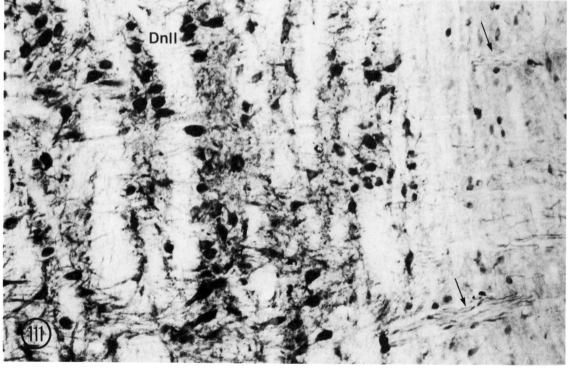

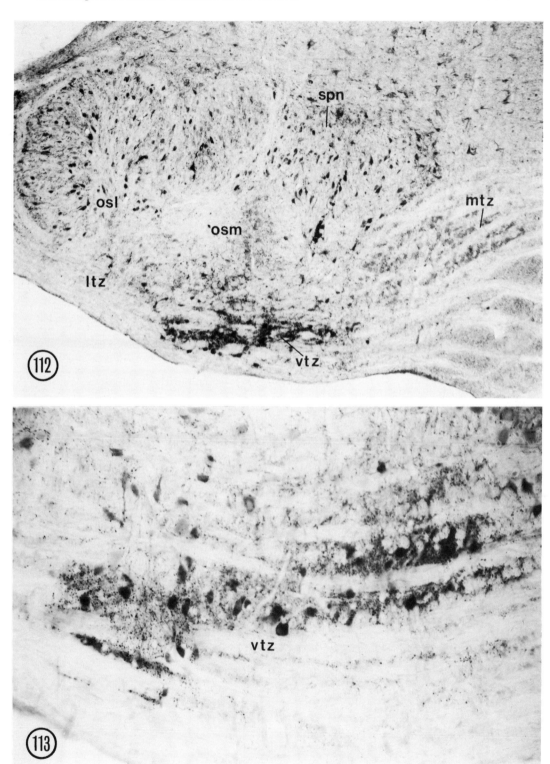

Nuclei cochleares

Figs 114–117. Bouton staining in the nuclei cochleares on the left-hand side (Fig. 114); radix nervi acoustico-vestibularis (VIII) (Fig. 115).

GABAergic cell bodies in the nucleus cochlearis dorsalis (right) (Fig. 116), and in the nucleus cochlearis ventralis (Fig. 117) after topical colchicine injection. All micrographs are taken from coronal sections.

Fig. 114. Lamina superficialis granularis (lg) of nucleus cochlearis ventralis (cov) and layers 1 and 2 of nucleus cochlearis dorsalis (cod) have the highest densities of boutons. At high magnification (not shown), the patterns of staining vary. A pericellular pattern predominates in the magnocellular region of nucleus cochlearis ventralis (see also Fig. 117) and around pyramidal neurons in layer 2 of nucleus cochlearis dorsalis; clustering of boutons occurs particularly in the regions containing granule cells, such as in lamina superficialis granularis (lg) of nucleus cochlearis ventralis and layer 2 of nucleus cochlearis dorsalis. GABAergic terminals tend to be larger in the anterior than in the posterior parts of nucleus cochlearis ventralis. In layer 1, 3 and 4 of nucleus cochlearis dorsalis diffusely distributed small boutons predominate. × 50.

Fig. 115. Immunoreactive boutons and fibers, some of which are directed to the periphery (Fex and Altschuler 1984), are present in the eighth nerve root (VIII). × 200.

Fig. 116. Layer 2 of nucleus cochlearis dorsalis (cod) is the region with the highest concentration of GABAergic neurons in nuclei cochleares. × 105.

Fig. 117. Nucleus cochlearis ventralis (cov): relatively low density of GABAergic neurons is present in the small cell cap area and in the granule cell domains (lg). GABAergic neurons occur sparsely in the magnocellular regions. × 50.

NUCLEI RAPHE AND OTHER MIDLINE STRUCTURES

Figs 118–120. The raphe system includes regions particularly rich in GABAergic neurons, demonstrated in these photographs from coronal sections processed for cell body staining.

Fig. 118. Raphe magnus (rm). Numerous neurons are GAD-immunoreactive in this region. × 86.

Fig. 119. GABAergic neurons in raphe linearis (rli). This photograph includes also GABAergic neurons in nucleus accessorius Darkschewitsch (aD) and nucleus interstitialis Cajal (ic). × 47.

Fig. 120. GABAergic neurons in nucleus raphe pallidus (rp). Note the superficial band of densely concentrated boutons continuous with the nucleus raphe pallidus. See also Figure 96. × 130.

Fig. 121. This detail from the sagittal section shown in Figure 20 illustrates the paramedian region of the brainstem from medullary to mesencephalic levels and includes portions of substantia grisea centralis (top), the transition between nuclei raphe and formatio reticularis paramediana (center), the nucleus interpeduncularis (ip) and the area ventralis tegmenti (vta) (bottom). Parts of the nuclei pontis (po) and the nucleus mamillaris medialis (mm) are also included. Regions of the nucleus originis nervi oculomotorii (nIII) and nucleus originis nervi trochlearis (nIV) are seen at the right above the fasciculus longitudinalis medialis (FLM). Substantia grisea centralis: the densities of GABAergic neurons in the substantia grisea centralis are particularly high in correspondence of the nucleus tegmenti dorsalis (Gudden) (ntd), nucleus tegmenti dorsalis lateralis (ntdl) and of the *lateral* aspect of nucleus raphe dorsalis (right upper corner). Note the band of GABAergic neurons extending from nucleus tegmenti ventralis (ntv) to nucleus interpeduncularis (ip). Numerous small GAD-immunoreactive neurons extend from the nucleus interpeduncularis (ip) in the caudal direction. This conspicuous wing of GABAergic cell bodies has been denominated with the arabic numeral *3*. See Figures 20 (p. 461) and 95. Cell body staining. × 55.

Fig. 122. Detail from the caudal aspect of Figure 20; sagittal section. Nucleus originis nervi vagi (nX) and nucleus originis nervi hypoglossi (nXII) have sparse GAD-immunoreactive neurons. A conspicuous band of GABAergic neurons is present at the ventral border of nXII. This 'area reticularis subhypoglossa' has been denominated by the arabic numeral *5*. High densities of GABAergic neurons are present in the area postrema (ap) (see Fig. 99), the nucleus tractus solitarii (nts), the nucleus vestibularis medialis (vm) and the nucleus praepositus hypoglossi (ph). Scattered GABAergic neurons are seen in the formatio reticularis, the nucleus intercalatus Staderini (nicS), and the nucleus gracilis (*gr*). See Figures 139–142. Cell body staining. × 62.

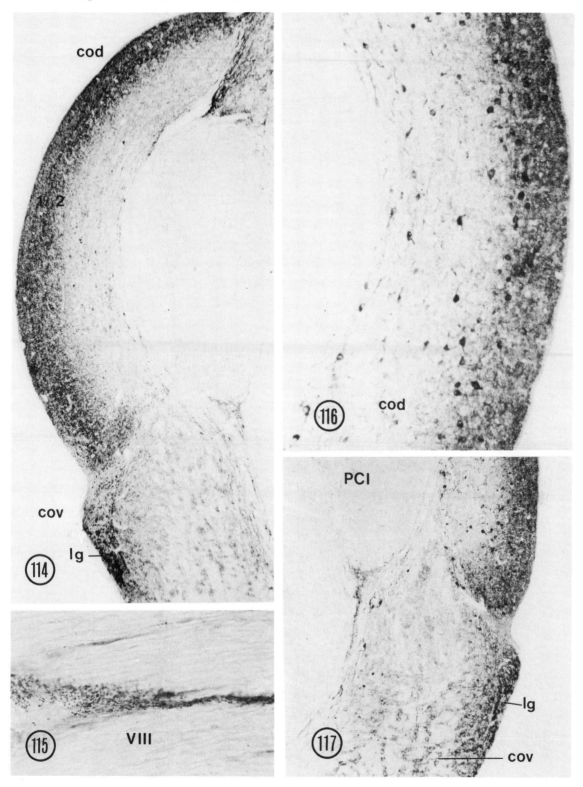

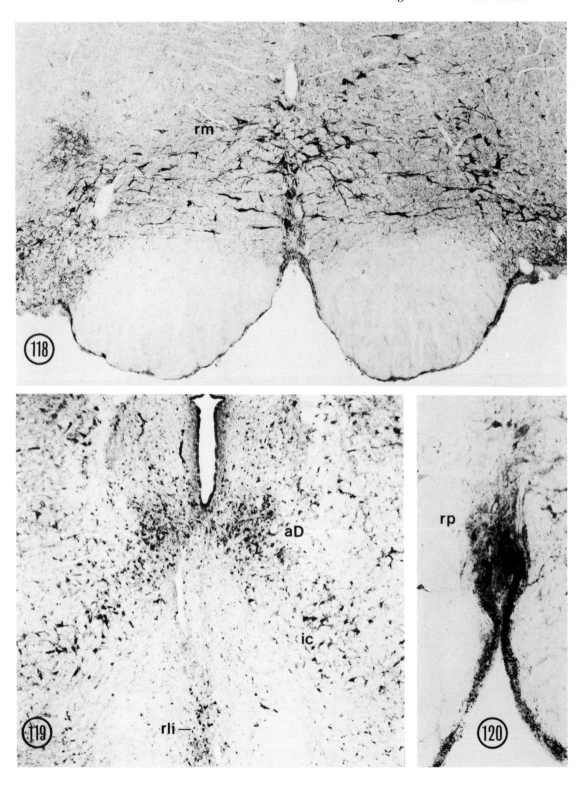

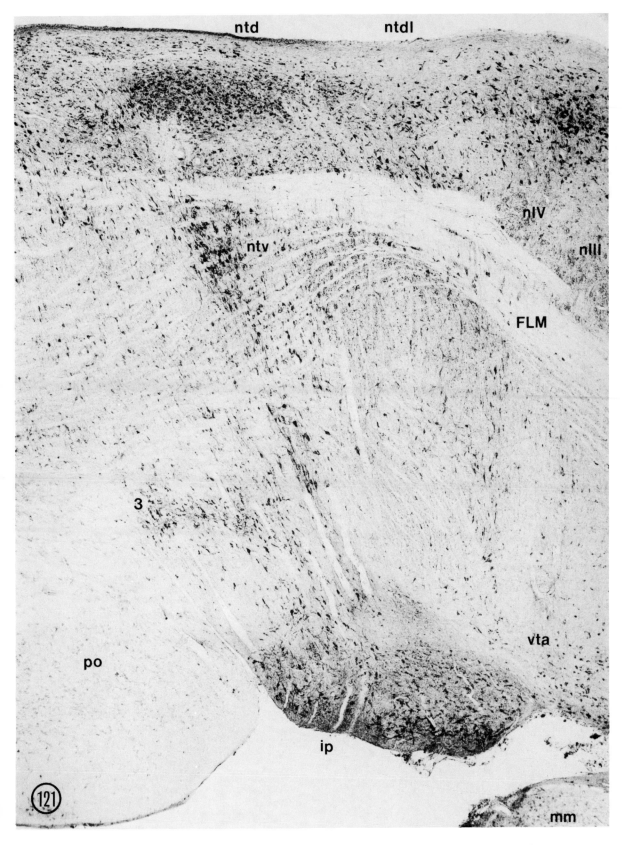

ntd　　　　　　ntdl

nIV

ntv

nIII

FLM

3

vta

po

ip

mm

121

555

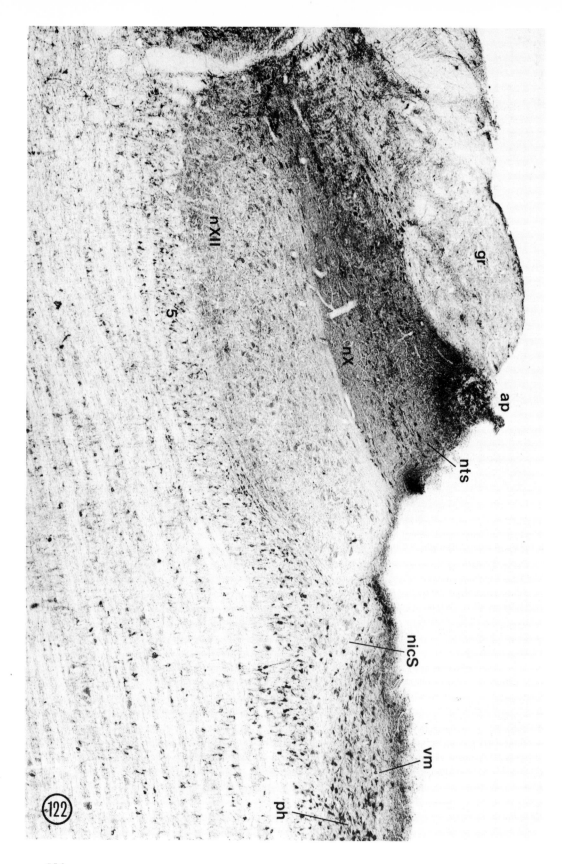

CEREBELLUM

Figs 123 and 124. All Purkinje cell bodies in the cortex cerebellaris are GAD-immunoreactive as seen in these photographs of horizontal sections stained for cell bodies.
Fig. 123. Folia 4 and 5 of vermis anterior are shown here across the midline. The level of this section corresponds approximately to Figure 65 in the atlas of Paxinos and Watson (1982). ×26.
Fig. 124. This section through the cerebral hemispheres and part of the vermis corresponds approximately to Figure 61 in the atlas of Paxinos and Watson (1982). Note the Purkinje cell axons in the white matter and the different patterns of bouton staining in lamina molecularis cerebelli and lamina granularis cerebelli. The dorsolateral protuberance of the nucleus medialis cerebelli appears grazed at center right. ×30.
Fig. 125. Cortex cerebellaris: Golgi cells in lamina granularis and basket/stellate neurons in lamina molecularis as well as Purkinje cells are GAD-immunoreactive in this sagittally sectioned vermal folium processed for cell body staining. Note that the axons of basket cells and Purkinje cells and the dendrites of Purkinje cells and Golgi cells are also immunoreactive without the use of colchicine. ×210.
Fig. 126. This detail of cortex cerebellaris shows that 3 different patterns of bouton staining distinguish the lamina molecularis cerebelli (left), the pinceau around the initial segment of the Purkinje cell axons (arrows), and the lamina granularis cerebelli (center right). Note that the primary dendrites of basket cells are also immunostained. ×609.

NUCLEI CEREBELLARES

Fig. 127. Dense bouton staining (largely pericellular) is present in all subdivisions of the nuclei cerebellares and the nucleus vestibularis lateralis (vl), as seen in this coronal section. The photograph includes also the nucleus vestibularis medialis (vm) and pars y nucleorum vestibulorum (y). ×35.
Fig. 128. GABAergic terminals of Purkinje cell axons outline cell bodies and main stem dendrites of the giant cells in the nucleus vestibularis lateralis (nucleus of Deiters) (vl). Bundles of myelinated GAD-immunoreactive Purkinje cell axons are also evident. *cf.* Figure 132. ×267.
Figs 129-132. GABAergic cell bodies in the nuclei cerebellares.
Fig. 129. Numerous small GABAergic neurons are present in the nuclei interpositi anteriores and posteriores (i). ×58.
Fig. 130. The nucleus lateralis cerebelli (l) contains also numerous small cell bodies. ×120.
Fig. 131. The nucleus medialis cerebelli (m) contains fewer GABAergic neurons. These are more numerous in the caudal portion (C) than in the rostral portion (R). ×58.
Fig. 132. Detail of the nucleus interpositus anterior (i(a)). The profiles of 6 small GABAergic cell bodies are illustrated. Note that all medium-size to large GAD-negative neurons in the nuclei cerebellares are outlined by GABAergic boutons. *cf.* Figure 128. ×500.

NUCLEI VESTIBULARES

Fig. 133. Different patterns of distribution of GAD-immunoreactive boutons in the 4 major nuclei vestibulares (medialis: vm, lateralis: vl, spinalis: vsp, and superior: vs) are evident in this horizontal section. Some of the differences might be due to the number and assembly of myelinated fibers in the nuclei, for example as in nucleus vestibularis medialis (vm) and nucleus vestibularis spinalis (vsp). Other patterns, such as the pericellular distribution of terminals in the nucleus vestibularis lateralis (vl) (see also Fig. 128) are due to peculiar GABAergic afferents. ×50.
Figs 134-136. Coronal sections of the nuclei vestibulares show the distribution of GABAergic vestibular neurons.
Fig. 134. Cell bodies of GABAergic neurons appear numerous in the nucleus vestibularis medialis (vm) and nucleus vestibularis spinalis (vsp). *cf.* Figure 122. ×53.
Fig. 135. A very high density of GAD-positive neurons is found in pars y nucleorum vestibulorum (y). The numerous GAD-immunoreactive neurons above pars y nucleorum vestibulorum correspond to the small-celled part of nucleus lateralis cerebelli (arrowhead). Immunostaining in nucleus vestibularis lateralis (vl), which contains scattered small GABAergic neurons, is mainly due to its complement of pericellular GABAergic boutons (left). (see Fig. 128). ×51.
Fig. 136. Numerous GAD-positive neurons are present in nucleus vestibularis superior (vs). Nucleus suprageniculatus facialis (sg) is devoid of GAD-positive perikarya. ×53.

557

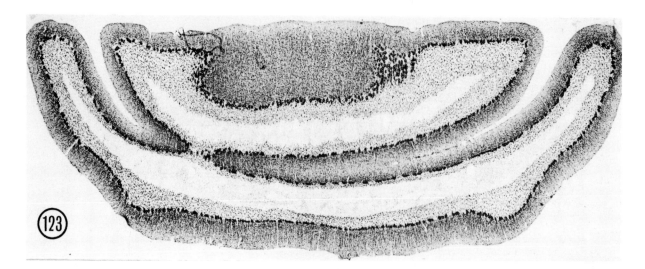

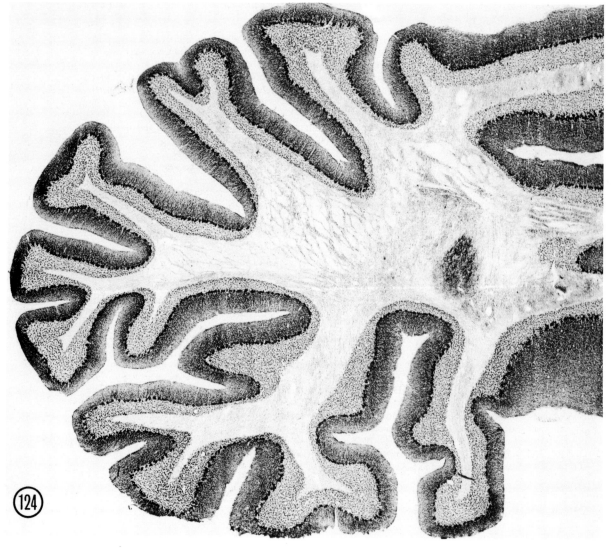

558

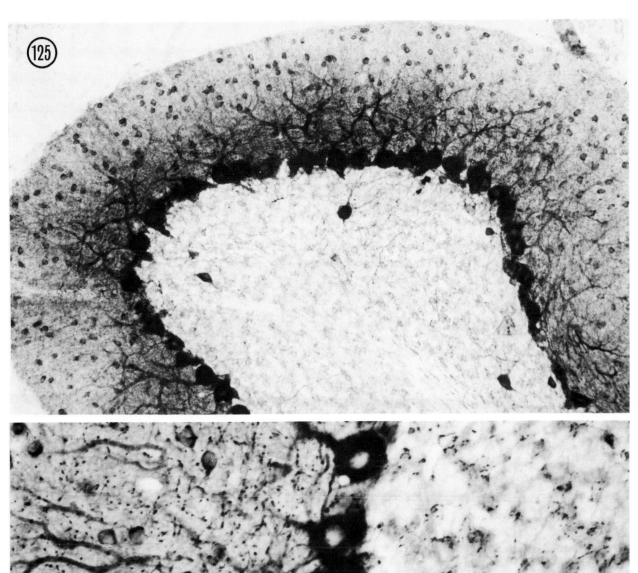

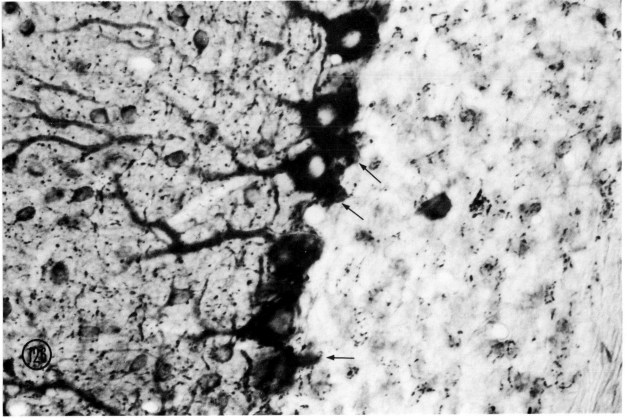

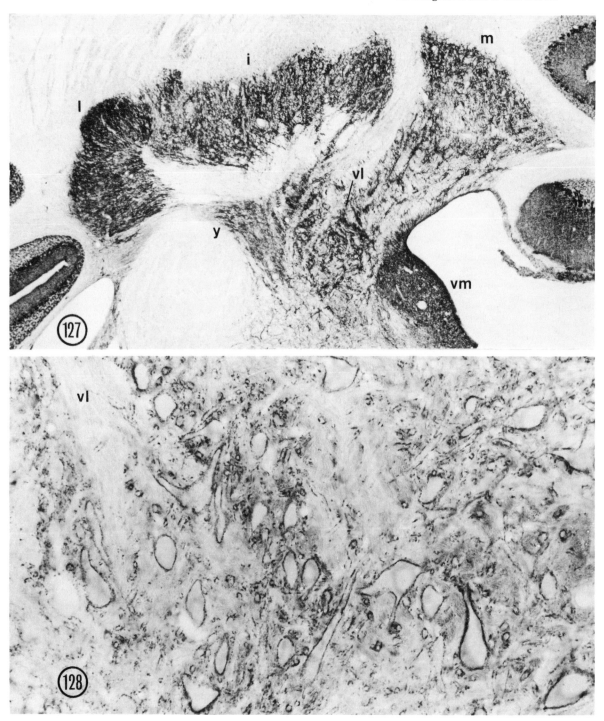

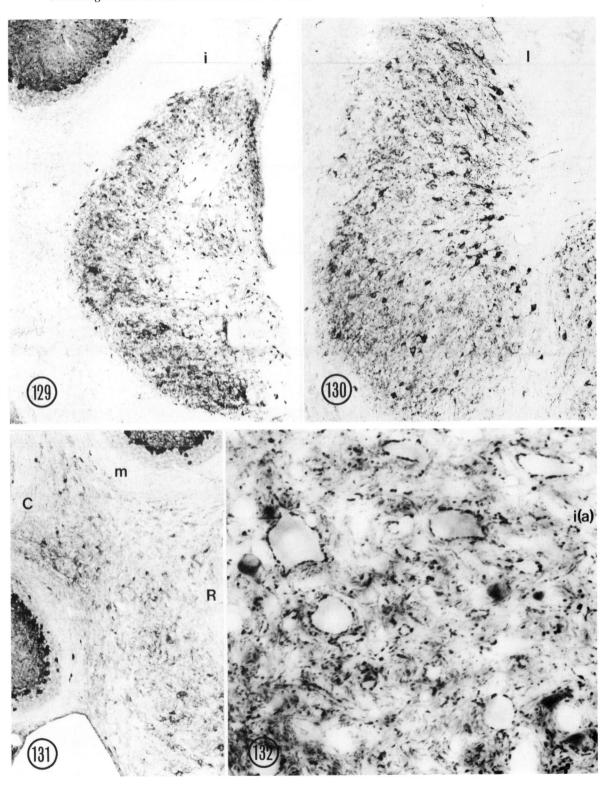

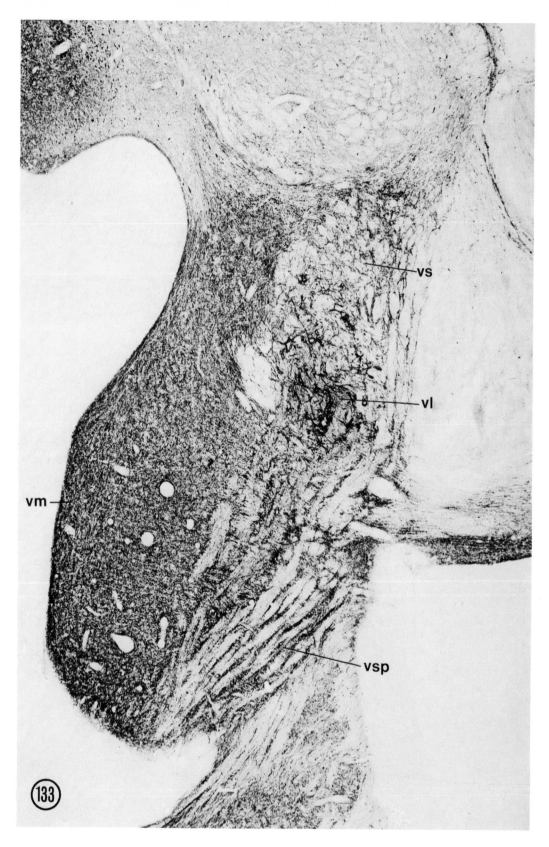

vs

vl

vm

vsp

⑬

562

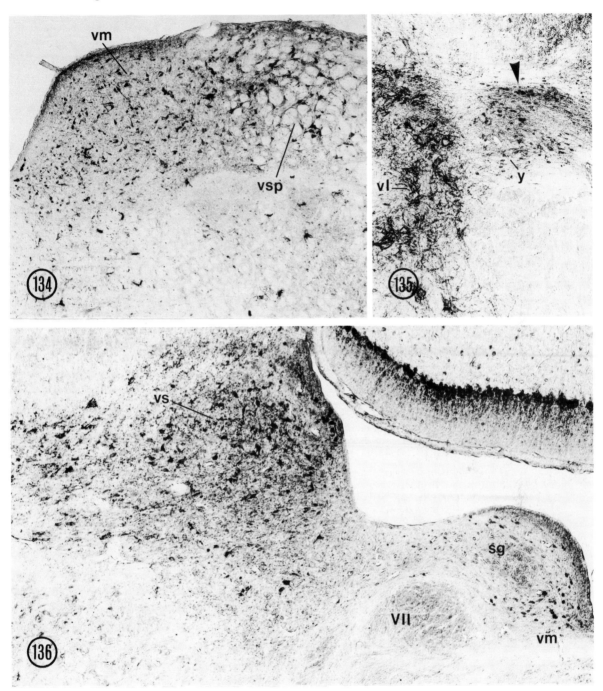

OLIVA INFERIOR

Fig. 137. The pattern of bouton staining varies in the different subdivisions of the oliva inferior (OI). Staining is densest in the β-subnucleus (β), in lateral and caudal portions of the oliva accessoria dorsalis (dao), and in the lateral band of the oliva principalis (po). At high magnification (not shown) boutons in the β-subnucleus are larger and more heavily stained than in the other subdivisions. $\times 47$.

Fig. 138. GABAergic cell bodies are absent or rare in all subdivisions of the oliva inferior (OI), while they abound in the nucleus reticularis paragigantocellularis (nrpg) in the reticular formation. Cell body staining. $\times 78$.

MEDULLA OBLONGATA

Figs 139 (most rostral) to 142 (most caudal). Distribution of GAD-immunoreactive nerve cell bodies in the medulla oblongata – processed for cell body staining – as shown in 4 coronal sections, spaced 250 μm apart. The nucleus gracilis (gr) and nucleus cuneatus (cu) contain scattered small GABAergic neurons. GABAergic neurons are particularly concentrated in subdivisions of the nucleus tractus solitarii (nts). A portion of the substantia grisea centralis is also rich in GABAergic neurons. Note the few GAD-positive neurons in the ependyma of canalis centralis (arrow) in Figures 140 and 142. *cf.* Figure 122. All Figs: $\times 67$.

NUCLEI TRIGEMINI

Fig. 143. The patterns of bouton staining seen in the dorsal most laminae of the medulla spinalis (sc) (see Figs 14–19, pp. 458-460) continue in corresponding regions of the nucleus tractus spinalis nervi trigemini, pars caudalis (ntV) but change rather abruptly at the beginning (arrow) of the nucleus tractus spinalis nervi trigemini, pars interposita. $\times 14$.

Fig. 144. Small GABAergic cell bodies are scattered in the pars interposita of nucleus tractus spinalis nervi trigemini (ntV) and adjacent regions of formatio reticularis. Portion of the nucleus reticularis paragigantocellularis (nrpg) is included in this micrograph. Inset shows numerous GABAergic cell bodies and terminals in the nucleus paratrigeminalis (npt). Cell body staining. $\times 31$. Inset: $\times 167$.

Figs 145 and 146. The nucleus originis nervi trigemini (motorius) (nV) is dorsally and caudally capped by a reticular area rich in GAD-immunoreactive neurons. This area presumably corresponds to the nucleus supratrigeminalis (Lorente de Nó 1922) and is shown here in the sagittal plane (Fig. 145) and transverse plane (Fig. 146). This area has been denominated by the arabic numeral *4*. Cell body staining. In Figure 145, *R* indicates the rostral direction. Figure 146 also illustrates locus ceruleus (lc). Figs 145 and 146 $\times 54$.

MEDULLA SPINALIS

Figs 147–149. Cell body staining in the medulla spinalis.

Fig. 147. Numerous GABAergic neurons are located in the commissural regions of the substantia grisea medullae spinalis (lamina Rexed X) and adjacent regions of lamina Rexed IV. $\times 200$.

Fig. 148. Few GABAergic neurons are scattered in the columna cellularis intermediolateralis (medullae spinalis) (iml) and also in lamina Rexed IX (not shown) among the motoneurons which have numerous pericellular GABAergic boutons. $\times 133$.

Fig. 149. Numerous, small GABAergic neurons are present in cornu dorsalis of laminae Rexed I to III. $\times 333$.

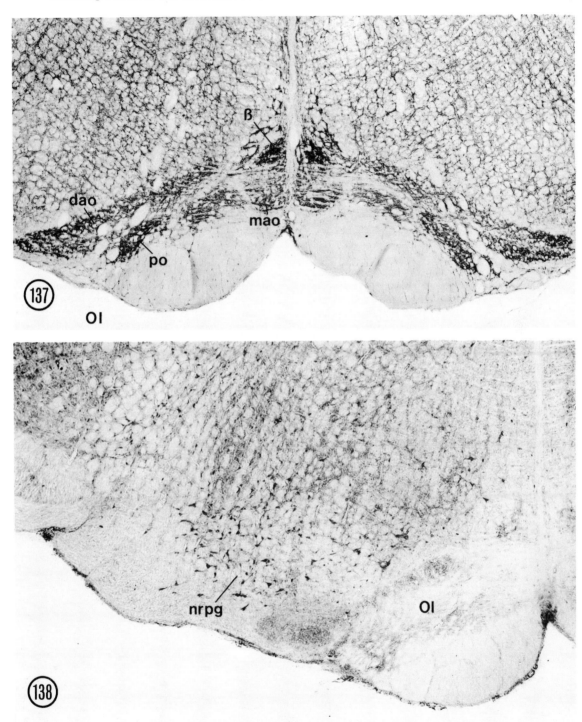

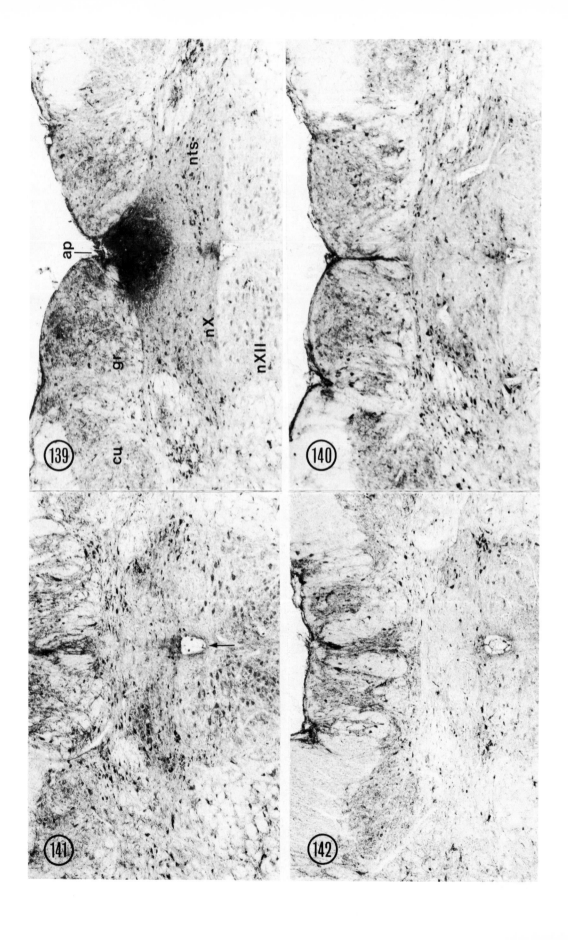

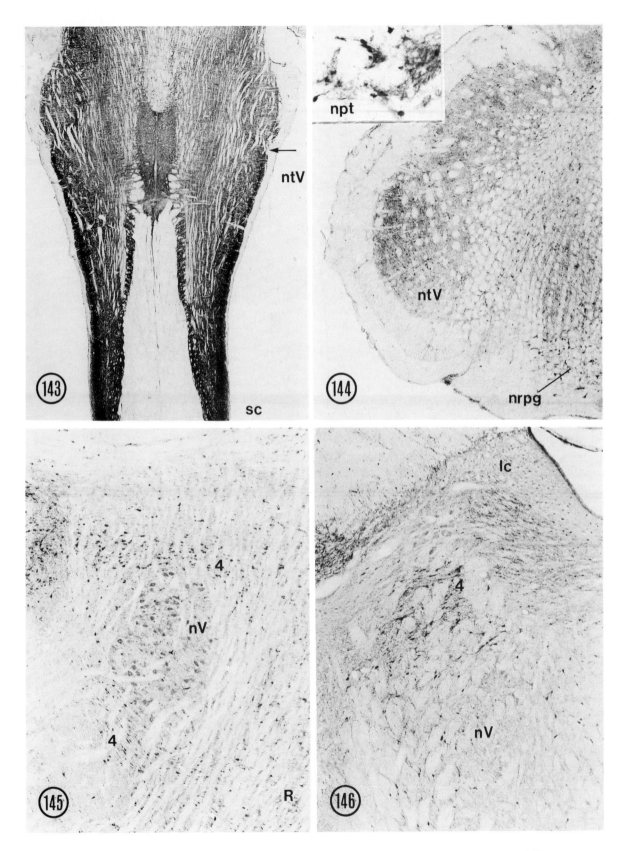

567

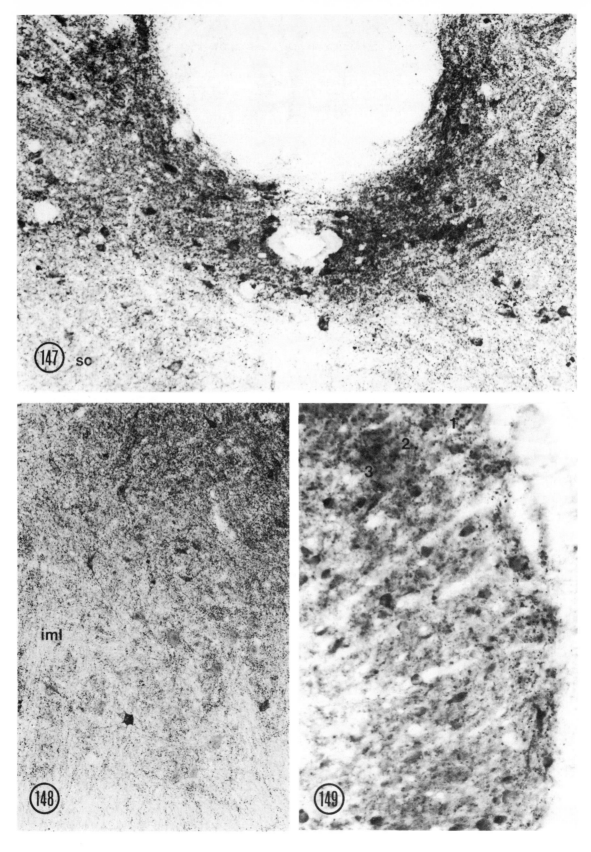

8. DISCUSSION

8.1. CELLULAR LOCALIZATION OF GAD

GAD immunoreactivity has so far been exclusively localized in neuronal profiles in the CNS, in certain neuroendocrine cells in peripheral organs and in some neurons of intestinal ganglia (Mirsky and Jessen, personal communication) (Section 8.11.). Glial cells are devoid of GAD immunoreaction.

Terminal staining: GABAergic axon terminals are easily demonstrated by GAD immunohistochemistry, as GAD is highly concentrated in synaptosomes (Salganikoff and De Robertis 1965). By contrast, axons, cell bodies and dendrites vary substantially in their degree of stainability, depending on cell type, brain area, fixation condition and antiserum employed (Oertel et al. 1983b). Degrees of immunoreactivity presumably reflect different concentrations of GAD enzyme.

Cell bodies: Intense GAD positivity is found in cell bodies and dendrites of neurons without an axon (such as granule cells of the bulbus olfactorius) and neurons provided with an axon and presynaptic dendrites (such as periglomerular cells of the bulbus olfactorius; Ribak et al. 1977; Mugnaini et al. 1984b) (Fig. 29). The level of GAD immunoreactivity ranges from dense to light in 'conventional' neurons with postsynaptic dendrites. Under optimal conditions, the cell bodies and the primary dendrites of a given class of conventional GABAergic neurons are readily visible in most brain regions in untreated animals (Section 4.4.) (Figs 2 (p. 443), 20–24 (pp. 461–465), 73, 74, 75, 111, 121, 125, 149).

Dendritic staining: Certain conventional neurons such as the cerebellar Purkinje cells show dendritic staining (including staining of the spines) also without colchicine pretreatment (Figs 42, 108, 111, 125).

The role of dendritic GAD in these cells is unclear. The enzyme could simply reach the peripheral dendritic branches by diffusion from the cell body without a specific functional correlate or be transported in the dendrites where it could synthesize GABA for release by a non-vesicular mechanism, as has been described for the dopaminergic neurons in the substantia nigra pars compacta (Geffen et al. 1976; Korf et al. 1976; Nieoullon et al. 1977; Wassef et al. 1981).

After topical colchicine injection all GABAergic neurons display GAD-immunoreactive dendrites and this fact facilitates the electron microscopic study of their synaptic connections as shown for the cartwheel neurons of the nucleus cochlearis dorsalis (Mugnaini 1985).

Ultrastructural level: At the ultrastructural level and without the use of colchicine the immunoreaction product is concentrated around synaptic vesicles, the Golgi apparatus, microtubules and mitochondria. This distribution may in part reflect an artifactual displacement of the antigen during and after the fixation.

GAD-IMMUNOREACTIVE CELL BODIES

8.2. TYPOLOGY OF GAD-IMMUNOREACTIVE NEURONS

Utilizing concepts and data of cellular typology already established by Golgi methods, electron microscopy, tract tracing and microelectrode techniques, a typological classification of GABA neurons can be established. GABA neurons can be classified by the morphological features of their cell processes, their internal structure, geometrical ar-rangements, afferent and efferent synaptic connections, and by their participation into circuits as interneurons or projection neurons.

Classifications of GABAergic neurons include amacrine (axonless) type cells, as known to exist in the retina (Brandon et al. 1979; Vaughn et al. 1981; Schnitzer and Rusoff 1985) and in the bulbus olfactorius (Ribak et al. 1977; Mugnaini et al. 1984b). GAD-positive local circuit neurons with presynaptic dendrites and an axon, as mention-ed above, exist for example in the bulbus olfactorius (Ribak et al. 1977; Mugnaini et al. 1984b), in nucleus dorsalis corporis geniculati lateralis (Hendrickson et al. 1983; Oha-ra et al. 1983; Fitzpatrick et al. 1984; Penny et al. 1984), in corpus geniculatum mediale (Adams and Mugnaini 1985c) and in colliculus superior (Houser et al. 1983b). The majority of GABAergic interneurons and GABAergic projection neurons, however, possess conventional, i.e. postsynaptic dendrites and an axon.

The cell body size of GABAergic neurons ranges from microneurons (Ribak et al. 1977; Vaughn et al. 1981; Mugnaini et al. 1984b) to medium-size spiny neurons (Fig. 43) (Ribak et al. 1979b; Oertel and Mugnaini 1984) up to the very large neurons in the nucleus caudalis magnocellularis hypothalami posterioris (Figs 80, 84) (Vincent et al. 1982a; Takeda et al. 1984). GAD-immunoreactive neurons include bipolar, fusiform, multipolar, spiny and aspiny neurons (Ribak 1978; Ribak et al. 1981; Somogyi et al. 1983c; Schmechel et al. 1984).

8.3. LOCAL CIRCUIT NEURONS

At the outset, GABA was considered as a transmitter of inhibitory interneurons. Exam-ples of GABAergic local circuit neurons have already been discussed in Sections 8.1. and 8.2. (see also Table 2). Immunolocalization of GAD in stratified gray matters – such as the bulbus olfactorius, the neocortex, the cortex entorhinalis, the hippocampus, the cortex cerebellaris, the colliculus superior and colliculus inferior, and the nucleus coch-learis dorsalis (for References and Illustrations, see Table 1) – indicate that each layer of these cortical structures is provided with GABAergic local circuit neurons. Golgi studies and electron microscopic data show that these interneurons often have morpho-logical features which are characteristic for each layer. However, in regions such as layer I of neocortex, where nearly all of the scattered cell bodies may represent GABAergic neurons, they even form different morphological subcategories (Schmechel et al. 1984). Thus, the neuronal morphological differentiation of GABAergic interneurons may be independent of the neurochemical transmitter type and may be determined by other fac-tors. A possible general property of neuronal circuits may be that *each major input*, for example to the cerebellum, cortex entorhinalis (see Wouterlood et al. 1985) or cortex occipitalis (visual cortex) *may be modulated by its own subclass of inhibitory interneurons*.

8.4. PROJECTION NEURONS

Known GABAergic projection neurons such as the cerebellar Purkinje cells (Ito and Yoshida 1964; Saito et al. 1974; Oertel et al. 1981d) and the striato-nigral neurons (Kim et al. 1971; Bunney and Aghajanian 1976; Ribak et al. 1980; Oertel and Mugnaini 1984) were thought to present the exception to the rule that GABA is a transmitter of inter-neurons. Over the last few years, however, other classes of GABAergic projection neu-rons have been discovered, for example in the basal ganglia (Penney and Young 1981), the hypothalamus (Vincent et al. 1982a) or the nuclei cerebellares (Nelson et al. 1984). In Table 3 examples of established GABAergic projection neurons are referenced.

TABLE 2. *Examples of GAD-immunoreactive interneurons*

Brain region	Cell type	Reference
Retina	amacrine cell	28, 29, 210, 242
Bulbus olfactorius	periglomerular cell	139, 140, 189, 191
	granule cell	
	short axon cell	
Cortex entorhinalis	non-pyramidal	260
Neocortex	non-pyramidal:	56, 79, 82, 89, 190,
	spiny and sparsely spiny	209, 216, 217, (219),
	axo-axonic cell	221, 257
	bitufted cell	
	basket-cell type	
	(double bouquet cell)	
Hippocampus	non-pyramidal:	58, 114, 161, 191, 209,
	axo-axonic cell	213, 218, 221, 245
	basket cell type	
Striatum	? medium-to-large	26, 166
	(aspiny) cell	
Thalamus		
Nucleus dorsalis corporis geniculati lateralis	small neuron	50, 80, 168, 180
Nucleus centralis corporis geniculati medialis	small neuron	5
Colliculus superior		90
Colliculus inferior		203, 244
Cerebellum	stellate cell	159, 161, 191, 205
	basket cell	
	Golgi cell	
Nucleus cochlearis dorsalis and ventralis	stellate cell cartwheel cell	2,141
Medulla spinalis		17,93

TABLE 3. *Examples of established and hypothetical (?) GAD-immunoreactive projection neurons*

Brain region	Projection to	References
Hippocampus		
Gyrus dentatus	? gyrus dentatus contralateralis	213
BASAL GANGLIA AND AMYGDALA COMPLEX		
*Striatum**		
N. caudatus/putamen	globus pallidus	41, 53, 66, 69, 107, 144,
	n. entopeduncularis	156, 166, 176, 185, 193,
	substantia nigra	194, 231
N. accumbens	globus pallidus	44, 102, 251,
	? pallidum ventrale	253, 270
	? substantia nigra	
	? area ventralis tegmenti	
? Tuberculum olfactorium		47 (132)

*Medium size spiny projection neurons in striatum possess extensive local axon collaterals (185).

TABLE 3 (*continued*)

Amygdala complex
  ? N. amygdaloideus centralis   ? n. interstitialis striae   14, 22, 30, 117, 122, 165,
                                    terminalis   167a, 211
                                    ? n. motorius dorsalis n.X
                                    ?n. tractus solitarius
  ? N. amygdaloideus medialis   ? n. ventromedialis hypothalami

Septum and diagonal band
  ? N. septi lateralis   ? n. septi medialis   232
                         ? diagonal band of Broca
  ? N. septalis fimbrialis   ? n.habenulae lateralis   232
  ? N. tractus diagonalis (Broca)   ? bulbus olfactorius   271
  ? N. interstitialis striae terminalis   ? n. tractus solitarii   121, 211

Pallidum
  Globus pallidus   n. subthalamicus   10, 30a, 54, 66, 69, 76,
                 n. ventralis anterior thalami   119a, 146, 167, 178,
                 n. ventralis lateralis thalami   204, 225, 226, 241
                 ? striatum
                 ? subst. nigra pars compacta
  N. entopeduncularis   n. habenulae lateralis   30a, 64, 143
                 ? n. ventromedialis thalami
                 ? n. pedunculopontinus tegmentalis
  Pallidum ventrale   n. mediodorsalis thalami   47, (132), 185a, 268
  substantia nigra pars   colliculus superior   34, 35, 36, 42, 43, 87,
  reticulata   ? formatio reticularis   106, 227, 246
                 ? n. parafascicularis thalami
                 n. ventromedialis thalami
                 ? tectum
                 ? tegmentum

Thalamus
  N. reticularis thalami   n. reticularis thalami contralateralis   57, 80, 88, 103, 163, 208
                 other thalamic nuclei
  ? Zona incerta   ? some thalamic nuclei   97, 198, 255
                 ? some hypothalamic nuclei
                 ? tectum
                 ? tegmentum
                 ? pons
                 ? oliva inferior
                 ? medulla oblongata

Hypothalamus
  ? Area preoptica   ? nuclei hypothalamici   39
  N. caudalis magnocellularis   neocortex   233, 250
  hypothalami posterioris   ? striatum
  Centro-hypophyseal neuron   lobus anterior, pars intermedia   160
                 lobus posterior (pars nervosa) of the hypophysis

Mesencephalon
  ? N. tractus optici   ? oliva inferior   104a
                 ? n. reticularis tegmenti pontis   125a
  ? N. terminalis tractus optici   ? caudal part of the ipsi-

TABLE 3 (*continued*)

accessorii (pars dorsalis)	lateral dorsal cap of the oliva inferior	
(pars medialis)	nuclei pretectales	23a
? N. dorsalis lemnisci lateralis	colliculus inferior contralateralis	1
? N. interpeduncularis	? area (n.) tegmenti dorsalis ? raphe dorsalis raphe magnus	68
Cerebellum		
Cortex cerebellaris	n. cerebellares	51, 52, 91, 95, 153, 159,
(Purkinje cell)	n. vestibularis lateralis	205
N. lateralis cerebelli	oliva inferior	150
N. interpositus cerebelli	oliva inferior	150
Substantia grisea centralis		
? N. accessorius Darkschewitsch	? oliva inferior	31, 243
? N. tegmenti dorsalis	? n. interpeduncularis	67
(area tegm. dorsalis)	? n. mamillares ? n. anterior thalami ? n. medialis thalami	
Rhombencephalon		
? N. vestibularis medialis	n. III, n. IV	152, 154, 184, 203a

The localization of many other GAD-immunoreactive neurons in areas of the forebrain and the brainstem – in the nucleus amygdaloideus centralis (Oertel et al. 1983c; Oertel and Mugnaini 1985), the zona incerta (Oertel et al. 1982c), in the nuclei terminales tractus optici accessorii (Penny et al. 1984; Ottersen and Storm-Mathisen 1984c), the nucleus interpeduncularis, the nucleus dorsalis lemnisci lateralis (Adams and Mugnaini 1984a), the nucleus accessorius Darkschewitsch (Penny et al. 1984), the oliva superior (Adams and Mugnaini 1985a), in the vestibular nuclei (Nomura et al. 1984), and the nucleus raphe magnus – suggests that these GABA neurons are valid candidates for additional projection neurons.

Such areas that *potentially* contain GABAergic projection neurons are included in Table 3 and are indicated by a question mark ('?'). The respective literature on tracing methods is listed.

A combination of available labeling techniques with immunohistochemistry is required in each case to test the nature of individual GABAergic cell classes. Nevertheless, even in the absence of a complete list, *the notion that GABAergic neurons represent predominantly local circuit neurons can now definitely be dispelled.*

Morphologically, projection neurons can be subdivided into projection neurons with extensive, or widespread axon collaterals, as found in the striatum (Preston et al. 1980; Ribak et al. 1981), and projection neurons with relatively scarce or highly concentrated axon collaterals, for example the Purkinje cell.

Some GABAergic projection neurons have a large cell body size (cerebellar Purkinje cell, principal cell of the nucleus caudalis magnocellularis hypothalami posterioris (Vincent et al. 1982a)). Other projection neurons are of medium size (striatal medium size spiny neurons; Ribak et al. 1979b; Oertel and Mugnaini 1984) and some of the proven GABAergic projection neurons are even small (cerebello-olivary projection neuron;

Nelson et al. 1984). *Cell size, therefore, cannot be taken as a general differential criterion between GABAergic local circuit and projection neurons.*

8.5. BRAIN AREAS WITH A HIGH OR LOW PROPORTION OF GABAERGIC NEURONS

Mapping of GABA neurons in rat brain has revealed that some brain areas contain a high proportion of GABAergic neurons (Table 4). Striking examples are: the bulbus olfactorius (Ribak et al. 1977; Mugnaini et al. 1984b), the cortex cerebellaris (Ribak et al. 1978; Oertel et al. 1981d, 1982b), the nucleus reticularis thalami (Houser et al. 1980; Oertel et al. 1983a), and the nucleus dorsalis lemnisci lateralis (Adams and Mugnaini 1984a), as in these regions nearly all members of certain cell classes exhibit GAD-like immunoreactivity; furthermore, the vast majority of the neurons in the striatum (Oertel and Mugnaini 1984), the nucleus amygdaloideus centralis (Oertel et al. 1983c; Oertel and Mugnaini 1985) and the nucleus amygdaloideus medialis (Oertel and Mugnaini 1985), the pallidum including the substantia nigra pars reticulata (Oertel et al. 1984), the nuclei terminales tractus optici accessorii (Penny et al. 1984), and certain subdivisions of the superior olivary complex or of the nucleus interpeduncularis appear GAD-positive.

Moreover, high densities of GAD-positive neurons sharing significant features such as cell body size, dendritic arborization and types of dendritic appendages, allow to subsume several topographically related nuclei under a common denominator as e.g.:

Striatum and striatum-like areas: Figs (36, 39) 43, 54, 55, 58, 59, 72
The nucleus amygdaloideus centralis and medialis and the massae intercalatae share the types and density of GAD-immunoreactive cell bodies with the 'classical' striatal areas, i.e. the nucleus caudatus/putamen, the nucleus accumbens and the tuberculum olfactorium (Heimer 1978; Oertel and Mugnaini 1985). These three amygdaloid areas are, therefore, considered as a part of the striatum (striatum-like). Striatum-like density of GAD-immunoreactive cell bodies are also found in the nucleus septi lateralis (Fig. 39) and the nucleus interstitialis striae terminalis (Fig. 36) including the 'bed of the stria terminalis' (Johnston 1923) (see Section 8.6.).

Pallidum: Figs 44, 45, 47, 48, 49, 50, 53
The regions globus pallidus, the nucleus entopeduncularis, the pallidum ventrale (Heimer et al. 1982) and the substantia nigra pars reticulata are suggested to constitute the 'pallidial system', as their neurons share cytological features and the vast majority of these neurons are GAD-immunoreactive (Oertel and Mugnaini 1984). The substantia nigra pars reticulata is contiguous with the zona incerta pars lateralis (Figs 64, 70, 71). The zona incerta pars lateralis is contiguous with the nucleus reticularis thalami as well as with the pars parvocellularis of the nucleus ventralis corporis geniculati lateralis. These latter brain regions also consist predominantly of GAD-immunoreactive neurons (Fig. 67). At present, however, the significance of this observation is unclear.

Similarly, the nucleus parafascicularis pars posterior and parts of the nucleus subparafascicularis may be subsumed under the denominator 'substantia grisea centralis' (periaquaeductal gray) (see Section 8.6.; Fig. 62).

On the other hand, numerous brain areas are characterized by a very low number of GAD-immunoreactive neurons such as the nuclei mamillares (Figs 20, 73, 121), the nucleus reticularis lateralis, the cranial (Figs 121, 122, 139–142, 145, 146) and spinal motor nuclei and most of the rat thalamic nuclei (Figs 21, 61) (but see Section 8.10. for

TABLE 4. *Summary of brain areas rich (Grade 4 and 5) in GABAergic cell bodies*

BULBUS OLFACTORIUS, RHINENCEPHALON

LG	lamina glomerulosa bulbi olfactorii
LGR	lamina granularis bulbi olfactorii

NEOCORTEX, PALEOCORTEX AND ARCHICORTEX

Neocortex
Lamina moleculare (I)
Substantia alba subcorticalis

Hippocampus
Stratum oriens
Stratum radiatum
Stratum lacunosum-moleculare
Stratum moleculare gyri dentati
Hilus gyri dentati

BASAL GANGLIA AND AMYGDALA COMPLEX

Striatum

a*	n. accumbens
cp(*)	n. caudatus/putamen
iC	insula Calleja (granule cell clusters)
iCm	insula Calleja magna (granule cell clusters)
tu	tuberculum olfactorium

Amygdala complex (striatum-like)

ac(*)	n. amygdaloideus centralis
am(*)	n. amygdaloideus medialis
mi*	massae intercalatae

Striatum-like areas, see also SEPTUM AND DIAGONAL BAND OF BROCA

Pallidum

ep	n. entopeduncularis
gp	globus pallidus
iC	insula Calleja (cap region)
iCm	insula Calleja magna (cap region)
npp	n. peripeduncularis
snr	substantia nigra pars reticulata
vp	pallidum ventrale

SEPTUM AND DIAGONAL BAND OF BROCA

Striatum-like

nist*	n. interstitialis striae terminalis
nistd*	n. interstitialis striae terminalis dorsalis
nistv*	n. interstitialis striae terminalis ventralis
sl*	n. septi lateralis
sf	n. septalis fimbrialis
shi	n. septohippocampalis
shy	n. septohypothalamicus
sm	n. septi medialis (Grade 3–4)
tdh	n. tractus diagonalis pars horizontalis (Grade 3–4)
tdv	n. tractus diagonalis pars ventralis (Grade 3–4)

THALAMUS

pf	see SUBSTANTIA GRISEA CENTRALIS
spf	see SUBSTANTIA GRISEA CENTRALIS

---

* = colchicine pretreatment necessary for reliable scoring of cell body density.

TABLE 4 (*continued*)

tr	n. reticularis thalami
vcgl	*n. ventralis corporis geniculati lateralis*
vcglmc	n. ventralis corporis geniculati lateralis, pars magnocellularis
vcglpc	n. ventralis corporis geniculati lateralis, pars parvocellularis

SUBTHALAMUS

zi	zona incerta [see tr, THALAMUS]

HYPOTHALAMUS

AHD	area hypothalamica dorsalis
AHL	area hypothalamica lateralis, pars intermedialis
cmc	n. caudalis magnocellularis hypothalami posterioris
na	n. arcuatus
ndmv	n. dorsomedialis hypothalami, pars ventralis
pef	n. perifornicalis (Grade 3–4)
pom	n. preopticus medialis
pos	n. preopticus suprachiasmaticus
tmc	n. tuberalis magnocellularis hypothalami posterioris
[smt]	n. supramamillothalamicus	in the mammillary complex only these two nuclei contain cell
[sum]	n. supramamillaris	bodies with a density Grade 2 and therefore stand out in this nuclear complex (*cf.* Table 5)

MESENCEPHALON

Dnll	n. dorsalis lemnisci lateralis
ipc	n. interpeduncularis pars centralis
ipp	n. interpeduncularis pars paramedianus (lateralis)
opt	n. olivaris praetectalis
pl	n. paralemniscalis
toa	n. terminalis tractus optici accessorii
toad	n. terminalis tractus optici accessorii, pars dorsalis
toal	n. terminalis tractus optici accessorii, pars lateralis
toam	n. terminalis tractus optici accessorii, pars medialis
tol	n. tractus optici, pars lateralis
tom	n. tractus optici, pars medialis
1	area commissuralis colliculi superioris and inferioris (Grade 3–4)

SUBSTANTIA GRISEA CENTRALIS

aD	n. accessorius Darkschewitsch
ntd	n. tegmenti dorsalis, pars rostralis
ntv	n. tegmenti ventralis, pars rostralis
pf	n. parafascicularis pars caudalis (posterior to fasciculus retroflexus) (*cf.* Table 5, THALAMUS)
spf	n. subparafascicularis

ORGANA CIRCUMVENTRICULARIA

ap	area postrema

CEREBELLUM

1	small celled part of n. lateralis cerebelli
mol	basket cells, stellate cells
pcl	Purkinje cells
	[Golgi cells]

576

TABLE 4 (*continued*)

RHOMBENCEPHALON

ltz	n. lateralis corporis trapezoidei
nts	n. tractus solitarius
ph	n. prepositus hypoglossi (Grade 3–4)
spn	n. paraolivaris superior
vm (r)	n. vestibularis medialis, pars rostralis
vm (c)	n. vestibularis medialis, pars caudalis
vsp	n. vestibularis spinalis
y	pars 'y' nucleorum vestibulorum
4	area supra/retrotrigeminalis n. motorii nervi trigemini
6	area reticularis paratrigeminalis ventralis (Grade 3–4)
7	area parapyramidalis ['B1–lateral']

FORMATIO RETICULARIS

nrpc	n. reticularis parvocellularis, pars caudalis (Grade 3)
nrpg	n. reticularis paragigantocellularis
pl	nucleus paralemniscalis
RR	area retrorubralis (Grade 3–4)
2	area parvocellularis paramedianus tegmentalis (Grade 3–4)
3	area parvocellularis parareticularis tegmentalis (Grade 3–4)
5	area reticularis subhypoglossus (Grade 3–4)

RAPHE NUCLEI

rli	n. raphe linearis, pars supramamillaris (Grade 3)
rm	n. raphe magnus, pars caudalis
rp	n. raphe pallidus, pars rostralis

MEDULLA SPINALIS

I-III	lamina Rexed I–III (Grade 3)
X	lamina Rexed X (Grade 3)

TABLE 5. *Summary of brain areas poor (Grade 0, 1 and 1–2) in GABAergic cell bodies (white matter not considered)*

BULBUS OLFACTORIUS, RHINENCEPHALON

LMA	lamina cellularum mitralium bulbi olfactorii accessorii
LP	lamina plexiformis externa bulbi olfactorii

BASAL GANGLIA AND AMYGDALA COMPLEX

bac	bed nucleus of the anterior commissure (Grade 1–2)
rmc	n. ruber pars magnocellularis
snc	substantia nigra pars compacta
sut	n. subthalamicus

EPITHALAMUS

hl	n. habenulae lateralis
hm	n. habenulae medialis

TABLE 5 (*continued*)

THALAMUS

cgm	*n. centralis corporis geniculati medialis*
cgmd	n. centr. corp. gen. med. pars dorsalis
cgmm	n. centr. corp. gen. med. pars medialis
cgmv	n. centr. corp. gen. med. pars ventralis
cm	n. centromedianus thalami
g	n. gelatinosus thalami
intg	n. intermedialis corporis geniculati
	(intermediate geniculate nucleus)
pf	n. parafascicularis pars rostralis (anterior to fasciculus retroflexus)
	(*cf.* Table 4, SUBSTANTIA GRISEA CENTRALIS)
pt	n. parataenialis
pv	n. paraventricularis
re	n. reuniens
rh	n. rhomboideus
sgt	n. suprageniculatus thalami
tad	n. anterior dorsalis thalami
tam	n. anterior medialis thalami
tav	n. anterior ventralis thalami
tl	n. lateralis thalami
tlp	n. lateralis thalami, pars posterior
tm	n. medialis thalami
tml	n. medialis thalami, pars lateralis
tmm	n. medialis thalami, pars medialis
tpo	n. posterior thalami
tv	n. ventralis thalami
tvl	n. ventrolateralis thalami
tvm	n. ventralis medialis thalami, pars magnocellularis
tvpl	n. ventroposterior lateralis thalami
tvpm	n. ventroposterior medialis thalami
tvppc	n. ventroposterior thalami, pars parvocellularis

HYPOTHALAMUS

AHL	area hypothalamica lateralis, pars caudalis
em	eminentia mediana
hy	hypophysis
ml	n. mamillaris lateralis
mml	n. mamillaris medialis, pars lateralis
mmm	n. mamillaris medialis, pars medialis
mmn	n. mamillaris medialis, pars medianus
mmp	n. mamillaris medialis, pars posterior
ndmc	n. dorsomedialis hypothalami, pars compacta
npmd	n. praemamillaris dorsalis
npmv	n. praemamillaris ventralis
npvm	n. paraventricularis hypothalami, pars magnocellularis
nso	n. supraopticus
nvm	n. ventromedialis hypothalami

MESENCEPHALON

dVnll	n. ventralis lemnisci lateralis, pars dorsalis	
ipa	n. interpeduncularis, pars apicalis	(Grade 2 (low cell body density compared to
ipip	n. interpeduncularis, pars inferior posterior	ipc and ipp))
N III	n. originis nervi oculomotorii	
N IV	n. originis nervi trochlearis	

TABLE 5 (*continued*)

pbg	n. parabigeminalis
pptg	n. pedunculopontinus tegmentalis
rmc	see BASAL GANGLIA AND AMYGDALA COMPLEX
SAM	stratum album mediale colliculi superioris
snc	see BASAL GANGLIA AND AMYGDALA COMPLEX

ORGANA CIRCUMVENTRICULARIA

ovlt	organum vasculosum laminae terminalis
pin	corpus pineale
sco	organum subcommissurale

CEREBELLUM

m	n. medialis cerebelli

RHOMBENCEPHALON

cov	n. cochlearis ventralis
cul	n. cuneatus lateralis
lc	locus ceruleus
mtz	n. medialis corporis trapezoidei
nRo	n. Roller
OI	oliva inferior
osm	n. olivaris superior, pars medialis
pbv	n. parabrachialis ventralis
po	n. pontis
sg	n. suprageniculatus facialis

RHOMBENCEPHALON – NUCLEI MOTORII CRANIALES

amb	n. ambiguus
N V	n. originis nervi trigemini
Np V	n. sensorius principalis nervi trigemini
Nt Vd	n. tractus spinalis nervi trigemini, pars dorsomedialis
N VI	n. originis nervi abducentis
N VII	n. originis nervi facialis
N X	n. originis nervi vagi (dorsal motor nucleus N X)
N XII	n. originis nervi hypoglossi
vl	n. vestibularis lateralis

FORMATIO RETICULARIS

nrd	n. reticularis medullae oblongatae, pars dorsalis
nrgc	n. reticularis gigantocellularis (Grade 1–2)
nrp	n. reticularis paramedianus
nrpc	n. reticularis parvocellularis, pars rostralis
nrv	n. reticularis medullae oblongatae, pars ventralis
rl	n. reticularis lateralis
rpoc	n. reticularis pontis, pars caudalis
rtp	n. reticularis tegmenti pontis

RAPHE NUCLEI

rd	n. raphe dorsalis
rpo	n. raphe pontis (Grade 1–2)

TABLE 5 (*continued*)

MEDULLA SPINALIS	
CeC	n. centralis cervicalis
d	n. dorsalis (medullae spinalis)
iml	columna cellularis intermediolateralis
IV	lamina Rexed IV (pars lateralis)
VIII	lamina Rexed VIII
IX	lamina Rexed IX

species difference in respect to the number of GABAergic thalamic interneurons).

Brain areas with a high proportion of GABAergic neurons (Grade 4 and 5) are listed in Table 4 and those with a low proportion of GABAergic neurons (Grade 0, 1, and 1–2) in Table 5. The above-mentioned common denominators have been used as sub-headings in these tables.

8.5.1. Nameless regions with a high density of GAD-immunoreactive neurons

Concentrations of GABAergic neurons exist in several regions that at present can be qualified only by their topographic situation. These discrete pools of GAD-positive neurons are particularly notable in poorly defined territories such as the region of the medial forebrain bundle, the 'substantia innominata', the hypothalamus, the ansa lenticularis, the anterior amygdaloid area, the substantia grisea centralis (periaqueductal gray matter), the area pretectalis, the peripeduncular zones and especially in the formatio reticularis. Some of these neuronal pools have been subsumed tentatively, and not necessarily correctly, into nuclei defined by the atlas to which we have adhered. Others, more difficult to allocate are listed on page 501 at the end of Table 1. The terms used by no means represent an attempt to introduce a new terminology but serve only the practical purpose to define topographically the regions pointed out by *arabic numerals* in the atlas drawings. In certain cases, these discrete GABAergic neuronal pools seem to be closely associated with other neurons to suggest a particular function. For example, area 4 ('area supra/retrotrigeminalis') (Figs 145, 146) and area 5 ('area reticularis subhypoglossa') (Fig. 122) are associated with motoneurons. Area 3 ('area parvocellularis parareticularis tegmenti') seems to be continuous with a lateral portion of nucleus interpeduncularis (Fig. 121). Furthermore, area 7 (area parapyramidalis) corresponds in location to the 'B1-lateral' area of serotonin-containing neurons (see Chapter III, *Vol. 3*, This Series). The significance of these GABAergic neuronal pools remains a matter of speculation.

GAD-IMMUNOREACTIVE TERMINALS

8.6. DENSITY OF GAD-IMMUNOREACTIVE AXON TERMINALS

A survey of the map presented above demonstrates the tremendous variation in GAD-positive axon terminal density. On the other hand, it emphasizes the existence of areas with much higher and much lower density of GAD-immunoreactive terminals and GABAergic nerve cell bodies than the average density. For schematic purposes these brain areas with a high (Grade 4 and 5) or low (Grade 0–1 and 1–2) density of axon terminals are listed in Tables 6 and 7.

TABLE 6. *Summary of brain areas rich (Grade 4 and 5) in GABAergic axon terminals*

BULBUS OLFACTORIUS, RHINENCEPHALON

LG	lamina glomerulosa bulbi olfactorii
LMA	lamina cellularum mitralium bulbi olfactorii accessorii
LP	lamina plexiformis externa bulbi olfactorii

BASAL GANGLIA AND AMYGDALA COMPLEX

	Striatum
a	n. accumbens (Grade 3–4)
tu	tuberculum olfactorium
	Amygdala complex
ac	n. amygdaloideus centralis (Grade 3–4)
am	n. amygdaloideus medialis
mi	massae intercalatae
	Pallidum
ep	n. entopeduncularis
gp	globus pallidus
iC	insula Calleja (cap region)
iCm	insula Calleja magna (cap region)
npp	n. peripeduncularis (Grade 3–4)
snl	substantia nigra pars lateralis
snr	substantia nigra pars reticulata
vp	pallidum ventrale

SEPTUM AND DIAGONAL BAND

	Striatum-like
nist	n. interstitialis striae terminalis
nistd	n. interstitialis striae terminalis dorsalis
nistv	n. interstitialis striae terminalis ventralis
sl	n. septi lateralis
nbm	n. basalis magnocellularis (Meynert) (Grade 3–4)
shi	n. septohippocampalis
shy	n. septohypothalamicus
sm	n. septi medialis (Grade 3–4)

THALAMUS

pf	see SUBSTANTIA GRISEA CENTRALIS
vcgl	n. ventralis corporis geniculati lateralis

HYPOTHALAMUS

AHD	area hypothalamica dorsalis (Grade 3–4)
ar	area retrochiasmatica
cmc	n. caudalis magnocellularis hypothalami posterioris
em	eminentia mediana pars externa
hpe	n. periventricularis hypothalami (Grade 3–4)
na	n. arcuatus
ndmd	n. dorsomedialis hypothalami pars dorsalis (Grade 3–4)
ndmv	n. dorsomedialis hypothalami pars ventralis
nha	n. hypothalamicus anterior
npl	n. mamillaris prelateralis
nsc	n. suprachiasmaticus (Grade 3–5)
pef	n. perifornicalis
pom	n. preopticus medialis

TABLE 6 (*continued*)

pos	n. preopticus suprachiasmaticus
smt	n. submamillothalamicus (Grade 3–4)
sum	n. supramamillaris
tmc	n. tuberalis magnocellularis hypothalami posterioris

MESENCEPHALON

Dnll	n. dorsalis lemnisci lateralis (Grade 3–4)
ipc	n. interpeduncularis pars centralis
ipip	n. interpeduncularis pars inferior posterior
pl	n. paralemniscalis
sgs	stratum griseum superficiale colliculi superioris
toad	n. terminalis tractus optici accessorii divisio dorsalis
toal	n. terminalis tractus optici accessorii divisio lateralis
toam	n. terminalis tractus optici accessorii divisio medialis
tol	n. tractus optici, pars lateralis
tom	n. tractus optici, pars medialis

SUBSTANTIA GRISEA CENTRALIS

[hpe	n. periventricularis hypothalami (see HYPOTHALAMUS)]
pf	n. parafascicularis pars caudalis (posterior to fasciculus retroflexus) (Grade 3–4)
[ph	n. prepositus hypoglossi (see RHOMBENCEPHALON)]
[pv	n. paraventricularis thalami (Grade 3–4)]
SGC	substantia grisea centralis (Grade 3)
[X	lamina Rexed X, substantia grisea centralis medullae spinalis, see MEDULLA SPINALIS

ORGANA CIRCUMVENTRICULARIA

ap	area postrema
sfo	organum subfornicale

CEREBELLUM

cn	nuclei cerebellares
i (a, p)	n. interpositus pars anterior and posterior
l	n. lateralis cerebelli including small celled part of n. lateralis cerebelli
m	n. medialis cerebelli
pcl	lamina cellularum Purkinje cerebelli

RHOMBENCEPHALON

ltz	n. lateralis corporis trapezoidei
nts	n. tractus solitarii (Grade 3–4)
OI	oliva inferior
ph	n. prepositus hypoglossus
sgv	n. tractus spinalis nervi trigemini, substantia gelatinosa
vl	n. vestibularis lateralis, pars dorsalis caudalis
vm	n. vestibularis medialis
y	pars 'y' nucleorum vestibulorum
7	area parapyramidalis ['B1–lateral']

RAPHE NUCLEI

rp	n. raphe pallidus, pars ventralis

MEDULLA SPINALIS

I	lamina Rexed I (Grade 3–4)
IIb, IIIa	laminae Rexed IIb and IIIa
IV	lamina Rexed IV
X	lamina Rexed X (Grade 3–4)

The distribution of GAD terminals – and also of GABAergic cell bodies (Section 8.5) – *often follows anatomical borders* and thus may facilitate the topographic identification of brain structures.

Cortical areas: Figs 5–11, 21, 22, 32
The borders of most subregions of the cortical areas are clearly demonstrated by variations in the densities of the terminals (see for example Figs 11, 32). Cortical areas including the hippocampal formation in general have a low-to-medium (Grade 2–3) density of GAD-positive terminals. In addition, those subnuclei of the amygdaloid complex thought to be of cortical origin – such as the nucleus amygdaloideus lateralis – also possess a similar low-to-medium density of terminals (Figs 8, 56, 68) as do the claustrum and the nucleus entorhinalis (Fig. 26).

Striatum and striatum-like areas: Figs 6, 7, 8, 22, 35, 56, 68
A medium-to-high density (Grade 3–4) is found in the striatal areas (Table 6) and is characteristic also for areas such as the nucleus amygdaloideus centralis, nucleus amygdaloideus medialis, the massae intercalatae, the nucleus septi lateralis and the nucleus interstitialis striae terminalis. Thus, according to the density of GAD-immunoreactive terminals – and cell body density (Section 8.5) – these areas are very similar to the striatal areas and have, therefore, been termed striatum-like areas (Tables 4 and 6).

Pallidum: Figs 7, 8, 44, 45, 52, 53, 54, 56
A very high density of large terminals is observed in the nuclei of the pallidum, including the deep fibrocellular layer of the pallidum ventrale dorsal to the tuberculum olfactorium, the so-called 'cap region' of the islands of Calleja (insula Callejae) and perhaps also parts of the area amygdaloidea anterior.

Thalamus-Hypothalamus: Figs 8, 9, 60, 63, 64, 69
In rat brain, the thalamus in general stands out as an area of low terminal density, as most thalamic nuclei express a very low to low density of terminals. This is in sharp contrast to the neighboring zona incerta and hypothalamus (Fig. 64) with their medium-to-high density of small terminals. Within the thalamus, the nuclei located at the midline (nucleus paraventricularis thalami, nucleus paratenialis, nucleus rhomboideus and nucleus reuniens) contain a higher terminal density (Grade 2–3) and are combined in a compartment that appears continuous at certain frontal planes where it assumes an 'hour-glass' shape (Fig. 68).

Substantia grisea centralis: Figs 10, 22, 63, 68, 92, 133, 143, 147
The periventricular regions are characterized by a medium-to-high density of axon terminals (Grade 3–4). Rostrally, they begin with the nucleus paraventricularis thalami and the nucleus periventricularis hypothalami (Fig. 68). They continue with the nucleus parafascicularis pars posterior (posterior to the fasciculus retroflexus) as the most rostral aspect of the periaquaeductal gray. The periventricular regions also include the nucleus tegmenti dorsalis (Gudden) (Figs 22, 121) and extend caudally via the nucleus vestibularis medialis (Fig. 133) and the nucleus prepositus hypoglossi (Fig. 122) to the substantia grisea centralis medullae spinalis (lamina Rexed X) (Figs 143, 147).

Nuclei cerebellares:
A high to very high density of mostly intensely stained axon terminals is characteristic for the nuclei cerebellares and the nucleus vestibularis lateralis (Figs 127, 128).

TABLE 7. *Summary of brain areas poor (Grade 0–1, 1 and 1–2) in GABAergic axon terminals (white matter with Grade 0 and 0–1 not considered)*

EPITHALAMUS

hm	n. habenulae medialis

THALAMUS

cgmd	n. centralis corporis geniculati medialis, pars dorsalis
cm	n. centromedianus thalami
g	n. gelatinosus thalami
intg	n. intermedialis corporis geniculati
pf	n. parafascicularis, pars anterior (anterior to fasciculus retroflexus)
tam	n. anterior medialis thalami
tav	n. anterior ventralis thalami
tl	n. lateralis thalami, pars caudalis
tlp	n. lateralis thalami, pars posterior
tm	n. medialis thalami
tml	n. medialis thalami, pars lateralis
tmm	n. medialis thalami, pars medialis
tpo	n. posterior thalami
tv	n. ventralis thalami
tvl	n. ventrolateralis thalami
tvm	n. ventromedialis thalami
tvpl	n. ventroposterior lateralis thalami
tvpm	n. ventroposterior medialis thalami
tvppc	n. ventroposterior thalami, pars parvocellularis

HYPOTHALAMUS

CSD	commissura supraoptica dorsalis
hy, pd	hypophysis, lobus anterior, pars distalis
ml	n. mamillaris lateralis, pars dorsalis

MESENCEPHALON

SAM	stratum album mediale colliculi superioris
SO	stratum opticum colliculi superioris

ORGANA CIRCUMVENTRICULARIA

pin	corpus pineale
sco	organum subcommissurale

FORMATIO RETICULARIS

nrgc	n. reticularis gigantocellularis (Grade 1–2)
rl	n. reticularis lateralis
rpoc	n. reticularis pontis caudalis

RHOMBENCEPHALON

pbd	n. parabrachialis dorsalis (Grade 1–2)
sg	n. suprageniculatus facialis
vl	n. vestibularis lateralis pars rostralis

MEDULLA SPINALIS

FDL	fasciculus dorsalis lateralis (medullae spinalis)
VII	lamina Rexed VII (Grade 1–2)
VIII	lamina Rexed VIII
IX	lamina Rexed IX

Density gradients: Figs 27, 29

Density gradients of GAD-positive dendritic presynaptic contacts are observed in the lamina plexiformis externa bulbi olfactorii and in the lamina granularis bulbi olfactorii with a higher density at the superficial parts. For tubercule-like distributions, see Figs 63, 68 and Section 8.7.

In several instances, a brain region with a low density of GAD-positive axon terminals *borders* a brain area with a high density of GAD-immunoreactive axon terminals. Especially striking are the border of the nucleus amygdaloideus centralis versus the nucleus amygdaloideus lateralis (Figs 8, 56) and the border of the thalamus proper versus the zona incerta and the preoptic/pretectal area (Figs 21, 22, 60, 61).

8.7. DISTRIBUTION PATTERNS OF GAD-IMMUNOREACTIVE TERMINALS

In addition to variations in their densities (Tables 6 and 7), the immunoreactive terminals show specific patterns that characterize well-defined regions because of the particular size of the terminals, their mode of distribution, or the relations between terminal fibers and target profiles.

Bands of terminals: In the retina, the GAD-immunoreactive punctate profiles form 7 to 9 bands in the inner nuclear layer (Vaughn et al. 1981). Other bands of terminals are seen in the nucleus olfactorius anterior and in the stratum moleculare gyri dentati.

Cluster patterns: These are rare. Cluster patterns are observed in the glomeruli of the bulbus olfactorius, in certain thalamic nuclei, the corpus geniculatum mediale (Adams and Mugnaini 1985c), the lamina granularis cerebelli (Figs 125, 126), the nuclei cochleares (Figs 114, 117) and the oliva inferior (Mugnaini et al. 1982).

Axonal perisomatic arrays: Axosomatic GABAergic boutons surround and represent a very prominent input to the following cell bodies:

– the pyramidal cells (including the initial axon segment) of lamina II–V in the neocortex (Freund et al. 1983), especially prominent in the motor cortex (Fig. 1, inset)

– the pyramidal cells (including their initial axon segment) of the hippocampal cortex (Somogyi et al. 1983c)

– the granule cells of the gyrus dentatus (Fig. 34)

– the Purkinje cell bodies in the cerebellar cortex (Oertel et al. 1981d)

– the large and medium size neurons of the nuclei cerebellares (Oertel et al. 1981d), and of the nucleus vestibularis lateralis (Fig. 128; Houser et al. 1984)

– certain large neurons of the formatio reticularis.

In addition, dense perisomatic arrays of GAD-terminals are observed inter alia in the pallidal nuclei (Ribak et al. 1976; 1979b; Oertel et al. 1984), in the anterior cochlear nucleus and in layer 2 of the dorsal cochlear nucleus (Mugnaini 1985).

Axonal peridendritic arrays: Axodendritic GAD terminals appear to be the most common type of GABAergic synapses in the central nervous system. The dendrites in the globus pallidus, the nucleus entopeduncularis, the substantia nigra pars reticulata, and the pallidum ventrale including the cap region of the island of Calleja are outlined by rows and rings of relatively large terminals which facilitate recognition of whether the dendrites run longitudinally or transversely to the plain of the section (Figs 44, 45, 53) (Ribak et al. 1976, 1979b; Oertel et al. 1984).

In the frontal plane, individual axonal peridendritic arrays, running radially from lateral to medial to the pallidal structures, are observed in striatal areas such as the nucleus caudatus/putamen and nucleus amygdaloideus centralis (Fig. 56). These patterns have been termed 'woolly fibers' (Haber and Nauta 1983) and seem to represent enkephalin-positive striatal GABAergic boutons monosynaptically contacting GABAergic pallidal dendrites. Apart from this characteristic 'woolly fiber' pattern, the striatal areas possess a random type distribution ('carpet-like image') of smaller, less intensely stained GAD-positive punctate profiles and therefore differ sharply from the pallidal areas with their high density and peridendritic and perisomatic patterns of GAD-immunoreactive terminals (Fig. 47).

GAD-negative dendrites of neocortical (Fig. 1) and hippocampal pyramidal neurons (Freund et al. 1983; Somogyi et al. 1983c) and of large neurons in the nuclei cerebellares (Fig. 132) (Oertel et al. 1981d) and in the nucleus vestibularis lateralis (Fig. 128) (Houser et al. 1984) also exhibit this peridendritic pattern of GAD-positive axodendritic contacts.

Dendritic peridendritic arrays: GAD-negative dendrites of tufted cells and mitral cells are outlined in the lamina plexiformis externa bulbi olfactorii by dendro-dendritic contacts (Rall et al. 1966) of GABAergic granule cells (Ribak et al. 1977; Mugnaini et al. 1984b). As mentioned in Section 8.6., the lamina plexiformis externa bulbi olfactorii exhibits a density gradient of these presynaptic GABAergic contacts with a higher density in its superficial part (Fig. 29; LPE).

Carpet-like image: The nucleus septi lateralis, the nucleus interstitialis striae terminalis, the nucleus accumbens and the nucleus caudatus/putamen (without white matter), most nuclei of the hypothalamus including the zona incerta pars lateralis, and the substantia grisea centralis contain a medium-to-high density of small terminals. Their distribution appears random as it fails to exhibit an obvious light microscopic relation to target neuronal profiles and therefore gives these regions a characteristic 'carpet-like image' of immunoprecipitate distribution.

Tubercule-like pattern: Dorsally located thalamic nuclei exhibit a higher axon terminal density (Grade 3) at their most dorsal aspect, where they contact the ventricle, than at their ventral (and medial) aspect (Grade 1) (Figs 60, 63, 68).

Certain subnuclei, such as the β-subnucleus of the oliva inferior (Figs 13, 137) contain larger axon terminals than others, and appear, therefore, as especially evident 'lumps' in the immunoreacted section.

8.8. SYNAPTIC RELATIONS OF GAD-IMMUNOREACTIVE TERMINALS

The terminal fibers giving rise to GABAergic boutons show different kinds of relation with the target cells:
– Crossing-over situations (for instance the preterminal portions of basket cells traversing a Purkinje cell arbor) establish the condition for a simple synaptic linkage
– Longitudinal relations (such as the striatal fibers on pallidal dendrites) provide for multiple and closely spaced contacts of boutons en passant of the same parent fiber on the same postsynaptic element
– Glomerular and synaptic nests arrays provide a means by which en passant boutons of the same fiber form multiple contacts on the same postsynaptic element and/or with a large number of postsynaptic elements (the latter may belong to cells of a single category, such as the granule cell dendrites in the cerebellar glomeruli)
– Certain GABAergic interneurons – for example in the retina, the hippocampus or nucleus cochlearis dorsalis – are coupled to one another by gap junctions (Vaughn et al. 1981; Wouterlood and Mugnaini 1984; Kosaka and Hama 1985; Mugnaini 1985)
– Synaptic contacts of GAD-positive terminals on neurosecretory cells as well as on pituicytes and GAD-immunoreactive terminals in the perivascular space have been de-

scribed in the pars intermedia and pars nervosa of the hypophysis (Oertel et al. 1982a). For further examples see Section 8.10.

In conclusion, *GABAergic neurotransmission involves practically all kinds of synaptic arrays known to occur in the vertebrate brain.*

Features of GABAergic synaptic structures, however, show less heterogeneity: GAD-immunoreactive terminals, whether they originate from axons or dendrites, usually contain pleomorphic synaptic vesicles and form symmetric (Gray II type) synaptic junctions. Boutons with pleomorphic vesicles and symmetric synaptic junctions are generally associated with inhibitory function. Asymmetric (Gray I type) synapses of GABAergic endings, however, have occasionally been observed to be formed, for example, by axon terminals of basket and stellate cells on Purkinje cell dendritic spines in the cerebellar cortex (Oertel et al. 1981d). The significance of these unorthodox synapses is uncertain in the substantia nigra (Ribak et al. 1976) and in the gyrus dentatus (Kosaka et al. 1984).

8.9. RELATION OF CELL BODY DENSITY AND AXON TERMINAL DENSITY

The relation between the cell body density and axon terminal density is complex. (For comparison, see Tables 4, 5, 6 and 7.) In some areas, the grades of scoring for cell bodies and axon terminals appear to correspond. One should note that even in these cases the biochemically determined GAD levels are mainly attributable to the synaptic endings, as the concentration of GAD in cell bodies is generally low.

Some examples of the relation between the density of GAD-immunoreactive cell bodies and nerve terminals are listed below:
– Low GABAergic cell body density and low GAD-positive axon terminal density is paired in numerous thalamic nuclei, the nucleus reticularis lateralis or the nucleus reticularis tegmenti pontis – to name a few
– Low-to-medium GABAergic cell body density is combined with a low-to-medium GAD-positive axon terminal density in cortical, hippocampal and cortico-amygdaloid regions
– Low GABAergic cell body density and high GAD-positive axon terminal density is found in the nucleus medialis cerebelli and the nucleus vestibularis lateralis
– High GABAergic cell body density is paired with a medium-to-high GAD-positive axon terminal density in the striatum and striatum-like areas
– High density of GABAergic cell bodies and of GAD-immunoreactive axon terminals is found in the nuclei terminales tractus optici accessorii
– High GABAergic cell body density is paired with a very high density of GAD-immunoreactive axon terminals in pallidal areas or in the nucleus interpeduncularis; the latter is so intensely stained, that it gives the impression of a 'GABAergic switchboard' in the raphe system
– In the hypothalamic regions marked differences in cell body density are found in neighboring nuclei – for example, in the nucleus dorsomedialis hypothalami pars ventralis with a high density of GAD-immunoreactive cell bodies *vs* the nucleus ventromedialis hypothalami with a very low number of GABAergic neurons – but the GAD-positive axon terminal density does not vary correspondingly.

8.10. INHIBITION AND DISINHIBITION

Neurophysiology has revealed different forms of GABAergic inhibition. In many of the cases the exact morphological description of the neuronal circuits and the details of GAD immunocytochemistry are not available. However, where circuits have been analyzed by GAD immunocytochemistry in relation to Golgi impregnations and electron microscopic studies the data suggest that GAD-immunoreactive neurons are involved in presynaptic and postsynaptic inhibition, recurrent (local) and/or lateral inhibition, feed-forward inhibition, feed-back inhibition and disinhibition.

INHIBITION

In most areas of the brain, postsynaptic inhibition morphologically predominates and is mediated by axodendritic and axosomatic GABAergic terminals (Section 8.7).

In the spinal cord, GAD-immunoreactive terminals are found presynaptic to primary afferents in serial synaptic arrays. They presumably represent the morphological correlate for presynaptic inhibition (McLaughlin et al. 1975a; Barber et al. 1978, 1982) and may modulate the release of transmitters from individual presynaptic terminals in the serial synapses.

Examples of recurrent or lateral inhibition can be found in the retina (Vaughn et al. 1981), the striatum (Ribak et al. 1979b, 1981) or the cerebellum (Saito et al. 1974; Oertel et al. 1981d).

Feed-forward inhibition of pyramidal cells in hippocampus (Alger and Nicoll 1982) may take place through GAD-positive non-pyramidal cells in the supra- and the sub-pyramidal layers, which receive monosynaptic commissural input (Frotscher et al. 1984). GABAergic neurons wired in a similar way are present in many regions. They also may form inhibitory contacts with one another (Wouterlood et al. 1985) and thus one mode of wiring is not exclusive of the others. In the retina, cerebral, hippocampal and cerebellar cortices, and nucleus cochlearis dorsalis GABAergic local circuit neurons are connected to one another by gap junctions, suggesting a tendency to fire synchronously and hence to increase inhibitory effectiveness with increased input size (Vaughn et al. 1981; Wouterlood and Mugnaini 1984; Kosaka and Hama 1985; Mugnaini 1985).

Participation of GABAergic elements in the input of strategic areas of the neurons may have a particularly powerful modulatory effect on the spiking activity of the target neuron. Such strategic areas include the initial axon segment, the cell body, the stems of spiny dendrites and of dendritic branching sites: for example, the axon hillock of pyramidal cells in the hippocampus (Somogyi et al. 1983c) and in the neocortex (Freund et al. 1983) are densely covered by axon terminals of which more than 90% are GAD-immunoreactive. A relatively large proportion of these axon terminals are derived from a single axo-axonic cell. In addition, each individual axo-axonic cell innervates the initial axon segment of several hundred pyramidal cells (Somogyi et al. 1983c). Thus, GABA-ergic axo-axonic cells in the neocortex and hippocampus may be capable of synchronizing inhibitory control of the output of pyramidal cells. In the cerebellar cortex, basket cell fibers form special assemblies of GABAergic terminals (pinceau formation) around the initial axon segment of Purkinje cells and can generate an electric field effect (Axelrad and Korn 1982). In the oliva inferior GABAergic terminals may modulate electrotonic coupling between neurons, which takes place in the synaptic nests and along dendrodendritic and dendrosomatic appositions (Llinas et al. 1974, personal observations).

Synapses of GABAergic neurons (for example, those formed on peripheral dendrites and their appendages, as well as on the general surface of non-spiny neurons) may also be involved in subtle modulation of local currents without the involvement of spiking activity (Shepherd 1983).

If *terminal density* were related to the potential degree of inhibitory control, the neurons with dendrites and cell bodies outlined by GAD-immunoreactive profiles – for example in the neocortex, the hippocampal formation, in the pallidum or in the nuclei cerebellares – could be influenced by a wide range of inhibition depending on the firing characteristics of the parent neurons and the particular GABA receptor populations.

In addition to the mode of distribution and the size of the individual terminals, the intensity of staining for the biosynthetic enzyme may represent another relevant aspect of GABAergic inhibitory control. If the *intensity of terminal staining* were related to the extent of GABA synthesis and/or release, the regions of the rat brain where terminals are most densely stained, may represent true 'heavy duty' regions of inhibitory modulation. Accordingly, the GAD-positive peridendritic boutons in the deep fibrocellular layer of the pallidum ventrale dorsal to the tuberculum olfactorium, the boutons in the neuropil of the nucleus interpeduncularis, in the nucleus habenulae lateralis, in the nucleus ventralis corporis trapezoidei, in the β-subnucleus of the oliva inferior or in the substantia gelatinosa of the nucleus tractus spinalis n. trigemini would be among the most active GABAergic elements in rat brain. Interestingly, in the nuclei of the subcollicular acoustic system the size and number of GAD-immunoreactive somatic terminals tend to correspond to the size of excitatory somatic terminals (Adams and Mugnaini 1985a).

With respect to the *intensity of cell body staining,* it is striking for instance, how the periglomerular cells in the main bulbus olfactorius and the neurons of the nucleus reticularis thalami are stained with fixation protocols that do not visualize the neurons in the pallidal areas or those in the zona incerta. What the various degrees of GAD immunoreactivity in neuronal cell bodies indicate, is still poorly understood. How high the concentration of GAD molecules is in a given neuron and therefore how intense a cell body is stained for GAD immunoreactivity, may involve the ratio between the synthesis of GAD and the rate of the axoplasmic transport of GAD, the relation of synthesis of GAD to the total cell volume, or may be related to the electrical properties of the pre- and postsynaptic neurons, including their firing characteristics, to the distribution of GABA receptors and to other unknown parameters.

DISINHIBITION – MULTIPLE INHIBITORY SYSTEMS

Disinhibition, as reviewed by Roberts (1978, 1979, 1984) is a major principle of information processing in the CNS. Disinhibition occurs when an inhibitory neuron innervates a second inhibitory neuron. GAD immunocytochemistry has revealed numerous examples of a presynaptic GAD-immunoreactive profile contacting a postsynaptic GAD-immunoreactive profile. In fact, *most brain areas appear to contain such a GABA–GABA interaction,* although quantitative differences of occurrence are marked.

In general, synaptic connections between two GABA neurons may involve:
1. Local circuit neurons belonging to the same cell class, to closely related subclasses or to different cell classes;
– example: olfactory bulb (Ribak et al. 1977; Mugnaini et al. 1984b)
2. Local circuit neurons and projection neurons;
– example: in the cerebellar cortex basket cell axon terminals synapse on Purkinje cell bodies and their initial axon segment (Oertel et al. 1981d). In this region, the interaction of inhibitory GABAergic neurons is electrophysiologically well documented (Eccles et al. 1967)

3. Different types of projection neurons;
– example: the pallidal areas of the basal ganglia, which represent the most striking (presently known) example of GABA-mediated disinhibition in the (rodent) brain (Oertel et al. 1984). Here, striatal GABAergic projection neurons terminate monosynaptically on pallidal GABAergic projection neurons.

The synaptic relationship between intrinsic GABAergic neurons and GABAergic projection neurons remains to be scrutinized in many other brain areas:
– The neocortex, for example, contains GABAergic interneurons, which can be subdivided into subclasses according to neuropeptide content (Hendry et al. 1984; Schmechel et al. 1984; Somogyi et al. 1984c). It also receives a GAD-positive/histidine-decarboxylase-immunoreactive projection from the nucleus caudalis magnocellularis hypothalami posterioris (Vincent et al. 1982a; Takeda et al. 1984).
– In the striatum, the vast majority of the GAD-positive cells corresponds to the medium size spiny projection neurons with extensive axon collaterals in the striatum, whereas the GAD-immunoreactive medium-to-large cell type most likely represents a small population of interneurons (Ribak et al. 1981; Bolam et al. 1983; Oertel and Mugnaini 1984). Whether the striatum additionally receives a GABAergic projection from pallidal areas (Arbuthnott et al. 1983; Staines and Fibiger 1984) remains to be investigated.
– The colliculus superior receives at least one GABAergic projection from the substantia nigra pars reticulata (Chevalier et al. 1981) and possesses numerous GABA interneurons (Houser et al. 1983b).

Some brain areas may be innervated by *multiple* GABAergic systems. For example, in the thalamus at least 3 different inhibitory GABAergic systems exist: the GABAergic input from the pallidal areas (Penney and Young 1981; Young et al. 1984; Kultas-Ilinsky et al. 1985), from the nucleus reticularis thalami to the thalamic relay nuclei (Frigyesi 1972; Houser et al. 1980; Hendrickson et al. 1983; Oertel et al. 1983a) and the thalamic interneurons (Penny et al. 1983, 1984; Kultas-Ilinsky et al. 1985). Their detailed interrelation needs further analysis. Interestingly, the number of GABAergic interneurons in the thalamus dramatically increases from rodents to primates, indicating some type of change in the role of intrinsic inhibitory control mechanisms at the thalamic level throughout the hierarchy of the species (Penny et al. 1983, 1984).

8.10.1. Example of complex circuits involving GABAergic neurons – zone concept of the telencephalon and basal ganglia

As an example of the contribution of GAD immunocytochemistry to the analysis of complex circuits, where inhibition and disinhibition seem to play an extraordinarily relevant role, we review here briefly the so-called 'zone concept' of the relations between telencephalon and basal ganglia. Based on cytological and histological data, Nauta Jr (1979b) proposed a subdivision of these areas into 3 zones: Zone No. I represents the allocortex and neocortex; Zone No. II (striatum) consists of the nucleus caudatus/putamen, nucleus accumbens and the tuberculum olfactorium including the granule cell clusters of the islands of Calleja; Zone No. III (pallidum) subsumes the globus pallidus, the nucleus entopeduncularis, the pallidum ventrale, and the (non-dopaminergic) substantia nigra pars reticulata.

In respect to GAD immunoreactivity, the cortical Zone No. I in the rat exhibits a low-to-medium axon terminal density and low-to-medium cell body density. The rat striatum (Zone II) is characterized by a medium-to-high density of randomly distributed GAD-positive puncta and by a very high density of cell bodies. Furthermore, striatum-like amygdaloid areas such as the nucleus amygdaloideus centralis and nucleus amygdaloideus medialis may be part of the striatal zone. All subnuclei of the pallidum (Zone III) exhibit a very high density of mainly large type terminals in the form of peridendritic and perisomatic arrays and a very high density of cell bodies.

When compared to morphological Golgi studies and tract-tracing experiments, the data so far obtained strengthen the 'zone concept' from the viewpoint of *classical transmitters:* a glutamatergic striato-cortical projection of Zone I would monosynaptically activate a hierarchical sequence of two monosynaptically connected GABAergic projection neurons in Zone II and III. Cortical activation would therefore result in *disinhibition* of the target neurons of Zone III projection neurons – under the assumption of a generally inhibitory action of GABA. Both, Zone II and III, may contain in addition modulatory GABAergic local circuit neurons.

Neuropeptides: In the striatal zone, several neuropeptides exist in projection neurons and probably in interneurons. Especially the projection neurons show a complex distribution in respect to neuropeptide staining of cell bodies, dendrites and axon collaterals in the striatal subnuclei (Zone II), and in respect to neuropeptide staining of their axon terminals in the pallidal subnuclei (Zone III). Recently, the coexistence (Section 8.11.) of opioid-peptide-like immunoreactivity (Oertel et al. 1983c), of Met-enkephalin- and Leu-enkephalin-like immunoreactivity (Aronin et al. 1984; Afsharpour et al. 1984) and/or of substance P-like-immunoreactivity (Afsharpour et al. 1984) has been demonstrated in numerous GAD-immunoreactive medium size spiny neurons of the striatum. Thus, the massive GABAergic striato-fugal projection may be dividable into subprojections containing different neuropeptides.

In summary, the classical transmitter glutamate in the cortico-striatal pathway and the classical transmitter GABA in the striato-fugal projection and pallido-fugal projection define quantitatively dominant projections in the basal ganglia. In the striatal zone, this simple scheme is overlayed by a complex distribution pattern of neuropeptides, which, at least in part, coexist in GABAergic medium size striatal projection neurons.

8.11. CO-LOCALIZATION OF NEUROPEPTIDES AND GAD IN THE SAME NEURON

Coexistence of classical transmitters and neuropeptide transmitters in the same neuronal/neuroendocrine cell may be a general principle in the nervous system, as reviewed by Hökfelt et al. (1980) and Lundberg and Hökfelt (1983). In respect to GAD, neuropeptide coexistence studies have dealt mainly with areas containing large individual classes of neurons, the majority of which exhibit GAD immunoreactivity (1) (Table 4). Neuropeptides may be present in all or virtually all neurons of a given class of GABAergic cells (for example, somatostatin-like immunoreactivity in the principal neurons of the nucleus reticularis thalami of the cat (Oertel et al. 1983a), or (2) only in part of a GABAergic neuronal population (for example, somatostatin in non-pyramidal neocortical and hippocampal neurons of the cat, monkey and rat (Hendry et al. 1984; Schmechel et al. 1984; Somogyi et al. 1984c)). For an overview of known co-localizations of GAD and neuropeptides/neuro-active substances or neurotransmitter synthesizing enzymes see Table 8, including the respective references.

Many more examples of coexistence of GABA and other neuroactive substances in the same neuron remain to be ascertained, but appear probable when one analyzes the respective available maps (see, for instance, the main bulbus olfactorius (Halász and

TABLE 8. *Coexistence*

Brain area	Neuropeptide/amino acid transmitter biosynthetic enzyme	Cell type	Subclass	Species	Reference
NEOCORTEX					
visual cortex	cholecystokinin	non-pyramidal	+	cat	221
			+	monkey	82
visual cortex, substantia alba subcorticalis	somatostatin	non-pyramidal	+	cat	209, 221
			+	monkey	82, 209
			+	rat	209
HIPPOCAMPUS	cholecystokinin	non-pyramidal	+	cat	221
				rat	245
	somatostatin	non-pyramidal	+	cat	209, 221
				monkey	209
				rat	209
				rat (tissue culture)	100
STRIATUM					
n. caudatus/ putamen	Leu-enkephalin	medium size spiny neuron	?	cat	6
			?	rat	6, 11
	Met-enkephalin	medium size spiny neuron	?	rat	11
	opioid peptides	medium size neuron	?	rat	165
	substance P	medium size spiny neuron	?	cat	6
			?	rat	6
AMYGDALA COMPLEX					
n. amygdaloideus centralis	opioid peptides	medium size neuron	?	rat	165
THALAMUS					
n. reticularis thalami	somatostatin	principal cell		cat (no coex. in rat)	163
HYPOTHALAMUS					
n. caudalis magnocellularis hypothalami posterioris	histidine decarboxylase	principal cell		rat	233
n. arcuatus	tyrosine hydroxylase		+	rat	46a
CEREBELLUM	motilin-related	Purkinje cell	+	rat	33
MESENCEPHALON					
n. raphe dorsalis	serotonin	few cells		rat	145
PANCREAS	insulin	β-cell		rat	46, 249

Shepard 1983)). Neuropeptide co-localization studies may allow the definition of sub-classes of GABAergic neurons. On the other hand, the same neuropeptide might co-localize in a given area in GABAergic nerve cells and non-GABAergic nerve cells.

The mode of action and the role of neuropeptides in respect to GABA neurotrans-mission needs to be explored for each particular cell type before the general principles of neurotransmitter-peptide combination are understood. An attractive hypothesis is that while GABA may have short-lasting effects, the neuropeptide may have long-lasting actions.

Co-localization of GABA with neuropeptides may vary with species and part of the nervous system investigated: for example, somatostatin-like immunoreactivity is present in the feline, but not in the rodent nucleus reticularis thalami (Oertel et al. 1983a).

GAD immunoreactivity does not exist in the somatostatin-positive D-cells in the pancreas, but is present in the insulin-positive β-cells (Vincent et al. 1983a; Elde et al. 1984). GAD immunoreactivity has been visualized in cells of the adrenal medulla (Kataoka et al. 1984). Furthermore, in the rat Fallopian tube 'neuronal' GAD activity of extrinsic origin has been demonstrated biochemically and immunochemically (Apud et al. 1984). These morphological studies in areas outside the CNS – in conjunction with biochemical reports – indicate that GABA synthesis via 'neuronal' GAD is not restricted to the CNS, but can take place in neuroendocrine cells (APUD system) and probably in peripheral nerves as well. (In addition, GAD enzyme activity has been reported to be present in a preparation of pia-arachnoid membranes containing cerebral blood vessels (Hamel et al. 1981).) Which role GABA plays in these areas remains to be clarified.

8.12. GABA NEURONS – GABA RECEPTORS – OTHER NEUROCHEMICALLY DEFINED NEURONS

Visualization of GABAergic neurons in combination with receptor localization – in particular with GABA-A and GABA-B receptors (Bowery et al. 1984) or benzodiazepine receptors (Moehler et al. 1981) – will be an important aspect of 'GABA' research. For studies on GABA-B receptors and GAD immunocytochemistry the nucleus interpedun-cularis is especially suited. This nucleus possesses the highest density of GABA-B receptors in the CNS (Bowery et al. 1981) and also contains a high density of GAD-positive nerve cell bodies and GAD-positive axon terminals. Other areas of high GAD-immuno-reactive axon terminal density and cell body density, such as the striatal areas or pallidal areas, are virtually devoid of GABA-B receptors.

Quantitative and qualitative studies on the synaptic connectivity of GABA neurons with other neurochemically defined neurons allow the correlation of morphological data with physiological and pharmacological effects of GABA in neuronal circuits. The regions of choice for such studies are the areas which either contain major classes of GABAergic neurons or receive a substantial input, delivering another neuroactive compound – or vice versa. Possible candidates, to name a few, are a noradrenergic input to Purkinje cells (Bloom et al. 1971), a GABAergic innervation of the locus ceruleus (Berod et al. 1984), a cholinergic input to neurons of the nucleus reticularis thalami (Kimura et al. 1981), a cortical glutamatergic innervation of medium size spiny striatal neurons (Kim et al. 1977) or nigrostriatal dopaminergic 'input' to medium size striatal neurons (Freund et al. 1985). In addition, a light-microscopic association of dopaminergic neurons and GABAergic neurons has been observed in several brain regions, including the bulbus olfactorius (Mugnaini et al. 1984a), the zona incerta and substantia nigra (Oertel et al. 1982c).

Double immunocytochemical studies on semi-thin sections have demonstrated a very close relationship of dopaminergic and GABAergic neuronal profiles in the substantia nigra, eminentia mediana and the periventricular–arcuate hypothalamic complex and propose a GABAergic innervation of noradrenergic neurons in the locus ceruleus (Berod et al. 1984; Tappaz et al. 1985). *Ultrastructural double labeling* experiments have provided definite evidence for a GABAergic monosynaptic input to neuropeptide Y-containing neurons in the nucleus accumbens (Massari et al. 1984) to LHRH-containing neurons in the area preoptica medialis (Leranth et al. 1985a), to catecholaminergic neurons of the nucleus mediales tractus solitarii (Pickel et al. 1984) and to dopaminergic neurons in the nucleus paraventricularis hypothalami (Van den Pol 1985) and in the periventricular–arcuate hypothalamic complex (Leranth et al. 1985b; Tappaz et al. 1985).

Other possibilities include synaptoid contacts of GAD terminals on vasopressin- or oxytocin-containing neurosecretory fibers in the neural lobe or on secretory α-MSH-containing neurons in the intermediate lobe of the rat pituitary gland (Oertel et al. 1982a). While it is apparent that GABAergic neurons interact with neurons using amino acid neurotransmitters and biogenic amines, these features differ, depending on specific brain regions.

The relation of the inhibitory amino acids GABA and glycine remains another intriguing subject. Presently available maps of the distribution of strychnine binding sites (Young and Snyder 1973) and glycine uptake studies in the spinal cord and other brain areas (Aprison and Daly 1978) suggest that inhibition, presumably mediated by glycine, appears to exist independently of the presence or absence of a dominant GABAergic system. In regions of the CNS above the brainstem, glycine neurotransmission seems hardly to exist. It remains open, whether areas with a relatively low density of GABAergic axon terminals and cell bodies possess a (presently) unknown inhibitory intrinsic and/or extrinsic transmitter system.

9. CONCLUSION

Looking through the 'window of GAD immunostaining' offers a peculiar view at the brain: this staining procedure highlights only one single aspect of chemical neuroanatomy, leaving all other neurochemical maps in the dark. On the one hand GAD-immunohistochemical patterns follow known anatomical borders of certain nuclei or brain regions (for example, thalamus *vs* hypothalamus). On the other hand, at places, one sees constellations of neurons that do not coincide with the nuclear borders established with the Nissl method during the last century. In these instances, GAD immunohistochemistry tempts the viewer to propose new subdivisions of brain regions, for example, in certain regions of the periaqueductal gray, or to subsume several regions under a common denominator due to similarities in patterns and density of GAD-immunoreactive cell bodies and/or nerve terminals, as is proposed for the striatum with its dorsal, ventral and amygdaloid subregions.

From the reference list in Table 1 (pp. 487–501), it is evident that numerous brain regions have not been studied with morphological techniques for GABAergic neuronal profiles. Extensive work, therefore, remains to be done, especially in regions where our map is rather crude, such as in the reticular formation or central gray in the mesencephalon and brainstem, which are presently parcellated on the basis of cell size and packing density. More precise and detailed maps for GABAergic neurons are needed in combination with methods labeling classical neurotransmitters, neuropeptides and receptors as well as with the Golgi method and the tract-tracing procedures to include cytological features, the synaptic relations of GABAergic neurons and the wiring diagram in a general plan of evaluation.

This wide combination of techniques may reveal not only aspects which we have incorrectly interpreted, but also others that we have insufficiently stressed or missed. Furthermore, precise quantitation of the density of GAD-positive cell bodies and nerve terminals was not carried out. This precise estimation of the proportion and relation of presynaptic to postsynaptic GAD-immunoreactive profiles and/or of the intrinsic GABAergic components to extrinsic GABAergic components in a given area may turn out important for understanding the significance of various constellations of GAD-immunoreactive neurons. Finally, GAD-immunohistochemical techniques have now been employed for the analysis of normal and pathological human brain tissue (Adams and Mugnaini 1985c; Braak et al. 1985) and may help to investigate changes of GABAergic neuronal circuits in certain diseases.

10. ACKNOWLEDGMENTS

The authors wish to thank Mrs Anne-Lise Dahl, Mrs Mary Wright-Goss, Mrs Angela Schulze-Lutum, Mr J. Best and Mr J. Osby for invaluable technical assistance and photography.

We express our gratitude to Dr Irwin J. Kopin and Prof. Albrecht Struppler for generous support, to Dr Walle Nauta for encouragement and advice, to Dr Wolfgang Fries, Dr Donald E. Schmechel, Prof. Joachim R. Wolff and Prof. Walter Zieglgänsberger for numerous comments on the manuscript.

Dr Joe Adams, Mr Ulrich März, Ms Barbara Nelson and Mr Dough Vetter are gratefully acknowledged for their permission to include unpublished data in this overview and for collaborative efforts and Mrs Dorothea Mitteregger for her assistance in typing the manuscript.

Finally, we thank the editors and the staff at Elsevier Science Publishers for their patient cooperation.

Due to our ignorance over numerous parts of the CNS we may have erred at several occasions. For such instances we apologize and hope that they will be kindly brought to our attention.

11. REFERENCES

GENERAL OVERVIEW

Bowery NG (Ed.) (1984): *Actions and Interactions of GABA and Benzodiazepines. A Biological Council Symposium.* Raven Press, New York.
DeFeudis FV, Mandel P (Eds) (1981): *Amino Acid Neurotransmitters.* Raven Press, New York.
Enna SJ, Gallagher JP (1983): Biochemical and electrophysiological characteristics of mammalian GABA-receptors. *Int. Rev. Neurobiol., 24,* 181-212.
Fagg GE, Foster AC (1983): Amino acid neurotransmitters and their pathways in the mammalian central nervous system. *Neuroscience, 9,* 701-719.
Hertz L, Kramme E, McGeer EG, Schousboe A (Eds) (1983): *Neurology and Neurobiology,* Vol. 7: *Glutamine, Glutamate and GABA in the Central Nervous System.* Alan R. Liss Inc., New York.
Kroksgaard-Larsen P, Scheel-Krüger J, Kofod H (Eds) (1979): *GABA-Neurotransmitters: Pharmacochemical, Biochemical and Pharmacological Aspects. Proceedings, Alfred Benzon Symposium 12.* Munksgaard, Copenhagen.
Mandel P, DeFeudis FV (Eds) (1979): *GABA-Biochemistry and CNS Functions.* Plenum Press, New York/London.
Roberts E, Chase TN, Tower DB (Eds) (1976): *GABA in Nervous System Function.* Raven Press, New York.
Tallman JF, Gallager DW (1985): The GABA-ergic system: locus of benzodiazepine action. *Annu. Rev. Neurosci., 8,* 21–44.

STUDIES ON THE DISTRIBUTION OF GABAERGIC NEURONS

GABA immunohistochemistry and [³H]GABA autoradiography

Ottersen OP, Storm-Mathisen J (1984a): Glutamate- and GABA-containing neurons in the mouse and rat brain as demonstrated with a new immunocytochemical technique. *J. Comp. Neurol., 229*, 374-392.

Ottersen OP, Storm-Mathisen J (1984b): Neurons containing or accumulating transmitter amino acids. In: Björklund A, Hökfelt T, Kuhar MJ (Eds), *Handbook of Chemical Neuroanatomy. Vol. 3: Classical Transmitters and Transmitter Receptors in the CNS, P. II*, pp. 141-246. Elsevier, Amsterdam/New York/Oxford.

Seguela P, Geffard M, Buijs RM, LeMoal M (1984): Antibodies against γ-aminobutyric acid: specific studies and immunocytochemical results. *Proc. Natl Acad. Sci. USA, 81*, 3888-3892.

Somogyi P, Hodgson AJ, Chubb IW, Penke B, Erdei A (1985): Antisera to γ-aminobutyric acid. II. Immunocytochemical application to the central nervous system. *J. Histochem. Cytochem., 33*, 240-248.

GAD immunohistochemistry

Oertel WH, Schmechel DE, Mugnaini E (1983): Glutamic acid decarboxylase (GAD): purification, antiserum production, immunocytochemistry. In: Barker JL, McKelvy JF (Eds), *Current Methods in Cellular Neurobiology*, pp. 63-110. John Wiley & Sons, New York.

Penny GR, Coneley M, Diamond IT, Schmechel DE (1984): The distribution of glutamic acid decarboxylase immunoreactivity in the diencephalon of the opossum and rabbit. *J. Comp. Neurol., 228*, 38-57.

Perez de la Mora M, Possani LD, Tapia R, Teran L, Palacios R, Fuxe K, Hökfelt T, Ljungdahl A (1981): Demonstration of central γ-aminobutyrate-containing nerve terminals by means of antibodies against glutamate decarboxylase. *Neuroscience, 6*, 875-895

Ribak CE, Vaughn JE, Barber RP (1981): Immunocytochemical localization of GABAergic neurons at the electron microscopic level. *Histochem. J., 13*, 555-582.

Wu J-Y (1983): Immunocytochemical identification of GABAergic neurons and pathways. In: Hertz L, Kramme E, McGeer EG, Schousboe A (Eds), *Glutamine, Glutamate and GABA in the Central Nervous System*, pp. 161–176. Alan R. Liss, New York.

GAD enzyme activity in brain nuclei (punching technique)

Massari VJ, Gottesfeld Z, Jacobowitz DM (1976): Distribution of glutamic acid decarboxylase in certain rhombencephalic and thalamic nuclei of the rat. *Brain Res., 118*, 147-151.

Nieoullon A, Dusticier N (1981): Glutamate decarboxylase distribution in discrete motor nuclei in the cat brain. *J. Neurochem., 37*, 202-209.

Tappaz ML, Brownstein MJ, Palkovits M (1976): Distribution of glutamate decarboxylase in discrete brain nuclei. *Brain Res., 108*, 371-379.

Tappaz ML, Brownstein MJ, Palkovits M (1977): Distribution of glutamate decarboxylase and γ-aminobutyric acid (GABA) in discrete nuclei of hypothalamus and substantia nigra. *Brain Res., 125*, 109-121.

GABA transaminase pharmacohistochemistry

Nagai T, McGeer PL, McGeer EG (1983): Distribution of GABA-T-intensive neurons in the rat forebrain and midbrain. *J. Comp. Neurol., 218*, 220-238.

REFERENCES FOR TEXT AND TABLES*

1. Adams JC, Mugnaini E (1984a): Dorsal nucleus of the lateral lemniscus: a nucleus of GABAergic projection neurons. *Brain Res. Bull., 13*, 585-590.   rat

2. Adams JC, Mugnaini E (1984b): GAD-like immunoreactivity in the ventral cochlear nucleus. *Soc. Neurosci. Abstr., 10*, 393.   rat

3. Adams JC, Mugnaini E (1985a): Relations of excitatory and inhibitory inputs in the auditory system. *Neurosci. Lett., Suppl.*, in press.   cat

4. Adams JC, Mugnaini E (1985b): GAD-like immunoreactivity in the ventral nucleus of the lateral lemniscus. *Anat. Rec., 211*, A5.   cat

5. Adams JC, Mugnaini E (1985c): GAD-like immunoreactivity in the medial geniculate body. In: *Abstract Volume, 8th Midwinter Research Meeting of the Association of Research in Otolaryngology, Clearwater Beach, FL.*   cat/human/rat

6. Afsharpour S, Penny GR, Kitai ST (1984): Glutamic acid decarboxylase, leucine-enkephalin, and sub-

---

*An indication of 'article on METHOD', 'REVIEW article', 'study on TISSUE CULTURE' and 'SPECIES studied' is given at the end of each reference.

stance P immunoreactive neurons in the neostriatum of the rat and cat. *Soc. Neurosci. Abstr., 10,* 702. cat/rat

7.   Aguera M, Belin MF, Nanopoulus D, Pujol JF, Gamrani H, Calas A (1981): Autoradiographic evidence for a GABAergic innervation of the habenula complex. *Neurosci. Lett., Suppl., 7,* 354. rat

8.   Alger BE, Nicoll RA (1982): Feed-forward dendritic inhibition in rat hippocampal pyramidal cells studied in vitro. *J. Physiol. (London), 328,* 105-123. rat

9.   Anderson KJ, Maley B, Scheff SW (1984): Immunocytochemical localization of GABA in the rat hippocampal formation. *Anat. Rec., 208,* A9. rat

9a.   Aprison MH, Daly EC (1978): Biochemical aspects of transmission at inhibitory synapses. The role of glycine. In: Agranoff BW, Aprison MH (Eds), *Advances in Neurochemistry, Vol. 3,* pp. 203-294. Plenum Press, London. review

9b.   Apud JA, Tappaz ML, Celotti F, Negri-Cesi P, Masotto C, Racagni G (1984): Biochemical and immunochemical studies on the GABAergic system in the rat Fallopian tube and ovary. *J. Neurochem., 43,* 120–125. rat

10.   Arbuthnott GW, Staines WA, Walker RH, Whale D (1983): Pallidostriatal neurons with branches to the mesencephalon; electrophysiological evidence in the rat. *J. Physiol. (London), 346,* 33P. rat

11.   Aronin N, DiFiglia M, Graveland GA, Schwartz WJ, Wu J-Y (1984): Localization of immunoreactive enkephalins in GABA synthesizing neurons of the rat neostriatum. *Brain Res., 300,* 376-380. rat

12.   Awapara J, Landua AJ, Fuerst R, Seale B (1950): Free γ-aminobutyric acid in brain. *J. Biol. Chem., 187,* 35-39.

13.   Axelrad H, Korn H (1982): Field effect and chemical transmission: dual inhibitory action of basket cells in the rat cerebellar cortex. In: Palay SL, Chan-Palay V (Eds), *The Cerebellum - New Vistas.* Springer, Berlin. *Exp. Brain Res., Suppl., 6,* 412-438. rat

14.   Barasi S, Sharon P (1980): Electrophysiological investigation of the connection between the substantia nigra and the amygdala in rat. *Neurosci. Lett., 17,* 265-269. rat

15.   Barber R, Saito K (1979): Light microscopic visualization of GAD and GABA-T in immunocytochemical preparations of rodent CNS. In: Roberts E, Chase TN, Tower DB (Eds), *GABA in Nervous System Function,* pp. 113-132, Raven Press, New York. rat

16.   Barber R, Vaughn JE, Saito K, McLaughlin BJ, Roberts E (1978): GABAergic terminals are presynaptic to primary afferent terminals in the substantia gelatinosa of the rat spinal cord. *Brain Res., 141,* 35-55. rat.

17.   Barber RP, Vaughn JE, Roberts E (1982): The cytoarchitecture of GABAergic neurons in rat spinal cord. *Brain Res., 238,* 305-328. rat

17a.   Barker JL, MacDonald JF, Mathers DA, McBurney RN, Oertel WH (1981): GABA receptor function in cultured mouse spinal neurons. In: DeFeudis FV, Mandel P (Eds), *Amino Acid Neurotransmitters, Advances in Biochemical Psychopharmacology, Vol. 29,* pp. 281-293. Raven Press, New York. mouse/tissue culture

18.   Basbaum AI, Glazer EJ, Oertel WH (1981): Light and EM analysis of immunoreactive glutamic acid decarboxylase (GAD) in spinal and trigeminal dorsal horn of cat. *Soc. Neurosci. Abstr., 7,* 528. cat

19.   Bear MF, Schmechel DE, Ebner FF (1985): Glutamic acid decarboxylase in the striate cortex of normal and monocularly deprived kittens. *J. Neurosci., 5,* 1262-1275. cat

19a.   Beart PM, Kelly JS, Shon F (1974): γ-Aminobutyric acid in the peripheral nervous system, pineal and posterior pituitary. *Biochem. Soc. Transact., 2,* 266-268. rat

20.   Belin MF, Aguera M, Tappaz ML, Degueurce A, Bobillier P, Pujol JF (1979): GABA accumulating neurons in the nucleus raphe dorsalis and periaquaeductal gray in the rat: a biochemical and radioautographic study. *Brain Res., 170,* 279-297. rat

21.   Belin MF, Gamrani H, Aguera M, Calas A, Pujol JF (1980): Selective uptake of [³H]γ-aminobutyrate by rat supra- and subependymal nerve fibers, histological and high resolution radioautographic studies. *Neuroscience, 5,* 241-254. rat

22.   Ben-Ari Y, Kanazawa I, Zigmond RE (1976): Regional distribution of glutamate decarboxylase and GABA within the amygdaloid complex and stria terminalis system of the rat. *J. Neurochem., 26,* 1279-1283. rat

23.   Berod A, Chat M, Paut L, Tappaz ML (1984): Catecholaminergic and GABAergic anatomical relationship in the rat substantia nigra, locus coeruleus and hypothalamic median eminence: immunocytochemical visualization of biosynthetic enzymes on serial semithin plastic-embedded sections. *J. Histochem. Cytochem., 32,* 1331-1338. rat

23a.   Blanks RHI, Giolli RA, Pham SV (1982): Projections of the medial terminal nucleus of the accessory optic system upon pretectal nuclei in the pigmented rat. *Exp. Brain Res., 48,* 228-237. rat

24.   Blessing WW, Oertel WH, Willoughby JO (1984): Glutamic acid decarboxylase immunoreactivity is

present in perikarya of neurons in nucleus tractus solitarius of rat. *Brain Res., 322,* 346-350.   rat

25. Bloom FE, Hoffer BJ, Siggins GR (1971): Studies on norepinephrine-containing afferents to Purkinje cells of rat cerebellum. I. Localization of the fibers and their synapses. *Brain Res., 25,* 501-521.   rat

26. Bolam JP, Clarke DJ, Smith AD, Somogyi P (1983): A type of aspiny neuron in the rat neostriatum accumulates [³H]γ-aminobutyric acid: combination of Golgi-staining, autoradiography, and electron microscopy. *J. Comp. Neurol., 213,* 121-134.   rat

27. Bowery NG, Price GW, Hudson AL, Hill DR, Wilkin GP, Turnbull MJ (1984): GABA receptor multiplicity. *Neuropharmacology, 23,* 219-231.

27a. Braak E, Olbrich HG, Braak H, Wieser HG, Oertel WH (1985): GAD-immunoreactive neurons in the human ammon's horn belong to the class of lipofuscin laden non-pyramidal cells. *Neurosci. Lett., Suppl.,* in press.   human

28. Brandon C, Lam DMK, Wu J-Y (1979): The γ-aminobutyric acid system in rabbit retina - localization by immunocytochemistry and autoradiography. *Proc. Natl Acad. Sci. USA, 76,* 3557-3561.   rabbit

29. Brandon C (1983): Retinal GABA neurons: immunocytochemical localization using a new antiserum against rabbit brain glutamate decarboxylase. *Soc. Neurosci. Abstr., 9,* 800.   cat/chick/goldfish/human/monkey/mouse/rabbit/rat/turtle

30. Bunney BS, Aghajanian GK (1976): The precise localization of nigral afferents in the rat as determined by retrograde tracing technique. *Brain Res., 117,* 423-435.   rat

30a. Carter DA, Fibiger HC (1978): The projections of the entopeduncular nucleus and globus pallidus in rat as demonstrated by autoradiography and horseradish peroxidase histochemistry. *J. Comp. Neurol., 177,* 113-124.   rat

31. Carlton SM, Leichnetz GR, Mayer DJ (1982): Projections from the nucleus parafascicularis prerubralis to medullary raphe nuclei and inferior olive in the rat: a horseradish peroxidase and autoradiography study. *Neurosci. Lett., 30,* 191-197.   rat

32. Chan-Palay V, Palay SL, Wu J-Y (1979): Gamma-aminobutyric acid pathways in the cerebellum studied by retrograde and anterograde transport of glutamic acid decarboxylase antibody after in vivo injections. *Anat. Embryol., 157,* 1-14.   rat

33. Chan-Palay V, Nilaver G, Zimmerman E, Wu J-Y, Palay SL (1981): Chemical heterogeneity in cerebellar Purkinje cells: on the existence and coexistence of glutamic acid decarboxylase and motilin like immunoreactivity. *Proc. Natl Acad. Sci. USA, 78,* 7787-7791.   rat

34. Chevalier G, Deniau JM, Thierry AM, Féger J (1981): The nigrotectal pathway. An electrophysiological reinvestigation in the rat. *Brain Res., 213,* 253-263.   rat

35. Chevalier G, Deniau JM (1982): Inhibitory nigral influence on cerebellar evoked responses in the rat ventromedial thalamic nucleus. *Exp. Brain Res., 48,* 369-376.   rat

36. Childs JA, Gale K (1983): Neurochemical evidence for a nigro-tegmental GABAergic projection. *Brain Res., 258,* 109-114.   rat

37. Chronwall BM, Wolff JR (1978): Classification and location of neurons taking up [³H]-GABA in the visual cortex of rats. In: Fonnum F (Ed.), *Amino Acids as Chemical Transmitters,* pp. 297-303. Plenum Press, New York.   rat

38. Chronwall BM, Wolff JR (1980): Prenatal and postnatal development of GABA-accumulating cells in the occipital neocortex of rat. *J. Comp. Neurol., 190,*187-208.   rat

39. Conrad LC, Pfaff DW (1976): Efferents from medial basal forebrain and hypothalamus in the rat. I. An autoradiographic study of the medial preoptic area. *J. Comp. Neurol., 169,* 185-220.   rat

40. Cuénod M, Bagnoli P, Beaudet A, Rustioni A, Wiklund L, Streit P (1982): Transmitter-specific retrograde labeling of neurons. In: Chan-Palay V, Palay SL (Eds), *Cytochemical Methods in Neuroanatomy,* pp. 297-329. Alan R. Liss, New York.   review

41. Deniau JM, Féger J, Le Guyader C (1976): Striatal evoked inhibition of identified nigrothalamic neurons. *Brain Res., 104,* 152-156.   cat/rat

42. Deniau JM, Lackner D, Féger J (1978): Effect of substantia nigra stimulation on identified neurons in the VL-VA thalamic complex. Comparison between intact and chronically decorticated cats. *Brain Res., 145,* 27-35.   cat

43. Di Chiara G, Porceddu ML, Morelli M, Mulas ML, Gessa GL (1979): Evidence for a GABAergic projection from the substantia nigra to the ventromedial thalamus and to the superior colliculus of the rat. *Brain Res., 176,* 273-284.   rat

44. Dray A, Oakley NR (1978): Projections from nucleus accumbens to globus pallidus and substantia nigra in the rat. *Experientia, 34,* 68-70.   rat

45. Eccles JC, Ito M, Szentágothai J (1967): *The Cerebellum as a Neuronal Machine.* Springer, Berlin.

46. Elde R, Seybold V, Sorenson RL, Cummings S, Holets V, Onstott D, Sasek C, Schmechel DE, Oertel WH (1984): Peptidergic regulation in neuroendocrine and autonomic systems. *Peptides, 5, Suppl. 1,* 101-107.   rat

46a. Everitt BJ, Hökfelt T, Wu J-Y, Goldstein M (1984): Coexistence of tyrosine hydroxylase-like and gamma-aminobutyric acid-like immunoreactivities in neurons of the arcuate nucleus. *Neuroendocrinology, 39*, 189-191. rat

47. Fallon JH (1983): The islands of Calleja complex of rat basal forebrain. II. Connections of medium and large sized cells. *Brain Res. Bull., 10*, 775-793. rat

48. Fallon JH, Loughlin SE, Ribak CE (1983): The islands of Calleja complex of rat basal forebrain. III. Histochemical evidence for a striatopallidal system. *J. Comp. Neurol., 218*, 91-120. rat

48a. Faye-Lund H, Osen KK (1985): Anatomy of the inferior colliculus in rat. *Anat. Embryol. (Berl.), 171*, 1-20. rat

49. Fex J, Altschuler RA (1984): Glutamic acid decarboxylase immunoreactivity of olivocochlear neurons in the organ of Corti of guinea pig and rat. *Hearing Res., 15*, 123-131. guinea pig/rat

49a. Finkelstein JA, Tappaz ML, Blessing WW, Oertel WH, Willoughby JO (1984): Localization of glutamic acid decarboxylase (GAD)-positive cells in the hypothalamus of the rat. *Soc. Neurosci. Abstr., 10*, 442. rat

50. Fitzpatrick D, Penny GR, Schmechel DE (1984): Glutamic acid decarboxylase-immunoreactive neurons and terminals in the lateral geniculate nucleus of the cat. *J. Neurosci., 4*, 1809-1829. cat

51. Fonnum F, Storm-Mathisen J, Walberg F (1970): Glutamate decarboxylase in inhibitory neurons. A study of the enzyme in Purkinje cell axons and boutons in the cat. *Brain Res., 20*, 259-275. cat

52. Fonnum F, Walberg F (1973): An estimation of the concentration of the γ-aminobutyric acid and glutamate decarboxylase in the inhibitory Purkinje axon terminals in the cat. *Brain Res., 54*, 115-127. cat

53. Fonnum F, Gottesfeld Z, Grofová I (1978a): Distribution of glutamate decarboxylase, choline acetyltransferase and aromatic amino acid decarboxylase in the basal ganglia of normal and operated rats. Evidence for striatopallidal, striatoentopeduncular and striatonigral GABAergic fibres. *Brain Res., 143*, 125-138. rat

54. Fonnum F, Grofová I, Rinvik E (1978b): Origin and distribution of glutamate decarboxylase in the nucleus subthalamicus of the cat. *Brain Res., 153*, 370-374. cat

55. Freed MA, Nakamura Y, Sterling P (1983): Four types of amacrine cells in the cat retina that accumulate GABA. *J. Comp. Neurol., 219*, 295-304. cat

56. Freund TF, Martin KAC, Smith AD, Somogyi P (1983): Glutamate decarboxylase-immunoreactive terminals of Golgi-impregnated axoaxonic cells and of presumed basket cells in synaptic contact with pyramidal neurons of the cat's visual cortex. *J. Comp. Neurol., 221*, 263-278. cat

56a. Freund TF, Powell JF, Smith AD (1984): Tyrosine hydroxylase-immunoreactive boutons in synaptic contact with identified striatonigral neurons with particular reference to dendritic spines. *Neuroscience, 13*, 1189-1215. rat

57. Frigyesi TL (1972): Intracellular recordings from neurons in the dorsolateral thalamic reticular nucleus during capsular, basal ganglia and midline thalamic stimulation. *Brain Res., 48*, 157-172. cat

58. Frotscher M, Léránth Cs, Lübbers K, Oertel WH (1984): Commissural afferents innervate glutamate decarboxylase immuno-reactive non-pyramidal neurons in the guinea pig hippocampus. *Neurosci. Lett., 46*, 137-143. guinea pig

59. Gamrani H, Calas A, Belin MF, Aguera M, Pujol JF (1979): High resolution radiographic identification of [³H]GABA labeled neurons in the rat nucleus raphe dorsalis. *Neurosci. Lett., 15*, 43-48. rat

60. Gamrani H, Belin MF, Aguera M, Calas A, Pujol JF (1981): Radioautographic evidence for an innervation of the subcommissural organ by GABA-containing nerve fibres. *J. Neurocytol., 10*, 411-424. rat

61. Gamrani H, Harandi M, Belin MF, Dubois MP, Calas A (1984): Direct electron microscopic evidence for the coexistence of GABA uptake and endogeneous serotonin in the same rat central neurons by coupled radioautographic and immunocytochemical procedures. *Neurosci. Lett., 48*, 25-30. rat

62. Geffen LB, Jessell TM, Cuello AC, Iversen LL (1976): Release of dopamine from dendrites in rat substantia nigra. *Nature (London), 260*, 258-260. rat

63. Goldowitz D, Vincent SR, Wu J-Y, Hökfelt T (1982): Immunohistochemical demonstration of plasticity in GABA neurons of the adult rat dentate gyrus. *Brain Res., 238*, 413-420. rat

64. Gottesfeld Z, Massari VJ, Muth EA, Jacobowitz DM (1977): Stria medullaris: a possible pathway containing GABA-ergic afferents to the lateral habenula. *Brain Res., 130*, 184-189. rat

65. Gottesfeld Z, Brandon C, Jacobowitz DM, Wu J-Y (1980): The GABA system in the mammalian habenula. *Brain Res. Bull., 5, Suppl. 2*, 1-6. rat

66. Graybiel AM, Ragsdale CW (1980): Fiber connections of the basal ganglia. In: Cuénod M, Kreutzberg GW, Bloom FE (Eds), *Development and Chemical Specificity of Neurons*, pp. 239-284. Elsevier, Amsterdam. review

67. Groenewegen HJ, Van Dijk CA (1984): Efferent connections of the dorsal tegmental region in the rat, studied by means of anterograde transport of the lectin phaseolus vulgaris leucoagglutinine PHAL. *Brain Res., 304*, 367-371. rat

68. Groenewegen HJ, Ahlenius S, Haber SN, Kowall NW, Nauta WJH (1985): Structure and fiber connections of the interpeduncular nucleus in the rat. An experimental study using neuroanatomical tracing techniques and immunohistochemistry. *J. Comp. Neurol.,* in press.   rat

69. Grofová I (1975): The identification of striatal and pallidal neurons projecting to substantia nigra. An experimental study by means of retrograde axonal transport of horseradish peroxidase. *Brain Res., 91* 286-291.   cat

70. Haber SN, Nauta WJH (1983): Ramifications of the globus pallidus in the rat as indicated by patterns of immunohistochemistry. *Neuroscience, 9,* 245-260.   (monkey)/rat

71. Halász N, Ljungdahl Å, Hökfelt T (1979): Transmitter histochemistry of the rat olfactory bulb. III. Autoradiographic localization of [³H]GABA. *Brain Res., 167,* 221-240.   rat

72. Halász N, Shepherd GM (1983): Neurochemistry of the vertebrate olfactory bulb. *Neuroscience, 10,* 579-619.   review

73. Hamel E, Krause DN, Roberts E (1981): Specific cerebro-vascular localization of glutamate decarboxylase activity. *Brain Res., 223,* 199-204.   rabbit

74. Hamos JE, Davis TL, Sterling P (1983): Four types of neurons in layer IVab of cat cortical area 17 accumulate 3H-GABA. *J. Comp. Neurol., 217,* 449-457.   cat

75. Harandi M, Nieoullon A, Calas A (1983): High resolution radioautographic investigation of [³H]GABA accumulating neurons in cat sensorimotor cortical areas. *Brain Res., 260,* 306-312.   cat

76. Hattori T, Fibiger HC, McGeer PL (1975): Demonstration of a pallidonigral projection innervating dopaminergic neurons. *J. Comp. Neurol., 162,* 487-504.   rat

77. Heimer L (1978): The olfactory cortex and the ventral striatum. In: Livingstone KE, Hornykiewicz O (Eds), *Limbic Mechanisms,* pp. 95-187. Plenum Press, New York.   rat

78. Heimer L, Switzer RD, Van Hoesen GW (1982): Ventral striatum and ventral pallidum: components of the motor system? *Trends Neurosci. 4,* 83-87.   rat/review

79. Hendrickson AE, Hunt SP, Wu J-Y (1981): Immunocytochemical localization of glutamic acid decarboxylase in monkey striate cortex. *Nature (London), 292,* 605-607.   monkey

80. Hendrickson AE, Ogren MP, Won JE Barber RP, Wu J-Y (1983): Light and electron microscopic immunocytochemical localization of glutamic acid decarboxylase in monkey geniculate complex: evidence for GABAergic neurons and synapses. *J. Neurosci., 3,* 1245-1262.   monkey

81. Hendry SHC, Jones EG (1981): Sizes and distribution of intrinsic neurons incorporating tritiated GABA in monkey sensory-motor cortex. *J. Neurosci., 1,* 390-408.   monkey

82. Hendry SHC, Jones EG, DeFilipe D, Schmechel D, Brandon C, Emson PC (1984): Neuropeptide containing neurons of the cerebral cortex are also GABAergic. *Proc. Natl Acad. Sci. USA,* 81, 6526-6530.   monkey

83. Hodgson AJ, Penke B, Erdei A, Chubb IW, Somogyi P (1985): Antisera to γ-aminobutyric acid. Production and characterization using a new model system. *J. Histochem. Cytochem., 33,* 229-239.   method

84. Hökfelt T, Ljungdahl Å (1970): Cellular localization of labeled gamma-aminobutyric acid (3H-GABA) in rat cerebellar cortex: an autoradiographic study. *Brain Res., 22,* 391-396.   rat

85. Hökfelt T, Ljungdahl Å (1972): Autoradiographic identification of cerebral and cerebellar cortical neurons accumulating labeled gamma-aminobutyric acid (3H-GABA). *Exp. Brain Res., 14,* 354-362.   rat

86. Hökfelt T, Johannson O, Ljungdahl Å, Lundberg JM, Schultzberg M (1980): Peptidergic neurons. *Nature (London), 284,* 515-521.   review

87. Hopkins DA, Niessen LW (1976): Substantia nigra projections to the reticular formation, superior colliculus and central gray in the rat, cat and monkey. *Neurosci. Lett., 2,* 253-259.   cat/monkey/rat

88. Houser CR, Vaughn JE, Barber RP, Roberts E (1980): GABA neurons are the major cell type of the nucleus reticularis thalami. *Brain Res., 200,* 341-354.   rat

89. Houser CR, Hendry SHC, Jones EG, Vaughn JE (1983a): Morphological diversity of immunocytochemically identified GABA neurons in the monkey sensory-motor cortex. *J. Neurocytol., 12,* 617-638.   monkey

90. Houser CR, Lee M, Vaughn JE (1983b): Immunocytochemical localization of glutamic acid decarboxylase in normal and deafferented superior colliculus: evidence for reorganization of γ-aminobutyric acid synapses. *J. Neurosci., 3,* 2030-2042.   rat

91. Houser CR, Barber RP, Vaughn JE (1984): Immunocytochemical localization of glutamic acid decarboxylase in the dorsal lateral vestibular nucleus: evidence for an intrinsic and extrinsic GABAergic innervation. *Neurosci. Lett., 47,* 213-220.   rat

92. Hsu SM, Raine L, Fanger H (1981): Use of avidin-biotin-peroxidase complex (ABC) in immunoperoxidase techniques: a comparison between ABC and unlabeled antibody (PAP) procedures. *J. Histochem. Cytochem., 29,* 577-580.   method

93. Hunt SP, Kelly JS, Emson PC, Kimmel JR, Miller RJ, Wu J-Y (1981): An immunohistochemical study

of neuronal populations containing neuropeptides or γ-aminobutyrate within the superficial layers of the rat dorsal horn. *Neuroscience, 6,* 1883-1898.   rat

94. Hwang BH, Wu J-Y (1984): Ultrastructural studies on catecholaminergic terminals and GABAergic neurons in nucleus tractus solitarius of the rat medulla oblongata. *Brain Res., 302,* 57-67.   rat

95. Ito M, Yoshida M (1964): The cerebellar-evoked monosynaptic inhibition of Deiters neurons. *Experientia, 20,* 515-516.   cat

96. Iversen LL, Bloom FE (1972): Studies on the uptake of 3H-GABA and [3H]glycine in slices and homogenates of rat brain and spinal cord by electron microscopic autoradiography. *Brain Res., 41,* 131-143.   rat

97. Iwahori N, Mizuma N (1980): A Golgi study on the zona incerta. *Anat. Embryol., 161,* 145-158.   mouse

98. Jennes L, Stumpf WE, Tappaz ML (1983): Anatomical relationships of dopaminergic and GABAergic systems with the GnRH-system in the septohypothalamic area. *Exp. Brain Res., 50,* 91-99   rat

99. Jessen KR, Hills JM, Dennison ME, Mirsky R (1983): Gamma-aminobutyrate as an autonomic neurotransmitter: release and uptake of [3H]gamma-aminobutyrate in guinea pig large intestine and cultured enteric neurons using physiological method and electron microscopic autoradiography. *Neuroscience, 10,* 1427-1442.   guinea pig

100. Jirikowsky G, Reisert I, Pilgrim Ch, Oertel WH (1984): Coexistence of glutamate decarboxylase and somatostatin immunoreactivity in cultured hippocampal neurons in the rat. *Neurosci. Lett., 46,* 35-39.   rat/tissue culture

101. Johnston JB (1923): Further contribution to the study of the evolution of the forebrain. *J. Comp. Neurol., 35,* 337-481.   human/opossum/rat

102. Jones DL, Mogenson GJ (1980): Nucleus accumbens to globus pallidus GABA projection: electrophysiological and iontophoretic investigations. *Brain Res., 188,* 93-105.   rat

103. Jones EG (1975): Some aspects of the organization of the thalamic reticular complex. *J. Comp. Neurol., 162,* 285-308.   cat/monkey/rat

104. Kataoka Y, Gutman Y, Guidotti A, Panula P, Wroblewski J, Cosenza-Murphy D, Wu J-Y, Costa E (1984): Intrinsic GABAergic system of adrenal chromaffin cells. *Proc. Natl Acad. Sci. USA, 81,* 3218-3222.   rat

104a Kawamura K, Onodera S (1984): Olivary projection from the pretectal region in the cat studied with horseradish peroxidase or tritiated amino acid axonal transport. *Arch. Ital. Biol., 122,* 155-168.   cat

105. Keeler JR, Chults CW, Chase TN, Helke CJ (1984): The ventral surface of the medulla in the rat: pharmacologic and autoradiographic localization of GABA-induced cardiovascular effects. *Brain Res., 297,* 217-224.   rat

106. Kilpatrick IC, Starr MS, Fletcher A, James TA, MacLeod NK (1980): Evidence for a GABAergic nigrothalamic pathway in the rat. *Exp. Brain Res., 40,* 45-54.   rat

107. Kim JS, Bak IJ, Hassler R, Okada Y (1971): Role of γ-aminobutyric acid (GABA) in the extrapyramidal motor system. II. Some evidence for the existence of a type of GABA rich strionigral neurons. *Exp. Brain Res., 14,* 95-104.   rat

108. Kim JS, Hassler R, Haug P, Paik KS (1977): Effect of frontal cortex ablation on striatal glutamic acid level in rat. *Brain Res., 132,* 370-374.   rat

109. Kimura H, McGeer PL, Peng JH, McGeer EG (1981): The central cholinergic system studied by choline acetyltransferase immunohistochemistry in the cat. *J. Comp. Neurol., 200,* 151-201.   cat

110. Köhler C, Chan-Palay V (1983a): Gamma-aminobutyric acid interneurons in the rat hippocampal region studied by retrograde transport of glutamic acid decarboxylase antibody after in vivo injections. *Anat. Embryol. (Berl.), 166,* 53-66.   rat

111. Köhler C, Chan-Palay V (1983b): Distribution of gamma aminobutyric acid containing neurons and terminals in the septal area. An immunohistochemical study using antibodies to glutamic acid decarboxylase in the rat brain. *Anat. Embryol. (Berl.), 167,* 53-55.   rat

112. König JFR, Klippel RA (1963): *The Rat Brain. A Stereotaxic Atlas of the Forebrain and Lower Parts of the Brain Stem.* Williams and Wilkins Co., Baltimore.   rat

113. Korf J, Zieleman M, Westerink BHC (1976): Dopamine release in substantia nigra? *Nature (London), 260,* 257-258.   rat

114. Kosaka T, Hama K, Wu J-Y (1984): GABAergic synaptic boutons in the granule cell layer of rat dentate gyrus. *Brain Res., 293,* 353-359.   rat

115. Kosaka T, Hama K (1985): Gap junctions between non-pyramidal cell dendrites in the rat hippocampus (CA1 and CA3 regions): a combined Golgi-electron microscopy study. *J. Comp. Neurol., 231,* 150-161.   rat

116. Krantis A, Kerr DIB (1981): Autoradiographic localization of [3H]γ-aminobutyric acid in the myenteric plexus of the guinea-pig small intestine. *Neurosci. Lett., 23,* 263-268.   guinea pig

117. Krettek JE, Price JL (1978): Amygdaloid projections to subcortical structures within the basal forebrain

601

and brainstem in the rat and cat. *J. Comp. Neurol., 178*, 225-254.   cat/rat

118. Krieger NR, Megill JR, Sterling P (1983): Granule cells in the rat olfactory tubercle accumulate 3H-γ-aminobutyric acid. *J. Comp. Neurol., 215*, 465-471.   rat

119. Krnjévic K, Schwartz S (1966): Is γ-aminobutyric acid an inhibitory transmitter? *Nature (London), 211*, 1372-1374.   cat

119a. Kultas-Ilinsky K, Ribak CE, Peterson GM, Oertel WH (1985): A description of the GABAergic neurons and axon terminals in the motor nuclei of the cat thalamus. *J. Neurosci., 5*, 1346-1369.   cat

120. Lanoir J, Soghomonian JJ, Cadenel G (1982): Radioautographic study of 3H-GABA uptake in the oculomotor nucleus of the cat. *Exp. Brain Res., 48*, 137-143.   cat

121. Le Gal La Salle G, Paxinos G, Emson P, Ben-Ari Y (1978): Neurochemical mapping of GABAergic systems in the amygdaloid complex and bed nucleus of the stria terminalis. *Brain Res., 155*, 397-403.   rat

121a. Legay F, Lecestre D, Oertel WH, Tappaz M (1985): GAD/CSD activities and taurine biosynthesis in vivo. *Neurosci. Lett., Suppl.*, in press.

122. Léránth Cs, MacLusky NJ, Sakamoto H, Shanabrough M, Naftolin F (1985a): Glutamic acid decarboxylase-containing axons synapse on LHRH neurons in the rat medial preoptic area. *Neuroendocrinology, 40*, 536-539.   rat

122a. Léránth Cs, Sakamoto H, MacLusky NJ, Shanabrough M, Naftolin F (1985b): Application of avidin-ferritin and peroxidase as contrasting electron-dense markers for simultaneous electron microscopic immunocytochemical labelling for glutamic acid decarboxylase and tyrosine hydroxylase in the rat arcuate nucleus. *Histochemistry, 82*, 1-4.   rat

123. Llinas R, Baker R, Sotelo C (1974): Electrotonic coupling between neurons in cat inferior olive. *J. Neurophysiol., 37*, 560-571.   cat

124. Lorente de Nó R (1922): Contribución al conocimiento del nervio trigémino. In: *Libro en Honor de D. Santiago Ramón y Cajal, Tomo II*, pp. 13-30. Jiménez y Molina-Impresores, Madrid.   rat

125. Lundberg JM, Hökfelt T (1983): Coexistence of peptides and classical neurotransmitters. *Trends Neurosci., 6*, 325-333.   review

125a. Maekawa K, Kimura M (1981): Electrophysiological study of the nucleus of the optic tract that transfers optic signals to the nucleus reticularis tegmenti pontis – the visual mossy fiber pathway to the cerebellar flocculus. *Brain Res., 211*, 456-462.

126. Maitre M, Blindermann JM, Ossola L, Mandel P (1978): Comparison of the structures of L-glutamate decarboxylases from human and rat brains. *Biochem. Biophys. Res. Commun., 85*, 885-890.   human/rat

126a. Massari VJ, Chan J, Chronwall B, O'Donohue TL, Pickel VM (1984): Neuropeptide Y in the rat nucleus accumbens: ultrastructure localization and synaptic interaction with GABA-ergic neurons. *Soc. Neurosci. Abstr., 10*, 537.   rat

127. McDonald AJ (1985): Immunohistochemical identification of γ-aminobutyric acid-containing neurons in the rat basolateral amygdala. *Neurosci. Lett., 53*, 203-207.   rat

128. McGeer PL, Eccles JC, McGeer EG (1978): *Molecular Neurobiology of the Mammalian Brain*. Plenum Press, New York/London.   review

129. McLaughlin BJ, Wood JG, Saito K, Barber R, Vaughn JE, Roberts E, Wu J-Y (1974): The fine structural localization of glutamate decarboxylase in synaptic terminals of rodent cerebellum. *Brain Res., 76*, 377-391.   rat

130. McLaughlin BJ, Barber R, Saito K, Roberts E, Wu J-Y (1975a): Immunocytochemical localization of glutamate decarboxylase in rat spinal cord. *J. Comp. Neurol., 164*, 305-322.   rat

131. McLaughlin BJ, Wood JG, Saito K, Roberts E, Wu J-Y (1975b): The fine structural localization of glutamate decarboxylase in developing axonal processes and presynaptic terminals of rodent cerebellum. *Brain Res., 85*, 355-371.   rat

131a. Meessen H, Olszewski J (1949): *A Cytoarchitectonic Atlas of the Rhombencephalon of the Rabbit*. S. Karger, Basel/New York.   rabbit

132. Millhouse OE, Heimer L (1984): Cell configuration in the olfactory tubercle of the rat. *J. Comp. Neurol., 228*, 571-597.   rat

133. Mize RR, Spencer RF, Sterling P (1981): Neurons and glia in cat superior colliculus accumulate [3H]gamma-aminobutyric acid (GABA). *J. Comp. Neurol., 202*, 385-396.   cat

134. Mize RR, Spencer RF, Sterling P (1982): Two types of GABA-accumulating neurons in the superficial gray layer of the cat superior colliculus. *J. Comp. Neurol., 206*, 180-192.   cat

135. Moehler H, Richards JG, Wu J-Y (1981): Autoradiographic localization of benzodiazepine receptors in immunocytochemically identified gamma-aminobutyrergic synapses. *Proc. Natl Acad. Sci. USA, 78*, 1935-1938.   rat

136. Morelli M, DiChiara G (1984): Coexistence of GABA and enkephalin striatal neurons and possible

coupling of GABA-ergic and opiatergic systems in the basal ganglia. *Neuropharmacology, 23/(7B),* 847. rat

137. Mugnaini E, Oertel WH (1981): Distribution of glutamate decarboxylase positive neurons in the rat cerebellar nuclei. *Soc. Neurosci. Abstr., 7,* 112. rat

137a. Mugnaini E, Barmack H, Oertel WH (1982): GABAergic innervation of the rabbit inferior olive studied by GAD-immunocytochemistry. *Soc. Neurosci. Abstr., 8,* 445. rabbit

138. Mugnaini E, Dahl A-L (1983): Zincaldehyde fixation for light microscopic immunocytochemistry of nervous tissues. *J. Histochem. Cytochem., 31,*1435-1438. rat

139. Mugnaini E, Oertel WH, Wouterlood FG (1984a): Immunocytochemical localization of GABA neurons and dopamine neurons in the rat main and accessory olfactory bulb. *Neurosci. Lett., 47,* 221-226. rat

140. Mugnaini E, Wouterlood FG, Dahl A-L, Oertel WH (1984b): Immunocytochemical identification of GABAergic neurons in the main olfactory bulb of the rat. *Arch. Ital. Biol., 122,* 83-113. rat

141. Mugnaini E (1985): GABA neurons in the superficial layer of the rat dorsal cochlear nucleus. Light and electronmicroscopic immunocytochemistry. *J. Comp. Neurol., 235,* 61-81. rat

142. Nagai T, McGeer PL, McGeer EG (1983): Distribution of GABA-T-intensive neurons in the rat forebrain and midbrain. *J. Comp. Neurol., 218,* 220-238. rat

143. Nagy JI, Carter DA, Lehmann J, Fibiger HC (1978a): Evidence for a GABA-containing projection from the entopeduncular nucleus to the lateral habenula in the rat. *Brain Res., 145,* 360-364. rat

144. Nagy JI, Carter DA, Fibiger HC (1978b): Anterior striatal projections to the globus pallidus, entopeduncular nucleus and substantia nigra in the rat: the GABA connection. *Brain Res., 158,* 15-29. rat

145. Nanopoulos D, Belin M-F, Maitre M, Vincendon G, Pujol JF (1982): Immunocytochemical evidence for the existence of GABAergic neurons in the nucleus raphe dorsalis. Possible existence of neurons containing serotonin and GABA. *Brain Res., 232,* 375-389. rat

146. Nauta HJW (1979a): Projections of the pallidal complex: an autoradiographic study in the cat. *Neuroscience, 4,* 1853-1873. cat

147. Nauta HJW (1979b): A proposed conceptual reorganization of the basal ganglia and telencephalon. *Neuroscience, 4,* 1875-1881. review

148. Nauta HJW, Cuénod M (1982): Perikaryal cell labelling in the subthalamic nucleus following the injection of 3H-gamma-aminobutyric acid into the pallidal complex: an autoradiographic study in cat. *Neuroscience, 7,* 2725-2734. cat

149. Neale EA, Oertel WH, Bowers LM, Weise VK (1983): Glutamate decarboxylase immunoreactivity and ³H-GABA accumulation within the same neurons in dissociated cell cultures of cerebral cortex. *J. Neurosci., 3,* 376-382. rat/tissue culture

150. Nelson B, Barmack NH, Mugnaini E (1984): A GABAergic cerebello-olivary projection in the rat. *Soc. Neurosci. Abstr., 10,* 539. rat

151. Nieoullon A, Cheramy A, Glowinsky J (1977): Release of dopamine in vivo from cat substantia nigra. *Nature (London), 266,* 375-377. cat

152. Nomura I, Senba E, Kubo T, Shiraishi T, Matsunaga T, Tohyama M, Shiotani Y, Wu J-Y (1984): Neuropeptides and γ-aminobutyric acid in the vestibular nuclei of the rat: an immunohistochemical analysis. I. Distribution. *Brain Res., 311,* 109-118. rat

153. Obata K, Takeda K (1969): Release of GABA into the fourth ventricle induced by stimulation of the cat cerebellum. *J. Neurochem., 16,* 1043-1047. cat

154. Obata K, Highstein SM (1970): Blocking by picrotoxin of both vestibular inhibition and GABA action on rabbit oculomotor neurones. *Brain Res., 18,* 538-541. rabbit

155. Oertel WH, Schmechel DE, Daly JW, Tappaz ML, Kopin IJ (1980): Localization of glutamate decarboxylase on line immunoelectrophoresis and two-dimensional electrophoresis by use of the radioactive suicide substrate [2-³H]-γ-acetylenic GABA. *Life Sci., 27,* 2133-2141. method

156. Oertel WH, Schmechel DE, Brownstein MJ, Tappaz ML, Ransom DH, Kopin IJ (1981a): Decrease of glutamate decarboxylase (GAD)-immunoreactive nerve terminals in the substantia nigra after kainic acid lesion of the striatum. *J. Histochem. Cytochem., 29,* 977-980. rat

157. Oertel WH, Schmechel DE, Tappaz ML, Kopin IJ (1981b): Production of a specific antiserum to rat brain glutamic acid decarboxylase by injection of an antigen-antibody complex. *Neuroscience, 6,* 2689-2700. rat

158. Oertel WH, Schmechel DE, Weise VK, Ransom DH, Tappaz ML, Krutzsch HC, Kopin IJ (1981c): Comparison of cysteine sulphinic acid decarboxylase (CSD) isoenzymes and glutamic acid decarboxylase (GAD) in rat brain and liver. *Neuroscience, 6,* 2701-2714. rat

159. Oertel WH, Schmechel DE, Mugnaini E, Tappaz ML, Kopin IJ (1981d): Immunocytochemical localization of glutamate decarboxylase in rat cerebellum with a new antiserum. *Neuroscience, 6,* 2715-2735. rat

160. Oertel WH, Mugnaini E, Tappaz ML, Weise VK, Dahl A-L, Schmechel DE, Kopin IJ (1982a): Central GABAergic innervation of neurointermediate pituitary lobe: biochemical and immunocytochemical study in the rat. *Proc. Natl Acad. Sci. USA, 79,* 675-679.   rat

161. Oertel WH, Mugnaini E, Schmechel DE, Tappaz ML, Kopin IJ (1982b): The immunocytochemical demonstration of GABAergic neurons – methods and application. In: Chan-Palay V, Palay SL (Eds), *Cytochemical Methods in Neuroanatomy,* pp. 297-329. Alan R. Liss, New York.   review

162. Oertel WH, Tappaz ML, Berod A, Mugnaini E (1982c): Two colour immunohistochemistry for dopamine and GABA neurons in rat substantia nigra and zona incerta. *Brain Res. Bull., 9,* 463-474.   rat

163. Oertel WH, Graybiel AM, Mugnaini E, Elde RP, Schmechel DE, Kopin IJ (1983a): Coexistence of glutamic acid decarboxylase-like immunoreactivity and somatostatin-like immunoreactivity in neurons of the feline nucleus reticularis thalami. *J. Neurosci., 3,* 1322-1332.   cat/rat

164. Oertel WH, Schmechel DE, Mugnaini E (1983b): Glutamic acid decarboxylase (GAD): purification, antiserum production, immunocytochemistry. In: Barker JL, McKelvy JF (Eds), *Current Methods in Cellular Neurobiology,* pp. 63-110. John Wiley & Sons, New York.   review

165. Oertel WH, Riethmüller G, Mugnaini E, Schmechel DE, Weindl A, Gramsch C, Herz A (1983c): Opioid peptide like immunoreactivity in GABAergic neurons of rat neostriatum and central amygdaloid nucleus. *Life Sci., 33, Suppl. I,* 76-79.   rat

166. Oertel WH, Mugnaini E (1984): Immunocytochemical studies of GABAergic neurons in rat basal ganglia and their relations to other neuronal systems. *Neurosci. Lett., 47,* 233-238.   rat

167. Oertel WH, Nitsch C, Mugnaini E (1984): The immunocytochemical demonstration of the GABAergic neurons in rat globus pallidus and nucleus entopeduncularis and their GABAergic innervation. *Adv. Neurol., 40,* 91-98.   rat

167a. Oertel WH, Mugnaini E (1985): Striatal(-like) GABA-ergic neuronal populations in rat olfactory tubercle, central and medial amygdaloid nucleus. *Soc. Neurosci. Abstr. 11,* in press.   rat

168. Ohara PT, Liebermann AR, Hunt SP, Wu J-Y (1983): Neural elements containing glutamic acid decarboxylase (GAD) in the dorsal lateral geniculate nucleus of the rat: immunohistochemical studies by light- and electron microscopy. *Neuroscience, 8,* 189-212.   rat

169. Olsen RW (1980): Review of GABA. *Science, 207,* 1196.

170. Ordronneau P, Lindstrom PB-M, Petrusz P (1981): Four unlabeled antibody bridge techniques. *J. Histochem. Cytochem., 29,* 1397-1404.   method

171. Osen KK, Mugnaini E, Dahl A-L, Christiansen AH (1984): Histochemical localization of acetylcholinesterase in the cochlear and superior olivary nuclei. A reappraisal with emphasis on the cochlear granule cell system. *Arch. Ital. Biol., 122,* 169-212.   rat

172. Ottersen OP, Storm-Mathisen J (1984a): Glutamate- and GABA-containing neurons in the mouse and rat brain, as demonstrated with a new immunocytochemical technique. *J. Comp. Neurol., 229,* 374-392.   mouse/rat

173. Ottersen OP, Storm-Mathisen J (1984b): Neurons containing or accumulating transmitter amino acids. In: Björklund A, Hökfelt T, Kuhar MJ (Eds), *Handbook of Chemical Neuroanatomy. Vol. 3: Classical Transmitters and Transmitter Receptors in the CNS, Part II,* pp. 141-246. Elsevier, Amsterdam/New York/Oxford.   mouse

174. Ottersen OP, Storm-Mathisen J (1984c): GABA-containing neurons in the thalamus and pretectum of the rodent. An immunocytochemical study. *Anat. Embryol. (Berl.), 170,* 197-207.   mouse/rat

174a. Panula P, Wu J-Y, Emson P (1981a): Ultrastructure of GABA-neurons in cultures of rat neostriatum. *Brain Res., 219,* 202-207.   rat/tissue culture

174b. Panula P, Wu J-Y, Emson P, Liesi P, Rechardt L (1981b): Demonstration of glutamate decarboxylase immunoreactive neurons in cultures of rat substantia nigra. *Neurosci. Lett., 2,* 303-307.   rat/tissue culture

175. Panula P, Revuelta AV, Cheney DL, Wu J-Y, Costa E (1984): An immunohistochemical study on the location of GABAergic neurons in rat septum. *J. Comp. Neurol., 222,* 69-80.   rat

176. Park MR, Falis WM, Kitai ST (1982): An intracellular HRP study of the rat globus pallidus. I. Responses and light microscopic analysis. *J. Comp. Neurol., 211,* 284-294.   rat

177. Paxinos G, Watson C (1982): *The Rat Brain in Stereotaxic Coordinates.* Academic Press, Sydney.   rat

178. Penney JB Jr, Young AB (1981): GABA as the pallido-thalamic neurotransmitter: implications for basal ganglia function. *Brain Res., 207,* 195-199.   rat

179. Penny GR, Conley M, Diamond IT, Schmechel DE (1984): The distribution of glutamic acid decarboxylase immunoreactivity in the diencephalon of the opossum and rabbit. *J. Comp. Neurol., 228,* 38-57.   opossum/rabbit

180. Penny GR, Fitzpatrick D, Schmechel DE, Diamond IT (1983): Glutamic acid decarboxylase-immunoreactive neurons and horseradish peroxidase-labeled projection neurons in the ventral posterior nucleus of the cat and Galago senegalensis. *J. Neurosci., 3,* 1868-1887.   cat/monkey

604

181. Perez de la Mora M, Possani LD, Tapia R, Teran L, Palacios R, Fuxe K, Hökfelt T, Ljungdahl Å (1981): Demonstration of central γ-aminobutyrate-containing nerve terminals by means of antibodies against glutamate decarboxylase. *Neuroscience, 6,* 875-895.   rat

182. Peterson GM, Ribak CE, Oertel WH (1984): Differences in the hippocampal GABAergic system between seizure-sensitive and seizure-resistant gerbils. *Anat. Rec., 208,* 173A.   gerbil

183. Pickel VM, Chan J, Joh TH, Massari VJ (1984): Catecholaminergic neurons in the medial nuclei of the solitary tracts receive direct synapses from GABA-ergic terminals: combined colloidal gold and peroxidase labeling of synthesizing enzymes. *Soc. Neurosci. Abstr., 10,* 537.   rat

184. Precht W, Baker R, Okada Y (1973): Evidence for GABA as the synaptic transmitter of the inhibitory vestibulo-ocular pathway. *Exp. Brain Res., 18,* 415-428.   cat

185. Preston RJ, Bishop GA, Kitai ST (1980): Medium spiny neuron projection from the rat striatum: an intracellular horseradish peroxidase study. *Brain Res., 183,* 253-263.   rat

185a. Price JL, Slotnick BM (1983): Dual olfactory representation in the rat thalamus: anatomical and electrophysiological study. *J. Comp. Neurol., 215,* 63-67.   rat

186. Rall W, Shepherd GM, Reese TS, Brightman MW (1966): Dendro-dendritic synaptic pathway for inhibition in the olfactory bulb. *Exp. Neurol., 14,* 44-56.   rat.

186a. Reisert I, Jirikowski G, Pilgrim C, Tappaz ML (1983): GABAergic neurons in dissociated cultures of rat hypothalamus, septum, and midbrain. *Cell Tissue Res., 229,* 685-694.   rat/tissue culture

187. Rexed B (1954): Cytoarchitectonic atlas of the spinal cord in cat. *J. Comp. Neurol., 100,* 297-379.   cat

188. Ribak CE, Vaughn JE, Saito K, Barber R, Roberts E (1976): Immunocytochemical localization of glutamate decarboxylase in rat substantia nigra. *Brain Res., 116,* 287-298.   rat

189. Ribak CE, Vaughn JE, Saito K, Barber R, Roberts E (1977): Glutamate decarboxylase localization in neurons of the olfactory bulb. *Brain Res., 126,* 1-18.   rat

190. Ribak CE (1978): Aspinous and sparsely-spinous stellate neurons in the visual cortex of rats contain glutamic acid decarboxylase. *J. Neurocytol., 7,* 461-478.   rat

191. Ribak CE, Vaughn JE, Saito K (1978): Immunocytochemical localization of glutamic acid decarboxylase in neuronal somata following colchicine inhibition of axonal transport. *Brain Res., 140,* 315-332.   rat

192. Ribak CE, Harris AB, Vaughn JE, Roberts E (1979a): Inhibitory GABAergic nerve terminals decrease at sites of focal epilepsy. *Science, 205,* 211-240.   monkey

193. Ribak CE, Vaughn JE, Roberts E (1979b): The GABA neurons and their axon terminals in rat corpus striatum as demonstrated by GAD immunocytochemistry. *J. Comp. Neurol., 187,* 261-284.   rat

194. Ribak CE, Vaughn JE, Roberts E (1980): GABAergic nerve terminals decrease in substantia nigra following hemitransections of striatonigral and pallidonigral pathways. *Brain Res., 192,* 413-420.   rat

195. Ribak CE, Vaughn JE, Barber RP (1981): Immunocytochemical localization of GABAergic neurones at the electron microscopical level. *Histochem. J., 13,* 555-582.   review

195a. Ribak CE, Bradburne RM, Harris AB (1982): A preferential loss of GABAergic inhibitory synapses in epileptic foci: a quantitative ultrastructural analysis of monkey neocortex. *J. Neurosci., 2,* 1725-1735.   monkey

196. Ribak CE (1985): Axon terminals of GABAergic chandelier cells are lost at epileptic foci. *Brain Res., 326,* 251-260.   monkey

196a. Ribak CE, Hunt CA, Bakay RA, Oertel WH (1985): A decrease in the number of GABAergic somata is associated with the preferential loss of GABAergic terminals at epileptic foci. *Brain Res.,* in press.   monkey

197. Ribeiro-Da-Silva A, Coimbra A (1980): Neuronal uptake of [3H]GABA and [3H]Glycine in laminae I-II (substantia gelatinosa Rolandi) of the rat spinal cord. An autoradiographic study. *Brain Res., 188,* 449-464.   rat

198. Ricardo JA (1981): Efferent connections of the subthalamic region in the rat. II. The zona incerta. *Brain Res., 214,* 43-60.   rat

199. Roberts E, Frankel S (1950): γ-Aminobutyric acid in brain: its formation from glutamic acid. *J. Biol. Chem., 187,* 55-63.

200. Roberts E (1978): Roles of GABA in neurons in information processing in the vertebrate CNS. In: Karlin A, Tennyson VM, Vogel HJ (Eds), *Neuronal Information Transfer,* pp. 213-239. P&S Biomedical Sciences Symposia, New York.   review

201. Roberts E (1979): New directions in GABA research. I: Immunocytochemical studies of GABA neurons. In: Krogsgaard-Larsen P, Scheel-Krüger J, Kofod H (Eds), *GABA-Neurotransmitters: Pharmacochemical, Biochemical and Pharmacological Aspects. Proceedings, Alfred Benzon Symposium 12,* pp. 28-45. Munksgaard, Copenhagen.   review

202   Roberts E (1984): GABA neurons in the mammalian central nervous system – model for a minimal basic neural unit. *Neurosci. Lett., 47,* 195-200.   review

203. Roberts RC, Ribak CE, Oertel WH (1985): Increased number of GABAergic neurons occur in the inferior colliculus of an audiogenic model of genetic epilepsy. *Brain Res.*, in press.   gerbil

203a. Roffler-Tarlov S, Tarlov E (1975): Reduction of GABA synthesis following lesions of inhibitory vestibulotrochlear pathway. *Brain Res.*, *91*, 326-330.   cat

204. Rouzaire-Dubois B, Hammond C, Hamon B, Féger J (1980): Pharmacological blockade of the globus pallidus-induced inhibitory response of subthalamic cells in the rat. *Brain Res.*, *200*, 321-329.   rat

205. Saito K, Barber R, Wu J-Y, Matsuda T, Roberts E, Vaughn JE (1974): Immunohistochemical localization of glutamic acid decarboxylase in rat cerebellum. *Proc. Natl Acad. Sci. USA*, *71*, 269-273.   rat

206. Saito K (1976): Immunochemical studies of GAD and GABA-T. In: Roberts E, Chase TN, Tower DB (Eds), *GABA in Nervous System Function*, pp. 102-112. Raven Press, New York.   rat

207. Salganikoff K, De Robertis E (1965): Subcellular distribution of the enzyme of the glutamic acid, glutamine and gamma-aminobutyric acid cycle in rat brains. *J. Neurochem.*, *12*, 287-309.   rat

208. Scheibel ME, Scheibel AB (1966): The organization of the nucleus reticularis thalami: a Golgi study. *Brain Res.*, *1*, 43-62.   rat

209. Schmechel DE, Vickrey BG, Fitzpatrick D, Elde RP (1984): GABAergic neurons of mammalian cerebral cortex: widespread subclass defined by somatostatin content. *Neurosci. Lett.*, *47*, 227-232.   cat/monkey/rat

210. Schnitzer J, Rusoff AC (1985): Glutamic acid decarboxylase in the developing mouse retina. *J. Neurosci.*, *4*, 2948-2955.   mouse

211. Schwaber JS, Kapp BS, Higgins GA, Rapp PR (1982): Amygdaloid and basal forebrain direct connections with the nucleus of the solitary tract and the dorsal motor nucleus. *J. Neurosci.*, *2*, 1424-1438.   rat

212. Seguela P, Geffard M, Buijs RM, LeMoal M (1984): Antibodies against γ-aminobutyric acid: specific studies and immunocytochemical results. *Proc. Natl Acad. Sci. USA*, *81*, 3888-3892.   method

213. Seress L, Ribak CE (1983): GABAergic cells in the dentate gyrus appear to be local circuit and projection neurons. *Exp. Brain Res.*, *50*, 173-182   rat

213a. Shepherd GM (1983): *Neurobiology*. Oxford University Press, New York.

214. Somogyi P, Cowey A, Halász N, Freund TF (1981a): Vertical organization of neurones accumulating 3H-GABA in visual cortex of rhesus monkey. *Nature (London)*, *294*, 761-763.   monkey

215. Somogyi P, Freund TF, Halász N, Kisvárday ZF (1981b): Selectivity of neuronal [3H]GABA accumulation in the visual cortex as revealed by Golgi staining of the labeled neurons. *Brain Res.*, *225*, 431-436.   rat

216. Somogyi P, Freund TF, Wu J-Y, Smith AD (1983a): The section Golgi impregnation procedure. 2. Immunocytochemical demonstration of glutamate decarboxylase in Golgi-impregnated neurons and in their afferent synaptic boutons in the visual cortex of the cat. *Neuroscience*, *9*, 475-490.   cat

217. Somogyi P, Kisvárday ZF, Martin AC, Whitteridge D (1983b): Synaptic connections of morphologically identified and physiologically characterized large basket cells in the striate cortex of cat. *Neuroscience*, *10*, 261-294.   cat

218. Somogyi P, Smith AD, Nunzi MG, Worio A, Takagi H, Wu J-Y (1983c): Glutamate decarboxylase immunoreactivity in the hippocampus of the cat: distribution of immunoreactive synaptic terminals with special reference to the axon initial segment of pyramidal neurons. *J. Neurosci.*, *3*, 1450-1468.   cat

219. Somogyi P, Cowey A (1984a): Double bouquet cells in the cerebral cortex. In: Jones EC, Peters A (Eds), *Cerebral Cortex, Vol. 1*, pp. 337-360. Plenum Press, New York.   review

220. Somogyi P, Freund TF, Kisvárday ZF (1984b): Different types of ³H-GABA accumulating neurons in the visual cortex of rat. Characterization by combined autoradiography and Golgi impregnation. *Exp. Brain. Res.*, *259*, 137-142.   rat

221. Somogyi P, Hodgson AJ, Smith AD, Nunzi MG, Gorio A, Wu J-Y (1984c): Different populations of GABAergic neurons in the visual cortex and hippocampus of cat contain somatostatin- or cholecystokinin-immunoreactive material. *J. Neurosci.*, *4*, 2590-2603.   cat

222. Somogyi P, Hodgson A, Chubb IW, Penke B, Erdei A (1985a): Antisera to γ-aminobutyric acid. II. Immunocytochemical application to the central nervous system. *J. Histochem. Cytochem.*, *33*, 240-248.   cat

223. Somogyi P, Hodgson A (1985b): Antisera to γ-aminobutyric acid. III. Demonstration of GABA in Golgi-impregnated neurons and in conventional electron microscopy sections of cat striate cortex. *J. Histochem. Cytochem.*, *33*, 249-257.   cat

224. Spreafico R, Schmechel DE, Ellis LC Jr, Rustioni A (1983): Cortical relay neurons and interneurons in the n. ventralis posterolateralis of cats: a horseradish peroxidase, electron microscopic, Golgi and immunocytochemical study. *Neuroscience*, *9*, 491-510.   cat

225. Staines WA, Admadhija S, Fibiger HC (1981): Demonstration of a pallido-striatal projection by retrograde transport of HRP-labelled lectin. *Brain Res.*, *206*, 446-450.   rat

226. Staines WA, Fibiger HC (1984): Collateral projections of the neurons of the rat globus pallidus to the striatum and substantia nigra. *Exp. Brain Res., 56*, 217-220.   rat

227. Starr MS, Kilpatrick IC (1981): Distribution of γ-aminobutyrate in the rat thalamus: specific decreases in thalamic γ-aminobutyrate following lesion or electrical stimulation of the substantia nigra. *Neuroscience, 6*, 1095-1104.   rat

228. Sterling P, Davis TL (1980): Neurons in cat lateral geniculate nucleus, that accumulate ³H]-γ-amino butyric acid (GABA). *J. Comp. Neurol., 192*, 737-749.   cat

229. Sternberger LA (1979): *Immunocytochemistry, 2nd Ed.* Wiley, New York.

230. Storm-Mathisen J, Leknes AK, Bore AT, Vaaland JL, Edminson P, Haug F-MS, Ottersen OP (1983): First visualization of glutamate and GABA in neurones by immunocytochemistry. *Nature (London), 301*, 517-520.   mouse

231. Streit P, Knecht E, Cuénod M (1979): Transmitter-specific retrograde in the striato-nigral and raphe-nigral pathways. *Science, 205*, 306-308.   rat

232. Swanson LW, Cowan M (1979): The connections of the septal region in the rat. *J. Comp. Neurol., 186*, 621-656.   rat

233. Takeda N, Inagaki S, Shiosaka S, Taguchi Y, Oertel WH, Tohyama M, Watanabe T, Wada H (1984): Immunohistochemical evidence for the coexistence of histidine decarboxylase-like and glutamate decarboxylase-like immunoreactivities in nerve cells of the magnocellular nucleus of the posterior hypothalamus of rats. *Proc. Natl Acad. Sci. USA, 81*, 7647-7650.   rat

234. Tappaz ML, Brownstein MJ, Palkovits M (1976): Distribution of glutamate decarboxylase in discrete brain nuclei. *Brain Res., 108*, 371-379.   rat

235. Tappaz ML, Brownstein MJ (1977a): Origin of glutamate decarboxylase (GAD) containing cells in discrete brain nuclei. *Brain Res., 132*, 95-106.   rat

236. Tappaz ML, Brownstein MJ, Kopin IJ (1977b): Glutamate decarboxylase (GAD) and γ-aminobutyric acid (GABA) in discrete nuclei of hypothalamus and substantia nigra. *Brain Res., 125*, 109-121.   rat

237. Tappaz ML, Aguera M, Belin MF, Oertel WH, Schmechel DE, Kopin IJ, Pujol JF (1981): GABA markers in the hypothalamic median eminence. In: Costa E, Di Chiara G, Gessa GL (Eds), *GABA and Benzodiazepine Receptors. Advances in Biochemistry and Psychopharmacology, Vol. 26*, pp. 229-236, Raven Press, New York.   rat

238. Tappaz ML, Oertel WH, Wassef M, Mugnaini E (1982): Central GABA-ergic neuroendocrine regulations: pharmacological and morphological evidences. In: Buijs RM, Pévet P, Swaab DF (Eds), *Chemical Transmission in the Brain. The Role of Amines, Amino acids and Peptides. Progress in Brain Research, Vol. 55*, pp. 77-96. Elsevier Biomedical, Amsterdam.   rat

239. Tappaz ML, Wassef M, Oertel WH, Paut L, Pujol JF (1983): Light- and electromicroscopic immunocytochemistry of glutamic acid decarboxylase (GAD) in the basal hypothalamus: morphological evidence for neuro-endocrine GABA. *Neuroscience, 9*, 271-287.   rat

239a. Tappaz ML, Bosler O, Pant L, Berod A (1985): GABAergic synaptic inputs on hypothalamic dopaminergic cells. *Neuroscience*, in press.   rat

240. Udenfriend S (1950): Identification of γ-aminobutyric acid in brain by the isotope derivate method. *J. Biol. Chem., 187*, 65-69.

241. Uno M, Yoshida M (1975): Monosynaptic inhibition of thalamic neurons produced by stimulation of the pallidal nucleus in cats. *Brain Res., 99*, 377-380.   cat

241a. Van den Pol AN (1985): Silver-intensified gold and peroxidase as dual ultrastructural immunolabels for pre- and postsynaptic neurotransmitters. *Science, 228*, 332-335.   rat

242. Vaughn JE, Famiglietti EV Jr, Barber RP, Saito K, Roberts E, Ribak CE (1981): GABAergic amacrine cells in rat retina: immunocytochemical identification and synaptic connectivity. *J. Comp. Neurol., 197*, 113-128   rat

243. Vertes RP (1984): A lectin horseradish peroxidase study of the origin of ascending fibers in the medial forebrain bundle of the rat. The upper brainstem. *Neuroscience, 11*, 669-690.   rat

244. Vetter DE, Mugnaini E (1984): Immunocytochemical localization of GABAergic elements in rat inferior colliculus. *Soc. Neurosci. Abstr., 10*, 1148.   rat

245. Vickrey BG, Schmechel DE, Haring JH (1983): Study of GABAergic non-pyramidal neurons in plexiform layers and deep white matters of rat hippocampus. *Soc. Neurosci. Abstr., 9*, 408.   rat

246. Vincent SR, Hattori T, McGeer EG (1978): The nigrotectal projection: a biochemical and ultrastructural characterization. *Brain Res., 151*, 159-164.   rat

247. Vincent SR, Hökfelt T, Wu J-Y (1982a): GABA neuron systems in hypothalamus and pituitary gland: immunohistochemical demonstration using antibodies against glutamate decarboxylase. *Neuroendocrinology, 34*, 117-125.   rat

248. Vincent SR, Kimura H, McGeer EG (1982b): GABA-transaminase in the basal ganglia: a pharmacohistochemical study. *Brain Res., 251*, 93-104.   rat

249. Vincent SR, Hökfelt T, Wu J-Y, Elde RP, Morgan LM, Kimmel JR (1983a): Immunohistochemical studies of the GABA system in the pancreas. *Neuroendocrinology, 36,* 197-204.   rat

250. Vincent SR, Hökfelt T, Skirboll LR, Wu J-Y (1983b): Hypothalamic gamma-aminobutyric acid neurons project to the neocortex. *Science, 220,* 1309-1311.   rat

251. Waddington JL, Cross AJ (1978): Neurochemical changes following kainic acid lesions of the nucleus accumbens: implications for a GABAergic accumbal-ventral tegmental pathway, *Life Sci., 22,* 1011-1014.   rat

252. Wagner GP, Oertel WH, Wolff JR (1983): Entorhinal lesions induce shrinkage and correlated increase of glutamate decarboxylase and cytochrom oxidase in the outer molecular layer of rat dentate gyrus. *Neurosci. Lett., 39,* 255-260.   rat

253. Walaas I, Fonnum F (1980): Biochemical evidence for γ-aminobutyrate containing fibers from the nucleus accumbens to the substantia nigra and ventral tegmental area in the rat. *Neuroscience, 5,* 63-72.   rat

254. Wassef M, Berod A, Sotelo C (1981): Dopaminergic dendrites in the pars reticulata of the rat substantia nigra and their striatal input. Combined immunocytochemical localization of tyrosine hydroxylase and anterograde degeneration. *Neuroscience, 6,* 2125-2139.   rat

255. Watanabe K, Kawana E (1982): The cells of origin of the incertofugal projections to the tectum, thalamus, tegmentum, and spinal cord in the rat: a study using the autoradiographic and horseradish peroxidase methods. *Neuroscience, 7,* 2389-2406.   rat

256. Wolff JR, Chronwall BM (1982): Axosomatic synapses in the visual cortex of adult rat. A comparison between GABA-accumulating and other neurons. *J Neurocytol., 11,* 409-425.   rat

257. Wolff JR, Böttcher H, Zetzsche T, Oertel WH, Chronwall BM (1984): Development of GABAergic neurons in rat visual cortex as identified by glutamate decarboxylase-like immunoreactivity. *Neurosci. Lett., 47,* 207-212.   rat

258. Wood JG, McLaughlin BJ, Vaughn JE (1976): Immunocytochemical localization of GAD in electron microscopic preparations of rodent CNS. In: Roberts E, Chase TN, Tower DB (Eds), *GABA in Nervous System Function,* pp. 133-148. Raven Press, New York.   rat

259. Wouterlood FG, Mugnaini E (1984): Cartwheel neurons of the dorsal cochlear nucleus: a Golgi-electron microscopic study in rat. *J. Comp. Neurol., 227,* 136-157.   rat

260. Wouterlood FG, Mugnaini E, Nederlof J (1985): GABAergic target neurons of olfactory bulb afferents in the entorhinal area of rat. Immunoelectron microscopy combined with anterograde degeneration. *Brain Res.,* in press.   rat

261. Wu J-Y, Matsuda T, Roberts E (1973): Purification and characterization of glutamate decarboxylase from mouse brain. *J. Biol. Chem., 248,* 3029-3034.   mouse

262. Wu J-Y (1976): Purification, characterization and kinetic studies of GAD and GABA-T from mouse brain. In: Roberts E, Chase TN, Tower DB (Eds), *GABA in Nervous System Function,* pp. 7-55. Raven Press, New York.   mouse

263. Wu J-Y (1982): Purification and characterization of cysteic/cysteine sulfinic acids decarboxylase and L-glutamate decarboxylase in bovine brain. *Proc. Natl Acad. Sci. USA, 79,* 4270-4274.   bovine

264. Wu J-Y (1983): Immunocytochemical identification of GABAergic neurons and pathways. In: Hertz L, Kramme E, McGeer EG, Schousboe A (Eds), *Glutamine, Glutamate and GABA in the Central Nervous System,* pp. 161-176. Alan R. Liss, New York.   review

265. Yazulla S, Mosinger J, Zucker C (1985): Two types of pyriform Ab amacrine cells in the goldfish retina: an EM analysis of [³H]GABA uptake and somatostatin-like immunoreactivity. *Brain Res., 321,* 352-356.   goldfish

266. Yoshida M, Nakajima N, Nijima K (1981): Effect of stimulation of the putamen on the substantia nigra in the cat. *Brain Res., 217,* 169-174.   cat

267. Young AB, Snyder SH (1973): Strychnine binding associated with glycine receptors of the central nervous system. *Proc. Natl Acad. Sci. USA, 70,* 2832-2836.   rat

268. Young WS, Alheid GF, Heimer L (1984): Ventral pallidal projection to mediodorsal thalamus: a study with fluorescent retrograde tracers and immunohistofluorescence. *J. Neurosci., 4,* 1626-1638.   rat

269. Záborszky L, Eckenstein F, Léránth Cs, Oertel WH, Schmechel DE, Alones V, Heimer L (1984): Cholinergic cells of the ventral pallidum – a combined electron microscopic immunocytochemical degeneration and HRP study. *Soc. Neurosci. Abstr., 10,* 63.   rat

270. Záborszky L, Zahm SD, Oertel WH, Heimer L (1985): Afferents to the GAD-containing cells in the ventral pallidum. *Anat. Rec., 211,* 221A.   rat

271. Záborszky L, Carlsen J, Oertel WH, Heimer L (1985): Cholinergic and GABAergic projections to the olfactory bulb in the rat. *Neurosci. Lett., Suppl.,* in press.   rat

272. Zucker C, Yazulla S, Wu J-Y (1984): Non-correspondence of [³H]GABA uptake and GAD localization in goldfish amacrine cells. *Brain Res., 298,* 154-158.   goldfish

608

List of abbreviations

The Rat Brain

a	nucleus accumbens
A	alveus
AA	area amygdala anterior
ab	nucleus amygdaloideus basalis
abl	nucleus amygdaloideus basalis, pars lateralis
abm	nucleus amygdaloideus basalis, pars medialis
ac	nucleus amygdaloideus centralis
aco	nucleus amygdaloideus corticalis
ACU	area cuneiformis
aD	nucleus accessorius Darkschewitsch
AHD	area hypothalamicus dorsalis
AHL(=lh)	area hypothalamicus lateralis
AHL	(Chapter X) area hypothalamica lateralis, pars caudalis
al	nucleus amygdaloideus lateralis
AL	ansa lenticularis
ala	nucleus amygdaloideus lateralis, pars anterior
alp	nucleus amygdaloideus lateralis, pars posterior
am	nucleus amygdaloideus medialis
AM	anteromedial dopamine terminal system
amb	nucleus ambiguus
ap	area postrema
apo	nucleus amygdaloideus posterior
APT	area pretectalis
APT	(Chapter X) area pretectalis, anterior
AR	area retrochiasmatica
AVT(=vta)	area ventralis tegmenti (Tsai)
BA	accessory olfactory bulb
BCI(=BCL)	brachium colliculi inferioris
BCL(=BCI)	brachium colliculi inferioris
BO	bulbus olfactorius
C I, II, V, VII	medulla spinalis, pars cervicalis, segmenta I, II, V and VII
CA	commissura anterior
CAI	capsula interna
CC	crus cerebri
CCA	corpus callosum
ccgm(=cgm)	nucleus centralis corporis geniculati medialis
Cci(=ci)	cortex cingularis
CCS	commissura colliculorum superiorum
CE	cortex entorhinalis
cel	nucleus centralis lateralis thalami
CF(=fc)	cortex frontalis
CFV	commissura fornicis ventralis (commissura hippocampi ventralis)
cgm(=ccgm)	nucleus centralis corporis geniculati medialis
cgm	(Chapter X) corpus geniculatum mediale
CH	commissura habenularum
ci(=Cci)	cortex cingularis
CI	colliculus inferior
cic	central nucleus of colliculus inferior
cie	external nucleus of colliculus inferior
cil	lateral nucleus of colliculus inferior

List of abbreviations

Cin(=inc)	cortex insularis
cipc	pericentral nucleus of colliculus inferior
cl	claustrum
cli	(Chapter X) nucleus raphe caudalis linearis
cm	nucleus centromedianus thalami
CN	cochlear nerve
cn	cochlear nucleus
Co I–III	medulla spinalis, pars coccygis, segmenta I–III
CO	chiasma opticum
COc(=oc)	cortex occipitalis
cod	nucleus cochlearis dorsalis
cov	nucleus cochlearis ventralis
cp	nucleus caudatus putamen
CP	commissura posterior
CPa(=pc)	cortex parietalis
CS	colliculus superior
CSD	commissura supraoptica dorsalis
ct(=ntb)	nucleus corporis trapezoidei
CT	corpus trapezoideum
CTe(=tc)	cortex temporalis
cu	nucleus cuneatus
cul	nucleus cuneatus lateralis
dcgl	nucleus dorsalis corporis geniculati lateralis
dcn	dorsal cochlear nucleus
dmpo	dorsomedial periolivary region
DP	decussatio pyramidis
DPCS	decussatio pedunculi cerebellarium superiorum
ep	nucleus entopeduncularis
F	fornix
fc(=CF)	cortex frontalis
FC	fasciculus cuneatus
FDL	fasciculus dorsalis lateralis of spinal cord
FH	fimbria hippocampi
FLD	fasciculus longitudinalis dorsalis (Schütz)
Flm(=FLM)	fasciculus longitudinalis medialis
FLM(=Flm)	fasciculus longitudinalis medialis
FMI	forceps minor
FMT	fasciculus mamillothalamicus
FMTG	fasciculus mamillotegmentalis
FOR	reticular formation
fpc(=FPC)	cortex frontopolaris
FPC(=fpc)	cortex frontopolaris
FR	fasciculus retroflexus
FS	fornix superior
g	nucleus gelatinosus thalami
G	granular cell layer of the hippocampus
G?	area in the ventral cochlear nucleus probably corresponding to area G of Webster and Trune
GC	granular layer of cerebellum
GCC	genu corporis callosi
gp	globus pallidus
gr(=grc)	nucleus gracilis
grc(=gr)	nucleus gracilis
H	cerebellum (hemispheres)

610

H1	Forel's field H1
HI	hippocampus
HIA	hippocampus, pars anterior
hl	nucleus habenulae lateralis
hm	nucleus habenulae medialis
hpe	nucleus periventricularis hypothalamicus
hpv	nucleus periventricularis (hypothalami)
i	nucleus interpositus cerebelli
ic	nucleus interstitialis Cajal
iCM	insula Callejae magna
IH	incertohypothalamic dopamine terminal system
inc(= Cin)	cortex insularis
io	nucleus olivaris inferior
ip	nucleus interpeduncularis
ipip	(Chapter X) nucleus interpeduncularis, pars inferior posterior
l	nucleus lateralis cerebelli
L	stratum lucidum of the hippocampus (mossy fiber zone)
L II, IV, VI	medulla spinalis, pars lumbalis, segmenta II, IV and VI
lai	lamina intercalaris
lc	locus ceruleus
LG	lamina glomerulosa bulbi olfactorii
LGA	lamina glomerulosa bulbi olfactorii accessorii
LGI	lamina granularis interna bulbi olfactorii
LGR	lamina granularis bulbi olfactorii
lh(=AHL)	area hypothalamicus lateralis
LL	lemniscus lateralis
lld	nucleus lemnisci lateralis dorsalis
llr	nucleus lemnisci lateralis rostralis
llv	nucleus lemnisci lateralis ventralis
Lm	stratum lacunosum-moleculare of the hippocampus
LM	lemniscus medialis
LMA	lamina cellularum mitralium bulbi olfactorii accessorii
LME	lamina medullaris externa thalami
LMI	layer of mitral cells
LMIN	lamina medullaris interna thalami
LMIO	lamina medullaris interna bulbi olfactorii
LMO	lamina molecularis bulbi olfactorii
LNO	lamina nervi olfactorii
LP	lamina plexiformis externa bulbi olfactorii
lso	lateral superior olive
m	nucleus medialis cerebelli
M	molecular layer of the fascia dentata, with sublaminae Mo, Mm, Mi
M?	area in the ventral cochlear nucleus probably corresponding to area M of Webster and Trune
mao	(Chapter X) oliva accessoria medialis
md	mediodorsal nucleus of the thalamus
me	median eminence
MFB	fasciculus medialis prosencephali (medial forebrain bundle)
mi	massae intercalatae
ml	lateral mammillary nucleus
MO	molecular layer of cerebellum
mml	nucleus mamillaris medialis, pars lateralis
mmm	nucleus mamillaris medialis, pars medialis
mr	nucleus raphe medianus

List of abbreviations

na	nucleus arcuatus
nco	nucleus commissuralis
ncs	nucleus centralis superior
ncu	nucleus cuneiformis
ndm	nucleus dorsomedialis hypothalami
nha	nucleus hypothalamicus anterior
nhp	nucleus hypothalamicus posterior
nic	nucleus intercalatus
nism	nucleus interstitialis striae medullaris
nist	nucleus interstitialis striae terminalis
nistd	nucleus interstitialis striae terminalis, pars dorsalis
nlo	nucleus linearis oralis
nmp	nucleus mamillaris posterior
np	nucleus parabrachialis ventralis
np V	nucleus sensorius principalis nervi trigemini
npd	nucleus parabrachialis dorsalis
npe	nucleus periventricularis
npf (= pef)	nucleus perifornicalis
npl	nucleus mamillaris prelateralis
npmd	nucleus premamillaris dorsalis
npmv	nucleus premamillaris ventralis
npv	nucleus paraventricularis hypothalami
nrd	nucleus reticularis medullae oblongatae, pars dorsalis
nrgc(= rgi)	nucleus reticularis gigantocellularis
nrm(= rm)	nucleus raphe magnus
nro(= ro)	nucleus raphe obscurus
nrp	nucleus reticularis paramedianus
nrpc(= rpc)	nucleus reticularis parvocellularis
nrpg	nucleus reticularis paragigantocellularis
nrpo(= rpo)	nucleus raphe pontis
nrv	nucleus reticularis medullae oblongatae, pars ventralis
nsc	nucleus suprachiasmaticus
nso	nucleus supraopticus
ntb(= ct)	nucleus corporis trapezoidei
ntd	nucleus tegmenti dorsalis (Gudden)
ntdl	nucleus tegmenti dorsalis lateralis
ntm	nucleus tractus mesencephali
nto	nucleus of the optic tract
nts	nucleus tractus solitarii
ntv	nucleus tegmenti ventralis (Gudden)
nt V	nucleus tractus spinalis nervi trigemini
ntVd	nucleus tractus spinalis nervi trigemini, pars dorsomedialis
nvm	nucleus ventromedialis hypothalami
nvma	nucleus ventromedialis anterior
n III	nucleus originis nervi oculomotorii
n IV	nucleus originis nervi trochlearis
n V	nucleus originis nervi trigemini
n VI	nucleus originis nervi abducentis
n VII	nucleus originis nervi facialis
n X	nucleus originis nervi vagi
n XII	nucleus originis nervi hypoglossi
O	stratum oriens of the hippocampus
O?	area in the ventral cochlear nucleus probably corresponding to area O of Webster and Trune

612

oa	nucleus olfactorius anterior
oad	nucleus olfactorius anterior, pars dorsalis
oae	nucleus olfactorius anterior, pars externa
oal	nucleus olfactorius anterior, pars lateralis
oam	nucleus olfactorius anterior, pars medialis
oap	nucleus olfactorius anterior, pars posterior
oc(=COc)	cortex occipitalis
OC	tractus olivocerebellaris
OI	oliva inferior
ol	nucleus tractus olfactorii lateralis
ope	nucleus preolivaris externus
os	nucleus olivaris superior
osp	nucleus parolivaris superior
ovlt(=OVLT)	organum vasculosum laminae terminalis
OVLT(=ovlt)	organum vasculosum laminae terminalis
p	nucleus pretectalis
P	tractus corticospinalis
pac	anterior pretectal nucleus, pars compacta
pag	periaqueductal gray matter
par	anterior pretectal nucleus, pars reticularis
pbc	parabrachial nucleus
pbd(=pbl)	nucleus parabrachialis lateralis (dorsalis)
pbl(=pbd)	nucleus parabrachialis lateralis (dorsalis)
pbm(=pbv)	nucleus parabrachialis medialis (ventralis)
pbv(=pbm)	nucleus parabrachialis medialis (ventralis)
pc(=CPa)	cortex parietalis
PCI	pedunculus cerebellaris inferior
PCM	pedunculus cerebellaris medius
PCMA	pedunculus corporis mamillaris
PCS	pedunculus cerebellaris superior
pef(=npf)	nucleus perifornicalis
pf	nucleus parafascicularis
ph	nucleus prepositus hypoglossi
pi	cortex piriformis
po	nuclei pontis
pol	nucleus preopticus lateralis
pom	nucleus preopticus medialis
pop	nucleus preopticus periventricularis
pos	nucleus preopticus suprachiasmaticus
pt	nucleus paratenialis
pv	nucleus periventricularis thalami
PVS	periventricular dopamine fiber system
r	nucleus ruber
R	stratum radiatum of the hippocampus
rd	nucleus raphe dorsalis
re	nucleus reuniens
rgi(=nrgc)	nucleus reticularis gigantocellularis
rh	nucleus rhomboideus
rl	nucleus reticularis lateralis
rm(=nrm)	nucleus raphe magnus
rm	(Chapter V) nucleus reticularis medullae
ro(=nro)	nucleus raphe obscurus
rp(=rpa)	nucleus raphe pallidus
rpa(=rp)	nucleus raphe pallidus

rpc(=nrpc)	nucleus reticularis parvocellularis
rpc	(Chapter V) nucleus reticularis pontis caudalis
rpo(=nrpo)	nucleus raphe pontis
rpo	(Chapter V) nucleus reticularis pontis oralis
rpoc	nucleus reticularis pontis caudalis
rpoo	nucleus reticularis pontis oralis
rtp	nucleus reticularis tegmenti
S	subiculum
S?	area in the ventral cochlear nucleus probably corresponding to area S of Webster and Trune
S II–IV	medulla spinalis, pars sacralis, segmenta II–IV
SA	striae acusticae
SAC(=SGC)	substantia grisea centralis
SAM	stratum album mediale colliculi superioris
sf	nucleus septalis fimbrialis
sfo	subfornical organ
sg	nucleus suprageniculatus facialis
sg V	nucleus tractus spinalis nervi trigemini, substantia gelatinosa
SG	supragenual dopamine terminal system
SGC(=SAC)	substantia grisea centralis
sgm	stratum griseum mediale colliculi superioris
SGPV	substantia grisea periventricularis
sgs	stratum griseum superficiale colliculi superioris
si	nucleus septalis intermedius
sin	substantia innominata
sl	nucleus septi lateralis
sm	nucleus septi medialis
SM	stria medullaris thalami
sn	substantia nigra
snc	substantia nigra, pars compacta
snl	substantia nigra, pars lateralis
snr	substantia nigra, pars reticularis
SO	stratum opticum colliculi superioris
SOD	supraoptic decussations
sor	(Chapter X) nucleus supraopticus retrochiasmaticus
spf	nucleus subparafascicularis
SR	sulcus rhinalis
SRH	suprarhinal dopamine terminal system
ssg	substriatal gray
st	nucleus triangularis septi
ST	stria terminalis
str	stria acustica
sut	nucleus subthalamicus
tad	nucleus anterior dorsalis thalami
tam	nucleus anterior medialis thalami
tav	nucleus anterior ventralis thalami
tc(=CTe)	cortex temporalis
td	nucleus tractus diagonalis (Broca)
TD	tractus diagonalis (Broca)
tdh	nucleus tractus diagonalis, horizontal limb
tdv	nucleus tractus diagonalis, vertical limb
Th I, IV, VII, IX, XII	medulla spinalis, pars thoracica, segmenta I, IV, VII, IX, XII
tl	nucleus lateralis thalami
tlp	nucleus lateralis thalami, pars posterior

tm	nucleus medialis thalami
TM	tractus mesencephalicus nervi trigemini
tml	nucleus medialis thalami, pars lateralis
tmm	nucleus medialis thalami, pars medialis
TO	tractus opticus
TOA	tractus opticus basalis (accessorius)
toam	(Chapter X) nucleus terminalis tractus optici accessorii, pars medialis
TOI	tractus olfactorius intermedius
tol	nucleus tractus optici, pars lateralis
TOL	tractus olfactorius lateralis
tom	nucleus tractus optici, pars medialis
tpm	nucleus posteromedianus thalami
tpo	nucleus posterior thalami
tr	nucleus reticularis thalami
TRS	tractus rubrospinalis
TS V	tractus spinalis nervi trigemini
TSHT	tractus septohypothalamicus (hypothalamoseptalis)
tu	tuberculum olfactorium
tv	nucleus ventralis thalami
tvd	nucleus ventralis thalami, pars dorsalis
tvm	nucleus ventralis medialis thalami, pars magnocellularis
tvpl	(Chapter X) nucleus ventroposterior lateralis thalami
tvpm	(Chapter X) nucleus ventroposterior medialis thalami
V	cerebellum (vermis)
V	(Chapter X) ventriculum laterale
vcgl	nucleus ventralis corporis geniculati lateralis
vcn	ventral cochlear nucleus
vl	nucleus vestibularis lateralis
vm	nucleus vestibularis medialis
vp(=VP)	ventral pallidum
VP(=vp)	ventral pallidum
vp	(Chapter X) fibrocellular layer of pallidum ventrale
vpo	ventral periolivary region
vs	nucleus vestibularis superior
vsp	nucleus vestibularis spinalis
vta(=AVT)	area ventralis tegmenti (Tsai)
zi(=ZI)	zona incerta
ZI(=zi)	zona incerta
zV	subnucleus zonalis nuclei tractus spinalis n. trigemini
V	nervus trigeminus
VII	nervus facialis
V M	nervus trigeminus, radix motoria
V S	nervus trigeminus, radix sensoria

615

List of abbreviations

The Rat Brain

accessory olfactory bulb	BA
alveus	A
ansa lenticularis	AL
anterior pretectal nucleus, pars compacta	pac
anterior pretectal nucleus, pars reticularis	par
anteromedial dopamine terminal system	AM
area amygdala anterior	AA
area cuneiformis	ACU
area hypothalamicus dorsalis	AHD
area hypothalamicus lateralis	AHL(=lh)
area hypothalamica lateralis, pars caudalis	AHL (Chapter X)
area postrema	ap
area pretectalis	APT
area pretectalis, anterior	APT (Chapter X)
area retrochiasmatica	ar
area in the ventral cochlear nucleus probably corresponding to area G of Webster and Trune	G?
area in the ventral cochlear nucleus probably corresponding to area M of Webster and Trune	M?
area in the ventral cochlear nucleus probably corresponding to area O of Webster and Trune	O?
area in the ventral cochlear nucleus probably corresponding to area S of Webster and Trune	S?
area ventralis tegmenti (Tsai)	AVT(=vta)
brachium colliculi inferioris	BCI(=BCL)
bulbus olfactorius	BO
capsula interna	CAI
central nucleus of colliculus inferior	cic
cerebellum (hemispheres)	H
cerebellum (vermis)	V
chiasma opticum	CO
claustrum	cl
cochlear nerve	CN
cochlear nucleus	cn
colliculus inferior	CI
colliculus superior	CS
commissura anterior	CA
commissura colliculorum superiorum	CCS
commissura fornicis ventralis (commissura hippocampi ventralis)	CFV
commissura habenularum	CH
commissura posterior	CP
commissura supraoptica dorsalis	CSD
corpus geniculatum mediale	cgm (Chapter X)
cortex cingularis	ci(=Cci)
cortex entorhinalis	CE
cortex frontalis	fc(=CF)
cortex frontopolaris	fpc(=FPC)
cortex insularis	inc(=Cin)
cortex occipitalis	oc(=COc)
cortex parietalis	pc(=CPa)

cortex piriformis	pi
cortex temporalis	tc(=CTe)
corpus callosum	CCA
corpus trapezoideum	CT
crus cerebri	CC
decussatio pedunculi cerebellarium superiorum	DPCS
decussatio pyramidis	DP
dorsal cochlear nucleus	dcn
dorsomedial periolivary region	dmpo
external nucleus of colliculus inferior	cie
fasciculus cuneatus	FC
fasciculus dorsalis lateralis of spinal cord	FDL
fasciculus longitudinalis dorsalis (Schütz)	FLD
fasciculus longitudinalis medialis	FLM(=Flm)
fasciculus mamillotegmentalis	FMTG
fasciculus mamillothalamicus	FMT
fasciculus medialis prosencephali (medial forebrain bundle)	MFB
fasciculus retroflexus	FR
fibrocellular layer of pallidum ventrale	vp (Chapter X)
fimbria hippocampi	FH
forceps minor	FMI
Forel's field H1	H1
fornix	F
fornix superior	FS
genu corporis callosi	GCC
globus pallidus	gp
granular cell layer of the hippocampus	G
granular layer of cerebellum	GC
hippocampus	HI
hippocampus, pars anterior	HIA
incertohypothalamic dopamine terminal system	IH
insula Callejae magna	iCM
lamina cellularum mitralium bulbi olfactorii accessorii	LMA
lamina glomerulosa bulbi olfactorii	LG
lamina glomerulosa bulbi olfactorii accessorii	LGA
lamina granularis bulbi olfactorii	LGR
lamina granularis interna bulbi olfactorii	LGI
lamina intercalaris	lai
lamina medullaris externa thalami	LME
lamina medullaris interna bulbi olfactorii	LMIO
lamina medullaris interna thalami	LMIN
lamina molecularis bulbi olfactorii	LMO
lamina nervi olfactorii	LNO
lamina plexiformis externa bulbi olfactorii	LP
lateral mammillary nucleus	ml
lateral nucleus of colliculus inferior	cil
lateral superior olive	lso
layer of mitral cells	LMI
lemniscus lateralis	LL
lemniscus medialis	LM
locus ceruleus	lc
massae intercalatae	mi
median eminence	me
mediodorsal nucleus of the thalamus	md

medulla spinalis, pars cervicalis, segmenta I, II, V, VII	C I, II, V, VII
medulla spinalis, pars coccygis, segmenta I–III	Co I–III
medulla spinalis, pars lumbalis, segmenta II, IV and VI	L II, IV, VI
medulla spinalis, pars sacralis, segmenta II–IV	S II–IV
medulla spinalis, pars thoracica, segmenta I, IV, VII, IX, XII	Th I, IV, VII, IX, XII
molecular layer of cerebellum	MO
molecular layer of the fascia dentata, with sublaminae Mo, Mm, Mi	M
nervus facialis	VII
nervus trigeminus	V
nervus trigeminus, radix motoria	V M
nervus trigeminus, radix sensoria	V S
nuclei pontis	po
nucleus accessorius Darkschewitsch	aD
nucleus accumbens	a
nucleus ambiguus	amb
nucleus amygdaloideus basalis	ab
nucleus amygdaloideus basalis, pars lateralis	abl
nucleus amygdaloideus basalis, pars medialis	abm
nucleus amygdaloideus centralis	ac
nucleus amygdaloideus corticalis	aco
nucleus amygdaloideus lateralis	al
nucleus amygdaloideus lateralis, pars anterior	ala
nucleus amygdaloideus lateralis, pars posterior	alp
nucleus amygdaloideus medialis	am
nucleus amygdaloideus posterior	apo
nucleus anterior dorsalis thalami	tad
nucleus anterior medialis thalami	tam
nucleus anterior ventralis thalami	tav
nucleus arcuatus	na
nucleus caudatus putamen	cp
nucleus centralis corporis geniculati medialis	ccgm(=cgm)
nucleus centralis lateralis thalami	cel
nucleus centralis superior	ncs
nucleus centromedianus thalami	cm
nucleus cochlearis dorsalis	cod
nucleus cochlearis ventralis	cov
nucleus commissuralis	nco
nucleus corporis trapezoidei	ct(=ntb)
nucleus cuneatus	cu
nucleus cuneatus lateralis	cul
nucleus cuneiformis	ncu
nucleus dorsalis corporis geniculati lateralis	dcgl
nucleus dorsomedialis hypothalami	ndm
nucleus entopeduncularis	ep
nucleus gelatinosus thalami	g
nucleus gracilis	gr(=grc)
nucleus habenulae lateralis	hl
nucleus habenulae medialis	hm
nucleus hypothalamicus anterior	nha
nucleus hypothalamicus posterior	nhp
nucleus intercalatus	nic
nucleus interpeduncularis	ip
nucleus interpeduncularis, pars inferior posterior	ipip (Chapter X)
nucleus interpositus cerebelli	i

nucleus interstitialis Cajal	ic
nucleus interstitialis striae medullaris	nism
nucleus interstitialis striae terminalis	nist
nucleus interstitialis striae terminalis, pars dorsalis	nistd
nucleus lateralis cerebelli	l
nucleus lateralis thalami	tl
nucleus lateralis thalami, pars posterior	tlp
nucleus lemnisci lateralis dorsalis	lld
nucleus lemnisci lateralis rostralis	llr
nucleus lemnisci lateralis ventralis	llv
nucleus linearis oralis	nlo
nucleus mamillaris medialis, pars lateralis	mml
nucleus mamillaris medialis, pars medialis	mmm
nucleus mamillaris posterior	nmp
nucleus mamillaris prelateralis	npl
nucleus medialis cerebelli	m
nucleus medialis thalami	tm
nucleus medialis thalami, pars lateralis	tml
nucleus medialis thalami, pars medialis	tmm
nucleus olfactorius anterior	oa
nucleus olfactorius anterior, pars dorsalis	oad
nucleus olfactorius anterior, pars externa	oae
nucleus olfactorius anterior, pars lateralis	oal
nucleus olfactorius anterior, pars medialis	oam
nucleus olfactorius anterior, pars posterior	oap
nucleus olivaris inferior	io
nucleus olivaris superior	os
nucleus of the optic tract	nto
nucleus originis nervi abducentis	n VI
nucleus originis nervi facialis	n VII
nucleus originis nervi hypoglossi	n XII
nucleus originis nervi oculomotorii	n III
nucleus originis nervi trigemini	n V
nucleus originis nervi trochlearis	n IV
nucleus originis nervi vagi	n X
nucleus parabrachialis dorsalis	npd
nucleus parabrachialis lateralis (dorsalis)	pbd(=pbl)
nucleus parabrachialis medialis (ventralis)	pbm(=pbv)
nucleus parabrachialis ventralis	np
nucleus parafascicularis	pf
nucleus paratenialis	pt
nucleus paraventricularis hypothalami	npv
nucleus parolivaris superior	osp
nucleus perifornicalis	npf (=pef)
nucleus periventricularis	npe
nucleus periventricularis (hypothalami)	hpv
nucleus periventricularis hypothalamicus	hpe
nucleus periventricularis thalami	pv
nucleus posterior thalami	tpo
nucleus posteromedianus thalami	tpm
nucleus premamillaris dorsalis	npmd
nucleus premamillaris ventralis	npmv
nucleus preolivaris externus	ope
nucleus preopticus lateralis	pol

619

nucleus preopticus medialis	pom
nucleus preopticus periventricularis	pop
nucleus preopticus suprachiasmaticus	pos
nucleus prepositus hypoglossi	ph
nucleus pretectalis	p
nucleus raphe caudalis linearis	cli (Chapter X)
nucleus raphe dorsalis	rd
nucleus raphe magnus	nrm(=rm)
nucleus raphe medianus	mr
nucleus raphe obscurus	ro(=nro)
nucleus raphe pallidus	rp(=rpa)
nucleus raphe pontis	rpo(=nrpo)
nucleus reticularis gigantocellularis	nrgc(=rgi)
nucleus reticularis lateralis	rl
nucleus reticularis medullae	rm (Chapter V)
nucleus reticularis medullae oblongatae, pars dorsalis	nrd
nucleus reticularis medullae oblongatae, pars ventralis	nrv
nucleus reticularis paragigantocellularis	nrpg
nucleus reticularis paramedianus	nrp
nucleus reticularis parvocellularis	nrpc(=rpc)
nucleus reticularis pontis caudalis	rpoc
nucleus reticularis pontis caudalis	rpc (Chapter V)
nucleus reticularis pontis oralis	rpoo
nucleus reticularis pontis oralis	rpo (Chapter V)
nucleus reticularis tegmenti	rtp
nucleus reticularis thalami	tr
nucleus reuniens	re
nucleus rhomboideus	rh
nucleus ruber	r
nucleus sensorius principalis nervi trigemini	np V
nucleus septalis fimbrialis	sf
nucleus septalis intermedius	si
nucleus septi lateralis	sl
nucleus septi medialis	sm
nucleus subparafascicularis	spf
nucleus subthalamicus	sut
nucleus suprachiasmaticus	nsc
nucleus suprageniculatus facialis	sg
nucleus supraopticus	nso
nucleus supraopticus retrochiasmaticus	sor (Chapter X)
nucleus tegmenti dorsalis (Gudden)	ntd
nucleus tegmenti dorsalis lateralis	ntdl
nucleus tegmenti ventralis (Gudden)	ntv
nucleus terminalis tractus optici accessorii, pars medialis	toam (Chapter X)
nucleus tractus diagonalis (Broca)	td
nucleus tractus diagonalis, horizontal limb	tdh
nucleus tractus diagonalis, vertical limb	tdv
nucleus tractus mesencephali	ntm
nucleus tractus olfactorii lateralis	ol
nucleus tractus optici, pars lateralis	tol
nucleus tractus optici, pars medialis	tom
nucleus tractus solitarii	nts
nucleus tractus spinalis nervi trigemini	nt V
nucleus tractus spinalis nervi trigemini, substantia gelatinosa	sg V

620

nucleus tractus spinalis nervi trigemini, pars dorsomedialis	ntVd
nucleus triangularis septi	st
nucleus ventralis corporis geniculati lateralis	vcgl
nucleus ventralis medialis thalami, pars magnocellularis	tvm
nucleus ventralis thalami	tv
nucleus ventralis thalami, pars dorsalis	tvd
nucleus ventromedialis anterior	nvma
nucleus ventromedialis hypothalami	nvm
nucleus ventroposterior lateralis thalami	tvpl (Chapter X)
nucleus ventroposterior medialis thalami	tvpm (Chapter X)
nucleus vestibularis lateralis	vl
nucleus vestibularis medialis	vm
nucleus vestibularis spinalis	vsp
nucleus vestibularis superior	vs
oliva accessoria medialis	mao (Chapter X)
oliva inferior	OI
organum vasculosum laminae terminalis	ovlt(=OVLT)
parabrachial nucleus	pbc
pedunculus cerebellaris inferior	PCI
pedunculus cerebellaris medius	PCM
pedunculus cerebellaris superior	PCS
pedunculus corporis mamillaris	PCMA
periaqueductal gray matter	pag
pericentral nucleus of colliculus inferior	cipc
periventricular dopamine fiber system	PVS
reticular formation	FOR
stratum album mediale colliculi superioris	SAM
stratum griseum mediale colliculi superioris	sgm
stratum griseum superficiale colliculi superioris	sgs
stratum lacunosum-moleculare of the hippocampus	Lm
stratum lucidum of the hippocampus (mossy fiber zone)	L
stratum opticum colliculi superioris	SO
stratum oriens of the hippocampus	O
stratum radiatum of the hippocampus	R
stria acustica	str
stria medullaris thalami	SM
stria terminalis	ST
striae acusticae	SA
subfornical organ	sfo
subiculum	S
subnucleus zonalis nuclei tractus spinalis n. trigemini	zV
substantia grisea centralis	SAC(=SGC)
substantia grisea periventricularis	SGPV
substantia innominata	sin
substantia nigra	sn
substantia nigra, pars compacta	snc
substantia nigra, pars lateralis	snl
substantia nigra, pars reticularis	snr
substriatal gray	ssg
sulcus rhinalis	SR
supragenual dopamine terminal system	SG
supraoptic decussations	SOD
suprarhinal dopamine terminal system	SRH
tractus corticospinalis	P

tractus diagonalis (Broca)	TD
tractus mesencephalicus nervi trigemini	TM
tractus olfactorius intermedius	TOI
tractus olfactorius lateralis	TOL
tractus olivocerebellaris	OC
tractus opticus	TO
tractus opticus basalis (accessorius)	TOA
tractus rubrospinalis	TRS
tractus septohypothalamicus (hypothalamoseptalis)	TSHT
tractus spinalis nervi trigemini	TS V
tuberculum olfactorium	tu
ventral cochlear nucleus	vcn
ventral pallidum	VP(= vp)
ventral periolivary region	vpo
ventriculum laterale	V (Chapter X)
zona incerta	zi(= ZI)

Subject index

Prepared by R. Warren, Ph.D., Edinburgh